Mosby's Emergency Nursing Reference

Mosby's Emergency Nursing Reference

second edition

PAMELA S. KIDD, PhD, ARNP, CEN
Associate Professor
College of Nursing
Director
Kentucky Injury Prevention and Research Center
University of Kentucky
Lexington, Kentucky

PATTY ANN STURT, RN, MSN, CEN
Staff Development Specialist
Department of Nursing Staff Development
University of Kentucky Hospital
Lexington, Kentucky

JULIA FULTZ, RN, BSN, CEN, CFRN
Flight Nurse
University of Kentucky Air Medical Service
Lexington, Kentucky

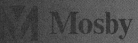

Mosby

Harcourt Health Sciences Company

St. Louis   London   Philadelphia   Sydney   Toronto

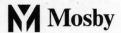

Mosby

A Harcourt Health Sciences Company

Editor-in-Chief and Vice-President: Sally Schrefer
Managing Editor: Lisa Potts
Editorial Assistants: Julia Koelsch, Amanda Sunderman
Project Manager: Patricia Tannian
Production Editor: Larry State
Designer: Amy Buxton
Cover Designer: E. Rohne Rudder

Mosby, Inc.
A Harcourt Health Sciences Company
11830 Westline Industrial Drive
St. Louis, Missouri 63146

Printed in the United States of America

International Standard Book Number
0-323-01108-X

00 01 02 03 04 TG/RRD 9 8 7 6 5 4 3 2 1

Contributors

MARY ROSE BAUER, RN, BSN
Staff Nurse
Emergency Department
University of Kentucky Hospital
Lexington, Kentucky

GREG BAYER, EMT-P
Lexington Fire Department
Lexington, Kentucky

BARBARA BLAKE, RN, BSN
Staff Nurse
Emergency Department
University of Kentucky Hospital
Lexington, Kentucky

CARLOS COYLE, AS, NR EMT-P
University of Kentucky Air Medical Service
University of Kentucky Hospital
Lexington, Kentucky

JANET COYLE, RN, CFRN
University of Kentucky Air Medical Service
University of Kentucky Hospital
Lexington, Kentucky

LISA L. CREECH, RN, BSN
Staff Nurse
Emergency Department
University of Kentucky Hospital
Lexington, Kentucky

LEE GARNER, RN, ADN, CEN
Divisional Charge Nurse
Emergency Department
University of Kentucky Hospital
Lexington, Kentucky

vi   Contributors

GEORGE P. GLESSNER III, NR, EMT-P
Flight Paramedic
University of Kentucky Air Medical Service
Lexington, Kentucky

THERESA M. GLESSNER, RN, MSN, ARNP-CS, CCRN, CEN
Vascular Nurse Practitioner/Case Manager
Department of Surgery
University of Kentucky Hospital
Lexington, Kentucky

REGINA M. HEISER, RN, MSN
Emergency Department Case Manager/Systems Coordinator
University of Kentucky Hospital
Lexington, Kentucky

DONNA ISFORT, RN, BSN
University of Kentucky Air Medical Service
University of Kentucky Hospital
Lexington, Kentucky

MARCIA G. MESSER, RN, BSN
Premier Inc.
Charlotte, North Carolina

ELIZABETH GAUDET NOLAN, RN, BSN, CEN
Clinical Staff Nurse
Emergency Department
University of Kentucky Hospital
Lexington, Kentucky

MARK B. PARSHALL, PhD, RN, CEN
Assistant Professor
College of Nursing
Health Sciences Center
University of New Mexico
Albuquerque, New Mexico

MARY PHILLIPS, RN, ARNP, CEN
Weekend Divisional Charge Nurse
Emergency Department
University of Kentucky Hospital
Lexington, Kentucky

MARY CELESTE SHAWLER, MSN, RN, CS
Psychiatric Clinical Nurse Specialist
University of Kentucky Hospital
Lexington, Kentucky

KIMOTHY SPARKS, RN, CEN, EMT-P
Staff Nurse
Emergency Department
University of Kentucky Hospital
Lexington, Kentucky

COLLEEN H. SWARTZ, RN, MSN, CCRN
Director, Emergency/Trauma Services
University of Kentucky Hospital
Lexington, Kentucky

STEVEN R. TALBERT, RN, MSN
University of Kentucky Air Medical Service
University of Kentucky Hospital
Lexington, Kentucky

DARLENE WELSH, RN, MSN, CS
Lecturer
University of Kentucky College of Nursing
Lexington, Kentucky

Contributors to the First Edition

Patricia L. Brisky, RN, BSN, CEN
Michele Nypaver, MD

NANCY A. BURTON, RN, CEN
Nursing Team Leader
Emergency Department
University of Wisconsin Hospital and Clinics
Madison, Wisconsin

CELESTE CHAMBERLAIN, RN, MS, CEN, CCRN
Unit Director
Emergency Center
Allegheny University Hospital
Philadelphia, Pennsylvania

SUSAN MCDANIEL HOHENHAUS, RN, CEN, SANE
Nursing Education Clinician
Emergency Department
University of North Carolina
Chapel Hill, North Carolina

MELINDA J. LAFLIN, RN, CEN
Flight Nurse
McKennan Careflight
McKennan Hospital
Sioux Falls, South Dakota

HELEN ROZNOWSKI, RNC, MSN
Nurse Manager
Emergency Department
Alpena General Hospital
Alpena, Michigan

ANNA M. SMITH, RN, MSN
Assistant Director
Emergency Services
University of Louisville Hospital
Louisville, Kentucky

This book is dedicated to emergency nurses everywhere for their ability to see the worst and make the best out of it. PSK

To God for His wonderful blessings. To Richard, who happens to be one of those blessings. PAS

To Skip and Trevor—the loves of my life. You two are the best! To Pam and Patty for your guidance and patience in teaching me how this is done. JHF

This book is still written by emergency nurses (and one "misplaced" nurse practitioner) for emergency nurses. Many of you wrote us after the first edition telling us how much you liked the format of the book and that you found the content useful and "right on" in terms of what we all need in the emergency setting. So, keeping true to the philosophy of, "If it isn't broke, don't fix it", the format of the second edition is basically unchanged.

The content, however, is a different matter. So much has changed over the course of the last few years that you will notice timely new nursing alerts, practice pearls, interventions, and evaluation criteria.

The new aspects of the second edition include additions and updates to the reference section including additional pediatric algorithms, updated pediatric immunization guidelines, additional new ACLS guidelines, the pediatric trauma score, and the inclusion of the pediatric and infant coma score.

The chapters have been revised to include updated material such as the new head injury guidelines in the Neurologic Conditions chapter and the newest information on the evaluation of abdominal trauma in the Trauma chapter. Information about rapid sequence induction in the Endotracheal Intubation procedure is one example of new information in the procedure section.

Pediatric reference material has been grouped together and the fluid and blood administration material has been moved to reference guides so it is easily accessible. The inside covers of the book now contain information that will be helpful to the practicing nurse such as pediatric and adult drug calculation formulas, a drug compatibility chart, and a temperature conversion table.

Triage sections are very similar to the first edition since airway, breathing, and circulation priorities remain the standard against which all patients are judged in terms of degree of acuity. Nursing diagnoses are very similar as well since there have been few modifications to the classification system that truly affect the emphasis of this book.

The editors and contributors to this book are currently practicing. They work in a variety of arenas, including but not limited to emergency departments (university affiliated as well as community non-profit and private facilities), urgent care centers, air medical and ground transport services, and across the acute care continuum in roles where they service patients from the ED to hospital discharge. We know the frustrations of caring for complex patients with few resources. Hopefully this book will promote your efficiency and effectiveness and offer suggestions that can improve the quality of your nursing care.

We welcome your ideas for future editions and your critique of this edition. We want this book to remain in every emergency nurse's lab coat pocket!

Pamela S. Kidd
Patty Ann Sturt
Julia Fultz

I would like to acknowledge my co-editors, Patty and Julia, for taking the ball and running with it—you scored! PSK

Contents

Contents

UNIT ONE

Reference
Guides

REFERENCE GUIDE 1
ACLS Algorithms: Adults

Ventricular Fibrillation and Pulseless Ventricular Tachycardia (VF/VT) Algorithms

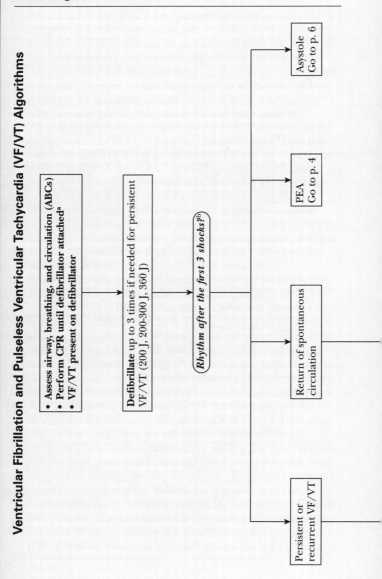

- Assess airway, breathing, and circulation (ABCs)
- Perform CPR until defibrillator attached[a]
- VF/VT present on defibrillator

Defibrillate up to 3 times if needed for persistent VF/VT (200 J, 200-300 J, 360 J)

Rhythm after the first 3 shocks?[b]

Persistent or recurrent VF/VT

Return of spontaneous circulation

PEA
Go to p. 4

Asystole
Go to p. 6

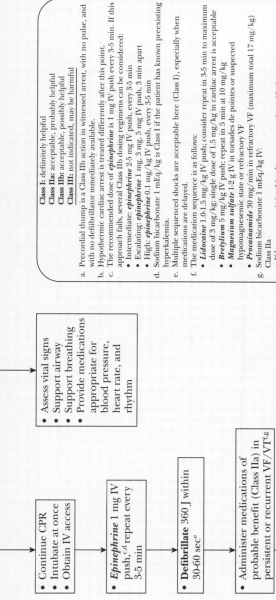

- Assess vital signs
- Support airway
- Support breathing
- Provide medications appropriate for blood pressure, heart rate, and rhythm

- Continue CPR
- Intubate at once
- Obtain IV access

- *Epinephrine* 1 mg IV push,[c,d] repeat every 3-5 min

- **Defibrillate** 360 J within 30-60 sec[e]

- Administer medications of probable benefit (Class IIa) in persistent or recurrent VF/VT[f,g]

- **Defibrillate** 360 J, 30-60 sec after each dose of medication[e]
- Pattern should be drug-shock, drug-shock

Class I: definitely helpful
Class IIa: acceptable, probably helpful
Class IIb: acceptable, possibly helpful
Class III: not indicated, may be harmful

a. Precordial thump is a Class IIb action in witnessed arrest, with no pulse, and with no defibrillator immediately available.

b. Hypothermic cardiac arrest is treated differently after this point.

c. The recommended dose of *epinephrine* is 1 mg IV push every 3-5 min. If this approach fails, several Class IIb dosing regimens can be considered:
- Intermediate: *epinephrine* 2-5 mg IV push, every 3-5 min
- Escalating: *epinephrine* 1 mg, 3 mg, 5 mg IV push, 3 min apart
- High: *epinephrine* 0.1 mg/kg IV push, every 3-5 min

d. Sodium bicarbonate 1 mEq/kg is Class I if the patient has known preexisting hyperkalemia.

e. Multiple sequenced shocks are acceptable here (Class I), especially when medications are delayed.

f. The medication sequence is as follows:
- *Lidocaine* 1.0-1.5 mg/kg IV push; consider repeat in 3-5 min to maximum dose of 3 mg/kg; single dose of 1.5 mg/kg in cardiac arrest is acceptable
- *Bretylium* 5 mg/kg IV push; repeat in 5 min at 10 mg/kg
- *Magnesium sulfate* 1-2 g IV in torsades de pointes or suspected hypomagnesemic state or refractory VF
- *Procainamide* 30 mg/min in refractory VF (maximum total 17 mg/kg)

g. Sodium bicarbonate 1 mEq/kg IV:
Class IIa
- If known preexisting bicarbonate-responsive acidosis
- If overdose with tricyclic antidepressants
- To alkalinize the urine in drug overdoses
Class IIB
- If intubated and continued long arrest interval
- Upon return of spontaneous circulation after long arrest interval
Class III
- Hypoxic lactic acidosis

Continued

Pulseless Electrical Activity (PEA)

Includes
- Electromechanical dissociation (EMD)
- Pseudo-EMD
- Idioventricular rhythms
- Ventricular escape rhythms
- Bradyasystolic rhythms
- Postdefibrillation idioventricular rhythms

- Continue CPR
- Intubate at once
- Obtain IV access

- Assess blood flow using Doppler ultrasound, end-tidal CO_2, echocardiography, or arterial line

Consider possible causes
(Parentheses = possible therapies and treatments)

- Hypovolemia (volume infusion)
- Hypoxia (ventilation)
- Cardiac tamponade (pericardiocentesis)
- Tension pneumothorax (needle decompression)
- Hypothermia
- Massive pulmonary embolism (surgery, *thrombolytics*)

- Drug overdoses such as tricyclics, digitalis, beta blockers, calcium channel blockers
- Hyperkalemia[a]
- Acidosis[b]
- Massive acute myocardial infarction

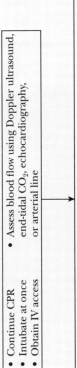

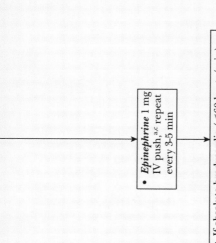

- *Epinephrine* 1 mg IV push,[a,c] repeat every 3-5 min

- If absolute bradycardia (<60 beats/min) or relative bradycardia, give *atropine* 1 mg IV
- Repeat every 3-5 min to a total of 0.03-0.04 mg/kg[d]

Class I: definitely helpful
Class IIa: acceptable, probably helpful
Class IIb: acceptable, possibly helpful
Class III: not indicated, may be harmful

a. *Sodium bicarbonate* 1 mEq/kg is Class I if the patient has known preexisting hyperkalemia.
b. *Sodium bicarbonate* 1 mEq/kg IV:
   Class IIa
   - If known preexisting bicarbonate-responsive acidosis
   - If overdose with tricyclic antidepressants
   - To alkalinize the urine in drug overdoses
   Class IIb
   - If intubated and continued long arrest interval
   - Upon return of spontaneous circulation after long arrest interval
   Class III
   - Hypoxic lactic acidosis
c. The recommended dose of *epinephrine* is 1 mg IV push every 3-5 min. If this approach fails, several Class IIb dosing regimens can be considered:
   - Intermediate: *epinephrine* 2-5 mg IV push, every 3-5 min
   - Escalating: *epinephrine* 1 mg, 3 mg, 5 mg IV push, 3 min apart
   - High: *epinephrine* 0.1 mg/kg IV push, every 3-5 min
d. The shorter *atropine* dosing interval (3 min) is possibly helpful in cardiac arrest (Class IIb).

Continued

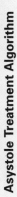

REFERENCE GUIDE 1

Asystole Treatment Algorithm

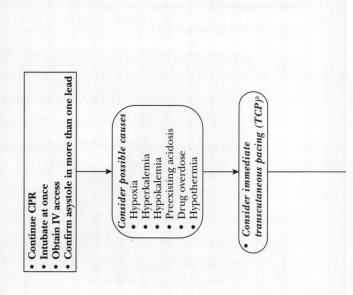

- **Continue CPR**
- **Intubate at once**
- **Obtain IV access**
- **Confirm asystole in more than one lead**

Consider possible causes
- Hypoxia
- Hyperkalemia
- Hypokalemia
- Preexisting acidosis
- Drug overdose
- Hypothermia

- *Consider immediate transcutaneous pacing (TCP)*[a]

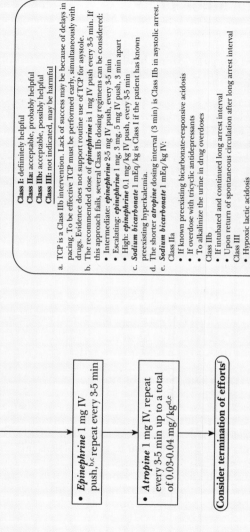

Class I: definitely helpful
Class IIa: acceptable, probably helpful
Class IIb: acceptable, possibly helpful
Class III: not indicated, may be harmful

a. TCP is a Class IIb intervention. Lack of success may be because of delays in pacing. To be effective TCP must be performed early, simultaneously with drugs. Evidence does not support routine use of TCP for asystole.

b. The recommended dose of *epinephrine* is 1 mg IV push every 3-5 min. If this approach fails, several Class IIb dosing regimens can be considered:
  • Intermediate: *epinephrine* 2-5 mg IV push, every 3-5 min
  • Escalating: *epinephrine* 1 mg, 3 mg, 5 mg IV push, 3 min apart
  • High: *epinephrine* 0.1 mg/kg IV push, every 3-5 min

c. *Sodium bicarbonate* 1 mEq/kg is Class I if the patient has known preexisting hyperkalemia.

d. The shorter *atropine* dosing interval (3 min) is Class IIb in asystolic arrest.

e. *Sodium bicarbonate* 1 mEq/kg IV:
   Class IIa
   • If known preexisting bicarbonate-responsive acidosis
   • If overdose with tricyclic antidepressants
   • To alkalinize the urine in drug overdoses
   Class IIb
   • If intubated and continued long arrest interval
   • Upon return of spontaneous circulation after long arrest interval
   Class III
   • Hypoxic lactic acidosis

f. If the patient remains in asystole or other agonal rhythm after successful intubation and initial medications, and if no reversible causes are identified, consider termination of resuscitative efforts by a physician. Consider the interval since arrest.

• *Epinephrine* 1 mg IV push,[b,c] repeat every 3-5 min

→ • *Atropine* 1 mg IV, repeat every 3-5 min up to a total of 0.03-0.04 mg/kg[d,e]

→ Consider termination of efforts[f]

Continued

Bradycardia Algorithm (Patient is not in cardiac arrest)

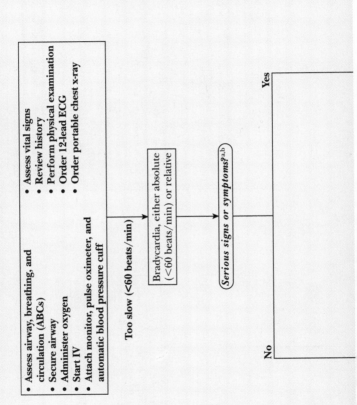

- Assess airway, breathing, and circulation (ABCs)
- Secure airway
- Administer oxygen
- Start IV
- Attach monitor, pulse oximeter, and automatic blood pressure cuff

- Assess vital signs
- Review history
- Perform physical examination
- Order 12-lead ECG
- Order portable chest x-ray

Too slow (<60 beats/min)

Bradycardia, either absolute (<60 beats/min) or relative

Serious signs or symptoms?[a,b]

No   Yes

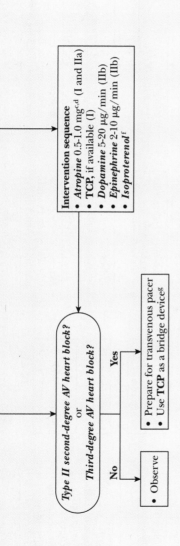

Intervention sequence
- *Atrophine* 0.5-1.0 mg[c,d] (I and IIa)
- **TCP**, if available (I)
- *Dopamine* 5-20 μg/min (IIb)
- *Epinephrine* 2-10 μg/min (IIb)
- *Isoproterenol*[f]

Type II second-degree AV heart block?
or
Third-degree AV heart block?

No
- Observe

Yes
- Prepare for transvenous pacer
- Use **TCP** as a bridge device[g]

a. Serious signs or symptoms must be related to the slow rate. Clinical manifestations include the following:
- Symptoms (chest pain, shortness of breath, decreased level of consciousness)
- Signs (low BP, shock, pulmonary congestion, CHF, acute MI)

b. Do not delay TCP while awaiting IV access or for *atrophine* to take effect if the patient is symptomatic.

c. Denervated transplanted hearts will not respond to *atrophine*. Go at once to pacing, *catecholamine* infusion, or both.

d. *Atrophine* should be given in repeat doses every 3-5 min up to a total of 0.03-0.04 mg/kg. Use the shorter dosing interval (3 min) in severe clinical conditions. It has been suggested that *atrophine* should be used with caution in atrioventricular (AV) block at the His-Purkinje level (type II AV block and new third-degree block with wide QRS complexes) (Class IIb).

e. Never treat third-degree heart block plus ventricular escape beats with *lidocaine*.

f. *Isoproterenol* should be used, if at all, with extreme caution. At low doses it is Class IIb (possibly helpful); at higher doses it is Class III (harmful).

g. Verify patient tolerance and mechanical capture. Use analgesia and sedation as needed.

TCP, Transcutaneous pacing.

Continued

Tachycardia Algorithm

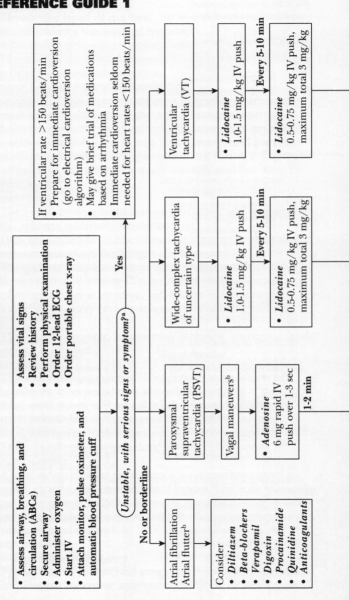

- Assess airway, breathing, and circulation (ABCs)
- Secure airway
- Administer oxygen
- Start IV
- Attach monitor, pulse oximeter, and automatic blood pressure cuff
- Assess vital signs
- Review history
- Perform physical examination
- Order 12-lead ECG
- Order portable chest x-ray

Unstable, with serious signs or symptom?[a]

No or borderline

Yes

Atrial fibrillation
Atrial flutter[b]

Consider
- *Diltiazem*
- *Beta-blockers*
- *Verapamil*
- *Digoxin*
- *Procainamide*
- *Quinidine*
- *Anticoagulants*

Paroxysmal supraventricular tachycardia (PSVT)

Vagal maneuvers[b]

- *Adenosine* 6 mg rapid IV push over 1-3 sec

1-2 min

Wide-complex tachycardia of uncertain type

- *Lidocaine* 1.0-1.5 mg/kg IV push

Every 5-10 min

- *Lidocaine* 0.5-0.75 mg/kg IV push, maximum total 3 mg/kg

Ventricular tachycardia (VT)

- *Lidocaine* 1.0-1.5 mg/kg IV push

Every 5-10 min

- *Lidocaine* 0.5-0.75 mg/kg IV push, maximum total 3 mg/kg

- If ventricular rate >150 beats/min
- Prepare for immediate cardioversion (go to electrical cardioversion algorithm)
- May give brief trial of medications based on arrhythmia
- Immediate cardioversion seldom needed for heart rates <150 beats/min

Continued

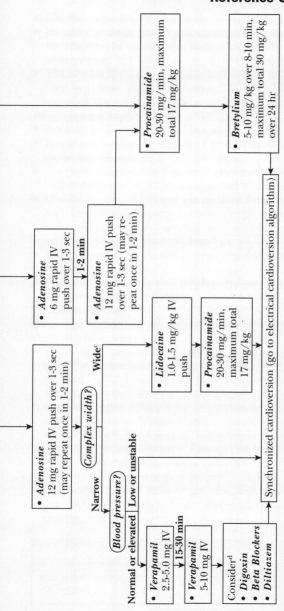

- **Procainamide** 20-30 mg/min, maximum total 17 mg/kg

- **Bretylium** 5-10 mg/kg over 8-10 min, maximum total 30 mg/kg over 24 hr

- **Adenosine** 6 mg rapid IV push over 1-3 sec

1-2 min

- **Adenosine** 12 mg rapid IV push over 1-3 sec (may repeat once in 1-2 min)

- **Adenosine** 12 mg rapid IV push over 1-3 sec (may repeat once in 1-2 min)

(*Complex width?*)

Narrow   Wide[c]

- **Lidocaine** 1.0-1.5 mg/kg IV push

- **Procainamide** 20-30 mg/min, maximum total 17 mg/kg

(*Blood pressure?*)

Normal or elevated | Low or unstable

- **Verapamil** 2.5-5.0 mg IV

15-30 min

- **Verapamil** 5-10 mg IV

Consider[d]
- **Digoxin**
- **Beta Blockers**
- **Diltiazem**

Synchronized cardioversion (go to electrical cardioversion algorithm)

a. Unstable condition must be related to the tachycardia. Signs and symptoms may include chest pain, shortness of breath, decreased level of consciousness, low blood pressure, shock, pulmonary congestion, congestive heart failure, or acute myocardial infarction.
b. Carotid sinus pressure is contraindicated for patients with carotid bruits; avoid ice water immersion with patients who have ischemic heart disease.
c. If the wide-complex tachycardia is known with certainly to be PSVT and blood pressure is normal or elevated, the sequence can include *verapamil*.
d. Use extreme caution with beta-blockers after *verapamil*.

Electrical Cardioversion Algorithm (Patient is not in cardiac arrest)

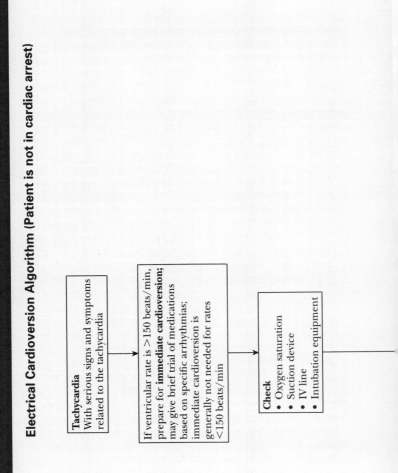

Tachycardia
With serious signs and symptoms related to the tachycardia

If ventricular rate is >150 beats/min, prepare for **immediate cardioversion;** may give brief trial of medications based on specific arrhythmias; immediate cardioversion is generally not needed for rates <150 beats/min

Check
- Oxygen saturation
- Suction device
- IV line
- Intubation equipment

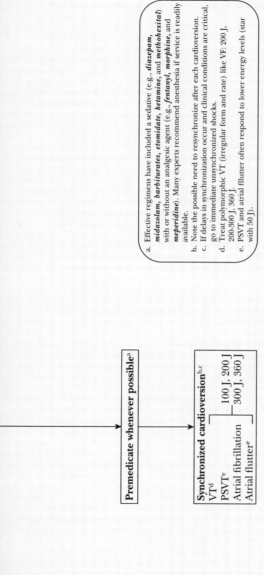

Premedicate whenever possible[a]

Synchronized cardioversion[b,c]
VT[d]
PSVT[e]   100 J, 200 J
Atrial fibrillation   300 J, 360 J
Atrial flutter[e]

a. Effective regimens have included a sedative (e.g., *diazepam, midazolam, barbiturates, etomidate, ketamine,* and *methohexital*) with or without an analgesic agent (e.g., *fentanyl, morphine,* and *meperidine*). Many experts recommend anesthesia if service is readily available.
b. Note the possible need to resynchronize after each cardioversion.
c. If delays in synchronization occur and clinical conditions are critical, go to immediate unsynchronized shocks.
d. Treat polymorphic VT (irregular form and rate) like VF: 200 J, 200-300 J, 360 J.
e. PSVT and atrial flutter often respond to lower energy levels (star with 50 J).

Continued

REFERENCE GUIDE 1

Algorithm for Suspected Stroke Patients

Immediate general assessment: <10 min from arrival
- Assess ABCs, vital signs
- Provide oxygen by nasal cannula
- Obtain IV access; obtain blood samples (CBC, electrolytes, coagulation studies)
- Check blood sugar; treat if indicated
- Perform general neurologic screening assessment
- Alert stroke team: neurologist, radiologist, CT technician

Immediate neurologic assessment: <25 min from arrival
- Review patient history
- Establish onset (<3 hours required for *thrombolytics*)
- Perform physical examination
- Perform neurologic examination
- Determine level of consciousness (Glasgow Coma Scale)
- Determine level of stroke severity (NIH stroke scale or Hunt and Hess scale)
- Order urgent noncontrast CT scan (door-to-CT scan performed; goal <25 min from arrival)
- Read CT scan (door-to-CT read; goal <45 min from arrival)
- Perform lateral cervical spine x-ray (if patient is comatose or has history of trauma)

Does CT scan show intracerebral or subarachnoid hemorrhage?

Probable acute ischemic stroke
- Review CT exclusions; are any observed?
- Repeat neurologic examination; are deficits variable or rapidly improving?
- Review *thrombolytic* exclusions; are any observed?
- Review patient data; is symptom onset now >3 hours?

No to All of Above

No

If high suspicion of subarachnoid hemorrhage remains despite negative findings on CT scan, perform lumbar puncture (lumbar puncture excludes use of *thrombolytic* therapy)

Yes

Consult neurosurgery

Blood on LP

Initiate actions for acute hemorrhage
- Reverse any *anticoagulants*
- Reverse any bleeding disorder
- Monitor neurologic condition
- Treat hypertension in awake patients

No Blood on LP

- Initiate supportive therapy as indicated
- Consider admission
- Consider anticoagulation
- Consider additional conditions needing treatment
- Consider alternative diagnoses

Patient remains candidate for thrombolytic therapy?

No

Yes

- Review risks and benefits with patient and family. If acceptable:
  Begin *thrombolytic* treatment (door-to-treatment goal <60 min):
- Monitor neurologic status; emergent CT if deterioration
- Monitor BP; treat as indicated
- Admit to critical care unit
- No anticoagulants or antiplatelet treatment × 24 hours

Continued

Hypothermia Algorithm

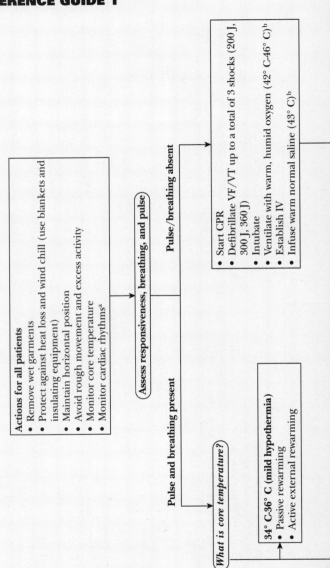

Actions for all patients
- Remove wet garments
- Protect against heat loss and wind chill (use blankets and insulating equipment)
- Maintain horizontal position
- Avoid rough movement and excess activity
- Monitor core temperature
- Monitor cardiac rhythms[a]

↓

Assess responsiveness, breathing, and pulse

Pulse and breathing present

What is core temperature?

34° C–36° C (mild hypothermia)
- Passive rewarming
- Active external rewarming

Pulse/breathing absent

- Start CPR
- Defibrillate VF/VT up to a total of 3 shocks (200 J, 300 J, 360 J)
- Intubate
- Ventilate with warm, humid oxygen (42° C–46° C)[b]
- Establish IV
- Infuse warm normal saline (43° C)[b]

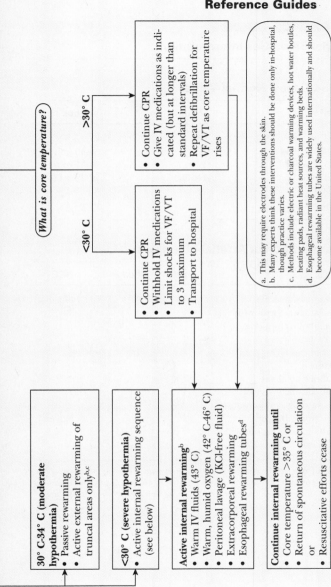

What is core temperature?

<30° C

- Continue CPR
- Withhold IV medications
- Limit shocks for VF/VT to 3 maximum
- Transport to hospital

>30° C

- Continue CPR
- Give IV medications as indicated (but at longer than standard intervals)
- Repeat defibrillation for VF/VT as core temperature rises

a. This may require electrodes through the skin.
b. Many experts think these interventions should be done only in-hospital, though practice varies.
c. Methods include electric or charcoal warming devices, hot water bottles, heating pads, radiant heat sources, and warming beds.
d. Esophageal rewarming tubes are widely used internationally and should become available in the United States.

30° C-34° C (moderate hypothermia)
- Passive rewarming
- Active external rewarming of truncal areas only[b,c]

<30° C (severe hypothermia)
- Active internal rewarming sequence (see below)

Active internal rewarming[b]
- Warm IV fluids (43° C)
- Warm, humid oxygen (42° C-46° C)
- Peritoneal lavage (KCl-free fluid)
- Extracorporeal rewarming
- Esophageal rewarming tubes[d]

Continue internal rewarming until
- Core temperature >35° C or
- Return of spontaneous circulation
or
- Resuscitative efforts cease

REFERENCE GUIDE 2

Arterial Blood Gas Interpretation

Blood Gases: Normal Values

Arterial	Value	Venous
7.35-7.45	pH	7.31-7.41
80-100 mm Hg	Po_2*	30-40 mm Hg
35-45 mm Hg	Pco_2	41-51 mm Hg
21-25 mEq/L	HCO_3^-	22-29 mEq/L
95%-99%	O_2 sat	60%-85%
−2 to +2	BE	0 to +4

Interpretation of Arterial Blood Gas Values

	pH	Pco_2	HCO_3^-
Respiratory acidosis	↓	↑	Normal
Respiratory acidosis with metabolic compensation	↓	↑	↑
Metabolic acidosis	↓	Normal	↓
Metabolic and respiratory acidosis	↓	↑	↓
Metabolic alkalosis	↑	Normal	↑
Metabolic alkalosis with respiratory compensation	↑	↑	↑
Respiratory alkalosis	↑	↓	Normal
Metabolic and respiratory alkalosis	↑	↓	↑

Modified from Lee G: *Quick emergency care reference,* St Louis, 1992, Mosby.
*In a patient over 60 years old, Pao_2 is equal to 80 mm Hg minus 1 mm Hg for every year over 60. Expected Pao_2 can be determined by multiplying the Fio_2 by 5.

REFERENCE GUIDE 3

Blood Component Administration Guidelines

Blood Component Administration Guidelines for Adults

Blood component	Infusion rate	Filter	Volume	Comments
Whole blood	2-4 hr Max: 4 hr	Required	500 ml	Rapid infusion if need is urgent
Packed red blood cells	2-4 hr Max: 4 hr	Required	250 ml	Hgb rises 1 g/dl; Hct rises 3% after 1 U
Leukocyte-poor red blood cells	2 hr	Required	Variable	—
Fresh frozen plasma	1-2 hr, rapidly if bleeding	Use component filter	250 ml	Notify blood bank—takes 20 min to thaw
Platelets	As rapidly as patient tolerates	Use component filter	35-50 ml U	Usually 6-10 U ordered; request that blood bank pool all units
Albumin	1-2 ml/min for normovolemic patients	Special tubing	Varies	Comes in 5% and 25%; can increase intravascular volume quickly; infuse cautiously
Cryoprecipitate	30 min	Use component filter	10 ml/U	Usually 6-10 U ordered; request that blood bank pool all units
Granulocytes	2-4 hr	Use component filter	300-400 ml	VS q15min during infusion; granulocytes have short life span; transfuse as soon after collection as possible

REFERENCE GUIDE 3

Blood Component Administration Guidelines for Children

Blood component	Usual dose	Rate of infusion	Comments
Whole blood	20 ml/kg initially	As rapidly as necessary to restore volume and stabilize the child	Administration is usually reserved for massive hemorrhage
Packed red blood cells	10 ml/kg, not to exceed 15 ml/kg	5 ml/kg/hr or 2 ml/kg/hr if congestive heart failure develops	1 ml/kg will increase Hct approximately 1%; infuse within 4 hr; if necessary, divide unit into smaller volumes for infusion
Platelets	1 unit for every 7-10 kg	Each unit over 5-10 min via syringe or pump	The usual dose will increase platelet count by 50,000/mm^3

Fresh frozen plasma	Hemorrhage: 15-30 ml/kg Clotting deficiency: 10-15 ml/kg	Hemorrhage: rapidly to stabilize the child Clotting deficiency: over 2-3 hr	Monitor for fluid overload
Granulocytes	Dependent on WBC counts and clinical condition, 10 ml/kg/day initially	Slowly over 2-4 hour because of fever and chills, side effects commonly associated with infusion	Granulocytes have short life span; transfuse as soon after collection as possible
Albumin 5%	1 g/kg or 20 ml/kg	1-2 ml/min or 60-120 ml/hr	Monitor for fluid overload; type and crossmatch not required
Albumin 25%	1 g/kg or 4 ml/kg	0.2-0.4 ml/min or 12-24 ml/hr	Monitor for fluid overload; type and crossmatch not required

REFERENCE GUIDE 4

Blood Transfusion Reaction Comparison

Transfusion reaction	Symptoms	Treatment
Acute hemolytic reaction	• Hypotension • Burning in vein • Flushed face • Headache • Diffuse pain	• Stop transfusion • Start NS or RL • Consider diuretics • Monitor BUN, serum creatinine, LDH, and bilirubin levels
Minor incompatibility	Symptoms occur after transfusion is completed • Mild jaundice • Failure to maintain expected hemo-globin level after transfusion	• No actions are indicated
Anaphylaxis	• Hypotension • Decreased respon-siveness • Severe dyspnea • Generalized edema may be present	• Stop transfusion • Airway and breathing support (anticipate intubation) • Administer epinephrine • Start NS or RL
Hypersensitivity	• Urticaria • Pruritus • Hives • Facial edema • Fever • Nausea and vomiting • Dyspnea	• Stop transfusion • Administer antihistamine • Administer steroids • Administer acetaminophen

BUN, blood urea nitrogen; *LDH,* lactate dehydrogenase; *NS,* normal saline; *RL,* lactate.

Steps in investigating transfusion reactions

1. Send (if available) prereaction recipient blood or get type and crossmatch results from prereaction recipient blood.
2. Send a postreaction recipient blood specimen.
3. Send donor blood being administered at time of reaction.
4. Send a posttransfusion urine sample.

Diagnosis is confirmed by direct antiglobulin testing (a positive result on the Coombs' test) and separation of the offending antibody from red blood cells.

REFERENCE GUIDE 5

Calculations and Conversions

Conversions
Volume

5 ml = 1 teaspoon (tsp)
15 ml = 1 tablespoon (T)
30 ml = 1 ounce (oz) = 2 T
500 ml = 1 pint (pt)
1000 ml = 1 quart (qt)

Length

2.5 centimeters (cm) = 1 inch

Pressure

1 mm Hg = 1.36 cm H_2O

Weight

1 kilogram (kg) = 2.2 pounds (lb)
1 gram (g) = 1000 milligrams (mg)
1 mg = 1000 micrograms (μg)
1 grain (gr) = 60 mg
$1/100$ gr = 0.6 mg
$1/150$ gr = 0.4 mg

Centigrade (C)/Fahrenheit (F)

$^\circ C = (^\circ F - 32) \times 5/9$
$^\circ F = (^\circ C \times 9/5) + 32$

Critical Care Calculations

Drug concentration
mg/ml = Drug in solution (mg)/Volume of solution (ml)
μg/ml = mg/ml $\times$ 1000

Delivery rate
ml/min = ml/hr/60

$$\mu g/kg/min = \frac{\mu g/ml \times ml/min}{Weight\ (kg)}$$

$$ml/hr = \frac{\mu g/kg/min\ prescribed \times kg \times 60\ min}{\mu g/ml}$$

From Keen J, Baird M, Allen J. *Mosby's critical care and emergency drug reference*, St Louis, 1994, Mosby.

Conversions and Estimates: Temperature

Centigrade (Celsius)	Fahrenheit	Centigrade (Celsius)	Fahrenheit
34.2	93.6	38.6	101.5
34.6	94.3	39.0	102.2
35.0	95.0	39.4	102.9
35.4	95.7	39.8	103.6
35.8	96.4	40.2	104.4
36.2	97.2	40.6	105.2
36.6	97.9	41.0	105.9
37.0	98.6	41.4	106.5
37.4	99.3	41.8	107.2
37.8	100.0	42.2	108.0
38.2	100.8	42.6	108.7

Adapted from Barkin R, Rosen P, editors: *Emergency pediatrics,* St Louis, 1994, Mosby. From *ENPC provider manual,* ed 2, Park Ridge, Ill, 1998, Emergency Nurses Association.

To convert centigrade to Fahrenheit:
$(\frac{9}{5} \times \text{temperature}) + 32$

To convert Fahrenheit to centigrade:
$(\text{temperature} - 32) \times \frac{5}{9}$

REFERENCE GUIDE 6

Diabetic Ketoacidosis (DKA): Adult

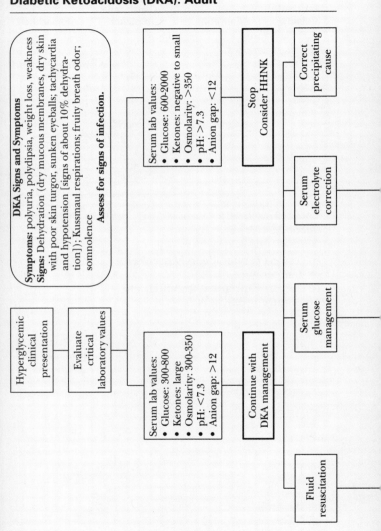

DKA Signs and Symptoms

Symptoms: polyuria, polydipsia, weight loss, weakness

Signs: Dehydration (dry mucous membranes, dry skin with poor skin turgor; sunken eyeballs; tachycardia and hypotension [signs of about 10% dehydration]); Kussmaul respirations; fruity breath odor; somnolence

Assess for signs of infection.

Hyperglycemic clinical presentation

Evaluate critical laboratory values

Serum lab values:
- Glucose: 600-2000
- Ketones: negative to small
- Osmolarity: >350
- pH: >7.3
- Anion gap: <12

Stop
Consider HHNK

Serum lab values:
- Glucose: 300-800
- Ketones: large
- Osmolarity: 300-350
- pH: <7.3
- Anion gap: >12

Continue with DKA management

Correct precipitating cause

Serum electrolyte correction

Serum glucose management

Fluid resuscitation

Goal: Attain normovolemia
Initial 1-2 hr: 0.9% NS at 1000 ml/hr
Maintenance: 0.9% NS at 250-400 ml/hr

When glucose ≤250, begin 5% dextrose/0.45% NS solution (see Glucose Correction)
IF
Glucose = 100-250 with ketones of moderate to large, consider starting 10% dextrose

Patient unstable:
Consider pulmonary artery catheter or CVP
If circulatory collapse, may administer plasma expanders

Regular insulin (IV) bolus:
0.3 U/kg or 10 U IV push (optional)
Followed by
Continuous IV regular insulin drip at 0.1 U/kg/hr (6-10 U/hr)
Increase insulin 2-10 fold if no response by 4 hr

Monitor serum:
Glucose: q1-2h
Acetone: q4h
Arterial pH: q4-12h
(Blood glucose should drop approximately 10%/hr)

Patient stable: Continue current therapy

Glucose: >300
Ketones: Moderate to large
pH: <7.30
Continue current therapy

Evaluate serum electrolytes:
K^+ = q1-2hr
Na^+ Cl^- = q4hr
PO_4 = q12-24hr
12-lead ECG: Continuous cardiac monitoring; phosphate therapy if hypophosphatemia; sodium or potassium phosphate at ≤10 mmol/hr
Cautious use of bicarbonate for correction of severe acidosis
K^+ replacement: initiate with second liter of IV fluid

Patient level/replacement	
3.5	40 mEq
3.5-5.5	20 mEq
>5.5	Hold replacement

Glucose: 200-300
Ketones: Negative to moderate
pH: 7.30-7.45
Initiate clear liquid diet and advance as tolerated
Initiate SQ insulin 30-60 min before DC of IV insulin
Placed on maintenance regular insulin q6hr or NPH with supplemental regular insulin SQ

Developed by Kathleen Wagner, RN, MSN, Critical Care CNS, University Hospital/University of Kentucky College of Nursing.

Electrocardiogram Changes in Myocardial Infarction

Type of infarction	Anatomical location	ECG patterns
Lateral		I, a V_L, V_5, V_6; abnormal Q wave, ST elevation, T wave inversion
Inferior		II, III, a V_F: abnormal Q wave, ST elevation, T wave inversion
Anterior		V_1-V_4: abnormal Q wave, loss of R wave progression, ST elevation, T wave inversion
Posterior		V_1, V_2: tall R wave, ST depression, tall symmetric T wave
Note: RV infarction		V_{4R}: ST elevation >1 mm

From Lee: *Quick emergency care reference*, St Louis, 1992, Mosby.

REFERENCE GUIDE 8

Fluid Resuscitation Summary*

Crystalloids	Description/indication	Action(s)
0.9% Normal saline (NS)	Isotonic	• May produce fluid overload† • 25% of volume administered will remain in vascular space
0.45% NS	Hypotonic, moves fluid from vascular space to interstitial and intracellular spaces	• Decreases blood viscosity • May promote hypovolemia • May promote cerebral edema
5% Dextrose	Hypotonic	• 7.5 cc/100 cc infused will remain in vascular space • Inadequate for fluid resuscitation
Ringers' lactate solution	Isotonic, contains multiple electrolytes and lactate	• May produce fluid overload† • May promote lactic acidosis in prolonged hypoperfusion with decreased liver function • Lactate metabolizes to acetate, may produce metabolic alkalosis when large volumes are transfused

*Dosages are not listed because of variability in patient response and need.
†Fluid overload may occur when these agents are used because of large amounts of fluid required for volume lost (3:1 ratio).

Continued

REFERENCE GUIDE 8

Fluid Resuscitation Summary—cont'd

Crystalloids	Description/indication	Action(s)
Hypertonic saline (7.5%)	Hypertonic, pulls fluid from interstitial and intracellular spaces into vascular space	• Requires smaller amount to restore blood volume • Increases cerebral oxygen while decreasing ICP • May promote hypernatremia • May promote intracellular dehydration • May promote osmotic diuresis • Controversial

Synthetic colloids	Description	Action(s)
Dextran	Comes in 40, 70, and 75 molecular weight	• Associated with anaphylaxis • Reduces factor VIII, platelets, and fibrinogen function, so increases bleeding time • May interfere with blood crossmatching and typing, glucose, and erythrocyte sedimentation levels • Risk of fluid overload‡
Hetastarch		• May increase serum amylase levels • Associated with coagulopathy • Risk of fluid overload‡

Natural colloids	Description	Action(s)
Fresh frozen plasma	Contains all clotting factors	• Potential to transmit blood-borne infection • Can cause hypersensitivity reaction • Blood volume expander
Plasma protein fraction (Plasmanate)	Does not contain clotting factors	• May cause hypersensitivity reaction • If given too rapidly, may cause hypotension • Blood volume expander
Albumin	5% isooncotic; 25% hyperoncotic; "salt poor"	• Preferred as volume expander when risk from producing interstitial edema is great (e.g., pulmonary and heart disease) • Hypocalcemia
Whole blood	Can be administered without normal saline; reduces donor exposure	• Hyperkalemia, hypothermia, and hypocalcemia • May require greater amount than packed RBCs to increase oxygen-carrying capacity of blood • Rarely used, not cost-effective

‡Fluid overload may occur when these agents are used in cases of preexisting pulmonary or heart disease.

Continued

REFERENCE GUIDE 8

Fluid Resuscitation Summary—cont'd

Natural colloids	Description	Action(s)
Packed RBCs	Administer with normal saline	• Deficient in 2,3-diphosphoglycerate, so may increase oxygen affinity to hemoglobin and may decrease oxygen delivery to tissue • Hypothermia, hyperkalemia, and hypocalcemia

Experimental agents	Description	Action(s)
Liposome-encapsulated hemoglobin/hypertonic saline (75%)	NOT APPROVED BY FDA	• Improves skeletal muscle oxygen tension • Expands vascular volume quickly • Improves tissue oxygenation
Hypertonic saline (75%) with Dextran 70	Combined crystalloid and colloid therapy	• Promotes rapid expansion of volume and promotes retention of volume in vascular space • Controversial

REFERENCE GUIDE 9
Formulas Used in Fluid Administration

Basal fluid maintenance

1500 cc/m^2 BSA/24 hr = cc/24 hr (calculate as cc/hr)

General guidelines: Up to 10 kg = 100 cc/kg/24 hr
11-20 kg = 50 cc/kg/24 hr plus 100 cc/kg for first 10 kg
>20 kg = 20-25 cc/kg/24 hr plus 50 cc/kg for each kg 11 through 20 plus 100 cc/kg for first 10 kg

Volume replacement with crystalloids

Administer 3 cc for every cc lost. For fluid challenges administer:
IV bolus 20 cc/kg RL in children and adult trauma patients
IV bolus of 200-300 cc RL in adult surgical patients
IV bolus of 200-300 cc NS in adult medical patients

Volume replacement with colloids

Administer 1 cc for every cc lost.

Volume replacement for measured losses

Gastric losses: Replace 1 cc for every cc lost q4hr. Use D$_5$ ½ NS plus 30 mEq K/L
Intestinal losses: Replace 1 cc for every cc lost q4hr. Use D5% RL.

Basal urine output

Up to 30 kg = 40 cc/kg/24 hr (2 cc/kg/hr)
>30 kg = 1200 cc/24 hr (17-18 cc/kg/hr)

*See Chapter 3 for burn resuscitation formulas.
NS, Normal saline; *RL*, Ringer's lactate.

REFERENCE GUIDE 10

Glasgow Coma Scale: Adult

Activity	Best response	Points
Eye opening	Spontaneous	4
	To verbal stimuli	3
	To pain	2
	No response to pain	1
Motor	Follows commands	6
	Localizes to pain/purposeful movement	5
	Withdrawal in response to pain	4
	Abnormal flexion in response to pain	3
	Abnormal extension in response to pain	2
	No response to pain	1
Verbal	Oriented and converses	5
	Confused and converses	4
	Inappropriate words	3
	Incomprehensible sounds	2
	No verbal response	1

Possible points of 3-15; score of <8 = coma.

REFERENCE GUIDE 11

Hemodynamic Values

Parameter	Formula	Normal range
Cardiac output (CO)	$HR \times SV$	4-8 L/min
Cardiac index (CI)	$\dfrac{CO}{BSA}$	2.5-4.0 L/min/m²
Stroke volume (SV)	$\dfrac{CO \times 1000}{HR}$	55-100 ml/beat
Stroke volume index (SVI)	$\dfrac{SV}{BSA}$	33-75 ml/m²/beat
Stroke index (SI)	$\dfrac{CI \times 1000}{HR}$	30-65 ml/m²/beat
Mean arterial pressure (MAP)	$\dfrac{2(DBP) + SBP}{3}$	70-105 mm Hg
Systemic vascular resistance (SVR)	$\dfrac{MAP - CVP \times 80}{CO}$	700-1600 dynes/sec/cm^{-5}
Pulmonary vascular resistance (PVR)	$\dfrac{PAM - PAWP \times 80}{CO}$	20-130 dynes/sec/cm^{-5}
Arterial oxygen content (Cao_2)	$Sao_2 \times Hgb \times 1.38 + (Pao_2 \times .0031)$	18-20 ml/100 ml or 20 vol %
Venous oxygen content (Cvo_2)	$Svo_2 \times Hgb \times 1.38 + (Pvo_2 \times .0031)$	15.5 ml/100 ml or 20 vol %
Arterial venous oxygen content difference (Co_2)$_{(a-v)}$	$Cao_2 - Cvo_2$	4-6 ml/100 ml or vol %
Arterial oxygen delivery (Dao_2)	$CO \times 10 \times Cao_2$	900-1200 ml/min
Venous oxygen delivery (Dvo_2)	$CO \times 10 \times Cvo_2$	775 ml/min
Oxygen consumption (Vo_2)	$CO \times 10 \times Co_{2(a-v)}$	200-250 ml/min
Mixed venous oxygen saturation (Svo_2)	$1 - Vo_2/Do_2$	60%-80%
Alveolar-arterial oxygen gradient (Do_2)$_{(A-a)}$	$PAo_2 - Pao_2$	<15 mm Hg
Respiratory quotient (RQ)	$\dfrac{O_2 \text{ consumption}}{CO_2 \text{ consumption}}$	0.8-1
Cerebral perfusion Pressure (CPP)	$MAP - ICP$	80-100 mm Hg

Modified from Keen J, Baird M, Allen J: *Mosby's critical care and emergency drug reference*, St Louis, 1994, Mosby.
BSA, Body surface area; *PAM*, pulmonary artery mean (pressure).

REFERENCE GUIDE 12

Laboratory Values

Test	Normal value
Blood studies	
RBC	Men: 4.7-6.1 million/mm^3
	Women: 4.2-5.4 million/mm^3
WBC	5000-10,000/mm^3
Hgb	Men: 14-18 g/dl
	Women: 12-16 g/dl (pregnancy: >11 g/dl)
Hct	Men: 42%-52%
	Women: 37%-47% (pregnancy: >33%)
Platelets	150,000-400,000/mm^3
PT	10-14 sec (pregnancy: 10% ↓)
PTT	30-45 sec (pregnancy: slight ↓)
Na	136-145 mEq/L
K	3.5-5.0 mEq/L
Cl	90-110 mEq/L
CO_2	23-30 mEq/L
BUN	5-20 mg/dl
Cr	Men: 0.7-1.5 mg/dl
	0.6-1.2 mg/dl (females; pregnancy: 0.4-0.9)
Glucose	70-115 mg/dl
Ca	9-10.5 mg/dl
Mg	1.6-3.0 mEq/L
Osmolality	275-300 mOsm/kg
Bilirubin	
Direct	0.1-0.3 mg/dl
Total	0.2-1.0 mg/dl
Indirect	0.2-0.8 mg/dl
Amylase	56-190 U/L
Anion gap	8-16 mEq/L
Lactate	0.6-1.8 mEq/L

Modified from *Mosby's medical, nursing, & allied health dictionary*, ed 5, St Louis, 1998, Mosby.

Laboratory Values—cont'd

Test	Normal value
AST (SGOT)	12-36 U/L
with MI elevations	
Onset:	12-18 hr
Peak:	24-48 hr
Duration:	3-4 days
CK	96-140 U/L (females)
	38-174 U/L (males)
with MI elevations	
Onset:	4-6 hr
Peak:	12-24 hr
Duration:	3-4 days
CK-MB	<5% total
with MI elevations	
Onset:	4-6 hr
Peak:	12-24 hr
Duration:	2-3 days
LDH	90-200 U/L
with MI elevations	
Onset:	24-48 hr
Peak:	3-6 days
Duration:	7-10 days
LDH$_1$	17%-27% of total LDH
LDH$_2$	28%-38% of total LDH
with MI	
LDH$_1$ >LDH$_2$	
Onset:	12-24 hr
Peak:	48 hr
Duration:	Variable

Continued

REFERENCE GUIDE 12

Laboratory Values—cont'd

Test	Normal value
Miscellaneous	
Urine Na	100-260 mEq/L
Urine K	25-100 mEq/L
Urine Cl	140-250 mEq/L
Digoxin level	Therapeutic: 0.5-2 ng/ml
	Toxic: >2.4 mg/ml
Phenytoin level	10-20 µg/ml toxic >20 mg/ml
Theophylline level	10-20 mg/ml toxic >20 mg/ml

Modified from *Mosby's medical, nursing, & allied health dictionary,* ed 5, St Louis, 1998, Mosby.

REFERENCE GUIDE 13
Organ Procurement Guideline

Medicare Conditions of Participation of August 21, 1998, require that all deaths and imminent deaths be referred to the Organ Procurement Organization (OPO) in a timely manner. For imminent deaths (potential brain deaths), the OPO must be notified when the Glasgow Coma Scale score is ≤4 and before brain death determination. The OPO will determine whether the patient is medically suitable for donation. If the patient is deemed suitable, the hospital in collaboration with the OPO must ensure that the family of each potential donor is informed of its options to donate. The individual designated by the hospital to make the request must be an organ procurement representative or a trained designated requester (an individual trained by the OPO on how to request a donation).

Criteria for Organ Donation Referral
Potential for brain death to occur
Any age
Need for ventilator to maintain respiration and circulation

Typical Causes of Brain Death
Head trauma (closed head injuries, gunshot wounds to the head, shaken child syndrome, etc.)
Massive bleeding in the brain (e.g., CVA, SAH, ICD, or SDH)
Anoxia (e.g., after CPR, near drowning, or prolonged seizures)
Brain tumors (primary CNS tumors or brain metastasis)
Infection (e.g., meningitis)
Encephalopathies (metabolic)

Preliminary Requirements to Make a Determination of Brain Death
Known mechanism of injury
Absence of toxic CNS depression (sedatives, ETOH, neuro-muscular blockades)
Absence of metabolic CNS depression (hypothermia, hypotension, acidosis)

REFERENCE GUIDE 13

One of the following three types of testing must be met to determine brain death:

Clinical Examination
(Cannot use if toxic or metabolic CNS depression exists)
Unresponsive to any verbal or painful stimuli
No pupil reflex
No doll's eyes (oculocephalic reflex)
No response to ice water calorics
No corneal reflex
No gag reflex
Apnea (Pco $\geq$60 mm Hg) after observation of no respiratory activity with no respiratory assistance given
NOTE: Spinal reflexes may be present, but all of the above reflexes must be absent.
OR

EEG Confirms Lack of Electrical Activity*
(Cannot use if toxic or metabolic CNS depression exists)
OR
No Blood Flow to the Brain Determined by One of the Following:
(Cannot use if systolic blood pressure $\leq$80 mm Hg)
Cerebral angiogram
Nuclear flow study
Transcranial Doppler

Provide Hemodynamic Support
Initiate IV crystalloid or colloids to maintain adequate intake
Administer dopamine or dobutamine to maintain systolic blood pressure $\geq$90 mm Hg
If possible, avoid potent vasoconstrictors (e.g., epinephrine); however, long-term hypotension is more damaging than the use of potent vasoconstrictors

---

*Must also have a clinical examination to confirm brain stem death, because EEG assesses only cerebral activity

Monitor the patient for diabetes insipidus (UOP >200 cc/hr, rising serum sodium level, specific gravity <1.005)

If the patient is in DI, treat with vasopressin or DDAVP to keep UOP ≥100 cc/hr and ≤200 cc/hr

Replace blood loss to maintain hematocrit ≥30

Treat DIC

Provide Temperature Support

Maintain temperature of 96° F to 100° F by using heating and cooling blankets, adequate room temperature, warm NG lavages, and head coverings or by increasing ventilator temperatures.

Provide Ventilatory Support

Maintain Po_2 ≥100 mm Hg

Use Fio_2 as appropriate to maintain Po_2 ≥100 mm Hg

Tidal volume 12-15 cc/kg of ideal body weight

Set rate to maintain Pco_2 35-45 mm Hg

Place all patients on PEEP of 5 cm H_2O

Turn and suction patient q1-2hr to maintain optimal lung clearance and function

Provide Supportive Care to Family

It is vital that donation not be mentioned to the family until they have been informed that their loved one is dead and they acknowledge an understanding of this. An OPO representative should be present when donation is **first** mentioned to the family.

Modified from Thacker D: *Organ and tissue donation*, Lexington, Ky, 1999, Kentucky Organ Donation Association.

REFERENCE GUIDE 14

Oxygen Delivery Devices

Supplemental adjunct	Flow rate	O₂ Concentration (%)	Indications
Nasal cannula	1-6 L/min	24-44	Patients with minimal or no respiratory distress or oxygenation problem
Face mask	8-10 L/min	40-60	Patients who require a higher O_2 concentration than a nasal cannula can provide
Nonrebreather face mask with O_2 reservoir	6-15 L/min	60 to almost 100	Patients who need the highest possible oxygen concentration but are not candidates for endotracheal intubation
Venturi mask	3-15 L/min	24-50	Useful in patients with COPD and moderate to severe hypoxemia

Data from American Heart Association: *Advanced cardiac life support textbook,* Dallas, Tx, 1997, The Association; Emergency Nursing Association: *Emergency nursing pediatric course provider manual,* Park Ridge, Ill, 1998, The Association.

Comments	Pediatric considerations
A low-flow system in which the tidal volume is mixed with room air; for each L/min of flow increase, O_2 concentration increases by approximately 4%	Lubricating the prongs may make cannula more tolerable for pediatric patient; to avoid scaring child, start flow of oxygen after cannula is in place
Tidal volume is mixed with room air; requires an oxygen flow of at least 5 L/min to prevent an accumulation of exhaled air in mask, which may be rebreathed	Allow child to hold mask before putting it in place; use correctly fitting mask; mask should extend from bridge of nose to cleft of chin
Mask needs to fit face snugly; monitor patient closely if level of consciousness is diminished; vomiting into mask may result in aspiration; mask has two flapper valve ports, one on each side, to allow exhaled air to escape	Not available for neonate; mask should extend from bridge of nose to cleft of chin; if child who needs oxygen is not tolerating a mask, blow-by oxygen through corrugated tubing held close to child's face may work
More controlled oxygen concentration delivery; oxygen diluter used dictates oxygen concentration delivered at specific oxygen flow rate; mask must fit snugly on patient's face; monitor for respiratory depression	Not used for children

Continued

REFERENCE GUIDE 14

Supplemental adjunct	Flow rate	O_2 Concentration (%)	Indications
Pocket mask	Room air	17	Support ventilations in the patient with inadequate or absent respiratory effort
	10 L/min	50	
	15 L/min	80	
Bag-valve mask	Room air	21	Need for ventilatory assistance secondary to shallow, ineffective respiratory effort or apnea
	15 L with reservoir	100	

Data from American Heart Association: *Advanced cardiac life support textbook,* Dallas, Tx, 1997, The Association; Emergency Nursing Association: *Emergency nursing pediatric course provider manual,* Park Ridge, Ill, 1998, The Association.

Comments	Pediatric considerations
Use head tilt/chin lift (providing there is no trauma) to open airway; must obtain good seal with mask; pocket mask has been shown to provide better tidal volumes than bag-valve-mask; gastric inflation common; applying cricoid pressure will help reduce possibility of regurgitation and subsequent aspiration	Must have mask that fits child's face; tidal volume should be 10-15 ml/kg; monitor rise and fall of the child's chest
Adult bag-valve-mask device has approximately 1600 ml volume; may provide less volume than mouth-to-mouth or mouth-to-mask; can be difficult to obtain effective seal to deliver appropriate tidal volume; gastric inflation common; applying cricoid pressure will help reduce possibility of regurgitation and subsequent aspiration; tidal volume should be 10-15 ml/kg	Pediatric BVM device has approximate volume of 650 ml; term infants need bag that delivers at least 450 ml; popoff valves should be easily bypassed; tidal volume should be 10-15 ml/kg; mask should fit correctly to decrease under-mask volume and thereby dead space

REFERENCE GUIDE 15

Pain Scales: Children

Pain scale/description	Instructions	Recommended age
Faces scale: Consists of six cartoon faces ranging from very happy, smiling face for "no pain," to tearful face for "worst pain"	*Original Instructions:* Explain to child that each face is for a person who feels happy because there is no pain (hurt) or sad because there is some or a lot of pain. FACE 0 is very happy because there is no hurt. FACE 1 hurts just a little bit. FACE 2 hurts a little more. FACE 3 hurts even more. FACE 4 hurts a whole lot, but FACE 5 hurts as much as you can imagine, although you don't have to be crying to feel this bad. Ask the child to choose the face that best describes own pain. Record the number under chosen face on pain assessment record.	Children as young as 3 yr Using same instructions without affect words, such as *happy* or *sad*, results in same pain rating, probably reflecting child's rating of pain intensity.

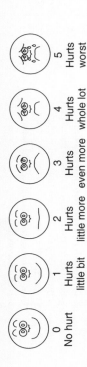

0	1	2	3	4	5
No hurt	Hurts little bit	Hurts little more	Hurts even more	Hurts whole lot	Hurts worst

Oucher: Consists of six photographs of child's face representing "no hurt" to "biggest hurt you could ever have"; also includes a vertical scale with numbers from 0 to 100; scales for African-American and Hispanic children have been developed.

Numeric Scale:
Point to each section of scale to explain variations in pain intensity:
"Zero means no hurt."
"This means little hurts" (pointing to lower part of scale, 1 to 29).
"This means middle hurts" (pointing to middle part of scale, 30 to 69).
"This means big hurts" (pointing to upper part of scale, 70 to 99).

Children 3 to 13 yr; use numeric scale if child can count to 100 by ones and identify larger of any two numbers, or by tens.
Determine whether child has cognitive ability to use photographic scale; child should be able to seriate six geometric shapes from largest to smallest.

Continued

From Wong DL, *Whaley and Wong's Essentials of Pediatric Nursing,* 5/e, St Louis, 1997, Mosby.

Pain scale/description	Instructions	Recommended age
	"One hundred means the biggest hurt you could ever have." Score is actual number stated by child. *Photographic Scale:* Point to each photograph on Oucher and explain variations in pain intensity using the following language: the first picture from the bottom is "no hurt," the second is "a little hurt," the third is "a little more hurt," the fourth is "even more hurt than that," the fifth is "pretty much a lot of hurt," and the sixth is the "biggest hurt you could ever have." Score pictures from 0 to 5, with the bottom picture scored as 0.	Determine which ethnic version of Oucher to use. Allow the child to select a version of Oucher, or use the version that most closely matches the physical characteristics of the child.

General:

Practice using Oucher by recalling and rating previous pain experiences (e.g., falling off a bike). Child points to number or photograph that describes pain intensity associated with experience. Obtain current pain score from child by asking, "How much hurt do you have right now?"

Numeric scale: Uses straight line with end points identified as "no pain" and "worst pain"; divisions along line are marked in units from "0" to "10" (high number may vary)

Explain to child that at one end of line is "0," which means that person feels no pain (hurt); at the other end is 10, which means person feels worst pain imaginable; numbers 1 to 9 are for very little pain to whole lot of pain; ask child to choose number that best describes own pain

Children as young as 5 yr, provided they can count and have some concepts of numbers and their values in relation to other numbers.

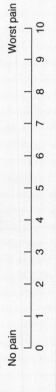

No pain 0 1 2 3 4 5 6 7 8 9 10 Worst pain

From Wong DL, *Whaley and Wong's Essentials of Pediatric Nursing*, 5/e, St Louis, 1997, Mosby.

Continued

Pain scale/description	Instructions	Recommended age
Poker Chip Tool: Uses four red poker chips placed horizontally in front of child.	Tell child, "These are pieces of hurt." Beginning at the chip nearest child's left side and ending at the chip nearest child's right side, point to chips and say, "This (the first chip) is a little bit of hurt and this (the fourth chip) is the most hurt you could ever have." For a young child or for any child who does not comprehend the instructions, clarify by saying, "That means this (the first chip) is just a little hurt; this (the second chip) is a little more hurt; this (the third chip) is more hurt; and this (the fourth chip) is the most hurt you could ever have." Ask the child, "how many pieces of hurt do you have right now?" Children without pain will say they don't have any. Clarify the child's answer with words such as, "Oh, you have a little hurt? Tell me about the hurt." Elicit descriptors, location, and cause. Ask the child, "What would you like me to do for you?" Record the number of chips selected.	Children as young as 4 to 4½ yr, provided they can count and have some concept of numbers

	Children ages 4 to 17 yr

Spanish Instructions: Follow the English instructions, substituting the following words. Tell the parent, if present, "Estas fichas son una manera de medir dolor. Usamos cuatro fichas." Say to the child, "Estas son pedazos de dolor: una es un poquito de dolor y cuatro son el dolor maximo que tu puedes sentir. Cuantos pedazos de dolor tienes?"

Word Graphic Rating Scale: Uses descriptive words (may vary according to scale) to denote varying intensities of pain

Explain to child, "This is a line with words to describe how much pain you may have." This side of the line means no pain and over here the line means worst possible pain." (Point with your finger where "no pain" is and run your finger along the line to "worst possible pain" as you say it.) "If you have no pain, you would mark somewhere along the line, depending on how much pain you have" (Show example). "The more pain you have, the closer to worst pain you should mark." The worst

Continued

From Wong DL, *Whaley and Wong's Essentials of Pediatric Nursing,* 5/e, St Louis, 1997, Mosby.

Pain scale/description	Instructions	Recommended age
	pain possible is marked like this" (Show example). "Show me how much pain you have right now by marking with a straight, up-and-down line anywhere along the line to show how much pain you have right now." With a millimeter rule, measure from the "no pain" end to the mark and record this measurement as the pain score.	

No pain · Little pain · Medium pain · Large pain · Worst possible pain

Pain scale/description	Instructions	Recommended age
Visual analogue scale: Uses 10-cm horizontal line with end points marked "no pain" and "worst pain"	Ask child to place mark on line that best describes amount of own pain; with centimeter ruler, measure from "no pain" end to mark and record this measurement as pain score	Children as young as 4½ yr; a vertical or horizontal scale may be used.

Color tool: Uses crayons or markers for child to construct own scale that is used with body outline	Present eight markers to the child in a random order. As the child, "Of these colors, which color is like _____?" (the event identified by the child as having hurt the most). Place the marker away from the other markers (represents severe pain). Ask the child, "Which color is like a hurt, but not as much as _____?" (the event identified by the child as having hurt the most). Place this marker with the marker chosen to represent severe pain. Ask the child, "Which color is like something that hurts just a little?" Place this marker with the other colors. Ask the child, "Which color is like no hurt at all?" Show the four marker choices to the child in order from the worst to the no-hurt color. Ask the child to show on the body outlines where he or she hurts, using the markers the child has chosen. After the child has colored the hurts, ask if they are current hurts or hurts from the past. Ask if the child knows why the area hurts if this is not clear.	Children as young as 4 yr, provided they know their colors, are not color blind, and are able to construct the scale if in pain

From Wong DL, *Whaley and Wong's Essentials of Pediatric Nursing*, 5/e, St Louis, 1997, Mosby.

REFERENCE GUIDE 16

Pain Treatment: Pediatrics and Adults

Drug	Usual adult dose	Usual pediatric dose*	Comments
Oral NSAIDs			
Acetaminophen	650-975 mg q4hr	10-15 mg/kg q4hr	Acetaminophen lacks the peripheral antiinflammatory activity of other NSAIDs
Aspirin	650-975 mg q4hr	10-15 mg/kg q4hr†	The standard against which other NSAIDs are compared; inhibits platelet aggregation; may cause postoperative bleeding
			Not first line for children due to increased risk of Reye syndrome in viral illness
Choline magnesium trisalicylate (Trilisate)	1000-1500 mg bid	25 mg/kg bid	May have minimal antiplatelet activity; also available as oral liquid
Diflunisal (Dolobid)	1000 mg initial dose followed by 500 mg q12hr		
Etodolac (Lodine)	200-400 mg q6-8hr		
Fenoprofen calcium (Nalfon)	200 mg q4-6hr		

Ibuprofen (Motrin, others)	400 mg q4-6hr	10 mg/kg q6-8hr	Available as several brand names and as generic; also available as oral suspension
Ketoprofen (Orudis)	25-75 mg q6-8hr		
Magnesium salicylate	650 mg q4hr		Many brands and generic forms available
Meclofenamate sodium (Meclomen)	50 mg q4-6hr		
Mefenamic acid (Ponstel)	250 mg q6hr		
Naproxen (Naprosyn)	500 mg initial dose followed by 250 mg q6-8hr	5 mg/kg q12hr	Also available as oral liquid
Naproxen sodium (Anaprox)	550 mg initial dose followed by 275 mg q6-8hr		
Salsalate (Disalcid, others)	500 mg q4hr		May have minimal antiplatelet activity
Sodium salicylate	325-650 mg q3-4hr		Available in generic form from several distributors

NOTE: Only the above NSAIDs have FDA approval for use as simple analgesics, but clinical experience has been gained with other drugs as well.

*Drug recommendations are limited to NSAIDs for which pediatric dosage experience is available.

†Contraindicated in presence of fever or other evidence of viral illness.

Continued

REFERENCE GUIDE 16

Drug	Usual adult dose	Usual pediatric dose*	Comments
Parenteral NSAIDs			
Ketorolac (Toradol)	IV: Begin with 30-60 mg IV Undiluted form through a Y-tube or three-way stop-cock of infusion set administered over 5 minutes; all succeeding doses are reduced by half (15-30 mg); 30 or 60 mg IM initial dose followed by 15 or 30 mg q6hr Oral dose following IM dosage: 10 mg q6-8hr		Intramuscular dose not to exceed 5 days

Drug	Approximate equianalgesic oral dose	Approximate equianalgesic parenteral dose	Recommended starting dose (adults >50 kg body weight)		Recommended starting dose (children and adults <50 kg body weight)*	
			Oral	Parenteral	Oral	Parenteral
Opioid agonist						
Morphine†	30 mg q3-4hr (around-the-clock doses); 60 mg q3-4hr single dose or intermittment dosage	10 mg q3-4hr	30 mg q3-4hr	10 mg q3-4hr	0.3 mg/kg q3-4hr	0.1 mg/kg q3-4hr

From Acute Pain Management Guideline Panel: *Acute pain management operative or medical procedures and trauma: clinical practice guidelines*, Rockland, Md, 1992, Agency for Health Care Policy and Research, Public Health Service, US Department of Health and Human Services.

NOTE: Published tables vary in the suggested doses that are equianalgesic to morphine. Clinical response is the criterion that must be applied for each patient; titration to clinical response is necessary. Because there is not complete cross-tolerance among these drugs, it is usually necessary to use a lower equianalgesic dose when changing drugs and to retitrate to response. CAUTION: Recommended doses do not apply to patients with renal or hepatic insufficiency or other conditions affecting drug metabolism and kinetics.
*CAUTION: Doses listed for patients with body weight less than 50 kg cannot be used as initial starting doses in infants younger than 6 months of age.
†For morphine, hydromorphone, and oxymorphone, rectal administration is an alternative route for patients unable to take oral medications, but equianalgesic doses may differ from oral and parenteral doses because of pharmacokinetic differences.

Continued

Drug	Approximate equianalgesic oral dose	Approximate equianalgesic parenteral dose	Recommended starting dose (adults >50 kg body weight)		Recommended starting dose (children and adults <50 kg body weight)*	
			Oral	Parenteral	Oral	Parenteral
Codeine†	130 mg q3-4hr	75 mg q3-4hr	60 mg q3-4hr	60 mg q2hr (IM, SC)	1 mg q3-4hr§	Not recommended
Hydromorphone† (Dilaudid)	7.5 mg q3-4hr	1.5 mg q3-4hr	6 mg q3-4hr	1.5 mg q3-4hr	0.06 mg q3-4hr	0.015 mg/kg q3-4hr
Hydrocodone (in Lorcet, Lortab, Vicodin, others)	30 mg q3-4hr	Not available	10 mg q3-4hr	Not available	0.2 mg q3-4hr	Not available
Levorphanol (Levo-Dromoran)	4 mg q6-8hr	2 mg q6-8hr	4 mg q6-7hr	2 mg q6-8hr	0.04 mg q3-4hr	0.02 mg/kg q6-8hr
Meperidine (Demerol)	300 mg q2-3hr	100 mg q3hr	Not recommended	100 mg q3hr	Not recommended	0.75 mg/kg q2-3hr
Methadone (Dolophine, others)	20 mg q6-8hr	10 mg q6-8hr	20 mg q6-8hr	10 mg q6-8hr	0.2 mg q6-8hr	0.1 mg/kg q6-8hr

| Oxycodone (Roxicodone, also in Percocet, Percodan, Tylox, others) | 30 mg q3-4hr | Not available | 10 mg q3-4hr | Not available | 0.2 mg q3-4hr§ | Not available |
| Oxymorphone† (Numorphan) | Not available | 1 mg q3-4hr | Not available | 1 mg q3-4hr | Not recommended | Not recommended |

From Acute Pain Management Guideline Panel: *Acute pain management operative or medical procedures and trauma: clinical practice guidelines*, Rockland, Md, 1992, Agency for Health Care Policy and Research, Public Health Service, US Department of Health and Human Services.

*CAUTION: Doses listed for patients with body weight less than 50 kg cannot be used as initial starting doses in infants younger than 6 months of age.

†For morphine, hydromomorphone, and oxymorphone, rectal administration is an alternative route for patients unable to take oral medications, but equianalgesic doses may differ from oral and parenteral doses because of pharmacokinetic differences.

‡CAUTION: Codeine doses above 65 mg are often inappropriate because of diminishing incremental analgesia with increasing doses but continually increasing constipation and other side effects.

§CAUTION: Doses of aspirin and acetaminophen in combination with opioid/NSAID preparations must also be adjusted to the patient's body weight.

Continued

REFERENCE GUIDE 16

Drug	Approximate equianalgesic oral dose	Approximate equianalgesic parenteral dose	Recommended starting dose (adults >50 kg body weight)		Recommended starting dose (children and adults <50 kg body weight)*	
			Oral	Parenteral	Oral	Parenteral
Opioid agonist-antagonist and partial agonist						
Buprenorphine (Buprenex)	Not available	0.3-0.4 mg q6-8hr	Not available	0.4 mg q6-8hr	Not available	0.004 mg/kg q6-8hr
Butorphanol (Stadol)	Not available	2 mg q3-4hr	Not available	2 mg q3-4hr	Not available	Not recommended
Nalbuphine (Nubain)	Not available	10 mg q3-4hr	Not available	10 mg q3-4hr	Not available	0.1 mg/kg q3-4hr
Pentazocine (Talwin, others)	150 mg q3-4hr	60 mg q3-4hr	50 mg q4-6hr	Not recommended	Not recommended	Not recommended

From Acute Pain Management Guideline Panel: *Acute pain management operative or medical procedures and trauma: clinical practice guidelines*, Rockland, Md, 1992, Agency for Health Care Policy and Research, Public Health Service, US Department of Health and Human Services.

Pediatric Pain Medications

Mild pain

Acetaminophen	10-15 mg/kg PO q4hr
Ibuprofen (Motrin, others)	5-10 mg/kg PO 6-8 hr

Moderate pain

Acetaminophen with codeine	1 mg/kg codeine PO q3-4hr

Severe pain

Morphine*	0.1 mg/kg IV/IM q3-4hr
Meperidine	0.75 mg/kg IV/IM q2-3hr
Hydromorphone Dilaudid)	0.015 mg/kg q3-4hr

From Acute Pain Management Guideline Panel: *Acute pain management, operative or medical procedures and trauma:* clinical practice guidelines, Rockland, Md, 1992, Agency for Health Care Policy and Research, Public Health Service, US Department of Health and Human Services.
*Fentanyl may be preferable when cardiovascular stability is an issue and patients are closely monitored or intubated. Meperidine should be used in exceptional circumstances.

REFERENCE GUIDE 17

PALS Algorithms: Pediatrics

Pediatric Bradycardia Algorithm

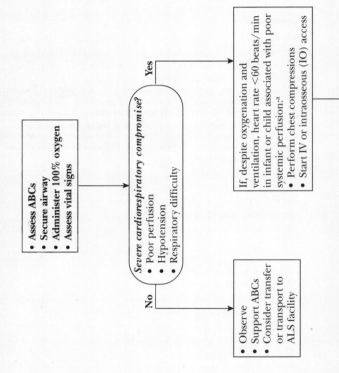

- Assess ABCs
- Secure airway
- Administer 100% oxygen
- Assess vital signs

Severe cardiorespiratory compromise?
- Poor perfusion
- Hypotension
- Respiratory difficulty

No

- Observe
- Support ABCs
- Consider transfer or transport to ALS facility

Yes

If, despite oxygenation and ventilation, heart rate <60 beats/min in infant or child associated with poor systemic perfusion:[a]
- Perform chest compressions
- Start IV or intraosseous (IO) access

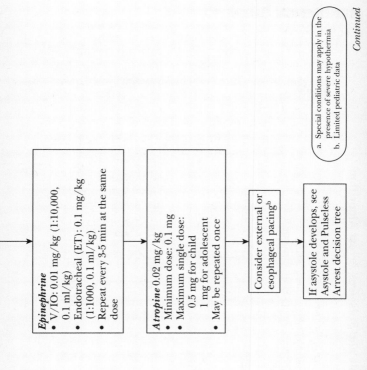

Epinephrine
- V/IO: 0.01 mg/kg (1:10,000, 0.1 ml/kg)
- Endotracheal (ET): 0.1 mg/kg (1:1000, 0.1 ml/kg)
- Repeat every 3-5 min at the same dose

Atropine 0.02 mg/kg
- Minimum dose: 0.1 mg
- Maximum single dose:
  0.5 mg for child
  1 mg for adolescent
- May be repeated once

Consider external or esophageal pacing[b]

If asystole develops, see Asystole and Pulseless Arrest decision tree

a. Special conditions may apply in the presence of severe hypothermia
b. Limited pediatric data

Continued

Pediatric Asystole and Pulseless Arrest Algorithm

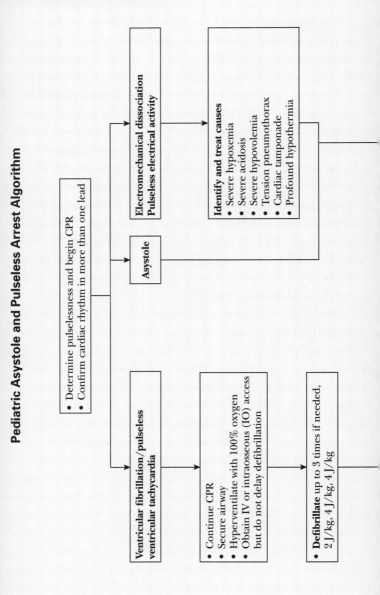

- Determine pulselessness and begin CPR
- Confirm cardiac rhythm in more than one lead

Ventricular fibrillation/pulseless ventricular tachycardia

- Continue CPR
- Secure airway
- Hyperventilate with 100% oxygen
- Obtain IV or intraosseous (IO) access but do not delay defibrillation

- **Defibrillate** up to 3 times if needed, 2 J/kg, 4 J/kg, 4 J/kg

Asystole

**Electromechanical dissociation
Pulseless electrical activity**

Identify and treat causes
- Severe hypoxemia
- Severe acidosis
- Severe hypovolemia
- Tension pneumothorax
- Cardiac tamponade
- Profound hypothermia

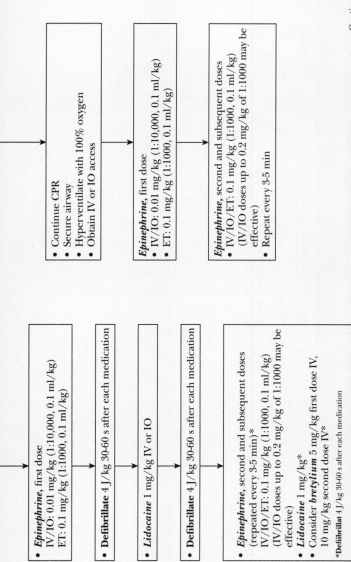

- ***Epinephrine,*** first dose
  IV/IO: 0.01 mg/kg (1:10,000, 0.1 ml/kg)
  ET: 0.1 mg/kg (1:1000, 0.1 ml/kg)

- **Defibrillate** 4 J/kg 30-60 s after each medication

- ***Lidocaine*** 1 mg/kg IV or IO

- **Defibrillate** 4 J/kg 30-60 s after each medication

- ***Epinephrine,*** second and subsequent doses
  (repeated every 3-5 min)*
  IV/IO/ET: 0.1 mg/kg (1:1000, 0.1 ml/kg)
  (IV/IO doses up to 0.2 mg/kg of 1:1000 may be
  effective)

- ***Lidocaine*** 1 mg/kg*

- Consider ***bretylium*** 5 mg/kg first dose IV,
  10 mg/kg second dose IV*

  ***Defibrillat** 4 J/kg 30-60 s after each medication

- Continue CPR
- Secure airway
- Hyperventilate with 100% oxygen
- Obtain IV or IO access

- ***Epinephrine,*** first dose
  - IV/IO: 0.01 mg/kg (1:10,000, 0.1 ml/kg)
  - ET: 0.1 mg/kg (1:1000, 0.1 ml/kg)

- ***Epinephrine,*** second and subsequent doses
  - IV/IO/ET: 0.1 mg/kg (1:1000, 0.1 ml/kg)
    (IV/IO doses up to 0.2 mg/kg of 1:1000 may be
    effective)
  - Repeat every 3-5 min

Algorithm for Pediatric Tachycardia with Poor Perfusion

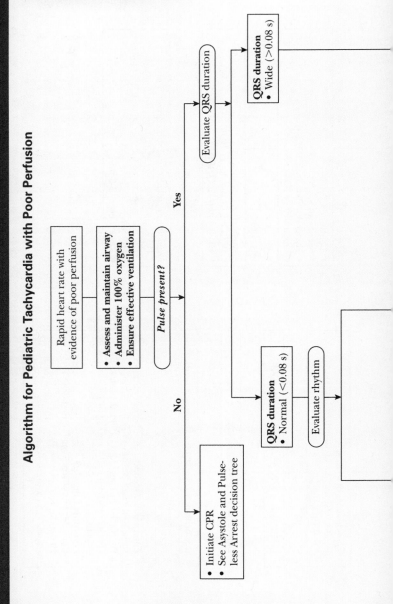

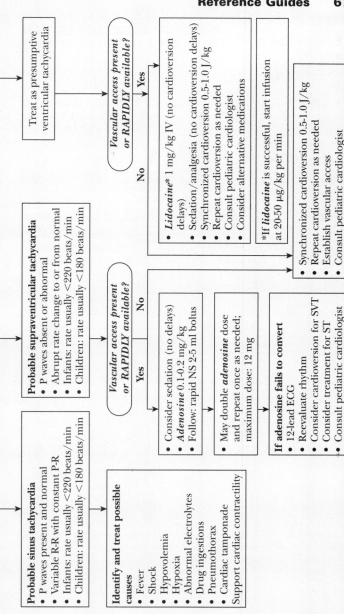

Probable sinus tachycardia
- P waves present and normal
- Variable R-R with constant P-R
- Infants: rate usually <220 beats/min
- Children: rate usually <180 beats/min

Identify and treat possible causes
- Fever
- Shock
- Hypovolemia
- Hypoxia
- Abnormal electrolytes
- Drug ingestions
- Pneumothorax
- Cardiac tamponade
- Support cardiac contractility

Probable supraventricular tachycardia
- P waves absent or abnormal
- Abrupt rate change to or from normal
- Infants: rate usually <220 beats/min
- Children: rate usually <180 beats/min

Vascular access present or RAPIDLY available?

Yes | **No**

- Consider sedation (no delays)
- *Adenosine* 0.1-0.2 mg/kg
- Follow: rapid NS 2-5 ml bolus

- May double *adenosine* dose and repeat once as needed; maximum dose: 12 mg

If adenosine fails to convert
- 12-lead ECG
- Reevaluate rhythm
- Consider cardioversion for SVT
- Consider treatment for ST
- Consult pediatric cardiologist

Treat as presumptive ventricular tachycardia

Vascular access present or RAPIDLY available?

No | **Yes**

- *Lidocaine** 1 mg/kg IV (no cardioversion delays)
- Sedation/analgesia (no cardioversion delays)
- Synchronized cardioversion 0.5-1.0 J/kg
- Repeat cardioversion as needed
- Consult pediatric cardiologist
- Consider alternative medications

*If *lidocaine* is successful, start infusion at 20-50 µg/kg per min

- Synchronized cardioversion 0.5-1.0 J/kg
- Repeat cardioversion as needed
- Establish vascular access
- Consult pediatric cardiologist

REFERENCE GUIDE 18
Pediatric and Infant Coma Scale

Activity	Best response Infant Coma Scale (<1 year)	Points	Best response Pediatric Coma Scale (>1 year)
Eye opening	Spontaneous	4	Spontaneous
	To voice/shout	3	To verbal command
	To pain	2	To pain
	No response to pain	1	No response to pain
Motor	Normal spontaneous movements	6	Obeys commands
	Localizes to pain/ purposeful movement	5	Localizes to pain/ purposeful movement
	Flexion—withdrawal in response to pain	4	Flexion—withdrawal in response to pain
	Abnormal flexion in response to pain	3	Abnormal flexion in response to pain
	Abnormal extension in response to pain	2	Abnormal extension in response to pain
	No motor response to pain	1	No motor response to pain
Verbal	Cries appropriately, to pain, coos, babbles	5	Appropriate words and phrases
	Irritable, appropriate crying	4	Inappropriate words
	Inappropriate crying, screaming	3	Persistent crying or screaming
	Grunts and moans to pain, agitated	2	Grunts or moans to pain
	No verbal response	1	No verbal response

Data from from Chiafery M: Life-threatening neurological emergencies. In Soud TE, Rogers JS, editors: *Manual of pediatric emergency nursing*, St Louis, 1998, Mosby, and Semonin-Holleran R: Trauma in childhood. In Neff JA, Kidd PS, editors: *Trauma nursing*, St Louis, 1993, Mosby.
Possible points of 3-15; score <8 = coma.

REFERENCE GUIDE 19

Pediatric Emergency Drugs Used in Advanced Life Support

Drug	Dose	Remarks
Adenosine	0.1-0.2 mg/kg; maximum single dose 12 mg	Rapid IV bolus
Atropine sulfate*	0.02 mg/kg per dose	Minimum dose: 0.1 mg; maximum single dose: 0.5 mg in child, 1 mg in adolescent
Bretylium	5 mg/kg; may be increased to 10 mg/kg	Rapid IV
Calcium chloride 10%	20 mg/kg per dose	Give slowly
Dopamine hydrochloride	2-20 µg/kg/min	alpha-adrenergic action dominates at ≥15-20 µg/kg/min
Dobutamine hydrochloride	2-20 µg/kg/min	Titrate to desired effect
Epinephrine*†		
For bradycardia	IV/IO: 0.01 mg/kg (1:10,000) ET: 0.1 mg/kg (1:1000)	

From Chameides L, Hazinski MF, editors: *Pediatric advanced life support,* Dallas, 1997, American Heart Association.

ET, Endotracheal route; *IO,* intraosseous route; *IV,* intravenous route.

*For ET administration, dilute drug with normal saline to a volume of 3 to 5 ml and follow with positive-pressure ventilations.

†Be aware of effective dose of preservative administered (if preservatives present in epinephrine preparation) when high doses are used.

Continued

REFERENCE GUIDE 19

Drug	Dose	Remarks
Epinephrine—cont'd	**First dose:**	
For asystolic or pulseless arrest	IV/IO: 0.01 mg/kg (1:10,000); doses as high as 0.2 mg/kg may be effective	
	ET: 0.1 mg/kg (1:1000)	
	Subsequent doses:	
	IV/IO/ET: 0.1 mg/kg (1:1000)	
	IV/IO doses as high as 0.2 mg/kg may be effective	
Epinephrine infusion	Initial at 0.1 µg/kg/min; higher infusion dose used if asystole present	Titrate to desired effect (0.1-1 µg/kg/min)
Lidocaine*	1 mg/kg per dose	
Lidocaine infusion	20-50 µg/kg per minute	Titrate to desired effect
	≤5 years old or ≤20 kg: 0.1 mg/kg	
Naloxone*	>5 years old or >20 kg: 2.0 mg	
Prostaglandin E_1	0.05-0.1 µg/kg/min	Monitor for apnea, hypotension, hypoglycemia
Sodium bicarbonate	1 mEq/kg per dose or 0.3 × kg × base deficit	Infuse slowly and only if ventilation is adequate

From Chameides L, Hazinski MF, editors: *Pediatric advanced life support,*
Dallas, 1997, American Heart Association.
*For ET administration, dilute drug with normal saline to a volume of 3 to
5 ml and follow with positive-pressure ventilations.

REFERENCE GUIDE 20

Pediatric Trauma Score

| | Category | | |
Component	+2	+1	−1
Size	≥20 kg	10-20 kg	<10 kg
Airway	Normal	Maintainable	Unmaintainable
Systolic BP	≥90 mm Hg	50-90 mm Hg	<50 mm Hg
CNS	Awake	Obtunded/LOC	Coma/decerebrate
Open wound	None	Minor	Major/penetrating
Skeletal	None	Closed fracture	Open/multiple fractures
Sum Total Points			

From Tepas JJ et al: The pediatric trauma score as a predictor of injury severity in the injured child, *J Pediatr Surg* 22(1):14-18, 1987.

Size
　≥20 kg or 44 lb = +2
　10-20 kg or 22-44 lb = +1
　<10 kg or 22 lb = −1
Airway
　Normal = requiring no additional supportive measures
　Maintainable = partially obstructed airway requiring
　　simple measures such as head positioning, oral airway,
　　mask oxygen
　Unmaintainable = requiring definitive management and
　　requiring intubation, cricothyrotomy, or other invasive
　　procedures
SPB—If BP cuff size inadequate, the following can be used
　Pulse at the wrist = +2
　Pulse at the neck or groin = +1
　Absence of palpable pulse = −1

Skeletal (fractures)

    None—no evidence = +2

    Minor—single closed fracture or suspicion thereof = +1

    Open multiple closed fractures = −1

Open wound

    No evidence of external trauma = +2

    Abrasions or minor cutaneous injury = +1

    Any penetrating injury or major avulsion or
       laceration = −1

Sum range is −6 to +12

REFERENCE GUIDE 21
Pediatric Tube Sizes

Equipment	Premature	Neonate	6 mo	1 yr	2 yr	3 yr
Airway						
Oral Airway (size)*	Infant	Infant/small	Small	Small	Small	Small
Endotracheal tube (mm)†	2.5-3.0	3.0-3.5	3.5-4.0	4.0-4.5	4.0-4.5	4.0-4.5
Laryngoscope blade* (s = straight c = curved)	0 s	1 s	1 s	1 s	1 s	1 s
Suction catheter (French)†	5	6	6	8	8	8
Breathing						
Face mask (size)*	Premie NB	NB	NB	Ped	Ped	Ped
Bag-valve device (size)*	Inf	Inf	Inf	Ped	Ped	Ped
Chest tube (French)*	10-14	12-18	14-20	14-24	14-24	14-24
Circulation						
Over-the-needle catheter (gauge)‡	22-24	22-24	22-24	20-22	20-22	20-22
Intraosseous device (gauge)	18	15	15	15	15	15
Gastrointestinal/ Genitourinary						
Nasogastric tube (French)§	5	5	8	8	10	10
Urinary catheter (French)*	5 feeding tubex	5-8 feeding tube	8	10	10	10

From Bernardo LM: *Pediatric emergency nursing procedures,* Sudbury, Mass, 1993, Jones & Bartlett. www.jbpub.com. Reprinted with permission.
This reference demonstrates suggested sizes only. Consider each child's size and health condition when selecting appropriate equipment for procedures.
*Committee on Trauma: *Advanced trauma life support student manual,* Chicago, 1989, American College of Surgeons.
†Motoyama E: *Endotracheal intubation.* In Motoyama E, Davis P, editors: *Smith's anesthesia for infants and children,* St Louis, 1990, Mosby.
‡Chameides L, editor: *Textbook of pediatric advanced life support,* Dallas, 1988, American Heart Association and American Academy of Pediatrics.
§Skale N: *Manual of pediatric nursing procedures,* Philadelphia, 1992, JB Lippincott.
Ad, Adult; *Inf,* infant; *NB,* newborn; *Ped,* pediatric.

4 yr	5 yr	6 yr	7 yr	8 yr	9 yr	10 yr	11-18 yr
Medium	Medium	Medium	Medium	Medium/ Large	Medium/ Large	Medium/ Large	Large
5.0-5.5	5.0-5.5	5.5-6.0	5.5-6.0	6.0-6.5*	6.0-6.5*	6.0-6.5*	7.0-8.0*
2 s/c	2 s/c	2 s/c	2 s/c	2-3 s/c	2-3 s/c	2-3 s/c	3 s/c
10	10	10	10	10	10	10	12
Ped	Ped	Ped	Ped	Ad	Ad	Ad	Ad
Ped	Ped	Ped	Ped/Ad	Ad	Ad	Ad	Ad
20-32	20-32	20-32	20-32	28-38	28-38	28-38	28-38
20-22	18-22	18-20	18-20	16-20	16-20	16-20	14-18
15	15	—	—	—	—	—	—
10	10	10	12	12	12	12	14-16
10-12	10-12	10-12	10-12	12	12	12	12-18

REFERENCE GUIDE 22
Vital Sign Norms: Pediatric

	6 mo	1 yr	3 yr	6 yr	10 yr
Heart rate (beats/min)	90-120	90-120	80-120	70-110	60-90
Respirations (breaths/min)	25-40	20-30	20-30	18-25	15-20
Systolic blood pressure (mm Hg)	80-100	80-100	80-110	80-110	90-120

From Stillwell SB: *Quick critical care reference guide,* ed 3, St Louis, 1998, Mosby.

REFERENCE GUIDE 23

Skin Rash Diseases

Disease	Type of rash	Incubation	Duration	Cause
Maculopapular rashes				
Rubella (German measles, measles)	Macular, pink to red. First appears on head and spreads downward	14-21 days; contagious from 7 days before to 5 days after rash appears	3-4 days	Viral; can cause joint pain; fever is uncommon
Rubeola (measles, red measles)	Preceded for 2-3 days by cough, coryza, and conjunctivitis; Koplik's spots appear on buccal mucosa (pinpoint white lesions on a red base) 12-24 hr before rash appears; rash consists of reddish macules and begins on face and spreads downward; within 1-2 days, rash is confluent	10-20 days; contagious from 4 days before to 5 days after rash appears	10-15 days	Viral

Continued

From Thomas DO: *Quick reference to pediatric emergency nursing*, Gaithersburg, Md, 1991, Aspen Publishers.

Disease	Type of rash	Incubation	Duration	Cause
Roseola	Maculopapular, small, pink, widely disseminated, and nonpruritic; onset follows 3-4 days of fever	1-2 days	1-2 days	Probably viral
Erythema infectiosum (fifth disease)	Macular; facial distribution ("slapped cheeks" appearance); lacy rash is found on flexor surfaces of arms and legs	Acute phase, 3-4 days; may recur for several weeks if exposed to strong sunlight	Acute phase, 3-4 days; may recur for several weeks if exposed to strong sunlight	Viral (parvovirus B19)
Scarlet fever	Fine, raised generalized maculopapular rash ("sandpaper rash"); may be absent around mouth and face; red "strawberry tongue," bright red lines found in axilla and antecubital fossae (Pastia's lines); may peel after 5 days	Up to 3 weeks, until treated	Up to 3 weeks, until treated	Bacterial: group A strep toxin

Rocky Mountain spotted fever	Systemic signs for 1-3 days, consists of fever, headache, vomiting, and myalgias; rash consists of pink macules on peripheral extremities that become papular after 1-2 days	2-10 days	Until treated	Tick-introduced *Rickettsia*
Scabies	Initial: linear, threadlike gray to brown lesions between fingers and toes and on ankles and axillae; advanced: pruritic red papules	Up to 30-60 days	Until treated	Parasitic mite that burrows under the skin
Contact dermatitis	Red maculopapular lesions; sharp demarcation exists between involved and uninvolved areas of skin; may develop into a secondary lesion (e.g., vesicles or wheals)	Lesions developing within a few hours after contact with allergen	Until treated; may gradually disappear without treatment	Irritating agents such as soaps, detergents, and rough sheets

From Thomas DO: *Quick reference to pediatric emergency nursing*, Gaithersburg, Md, 1991, Aspen Publishers.

Continued

REFERENCE GUIDE 23

Disease	Type of rash	Incubation	Duration	Cause
Varicella (chickenpox)	Rash begins as small red macules and then progresses to papules and then vesicles; after the vesicles rupture, a dry crust forms over the lesion; may have all types of lesions present at the same time	14-21 days; contagious from 1 day before eruption of lesions until 6-7 days after all lesions are crusted over	5-20 days	Viral; scratching may cause a secondary infection
Tinea corporis (ringworm)	Round or oval, red scaly patch that spreads peripherally and clears centrally	N/A	Until treated	Fungus through direct or indirect contact
Impetigo	Rash begins as vesicular lesions, advances to yellow crusts on a red base; usually seen on feet and hands and around the mouth; may cause cellulitis	N/A	Until treated	Bacterial (staphylococcal or streptococcal)

Candida (Monilia)	Oral: white patches on mucous membranes; will not scrape off; Skin: red lesions with serous drainage, white crust (usually in diaper area)	N/A	Until treated	Yeast infection, which proliferates in warm, moist environments
Kawasaki syndrome	Rash begins as red maculopapular lesions, commonly in the perineum area; progresses to confluent pruritic wheals; desquamation of lesions occurs within 2-7 days	Unknown	6-8 weeks	Unknown

From Thomas DO: *Quick reference to pediatric emergency nursing*, Gaithersburg, Md, 1991, Aspen Publishers. *Continued*

REFERENCE GUIDE 23

Rash type	Appearance	Disease(s)
Associated with hemorrhagic lesions		
Petechiae	Small (1-2 mm) pinpoint reddish purple macular lesions that do not blanch with pressure	Platelet disorders, leukemia, meningococcemia, bacterial meningitis
Purpura (ecchymoses)	Larger ecchymotic lesions that are macular and do not blanch with pressure	Henoch-Schönlein purpura, idiopathic thrombocytic purpura, hemophilia, trauma, viral infections

From Thomas DO: *Quick reference to pediatric emergency nursing,* Gaithersburg, Md, 1991, Aspen Publishers.

REFERENCE GUIDE 24

Tetanus and Immunization Guidelines

Tetanus Guidelines

History of adsorbed tetanus toxoid (doses)	Clean, minor wounds		All other wounds*	
	Td†	TIG	Td†	TIG
Unknown or <3	Yes	No	Yes	Yes
≥3‡	No§	No	No‖	No

Adapted from Centers for Disease Control: MMWR 34(27):422, 1985. In Keen J, Baird M, Allen J: *Mosby's critical care and emergency drug reference,* St Louis, 1994, Mosby.

*Such as, but not limited to, wounds resulting from missiles, crushing, burns, frostbite.

†For children <7 yr; DPT (DT, if pertussis vaccine contraindicated) preferred to tetanus toxoid alone. For persons ≥7 yr, Td preferred to tetanus toxoid alone.

‡If only 3 doses of fluid toxoid received, fourth dose of toxoid, preferably adsorbed toxoid, should be given.

§Yes, if <10 yr since last dose.

‖Yes, if >5 yr since last dose (more frequent boosters not needed; can accentuate side effects).

Recommended Childhood Immunization Schedule

Age	Vaccine
Newborn	Start Hepatitis B series if high-risk
2 mo	DPT #1
	HIB #1
	IPV #1
4 mo	DPT #2
	HIB #2
	IPV #2
6 mo	DPT #3
	HIB #3
	Hepatitis B #1
9 mo	Hepatitis B #2
12 mo	Hepatitis B #3
	Varicella vaccine*
	Polio vaccine #3
15 mo	MMR #1
	DPT #4
	HIB #4
24 mo	Hepatitis A†
4 yr	DPT #5
	Hepatitis A†
	Polio vaccine #4
	MMR #2
Middle School	MMR #2 (if not already given)
	Hepatitis A†
	Hepatitis B series (if not already given
	Varicella vaccine (if not already given)
14-16 yr	dT

From Centers for Disease Control and Prevention: *Recommended Childhood Immunization Schedule* 49(2):35-38, 47, 2000.

*Varicella vaccine is recommended at any visit on or after the first birthday for susceptible children (those who lack a reliable history of chickenpox, as judged by a health care provider and who have not been immunized). Susceptible persons 13 years of age or older should receive 2 doses, given at least 4 weeks apart.

†Hepatitis A (Hep A) is recommended in selected states and/or regions; consult your local public health authority.

REFERENCE GUIDE 25
Trauma Score (Revised): Adults

Find a subtotal for GCS. Use this subtotal to obtain a corresponding revised trauma score (RTS). Add this value to the score of the two other categories.

Glasgow Coma Scale

Eye opening	Spontaneous	4
	To voice	3
	To pain	2
	None	1
Verbal response	Oriented and converses	5
	Confused and converses	4
	Inappropriate words	3
	Incomprehensible sound	2
	None	1
Motor response	Obeys command	6
	Purposeful movement in response to pain	5
	Withdrawal in response to pain	4
	Abnormal flexion in response to pain	3
	Abnormal extension in response to pain	2
	None	1
GCS subtotal		3-15

REFERENCE GUIDE 25

Revised Trauma Score (RTS)

Glasgow Coma Scale

Find a subtotal for GCS. Use this subtotal to obtain a corresponding RTS. Add this value to the scores of the other two categories.	13-15	4
	9-12	3
	6-8	2
	4-5	1
	3	0

Respiratory rate

Number of respirations in 15 seconds multiplied by 4	10-29	4
	>29	3
	6-9	2
	1-5	1
	0	0

Systolic blood pressure

Systolic cuff pressure obtained from either arm palpitation or auscultation	>89	4
	76-89	3
	50-75	2
	1-49	1
	No pulse	0
	Total RTS	1-12

From Lee G: *Quick emergency care reference,* St Louis, 1992, Mosby.

REFERENCE GUIDE 26

Ventilator Alarms Troubleshooting

Alarm	Possible Causes
High pressure	Secretion buildup, kinked airway tubing, bronchospasm, coughing, fighting the ventilator, decreased lung compliance
Low exhaled volume	Disconnection from ventilator, loose ventilator fittings, leaking airway cuff
Low inspiratory pressure	Disconnection from ventilator, loose connections, low ventilating pressure
High respiratory rate	Anxiety, pain, hypoxia, fever
Apnea alarm	No spontaneous breath within preset time interval

From Stillwell SB: *Mosby's critical care nursing reference,* ed 2, St Louis, 1996, Mosby.

REFERENCE GUIDE 27
Ventilator Support

Modes of Ventilatory Support

Type	Description
Assist-controlled mode ventilation (ACV)	Patient triggers a breath and ventilator delivers a preset volume; control mode takes over at preset backup rate if patient becomes apneic
Bilevel CPAP (BiPAP)	Positive pressure applied during spontaneous breathing that allows inspiratory positive airway pressure (IPAP) and expiratory positive airway pressure (EPAP) to be independently adjusted
Continuous positive-airway pressure (CPAP)	Positive pressure applied during spontaneous breathing and maintained throughout the entire respiratory cycle; decreases intrapulmonary shunting
Controlled mandatory ventilation (CMV)	Ventilator delivers preset tidal volume at fixed rate regardless of patient's efforts to breathe
Intermittent mandatory ventilation (IMV)	Patient may be able to breathe spontaneously but receives intermittent ventilator breaths at preset rate and tidal volume; tidal volume stacking can occur
Inverse-ratio ventilation	Provides inspiratory time greater than expiratory time, thereby improving distribution of ventilation and preventing collapse of stiffer alveolar units

Modes of Ventilatory Support—cont'd

Type	Description
Positive end-expiratory pressure (PEEP)	Positive pressure applied during machine breathing and maintained at end-expiration; decreases intrapulmonary shunting
Pressure support ventilation (PSV)	Clinician-selected amount of positive pressure applied to airway during patient's spontaneous inspiratory efforts; PSV decreases work of breathing caused by demand flow valve, IMV circuit, and narrow inner diameter of ETT
Synchronized IMV (SIMV)	Intermittent ventilator breaths synchronized to spontaneous breaths to reduce competition between ventilator and patient

Modes of High-Frequency Ventilation

Type	Description
HF positive-pressure ventilation (HFPPV)	Extremely short inspiratory times with V_T equivalent to deadspace at a rate of 60-100 cycles/min
HF jet ventilation (HFJV)	Small volumes, ≤anatomic deadspace, are pulsed through jet injector catheter at rates of 60-600 cycles/min
HF oscillation (HFO)	Small volume of gas is continually vibrated in airways at rates of 900-3000 cycles/min

From Stillwell SB: *Mosby's critical care nursing reference,* ed 2, St Louis, 1996, Mosby.

UNIT TWO

Clinical Conditions

Chapter 1

Abdominal Conditions

Regina Heiser

CLINICAL CONDITIONS
Appendicitis
Bowel Obstruction
Cholecystitis
Crohn's Disease
Dehydration
Esophageal Varices
Gastritis and Gastroenteritis
Fulminant Hepatic Failure
Acute Pancreatitis

TRIAGE ASSESSMENT

Two of the most common reasons patients seek treatment
in the emergency department (ED) are abdominal pain
and abdominal conditions. Abdominal pain is estimated to
account for up to 10% of all ED visits. Pain can be indicative of an acute or chronic problem and may or may not be
accompanied by other associated symptoms such as nausea,
vomiting, fever, or diarrhea.

The initial triage assessment should focus on a general
observation of the patient. The primary survey should assess airway, breathing, and circulation (ABCs). Any condition that causes an alteration in the patient's ability to
maintain a patent airway, breathe normally, or maintain adequate circulation must be corrected before a focused or
secondary survey begins. Symptoms at triage that warrant
immediate treatment include severe, debilitating pain (the
patient is unable to sit or stand), protracted vomiting or diarrhea, and signs that indicate early shock (tachycardia,
tachypnea, and anxiety).

The triage history and assessment are invaluable tools that can direct an accurate workup and diagnosis in this population. A brief history should include the following:

1. **Chief complaint**

   Nausea and vomiting—suspect appendicitis or a bowel obstruction; colicky, epigastric pain—suspect gastritis or gastroenteritis; anorexia with diarrhea—suspect Crohn's disease

2. **Social and medical history**

   History of alcohol use and abuse—suspect liver disease; intravenous (IV) drug use—suspect withdrawal; previous abdominal surgeries—suspect bowel obstruction; prolonged salicylate or ibuprofen use—suspect liver disease or gastritis; antibiotic use—suspect dehydration or gastroenteritis

3. **Reason for seeking treatment**

   Identify changes in symptoms; identify contact with other health care providers for this illness

4. **Treatment before arrival**

   Identify use of home remedies, alteration in diet, use of over-the-counter medicines

5. **Pain**

   Record history and duration of pain; use the "PQRST" mnemonic as a systematic way to obtain information about pain:

   P (provoke): What provokes the pain? What makes it better or worse? What are positions of comfort and discomfort?

   Q (quality or character): What type of pain is it (burning, tight, crushing, tearing, pressure)?

   R (radiation): Where does the pain start? Where does it go? Have the patient point with one finger to where the pain is the most uncomfortable.

   S (severity): How severe is the pain on a scale of "0" to "10" ("0" representing no pain and "10" representing the worst pain)?

   T (time): When did the pain start? How long did it last? What time did the intensity change?

CHARACTERISTICS AND TYPES OF PAIN

There are three types of abdominal pain: primary, somatic, and referred. *Primary,* or visceral, pain originates in the organ itself and is experienced with conditions such as appendicitis, pancreatitis, and bowel obstruction. The pain is cramping and gaslike, and it intensifies and then decreases. This pain is usually periumbilical. *Somatic,* or secondary, pain results from irritation of surrounding structures and nerve fibers because of bacterial or chemical causes. Somatic pain is described as sharp and localized, and patients frequently assume a knee-chest position for comfort. This type of pain is experienced with conditions such as peritonitis or gastroenteritis. *Referred* pain is located distant from the affected organ and results from irritation of the same dermatome of the affected organ (such as in the case of cholecystitis and renal colic).

FOCUSED NURSING ASSESSMENT

A focused assessment should briefly reassess the ABCs for changes and necessary interventions. Ruptured esophageal varices, an aortic aneurysm, hemorrhagic pancreatitis, and severe gastroenteritis may produce sudden and severe hypotension with resultant shock. Nursing assessment should focus on ventilation, perfusion, cognition, elimination patterns, and associated signs and symptoms.

Ventilation
Breath sounds and breathing patterns
Atelectasis, pleural effusions, and crackles are common in pancreatitis and hepatic failure. In pancreatitis, left-sided effusions are most common. Although the exact cause is unknown, effusions are believed to be a result of diaphragmatic inflammation that occurs when enzymes are released from the ascitic abdomen.[1] The respiratory problems associated with liver failure are caused by arterial hypoxemia secondary to intrapulmonary dilation and noncardiogenic pulmonary edema.[2] Acute pain may cause an increased respiratory rate or splinting respirations because of an effort to decrease pressure on the abdomen. Patients who receive narcotics for pain management are at risk for respiratory depression.

Perfusion
Apical heart rate
Obtain an apical heart rate and compare the rate to all peripheral pulses. Moderate to severe dehydration that is a result of gastroenteritis or shock states causes weak, thready,

and rapid pulse rates. Tachycardia is the most common dysrhythmia in cases of pancreatitis and fulminant hepatic failure.[1,2]

Blood pressure

As dehydration or shock progresses from fluid volume loss, peripheral vasoconstriction increases and blood pressure (BP) decreases. Fifty percent of patients with fulminant hepatic failure have a systolic BP less than 90 mm Hg.[2]

Skin

Assess skin color, temperature, and capillary refill. Nausea, vomiting, and severe pain may produce diaphoresis. Pancreatitis and appendicitis are associated with fever.

Cognition

Severe hepatic failure causes decreased carbohydrate metabolism and increased circulating ammonia and bilirubin, which together produce encephalopathic changes. Within hours, hepatic encephalopathy may progress from mild confusion to coma. The patient's level of consciousness (LOC) is regarded as the most critical indicator of encephalopathic changes.[2] A decreased LOC is also a warning sign of early shock, which can be a result of hypovolemia caused by gastrointestinal bleeding, dehydration caused by vomiting and diarrhea, or sepsis secondary to peritonitis.

Elimination and Bowel Patterns

In cases of small bowel obstruction, stool initially passes and then stops. Dehydration and large bowel obstruction cause constipation. Pancreatitis produces steatorrheic (fatty, frothy, and foul-smelling) stools. Diarrhea is associated with gastroenteritis, gastritis, and appendicitis. Tarry stools or occult blood in the stool may be found in cases of diverticulitis, ulcerative colitis, and dysentery. Clay-colored stools are common with biliary tract obstructions.

Associated Signs and Symptoms
Emesis

Vomiting is one of the major gastrointestinal symptoms. If vomiting is significant, gastritis, gastroenteritis, diverticulitis, pancreatitis, and small bowel obstruction are likely. Cholecystitis is associated with anorexia.

Women of childbearing age who complain of abdominal pain present an additional challenge. Pelvic inflammatory disease, ectopic pregnancy, and ovarian cysts and abscesses are conditions that mimic other abdominal conditions. Classic symptoms of pelvic inflammatory disease include lower abdominal pain that increases with ambulation, pain on manual palpation of the cervix, and foul-smelling vaginal discharge. A right-sided ectopic pregnancy mimics the pain patterns of appendicitis. Pain may radiate to one or both shoulders with a ruptured ovarian cyst or ruptured ectopic pregnancy. In addition, patients may complain of vaginal bleeding that may be intermittent or significant. Missed or abnormal menses are key indications of ectopic pregnancy if the patient is sexually active. Patients with ovarian cysts complain of the same symptoms as patients with an ectopic pregnancy, but laboratory test results are negative for pregnancy in these instances.

NURSING ALERT

Patients with a ruptured ectopic pregnancy or a ruptured ovarian cyst may immediately display symptoms of or develop hemorrhagic shock. Patients with ruptured ovarian abscesses may develop septic shock (see Chapter 15).

Focused Abdominal Assessment

A focused abdominal assessment includes four components: inspection, auscultation, percussion, and palpation. These components should be performed in the order listed.

1. **Inspection**
   Inspection is best done from the patient's right side. Note symmetry and the presence or absence of movement, distention, dilated veins, ascites, and bruises. Coughing may elicit bulges or pain. Hemorrhagic pancreatitis has signs and symptoms consistent with abdominal trauma (blood and bruising periumbilically or on the left lower flank). An asymmetric abdominal wall may indicate the presence of masses, air, or fluid. A palpable, visible mass may indicate an abdominal aneurysm.

2. **Auscultation (abdominal sounds)**
   Auscultation should be performed in all four quadrants for a minimum of one full minute in each quadrant. Frequency, quality, and pitch should be noted. Most bowel sounds originate in the small intestine, located

A

in the right lower quadrant. Bowel sounds may be hyperactive in cases of gastroenteritis and may be accompanied by nausea, vomiting, and diarrhea. Abdominal
bruits may be noted with dissecting aneurysms and renal artery stenosis. Friction rubs may indicate inflammation of an organ surface or the presence of fluid. Early
bowel obstruction and complete obstruction produce
high-pitched, frequent, peristaltic bowel sounds. The
absence of bowel sounds may indicate a paralytic ileus
or peritonitis.

3. **Percussion**
   Tympanic sounds occur when air masses are percussed.
   Dull sounds are noted over solid structures such as tumors or organs. The liver should be percussed separately and its size should be noted. Borders of the liver
   can be obscured by right-sided pleural effusions, commonly a result of fulminant hepatic failure and less commonly secondary to acute pancreatitis.

4. **Palpation**
   Note tenderness, masses, guarding, rigidity, or rebound
   tenderness. Ask the patient to cough, and note where
   pain occurs. Gentle palpation is recommended in suspected cases of appendicitis because frequent deep palpation can result in perforation. The area reported to
   be the most painful should be palpated last.

Risk Factors

The following risk factors may precipitate an abdominal
condition:

1. Ingestion of noxious substances such as alcohol or caffeine: risk for acute gastritis
2. Overeating, rapid food intake, or high-fat diet: risk for
   gastritis, pancreatitis, and cholecystitis
3. Improperly prepared foods and water: risk for
   gastroenteritis
4. Over-the-counter medication (e.g., antacids, aspirin, and
   ibuprofen) abuse: risk for gastrointestinal bleeding and
   gastritis
5. Pregnancy: risk for gastritis
6. Chronic bowel problems, laxative abuse, and multiple
   abdominal surgeries with adhesions: risk for bowel obstruction and Crohn's disease
7. Parous women who smoke: risk for cholecystitis[3]

Life Span Issues

1. Pain assessment can be problematic with pediatric and geriatric patients. With pediatric patients, pain assessment may require the use of more than one method (smiley faces, numerical scales, or color intensity scales may each work with children of different ages—see Reference Guide 15). Geriatric patients have pain from multiple causes and are at increased risk for drug-drug and drug-disease interactions.[4] Drug absorption is least affected by age. Drug distribution, however, is affected by changes in the level of serum albumin, which decreases with age. In addition, total body water and lean muscle mass decrease with age, whereas fat increases. Drugs that distribute to lean mass compartments (e.g., antimicrobials, digoxin, lithium, alcohol) will have less absorption and may result in toxicity. Drugs that distribute to fatty mass compartments (e.g., psychotropic drugs) may have a prolonged effect and more of the drug may be needed to obtain therapeutic levels. Finally, metabolism and excretion are factors that affect drug-drug interactions and drug-disease interactions in geriatric patients.[4]

2. Geriatric patients are at risk for undertreatment and overtreatment. Intraabdominal infections are clinically worse in geriatric patients. This is attributed to delayed recognition and delayed surgical intervention. Cholecystitis, appendicitis, and intraabdominal sepsis, which are a result of diverticular leaks and cancers, are the most common infections and cause greater morbidity and mortality in geriatric patients because of delays in recognition and treatment.[5] Geriatric patients require more time and resources for evaluation because their complaints are generally more diffuse and nonspecific. Sixty-five percent of the geriatric patients have a preexisting condition that complicates the presentation of their symptoms to the ED. Routine signs and symptoms (nausea, vomiting, and diarrhea) are often milder and of longer duration than those of their younger cohorts. There is often an absence of peritoneal signs despite a serious disease process. Because of these factors, geriatric patients are at risk for overtreatment in the attempt to identify a disease process and they are also at risk for undertreatment, because signs and symptoms frequently appear benign.

3. Both the geriatric and pediatric populations are at risk for infection because of their immune systems. Changes in the geriatric patient include a reduction of polymorphonuclear leukocytes with a resultant decrease in phagocytosis.[5] An immature immune system and gut can result in infection in the pediatric patient.[6]

4. Pain management can be difficult with the geriatric population because of the patients' cognitive impairment, inability to express pain, and problems with chronic pain.[7]

5. Both the pediatric and geriatric populations are more susceptible to hypothermia. For the pediatric patient, less body fat and a larger surface area result in a higher basal metabolic rate to maintain a normal body temperature.[6] When affected by a known abdominal condition, the geriatric population is four times more likely to be hypothermic ($<36°$ C) because of a diminished sensation to cold, impaired sensation to temperature changes, impaired shiver, abnormal autonomic vasoconstriction in response to cold, and diminished thermogenesis.[4,8] Rapid rehydration with room-temperature fluids and repeated abdominal examinations can cause hypothermia and acidosis in these groups.

6. Both populations are more susceptible to dehydration. Infants have greater surface areas related to mass, with a greater proportion of extracellular fluid. The geriatric population has decreased thirst perception and diminished urine-concentrating capabilities (decreased renal blood flow and decreased glomerular filtration rates).[9]

INITIAL INTERVENTIONS

Most abdominal conditions in the ED will require similar treatment. *REMEMBER:* interventions are based on acuity and many abdominal conditions may be life threatening.

1. Maintain NPO status. Record the time and type of last oral intake.
2. Anticipate a diagnostic workup, including laboratory tests and radiography.
3. Anticipate and prepare for IV rehydration (see Procedure 18).
4. Provide comfort measures (e.g., positioning, access to bathroom, and an emesis basin).
5. Provide for and monitor pain needs.

PRIORITY NURSING DIAGNOSES

Risk for fluid volume deficit
Risk for pain
Risk for anxiety
Risk for impaired gas exchange
Risk for knowledge deficit

◆ **Fluid volume deficit** related to anorexia, nausea, vomiting, and diarrhea as demonstrated by delayed capillary refill, an elevated heart rate, altered mental status, decreased urine output, dry mucous membranes, furrowed tongue, decreased skin turgor, depressed fontanel in infants, or pale or flushed color:

INTERVENTIONS

• Monitor vital signs, including orthostatic vital signs.
• Monitor intake and output.
• Check specific gravity and color of urine.
• Perform hemoccult test on all vomitus and stool.
• Assess for signs and symptoms of dehydration.
• Assess neck veins (collapsed when lying flat).

◆ **Pain** related to cramping, burning, vomiting, diarrhea, and distention, as demonstrated by complaints of pain, crying, moaning, irritability, facial grimacing, restlessness, or hostility:

INTERVENTIONS

• Provide pain medications as ordered, preferably intravenously.
• Monitor oxygen saturation with pulse oximetry (maintain saturation above 94%).
• Monitor vital signs after pain medication administration.
• Reassess pain using a pain scale.
• Insert a nasogastric tube, if ordered, for protracted nausea, vomiting, or ileus.

◆ **Anxiety** related to potential surgery, hospitalization, and invasive procedures, as demonstrated by inability to relax, nervousness, increased heart rate, increased respiratory rate, and elevated blood pressure:

INTERVENTIONS

• Explain all procedures and answer questions.
• Provide reassurance and comfort.
• Provide a calm, quiet environment.
• Involve the family in patient teaching.

◆ **Impaired gas exchange** related to electrolyte imbalance, acid-base imbalance, and altered respiratory pattern because of pain and distention (Table 1-1), as demonstrated by dyspnea on exertion, tendency to assume a three-point position (sitting, bending forward, fetal position), lethargy, and fatigue:

INTERVENTIONS
- Monitor oxygen saturation.
- Administer oxygen as needed.
- Assess the patient's respiratory effort and pain-relief methods.
- Replace electrolytes as ordered.

TABLE 1-1 Electrolyte and Acid-base Imbalances and Associated Abdominal Conditions

Laboratory	Condition
Elevated glucose	Pancreatitis
Decreased glucose	Fulminant hepatic failure
Decreased calcium	Pancreatitis
	Fulminant hepatic failure
Elevated ammonia	Fulminant hepatic failure
Decreased magnesium	Pancreatitis
	Fulminant hepatic failure
Decreased phosphorus	Fulminant hepatic failure
Elevated potassium	Pancreatitis with acute renal failure
Decreased potassium	Pancreatitis with vomiting
	Fulminant hepatic failure
	Bowel obstruction
	Cholecystitis with vomiting
	Gastritis with vomiting and dehydration
Decreased sodium	Fulminant hepatic failure
	Hyponatremic dehydration
Elevated sodium	Dehydration
Acidosis—metabolic	Fulminant hepatic failure secondary to lactic acid from necrosis
	Bowel obstruction (lower small intestine)
Alkalosis—respiratory	Pancreatitis
Alkalosis—metabolic	Fulminant hepatic failure with hypokalemia
Elevated BUN	Dehydration
	Esophageal varices with hypovolemia
Elevated creatinine	Dehydration
	Fulminant hepatic failure

✦ **Knowledge deficit** related to diet, fluid intake, and med-ication use, as demonstrated by a lack of integration of the treatment plan into activities and by requests for informa-tion or by skill:

INTERVENTIONS
- Initiate patient teaching.
- Use the family to reinforce teaching whenever possible.
- Plan a dietary consultation or nutritionist visit.

PRIORITY DIAGNOSTIC TESTS

Laboratory

Serum electrolytes (including BUN and creatinine): Blood urea nitrogen (BUN) will be abnormal in moderate to severe dehydration states and with fluid shifts that ac-company bowel obstruction, hepatic failure, and pancre-atitis. Pancreatitis, severe gastroenteritis, and the severe vomiting and diarrhea that accompany fulminant hepatic failure can all cause hypokalemia.

Complete blood count with differential: The white count may be elevated because of the stress response secondary to infection.

Platelets: The patient will have immature platelets and a decreased platelet count in cases of fulminant hepatic failure.

PT/PTT and fibrinogen: The patient will have abnormal values in cases of hepatic failure and disease.

Serum amylase and lipase: The serum amylase and lipase levels will be elevated in cases of pancreatitis.

Serum bilirubin, aspartate aminotransferase (AST), alanine aminotransferase (ALT), and alkaline phosphatase (ALP): The levels of AST, ALT, and ALP will be mildly el-evated in cases of acute cholecystitis.

Serum ammonia: The serum ammonia level will be ele-vated in fulminant hepatic failure and states of severe hypokalemia.

Urinalysis: A baseline urinalysis should be done to rule out any genitourinary problems, especially with patients who complain of lower abdominal pain. A urine pregnancy screen should be done on all women of childbearing age.

Type and crossmatch: Blood and blood products may be needed for patients who do not respond to fluid resuscitation.

Radiographic Studies

Flat and upright abdominal film: These are done to detect air, dilation, looped bowel, thickening of the bowel wall, and foreign bodies. No preparation is needed.

Upright chest film: This is helpful in diagnosing pleural effusions. No preparation is needed.

Abdominal ultrasound and abdominal CT scan: These are useful in pancreatitis and in identifying gallstones in acute cholecystitis. Oral or IV administration contrast may be needed before the study.

Patients who are to be discharged from the ED with follow-up tests scheduled on an outpatient basis may need instructions regarding the test (see the "General Discharge Instructions" box).

GENERAL DISCHARGE INSTRUCTIONS FOR OUTPATIENT ABDOMINAL TESTS

Upper GI series

An upper GI series is used to identify patency and motility of the esophagus, stomach, and small intestine through serial radiographs over 4 to 6 hours after barium is ingested.

Preparation: The patient is placed on a low-residue diet two days before test and is NPO after midnight the night before examination. There is no need for a laxative or enema.

Lower GI series

A barium enema is used to reveal the contour and motility of the colon, cecum, and appendix.

Preparation: The patient is placed on a minimal-residue diet 2 days before the examination and given a cathartic (mineral oil) 24 hours before the examination. A cleansing enema is given the night before and the morning of the examination. The patient is NPO after midnight the night before the test.

Cholecystography

A cholecystography detects gallstones and estimates the ability of the gallbladder to fill and empty.

Preparation: The patient receives an iodine-containing contrast (e.g., Telepaque) 3.6 g orally 12 hours before the radiograph and then nothing else by mouth. The patient must *not* be allergic to iodine or iodine products.

GI, Gastrointestinal.

COLLABORATIVE INTERVENTIONS
Overview
1. Initiate IV access with a large-bore catheter and usually Ringer's lactate, except in cases of liver disease (including variceal bleeding). Isotonic solutions are the fluids of choice in these cases because of the inability of the liver to break down lactate into sodium bicarbonate. Fluid resuscitation, antibiotics, antiemetics, and pain medications may all be required intravenously (Table 1-2). Conduct the appropriate laboratory tests (e.g., chemistry, hematology, and coagulation studies and holding a clot tube of blood) with initiation of IV access.
2. Initiate continuous cardiac monitoring, pulse oximetry, and frequent hemodynamic monitoring for patients with severe fluid volume loss, active bleeding, or a decreased LOC. Anticipate the need for blood and blood product replacement.
3. Initiate the replacement of electrolytes.
4. Place a nasogastric tube and indwelling urinary catheter.
5. Anticipate and prepare to place an esophagogastric tamponade tube in cases of ruptured esophageal varices.

Clinical Conditions
Appendicitis
Appendicitis is the most common cause of abdominal pain requiring surgical intervention. It occurs when the appendix becomes obstructed from an increase in bacteria and mucus, causing distention and potential perforation.
Symptoms
- The patient experiences a classic progression of nausea and vomiting, followed by pain, and, finally, fever. Classic symptoms occur in one half to two thirds of patients.
- The pain starts periumbilically, then localizes at McBurney's point (midway between the anterior iliac crest and umbilicus) between 2 and 12 hours after the onset of the obstruction.
- The pain is steady and severe and increases with movement and perforation. An abrupt increase in pain with resultant confirming abdominal examination is indicative of perforation.
- Men may report right testicular pain.

TABLE 1-2 Drug Summary*

Drug	Dose/Route	Special considerations
Phenergan	**Adult:** 12.5-25 mg IV q4h	Should not be ambulatory
	Child: 0.25-1 mg/kg PO/IM/IV/PR q4-6h	Rate not to exceed 25 mg/min
Morphine sulfate	**Adult:** 4-15 mg IV over 5 minutes q2-4hr	Respiratory depression
	Child: 0.1-0.2 mg/kg IV q2-4hr; maximum dose 10 mg	
Meperidine	**Adult:** 50-100 mg q3-4hr	Not to be used in patients with glaucoma, closed head injury, liver disease
	Child: 1-1.5 mg/kg q3-4hr	
Fentanyl	0.025-0.1 mg/kg	Shorter acting respiratory depression
Vasopressin	Bolus: 20 U over 20 min	Reduction in coronary blood flow
	IV infusion: 0.2-0.8 U/min	Monitor for dysrhythmia and ST segment changes
Nitroglycerin	5-20 μg/min to counteract vasopressin	Monitor for hypotension
Neomycin	4-12 g/day in divided doses over 5-6 days	Ototoxicity Nephrotoxicity
Lactulose	20-30 g tid PO	—
Mannitol	12.5 g of 15%-20% over 3-5 min	Not to be used in anuric or dehydrated patients Monitor electrolytes

Information provided is for the adult patient unless otherwise specified.

DIAGNOSIS

- The white blood cell count is usually elevated but may not be with geriatric patients or patients who are immunocompromised (e.g., patients with AIDS and patients receiving chemotherapy).
- Vital signs may reveal mild tachypnea and a slight elevation in temperature.

- Radiography is not always diagnostic but is useful in ruling out other conditions.
- Ultrasound tests show a thickened cecum.[10] An abdominal sonogram has a 99.3% sensitivity, a 68.1% specificity, and a 91.6% accuracy for identifying appendicitis.
- The diagnosis is usually based on a physical examination.
- A computed tomography (CT) scan is 87% to 98% sensitive, 83% to 97% specific, and 93% to 94% accurate for identification of an abnormal appendix or appendocolith.[11] Suggestive findings include fluid collections or pericecal inflammation.

TREATMENT
- The treatment for a patient who does not "rule in" for appendicitis consists of observation with serial examinations (physical and white count) and IV rehydration.
- With classic symptoms, treatment involves hydration by IV fluids, broad-spectrum antibiotics, and laparoscopic surgery with removal of the appendix.

Bowel obstruction

One of the two most common causes of abdominal pain is a bowel obstruction. A bowel obstruction may result from one of many causes: ileus, impaction, stricture, volvulus, worms, or malignancy. The obstruction may be partial or complete and is most commonly located in the area of the duodenum or small or large bowel. A bowel obstruction is an extremely dangerous condition resulting in a high incidence of infection and perforation with consequent peritonitis, especially for the geriatric patient.

SYMPTOMS
- Symptoms include nausea and vomiting (frequently fecal-smelling emesis), abdominal pain that is localized and colicky, constipation, and abdominal distention.

DIAGNOSIS
- A radiographic examination shows dilated, fluid-filled loops of bowel proximal to the obstruction.
- Serum electrolyte levels are abnormal because of the massive loss of fluid and electrolytes from accumulated abdominal contents.

TREATMENT
- Treatment includes rehydration with Ringer's lactate solution, electrolyte replacement, insertion of a nasogastric tube and indwelling urinary catheter, antibiotics, and hospital admission.

- Patients may require intensive care, based on the degree of dehydration and electrolyte abnormality.
- Surgical intervention is considered in cases of perforation and ischemic bowel.

Cholecystitis

Cholecystitis is the second most common cause of abdominal pain. Pain is produced primarily from obstruction of the cystic duct in the gallbladder because of gallstones or, secondarily, from staphylococcal or streptococcal infection. The incidence of cholecystitis is increased for women less than 40 years of age and for all patients over 70 years of age.

SYMPTOMS

- Patients experience an acute onset of steady, noncramping right upper quadrant pain and tenderness, with nausea, anorexia, vomiting, and fever.

DIAGNOSIS

- An ultrasonographic examination of the right upper quadrant will usually identify gallstones. An ultrasound is 90% to 95% accurate in diagnosing cholecystitis.
- Serum laboratory test results are positive for leukocytosis with increased polymorphonuclear cells (basophils, eosinophils, granulocytes, and neutrophils) and bands, and elevations on bilirubin and liver function studies.
- Imaging studies (cholescintigraphy), although highly accurate, remain controversial because of cost, availability, and specificity to cystic duct obstruction.[12]

TREATMENT

- Treatment is usually conservative for the first 24 to 48 hours, consisting of IV fluid therapy, pain control, and antibiotic and antiemetic therapy.
- Nasogastric tube insertion may be indicated for the patient with vomiting, gastric distention, or ileus.
- Early surgery can be anticipated for patients for whom medical management is not successful.
- Laparoscopic cholecystectomy, as opposed to open laparotomy, has become the procedure of choice for this condition.
- Laparoscopic cholecystectomy has been shown to be successful in decreasing hospital stay and expediting recovery, resulting in an earlier return to work and an earlier return of the ability to perform the activities of daily living.[13]

Crohn's disease

Crohn's disease is an inflammatory process of the bowel that produces a thickened, incompressible bowel wall. This disease tends to occur in families and among Eastern European Jews between the ages of 15 and 35 years.

SYMPTOMS

- Symptoms and onset are varied.
- Patients may complain of localized pain; typically, the pain is worse after eating, especially after ingestion of milk products or mechanically or chemically irritating foods.
- The patients are usually anorexic and febrile and have frequent loose stools.
- Symptoms are insidious and sporadic, but episodes gradually become more severe and more frequent.

DIAGNOSIS

- A barium enema is diagnostic for thickened bowel walls with a narrowed passage through which a thin trickle of barium is able to pass.

TREATMENT

- Treatment is aimed at palliation, not cure. Therapy is directed toward pain control, the reduction of inflammation through steroid treatment, hydration, antibiotic therapy, the replacement of electrolytes, and dietary changes.

Dehydration

Many patients with abdominal conditions may exhibit some degree of dehydration and electrolyte imbalance, based on the severity of the illness. The most susceptible groups are geriatric and pediatric patients.

SYMPTOMS

- Symptoms vary with the degree of dehydration.
- In cases of mild (5%) dehydration, the skin is pale and cool, skin turgor decreases, mucous membranes are normal to slightly dry, and urinary output is diminished.
- As the degree of dehydration increases, signs and symptoms of shock are more marked.
- The patient becomes anuric, the pulse becomes increasingly rapid, weak, and thready, the skin color changes and becomes gray and mottled with a loss of elasticity (positive "tenting" sign), and the patient's LOC decreases.
- For the pediatric patient, the determination of dehydration is based on the percent of body weight loss and is most often caused by gastroenteritis.
- Additional causes include antibiotic intolerance, ingestion, food or formula allergies, and the improper handling of formula.

- The most common form of dehydration for the pediatric population is isotonic (defined as a serum sodium level of 130 to 150 mEq/L).
- Hyponatremic dehydration (a serum sodium level <130 mEq/L) and hypernatremic dehydration (a serum sodium level >150 mEq/L) are both less common.

DIAGNOSIS

- Diagnosis for adults is confirmed by a change in baseline weight, an increased hematocrit, a serum sodium level >148 mm/L, and a serum BUN/creatinine ratio >25.[9]
- For pediatric patients, diagnosis is confirmed by a change in weight, the serum sodium level, the amount of fluid intake, and the number of wet diapers in the past 6 hours with the percent each diaper was saturated.

TREATMENT

- Treatment varies with the degree of dehydration and electrolyte imbalance.
- Mild dehydration is treated with fluids and observation. Severe dehydration requires rapid IV rehydration, cardiac monitoring, hospitalization, electrolyte replacement over 2 to 3 days, accurate intake and output, and supportive care.
- In mild to moderate cases of dehydration with the pediatric population, the American Academy of Pediatrics recommends oral rehydration with an oral glucose-electrolyte solution in the first 4 to 6 hours, followed by diluted formula or milk.[14]
- In older children, after oral rehydration, a "BRATT" (*B*ananas, *R*ice, *A*pplesauce, *T*ea, *T*oast) diet is recommended (Table 1-3).
- In cases of severe dehydration, boluses of warm Ringer's lactate are given at a rate of 20 ml/kg and repeated until the heart rate is within normal range.
- Maintenance fluids are based on weight at a ml/kg/hr dosage.

Esophageal varices

Esophageal varices are dilated lower esophageal veins that are caused by portal hypertension. Ninety percent of portal hypertension cases are caused by cirrhotic changes.[15] It is the rupture and subsequent bleeding of these vessels that constitute a life-threatening emergency. Mortality within 1 year of the first episode of hemorrhage is 70%[16]; however, 50% of patients die within 6 weeks of the onset of symptoms.[15] The rupture of esophageal varices accounts for

TABLE 1-3 Special Diets for Abdominal Conditions

Condition	Diet	Special considerations
Crohn's disease	Low residue	Avoid milk, milk products, vegetable fiber (salads, fruit peels), nuts
Prep for upper and lower gastrointestinal series	Low fiber	
	Low fat	
	High calorie	
	High carbohydrate	
	High protein	
Chronic pancreatitis	Bland, low fat with six meals per day	Avoid alcohol
		Use antacid with meals
Dehydration in older pediatric patients	BRATT (Bananas, Rice, Applesauce, Tea, Toast)	—
Mild to medium dehydration, gastritis, gastroenteritis	Clear liquids (broth, gelatin, Jell-O, water, Pedialyte)	Avoid orange juice

10% of all upper gastrointestinal (UGI) bleeding and occurs more often in men.[8] There has been an increase in the incidence of UGI bleeding in the past 15 years because of use of over-the-counter pain medicines such as nonsteroidal antiinflammatory drugs (NSAIDs).

SYMPTOMS
- Patients have sudden painless hemorrhaging associated with nausea.
- The hematocrit is low and usually requires transfusion.
- On physical examination the spleen is enlarged.
- In serious cases of active bleeding the patient is in shock.

DIAGNOSIS
- Diagnosis is based on history, laboratory values (a decreased hematocrit and abnormal liver function studies), angiography, and esophagoscopy.

TREATMENT
- Treatment ranges from conservative management to aggressive resuscitation. Patients are hospitalized for fluid resuscitation with isotonic fluids and blood. The goal of blood administration is to maintain the hematocrit value near 30%. Overtransfusion can increase portal hypertension and cause rebleeding.[15] Ringer's lactate is not recommended for volume replacement in patients who experience this rebleeding, because of the inability of the diseased liver to convert lactate to sodium bicarbonate for excretion (which causes metabolic alkalosis). Procedures that have been effective in the ED include insertion of an esophagogastric balloon tamponade tube (Figure 1-1). Emergent endoscopy with sclerotherapy is the most effective treatment and is effective in up to 95% of cases.[15] Temporizing measures also include vasopressin infusion with concomitant nitroglycerin infusion to lower portal pressure by reducing blood flow in the arterial bed.[15] Surgical intervention may include placement of a portal-systemic shunt or a devascularization procedure to arrest bleeding. An ice water lavage with or without epinephrine is no longer recommended in cases involving acute bleeding.

Gastritis and gastroenteritis
Gastritis occurs when food is ingested too quickly or when noxious agents (e.g., coffee or alcohol) are ingested. Gastroenteritis is an infection that may be bacterial (e.g., food poisoning—causative agents: *Campylobacter, Salmonella,*

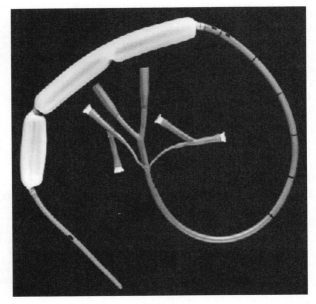

Figure 1-1 Minnesota Four Lumen Tube. (Courtesy Bard Medical Division and Davol, Inc.)

Shigella), viral, protozoan (e.g., *Giardia lamblia*, "amoebic dysentery"), or parasitic (e.g., worms).

SYMPTOMS
- Symptoms are similar for both conditions.
- Pain is colicky and epigastric in origin.
- Patients frequently complain of nausea, vomiting, and diarrhea within 6 to 8 hours after eating.

DIAGNOSIS
- Diagnosis is based on history and stool culture results.

TREATMENT
- Treatment is related to the severity of the incident.
- Patients with gastritis should alter the frequency and composition of meals.
- Gastroenteritis is treated by identifying and correcting the causative agent, by IV rehydration, and by electrolyte replacement.
- Severe episodes necessitate hospitalization for observation and monitoring.

Fulminant hepatic failure

Most cases of hepatic failure are caused by an acute episode of viral hepatitis, although use of common drugs such as acetaminophen, valproate, methyldopa, tetracycline, and NSAIDs can also cause failure. Massive cellular liver necrosis and disruption of all metabolic functions of the liver occur, producing neurologic, cardiopulmonary, renal, hematologic, and metabolic deficiencies.

SYMPTOMS
- Symptoms include encephalopathy (mild confusion to coma), jaundice, edema, dehydration, bleeding and bruising, acute tubular necrosis (ATN) and renal failure, fever, and anorexia.

DIAGNOSIS
- Diagnosis is based on history, a physical examination, and laboratory values (abnormal coagulation studies and liver function studies).

TREATMENT
- Acetaminophen toxicity is the only cause of fulminant hepatic failure that may be reversible (see Chapter 19). Patients with hepatic failure are admitted to an intensive care unit and treated with supportive care that includes cardiac monitoring, strict intake and output, fluid and electrolyte replacement, treatment of coagulopathy, routine culture and sensitivity of body secretions to identify sepsis (fever and leukocytosis occur with liver failure and cannot be used as a sign of sepsis), routine chest radiography, and restriction of dietary protein (to decrease the nitrogen load). Hypotension is treated with blood, fresh frozen plasma, platelets, albumin, and isotonic fluids.

Acute pancreatitis

The pancreas becomes inflamed as a result of alcohol intake or a blockage of the ampulla of Vater because of gallstones. A blockage causes pancreatic autodigestion. Pancreatitis is uncommon in children. Incidence increases with age.

SYMPTOMS
- The patient experiences the onset of excruciatingly sharp, upper abdominal pain that increases with supination and radiates to the back, chest, and epigastric, or flank, area.
- The pain is knifelike, severe, and twisting.

- The pain usually occurs after drinking large quantities of alcohol or ingesting a high-fat meal.
- Other symptoms include fever, signs of shock, vomiting, abdominal distention, ascites, and diminished to absent bowel sounds.

DIAGNOSIS

- Pancreatitis mimics other conditions.
- Diagnosis is based on laboratory and radiographic studies.
- The chest film is positive for pleural effusions.
- Increased serum lipase and serum amylase levels are present.
- There is marked general tenderness over the upper abdomen without true rigidity.
- An ultrasonographic examination, in combination with laboratory studies, has the best specificity and sensitivity for diagnosis.[12]
- An abdominal CT scan with contrast may also be performed.

TREATMENT

- Treatment is supportive, including admission to an intensive care unit, invasive monitoring, and aggressive fluid replacement with Ringer's lactate, normal saline, and colloids. High doses of fresh frozen plasma, in theory, may be of value by inhibiting further proteolytic activity.[1] Pain management with IV narcotics is preferred; however, controversy exists over the narcotic of preference. Analgesics that do not contain opioids (meperidine and fentanyl) have been preferred because they do not produce spasm at the sphincter of Oddi, which is thought to be the pain source. Morphine, initially avoided, is currently thought to have minimal effect on the sphincter.[1] Until the serum amylase level returns to normal, strict NPO maintenance is critical to preventing the recurrence of autodigestion. A nasogastric tube should be placed if the patient is vomiting or has abdominal distension, a decreased LOC, or an ileus.[17] Between 85% and 90% of patients respond to medical management. There is considerable debate about delayed versus early surgical intervention for the removal of gallstones.[12] Surgical intervention is based on clinical and morphologic criteria such as renal failure, sepsis, persistent acute abdomen, or intestinal perforation.[1] Surgery is necessary in these cases. The severity of the disease is related to the amount of tissue necrosis, and treatment is based on severity. Hemorrhagic pancreatitis necessitates immediate surgical intervention. Signs of hemorrhagic pancreatitis include Cullen's sign (periumbilical bruising) and Grey Turner's sign (bruising in the flank region and lower back). Hemorrhagic pancreatitis is frequently missed, and diagnosis occurs during autopsy in 30% to 40% of the cases.[18]

NURSING SURVEILLANCE

1. Monitor the severity of the condition based on changes in ABCs.
2. Monitor the level and type of pain and the response to pain management strategies.
3. Monitor intake and output and check gastric and rectal secretions for occult or gross bleeding.
4. Monitor the patient for cardiac dysrhythmia.
5. Monitor the patient for signs and symptoms of decreased perfusion.
6. Assess changes in the LOC (as appropriate).

EXPECTED PATIENT OUTCOMES

1. Rehydration and volume replacement will support a mean arterial pressure between 90 and 105 mm Hg.
2. Antibiotic therapy will be initiated as appropriate.
3. Pain management will be initiated as appropriate.

DISCHARGE IMPLICATIONS

1. Check orthostatic vital signs before discharge (pulse within normal limits of 50 to 100 beats/min, no hypotension when transferred from lying to standing).
2. Dietary instructions should be given to the family and patient (e.g., clear liquids, bland diet, small, frequent meals, and BRATT diet) (Table 1-3).
3. Teach the family and patient the signs and symptoms of dehydration. Caretakers of pediatric and geriatric patients may need teaching about the potential for aspiration with recurrent vomiting.
4. Instruct the patient and family about the need for follow-up (for fever over 101° F, vomiting more than six times in 24 hours, more than eight diarrheal stools in 24 hours, and cultures and sensitivities pending from ED laboratory work).

References

1. Krumberger JM: Acute pancreatitis, *Crit Care Nurs Clin North Am* 5(1):185-201, 1993.
2. Kucharski SA: Fulminant hepatic failure, *Crit Care Nurs Clin North Am* 5(1):141-149, 1993.
3. Murray FE et al: Cigarette smoking and parity as risk factors for the development of symptomatic gall bladder disease in women: results of the Royal College of General Practitioner's oral contraception study, *Gut* 35:107-111, 1994.
4. Kane RL, Ouslander JG, Abrass IB: *Essentials of clinical geriatrics,* ed 3, New York, 1994, McGraw-Hill.
5. Louria DB et al: Infections in older patients: a systematic clinical approach, *Geriatrics* 48(1):28-34, 1993.
6. Huddleston KC, Ferraro-McDuffie A, Wolff-Small T: Nutritional support of the critically ill child, *Crit Care Nur Clin North Am* 5(1):65-77, 1993.
7. Agency for Health Care Policy and Research: *Acute pain management: operative or medical procedures and trauma,* 1992, Rockville, MD, U.S. Department of Health and Human Services.
8. Sanson TG, O'Keefe KP: Evaluation of abdominal pain in the elderly, *Emerg Med Clin North Am* 14(3):615-627, 1996.
9. Hoffman NB: Dehydration in the elderly: insidious and manageable, *Geriatrics* 46(6):35-38, 1991.
10. Spiro HM: An internist's approach to acute abdominal pain, *Med Clin North Am* 77(5):963-971, 1993.
11. Graffeo CS, Counselman FL: Appendicitis, *Emerg Med Clin North Am* 14(4):653-671, 1996.
12. Kadakia SC: Biliary tract emergencies: acute cholecystitis, acute cholangitis, and acute pancreatitis, *Med Clin North Am* 77(5):1015-1030, 1993.
13. Kelley JE et al: Safety, efficacy, cost and morbidity of laparoscopic versus open cholecystectomy: a prospective analysis of 228 consecutive patients, *Am Surg* 59(1):23-27, 1993.
14. Bezerra JA et al: Treatment of infants with acute diarrhea: what's recommended and what's practiced, *Pediatrics* 90(1):1-4, 1992.
15. Kerber K: The adult with bleeding esophageal varices, *Crit Care Nurs Clin North Am* 5(1):153-161, 1993.
16. Schwartz SI et al: *Principles of surgery,* ed 4, New York, 1984, McGraw-Hill.
17. Melander S: *Review of critical care case studies and applications,* Philadelphia, 1992, WB Saunders.
18. Ransen JHC: Diagnostic standards for acute pancreatitis, *World J Surg* 21(2):136-142, 1997.

Abuse

Patty Sturt

CLINICAL CONDITIONS
Child Abuse
   Physical Abuse
      Injuries to Skin and Subcutaneous Tissues
      Burns
      Head Injuries
      Shaken Impact (or Baby) Syndrome
      Abdominal Injuries
      Münchausen Syndrome by Proxy
   Sexual Abuse
Battered Women
Elder Abuse
Physical Abuse
Psychologic and Emotional Abuse
Neglect
Exploitation

TRIAGE ASSESSMENT

Abuse occurs among people of all ages, races, religions, socioeconomic and educational levels, and religious backgrounds. The individuals most vulnerable to abuse are children, women, and the elderly; however, abuse can also occur to men.

The emergency department (ED) nurse may be the first health care professional to interact with the patient. Individuals reporting rape, sexual assault, or abuse should not be questioned at triage. This may increase the emotional trauma (guilt and embarrassment) the person may be experiencing. If no life-threatening injuries are present, escort the patient immediately to a private treatment area to obtain the triage assessment data.

Abuse is not always apparent. The triage nurse must have a high index of suspicion anytime an injury is not congruent with the patient's history. If life-threatening injuries are absent, the following data should be obtained.

Children
Deficits
Determine if there is a history of physical, mental, or psychosocial deficits. Increased stress within the family may be associated with children who have a variety of problems or who are perceived as "different" or difficult by their parents. These problems may be physical (e.g., cerebral palsy), mental (e.g., retardation), temperamental (e.g., moodiness and difficulty), or behavioral (e.g., hyperactivity).

Stressors
Ask about recent or multiple stressors in the family. Factors such as unemployment, poverty, parental discord, and a family crisis can create a stressful environment where abuse can occur.

Caregiver
Determine who the primary caregiver is. Who does the child live with? Where do they live? Single parents are more likely to experience social isolation and poverty, which may place the child at greater risk of being abused. Parents may drive great distances and bypass hospitals closer to home for fear of detection. See the "Risk Factors" box for a summary of risk factors for child abuse.

RISK FACTORS FOR CHILD ABUSE

Child risk factors
Physical disability
Mental or psychosocial
  deficits (e.g., mental
  retardation)
Parents' perceptions of the
  child as different or
  difficult
Prematurity
Product of a multiple birth
Chronic illness

Parental risk factors
Childhood history of abuse
Drug or alcohol dependency
Unmet emotional needs
Single parent
Social isolation
Low self-esteem
Inadequate social supports or
  role models
Belief in use of corporal
  punishment
Unemployment or poverty
Parental discord
Unrealistic expectations of child

Injury

If an injury (or injuries) is present, determine the following:
- Where is the pain the child describes?
- How did the injury occur?
- Where did the injury occur?
- Who was present or witnessed the injury?
- When did the injury occur?

This information is important to determining if the injury is consistent or possible with the history. The following are cues of possible abuse:
- There are inconsistencies in the history obtained from the parents or child.
- The parent is reluctant to describe the circumstances surrounding the injury.
- The parent denies any knowledge of how the injury occurred.
- A sibling, another child, or the baby-sitter is blamed for the injury.
- The child is developmentally incapable of causing the injury (e.g., a parent claims that a 6-month-old pulled down a pan of hot water from the stove).
- There is a delay in the seeking of medical treatment.

Immunizations

Determine if childhood immunizations are up to date. If they are not, this may indicate a lack of appropriate health care.

History

- History of repeated injuries or hospitalizations
- History of failure to gain weight at home; failure to gain weight, particularly in infants, possibly because of underfeeding
- History of genital or rectal discharge, bleeding, or pain (consider sexual abuse)
- History of dysuria or frequency of urination (consider sexual abuse)

Vital Signs

- *Tachycardia and hypotension:* May result from blood loss secondary to vaginal-cervical tears from sexual abuse, internal injuries from physical abuse, or dehydration secondary to malnourishment
- *Fever:* May be noted in children with genital-pelvic or urinary tract infections secondary to sexual abuse

General Observations

The following should increase the nurse's suspicion of possible abuse:

- The child appears frightened of the parent or caregiver.
- The child easily goes to strangers.
- The child exhibits extreme apprehension when hearing other children cry.
- The child has human bite marks.
- The child has bruises in various stages of healing.
- The child has bruises suggestive of being struck by an object, such as a looped cord or belt buckle, or a hand imprint.
- Cigarette burns are visible on the child.
- The child has burns in the configuration of the object used to cause the harm.
- The child has rectal burns and burns with a clear line of demarcation (dunking burns).
- The child is wearing inappropriate clothing.

Women

Privacy is a "must" when interviewing a suspected battered woman. Escort the woman to a private treatment room to obtain the needed history. The husband, friend, or family member should remain in the lobby.

Anxiety

Anxiety, nervousness, difficulty sleeping, and depression are common complications associated with battering.

Vague complaints

Frequent visits to the ED with vague complaints or chronic pain are suggestive of battering. Women who are beaten at regular intervals may come to the ED with psychosomatic or emotional complaints just before they expect another beating.

History of suicide attempts

Attempted suicide has been associated with battering.

Past injuries

Determine if there is a history of ED visits as a result of injuries. Repeated ED visits with injuries becoming more severe is highly suggestive of battering.

Present injuries

If an injury is present, determine the following:

- Location of the injury and pain

- How the injury occurred
- Time the injury occurred

Many times the extent or type of injury will be inconsistent with the explanation the patient gives. There may be a substantial delay between the time of the injury and the patient's visit for treatment. Common sites of injury are the face, head, neck, chest, breasts, abdomen, and genitals.

Menstruation

Determine the last menstrual period and ask about the possibility of pregnancy. A significant number of pregnant women are beaten, often in the breasts and abdomen.

NURSING ALERT

When a woman has one injury from abuse, there may be multiple old and new injuries that may be overlooked, especially if the presenting problem is a painful, obvious facial injury. The more subtle injury, such as in the abdomen, may be hidden by clothing and may be life threatening.

Vital Signs

- *Tachycardia:* Often present as a result of pain, anxiety, and fear secondary to abusive episodes from husband or male partner
- *Tachycardia and hypotension:* May result from blood loss secondary to inflicted blunt or penetrating trauma (see Chapter 20)

General Observations

The following observations should increase the nurse's index of suspicion for battering:

- The patient has unexplained lacerations, abrasions, burns, or bruises in various stages of healing.
- The patient minimizes the frequency or seriousness of the injuries.
- The patient describes the circumstances around the event in a hesitant, embarrassed, or evasive manner.
- The husband or male partner accompanying the patient insists on staying with her, makes hostile or threatening statements to her, answers the triage nurse's questions, makes defensive or derogatory comments to the triage

nurse, or appears to be under the influence of alcohol or other drugs.

NURSING ALERT

Any trauma without a clear indication of cause in a female patient needs to be considered battering until battering is ruled out.[1]

Elderly Patients
Age and gender
Note the patient's age and gender; the typical abused elder is female and more than 70 years of age.[2]
Caregiver
Determine with whom the patient lives. Does the patient have a history of any mental or physical impairments? Often the abused elder will have a physical impairment such as difficulty walking, hearing or vision deficits, or incontinence. Mental impairments may include confusion and senility secondary to Alzheimer's disease, previous strokes or head injuries, and organic brain syndrome. Daughters and daughters-in-law frequently have the responsibility of caring for aged parents. The abuser is often a middle-aged female.[3]
Transportation to the ED
Determine who brought the patient to the ED. The abused elder is often brought to the ED by someone other than the caregiver.
Medications
Determine current medications. Ask to look at the bottles. Try to determine if medications are being given as prescribed.
Past injuries
Frequent hospitalization from injuries is suggestive of abuse.
Time of injury or illness
Determine the interval between the injury or illness and the patient's appearance at the ED. Often this interval will be prolonged.
Chief complaint
Determine the chief complaint or reason for transfer to the ED. Although hip and proximal femoral fractures are common after unintentional falls, identical injuries can occur if

the patient has been pushed or tripped. The presence of multiple, untreated, or poorly treated decubiti is an important physical indicator of elder neglect.[4]

Weight loss

Excessive weight loss can occur as a result of malnourishment.

Vital Signs

• *Tachycardia and hypotension:* May result from blood loss secondary to inflicted trauma (usually chest, abdominal, or femur) or severe dehydration secondary to malnourishment

• *Fever:* May occur in patients with untreated decubiti

NURSING ALERT

Hypovolemic elderly patients may not experience tachycardia if they are taking beta-blockers.

General Observations

The following observations should increase the triage nurse's index of suspicion for abuse:

• The patient exhibits symptoms of severe dehydration such as pallor, poor skin turgor, sunken eyes and cheeks, and dry lips.
• The patient appears very nervous or fearful.
• The patient is notably passive and withdrawn.
• The caregiver verbalizes or demonstrates overt hostility, frustration, defensiveness, denial, or concern over the patient's "behavior."
• The caregiver demonstrates a lack of eye contact with the patient.

FOCUSED NURSING ASSESSMENT

Nursing assessment for all individuals of suspected abuse should focus on oxygenation and ventilation, perfusion, cognition, sexuality, and safety and security.

Oxygenation and Ventilation
Airway

Stridor and respiratory distress may be present in cases where the victim was strangled by hands or by rope or other objects. Patients with a decreased level of consciousness (LOC), such as infants with shaken impact syndrome (shaken baby syndrome), are at increased risk for airway compromise.

Breath sounds

Absent or decreased breath sounds may occur with inflicted blunt or penetrating injuries to the chest. Suspect a pneumothorax or hemothorax. Breath sounds may be decreased if the patient is hypoventilating secondary to increased intracranial pressure (ICP) from a head injury.

Perfusion

Assess skin color and temperature, capillary refill, and peripheral pulses. Pale, cool skin may indicate hemorrhage from inflicted blunt or penetrating abdominal trauma to the spleen or liver. Delayed capillary refill is a reliable indicator of hypovolemia and hemorrhage in infants and children. A weak or absent pulse distal to an injured extremity is indicative of impingement on vascular structures.

Cognition

Perform a neurologic assessment. An alteration in the LOC may be seen in cases of head injuries caused by abuse. Some examples would include infants exhibiting shaken impact syndrome, children repeatedly hit across the head, and women who are forcibly thrown against an object and strike their heads. Obtain a Glasgow Coma Scale score (see Reference Guide 10) and assess pupil size and reaction (see Chapter 14).

Sexuality

Sexual abuse can occur in both sexes and at any age. Assess the patient for any trauma to, or discharge or drainage from, the genitals or rectum. Determine the last menstrual period. Ask the patient about the use of birth control and the possibility of pregnancy (see Sexual Assault Evidence Collection Procedure 27, and Child Sexual Abuse under Collaborative Interventions in this chapter).

NURSING ALERT

Any patient with suspected sexual abuse should be interviewed and examined in a private area.

Safety and Security

- Assess the potential for suicide. Approximately 25% of battered women attempt suicide (see Chapter 3).
- Assess the potential for homicide. Battering is considered the most important precipitant for women killed by men and for men killed by women. Determine if the partner has threatened to kill the victim of the battering. Risk factors for homicide include sexual abuse, guns in the home, the partner being addicted to cocaine or intoxicated daily, the woman making plans to leave, and either partner having threatened or attempted suicide.

Risk Factors
Child abuse
See the "Risk Factors for Child Abuse" box.
Battering
- *Characteristics of the batterer*
  1. The batterer engages in heavy drinking. Experts report that 40% to 95% of wife beating involves drinking.
  2. He engaged in physical abuse during dating and courtship.
  3. He demonstrates cruelty to animals. Any man who savagely beats a dog or other pet should be considered a potential abuser.
  4. He comes from a violent home environment. Men who were abused as children or who have grown up seeing their mothers beaten by their fathers are apt to think that family violence is normal behavior.
  5. He has a poor self-image; men often attack their mates when they feel their masculinity is threatened.
  6. He exhibits excessive jealousy. Battered women often report that their husbands isolate them from social contacts (e.g., friends, neighbors, and relatives) and sources of transportation (e.g., take away car keys).
  7. He lacks the ability to differentiate feelings; emotions such as fear and loneliness are expressed as anger.
  8. He has rigid expectations of his wife; the mate must conform to his definitions of her role.
  9. He has a negative and derogatory opinion of women in general.
- *Characteristics of the battered mate*
  1. The battered mate engages in excessive minimization and denial.

2. She has a high economic and emotional dependency on the batterer.

3. She is unsure of her own ego needs; she defines herself only in terms of her roles as a wife and mother.

4. She has unlimited patience in hopes for the discovery of a magic combination in solving marital problems.

5. She has a family history of abuse; she witnessed her mother being abused by her father.

6. She constantly seeks approval from her spouse.

Elder abuse

Victims of elder abuse are likely to be individuals with characteristics that render them vulnerable. They are female and more than 70 years of age; they have limited economic resources and a lack of alternative living arrangements; they are physically or mentally impaired (inability to walk or need for assistance to walk, hearing or visual impairments, partial or total confusion, and incontinence); or they are living in the community with an adult child or other family member.

- *Characteristics of the elder abuser*

  1. The abuser has a violent background; he or she grew up being abused by a parent or witnessing abuse.

  2. The abuser has a history of alcohol or other drug addiction.

  3. The abuser has long-term financial problems.

  4. The abuser displaces anger; anger meant for some authority figure is often displaced onto a family member.

  5. The abuser confuses roles, expecting the victim to meet a wide range of his or her needs.

- *Characteristics of the elderly victim*

  1. The victim has a tendency to internalize blame and a belief that he or she causes the assaults.

  2. The victim demonstrates passivity and compliance and does not usually fight back.

  3. The victim exhibits loyalty and defends the abuser despite pain and anger.

Life Span Issues

1. Approximately 25% of obstetric patients, 45% of mothers of abused children, 25% of women who attempt suicide, and 30% to 50% of female psychiatric patients are abused women.[5]

2. Domestic assaults account for approximately 99,800 hospital days and 28,700 ED visits each year.
3. Violence occurs even after a relationship has ended. Approximately one fifth of both fatal and nonfatal incidents involve relationships that have been terminated or estranged.
4. Studies indicate that 2% to 5% of people over the age of 65 have been abused.

INITIAL INTERVENTIONS

Regardless of the victim's age or the type of suspected abuse, the following interventions must be considered:

1. Perform a primary survey to identify all life-threatening injuries.
2. Implement measures to maintain a patent airway (see Chapter 16). Always consider the possibility of a spine injury in patients with inflicted trauma to the head and upper torso.
3. If the patient exhibits signs and symptoms of hypovolemic shock, initiate 100% oxygen per nonrebreather mask and two large-bore IVs of Ringer's lactate or normal saline.
4. Perform a secondary survey (see Chapter 20) to identify all injuries.
5. Splint and immobilize all extremities as indicated.
6. Implement measures to decrease and control increased ICP for patients with a brain injury sustained from physical abuse (see Chapter 14).
7. Maintain confidentiality and privacy for any patient with injuries from suspected abuse.
8. Use words appropriate to the developmental level of the patient. For example, a four-year-old may not understand the word "urine" but will understand "pee."
9. Treat the abused individual with respect and empathy. Many abused victims experience embarrassment, guilt, and shame.
10. Determine the tetanus and diphtheria immunization status of any patient with impaired skin integrity as a result of suspected abuse.

PRIORITY NURSING DIAGNOSES

Risk for ineffective airway clearance
Risk for impaired gas exchange

Risk for fluid volume deficit
Risk for injury
Risk for rape trauma syndrome
Risk for violence
Risk for knowledge deficit (caregiver)

♦ **Ineffective airway clearance** related to a decreased LOC secondary to inflicted head trauma:
   INTERVENTIONS
   • Maintain a patent airway (see Chapter 16).

♦ **Impaired gas exchange** related to injury of the airway structures or lungs secondary to strangulation, or inflicted penetrating or blunt trauma to the chest:
   INTERVENTIONS
   • Provide 100% oxygen per nonrebreather mask.
   • Anticipate the need for an immediate chest x-ray examination.
   • Prepare for chest tube insertion if a pneumothorax or hemothorax is present (see Chapter 20).

♦ **Fluid volume deficit** related to severe malnutrition or hemorrhage because of chest, abdominal, or genital trauma secondary to neglect, physical abuse, or sexual abuse (large vaginal tears with vascular involvement in children):
   INTERVENTIONS
   • Initiate two large-bore IVs with Ringer's lactate or normal saline.
   • Obtain type and crossmatch for blood.
   • Administer blood products as ordered.
   • Prepare the patient for surgery.

♦ **Injury** related to an abusive home environment:
   INTERVENTIONS
   • Report abuse to the appropriate authorities according to hospital policy and state laws.
   • Provide abused women with written and oral information about a safety plan and community resources.
   • Provide information on spouse abuse shelters.
   • Give parents information on support services for children with physical, developmental, or mental impairments (e.g., support groups for parents with children with cerebral palsy).
   • Provide telephone numbers of community agencies that assist with child care and elder care.

- Provide information on coping techniques to deal with stressful situations.
- ◆ **Rape trauma syndrome** related to child sexual abuse, marital rape, or sexual assault: see Procedure 27.
- ◆ **Violence (either self-directed or directed at others)** related to suicide or homicide potential secondary to history of battering:
  INTERVENTIONS
  - Discuss removing or disabling any guns in the home.
  - Determine if the victim has a plan to harm himself or herself or his or her mate.
  - Use suicide precautions (see Chapter 3).
- ◆ **Knowledge deficit (caregiver)** related to normal child development, parental skills, management, and nonphysical methods of discipline:
  INTERVENTIONS
  - Provide the parent or other caregiver with information regarding child development, social and community agencies for support and therapy, and alternatives to corporal punishment.

PRIORITY DIAGNOSTIC TESTS

Laboratory Tests

Complete blood count (CBC): Obtain a CBC to assess hemoglobin and hematocrit of patients when symptoms of hemorrhage (hypovolemic shock) are present. Also use a CBC to assess the white blood cell (WBC) count in children and the elderly to determine if weight loss is related to an infectious process or malnutrition. Malnutrition increases the individual's susceptibility to an infection.

Type and crossmatch: Obtain a type and crossmatch when symptoms of hypovolemic shock are present.

Electrolytes and glucose: Hypokalemia and hypoglycemia, as well as other electrolyte abnormalities, may be present in malnourished children and elderly persons.

Coagulation profile: Obtain a coagulation profile to determine if any multiple unexplained bruises are from a bleeding disorder.[3]

Radiographic Tests

Radiographs: A complete skeletal survey is usually indicated for infants less than 2 years of age who have evidence of abuse or for infants less than 1 year of age who show evidence of significant neglect.[6] Fractures are rare with infants less than 1 year of age and suggest abuse. Bone injuries are more common with abused children less than 4 years of age, whereas accidental fractures occur more commonly with school-age children.[7] In the absence of major identifiable trauma or intrinsic bone disease, unexplained fractures of the ribs, sternum, skull, humerus, and femur may indicate abuse. Other skeletal radiologic findings suggestive of abuse include multiple and often symmetric fractures of the limbs and multiple fractures at different stages of healing. With the elderly, unexplained fractures of the skull, nose, or facial bones, multiple fractures in various stages of healing, or spinal fractures are suggestive of abuse.

Computed tomography (CT) scan: A CT scan may reveal skull fractures. Bilateral skull fractures or skull fractures in an infant are suggestive of abuse. Cerebral edema may occur in cases involving shaken impact syndrome. With adults, CT scans may reveal skull fractures, contusions, or intracranial bleeds from inflicted head trauma.

Sexual Abuse or Assault (Laboratory)

- Perform a Venereal Disease Research Laboratory (VDRL) test.
- Perform a serum pregnancy test.
- Obtain gonococcal and Chlamydia cultures of the oropharynx, rectum, or vagina, depending on the history. Obtain all three cultures in young children.
- Obtain vaginal swabs to test for spermatozoa and seminal plasma contents.
- Obtain saliva swabs to test for ABO-antigen typing. The swabs determine whether the patient secretes properties of his or her blood type in body fluids.[8]
- Obtain head and vaginal hair for forensic analysis under a microscope to compare with the suspected abuser's hair. Head hair should be pulled from different areas. Vaginal hair should be combed and then pulled.
- HIV antibody testing of adult abuse victims in the ED is controversial, since most EDs do not provide private counseling to individuals with a positive test result. Patients can be referred to health departments or clinics that specialize in sexually transmitted diseases.

COLLABORATIVE INTERVENTIONS

A

Clinical Conditions

Child Abuse

Child abuse can entail one or more of the following:

1. **Physical abuse:** Any intentionally inflicted injury to a child by a caregiver
2. **Sexual abuse:** Any sexual activity or contact between a child and adult (or older child), whether by physical force, persuasion, or coercion
3. **Emotional abuse**: Parental behaviors that are degrading, terrorizing, belittling, isolating, and threatening, or exposure to spouse abuse
4. **Neglect:** Usually involves acts of omission or failure to meet basic needs of child; basic needs include food, clothing, medical care, and safe environment

Physical abuse in children

Injuries to skin and subcutaneous tissues

Injuries to the skin and subcutaneous tissue are seen in 90% of abused children.[4] Children who fall and injure themselves and are not abused usually have bruises over bony prominences such as the chin, forehead, elbow, knee, and shin.

SYMPTOMS

- Often bruises will represent the configuration of the object used to cause the harm, such as the outline of fingers, belt straps, or buckles, or circumferential bruises around the ankles or wrists from cords or rope (Figures 2-1 to 2-3).
- Stages and colors of bruising include purple for 1 to 5 days; green in 5 to 7 days; yellow in 7 to 10 days; and brown in >10 days. Multiple bruises in various stages of healing are suggestive of abuse. Document the size, location, and color of the bruise. Do not document the suspected age of the bruise.

DIAGNOSIS

- Diagnosis is based on an examination and history that are not consistent with the injuries.

TREATMENT

- Apply ice packs and elevate the injured extremity. Monitor the amount of swelling.
- Immobilize the area for comfort.

Burns

Death rates from abuse-related burns are high, and children with inflicted burns are likely to be injured again.

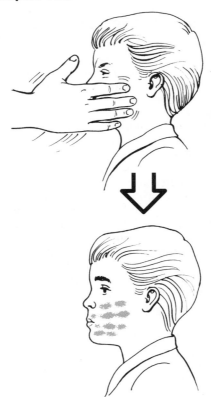

Figure 2-1 Typical slap pattern.

SYMPTOMS

- Tap water scalding is a common abusive burn. Splash injuries occur when hot water, liquid, or food is thrown or poured on the victim. The burns will not be uniform in depth and will involve different body areas. The top of the head and the anterior face, chest, and abdomen are most likely to be involved if a child pulls a pot of hot liquid on himself or herself.
- In immersion injuries the burn depth is uniform and wound boundaries are distinct. Inflicted immersion injuries from dipping or dunking generally involve the per-

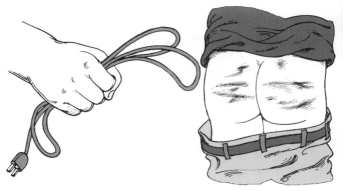

Figure 2-2 Loop or cord marks on buttocks.

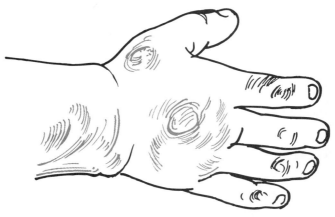

Figure 2-3 Blistering and edema in acute binding injury.

ineum, buttocks, external genitalia, or the face or hands (Figure 2-4).
- Circular burns to the soles of the feet and palms of the hands may be seen when cigarettes are intentionally placed on those areas.

DIAGNOSIS
- Diagnosis is based on an examination and history.

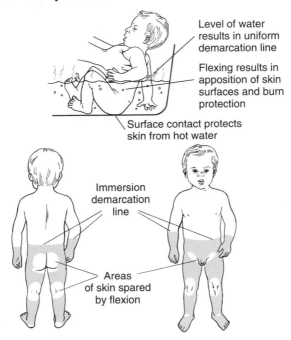

Figure 2-4 Typical immersion burn. Uniform degree of injury with interspersed protected areas.

TREATMENT
See Chapter 4.
Head injuries
Head injuries are the leading cause of death among children who are physically abused.[3]
SYMPTOMS
- Scalp bruises, subgaleal hematomas, and bald patches are common signs of abuse involving the head. The most common abuse-related intracranial injuries are subdural and subarachnoid hemorrhages.
- There may be serious intracranial injury without evidence of an external injury. Symptoms will include an altered LOC, pupillary and respiratory changes, seizures, and other signs of increased ICP.
DIAGNOSIS
- Diagnosis is based on an examination and history that do not correlate with the injury.

TREATMENT
- Monitor the patient for symptoms of increased ICP.
- Initiate nursing interventions to decrease ICP (see Chapter 14).
- Maintain a patent airway and cervical spine immobilization.
- Provide 100% oxygen.
- Intubate as necessary.
- Initiate an IV line.
- Prepare the patient for surgery.

Shaken impact syndrome

Shaken impact syndrome is a result of the vigorous shaking of an infant or small child.

SYMPTOMS
- Symptoms include retinal hemorrhaging, an altered LOC (usually from increased ICP from an epidural or subdural hematoma), a full or bulging anterior fontanel, seizure activity, fixed dilated pupils, decerebrate posturing, an abnormal respiratory rate and pattern, and bruising of the upper extremities.

DIAGNOSIS
- Diagnosis is based on an examination and history.

TREATMENT
- Initiate nursing interventions to decrease ICP (see Chapter 14).

Abdominal injuries

Bruises over the abdomen are not common in children. Children with abuse-related abdominal injuries are usually less than 2 years of age. A blow to the middle abdomen can cause a blowout rupture of the stomach or intestines. The liver and spleen may be injured because of compressing forces against the abdomen such as kicking (see Chapter 20).

SYMPTOMS
- Symptoms include a distended or rigid abdomen, persistent vomiting and abdominal pain, and symptoms of hypovolemic shock.

DIAGNOSIS
- Diagnosis is based on the results of a CT scan, a CBC, abdominal films, and an examination.

TREATMENT
- Administer 100% oxygen per nonrebreather mask.
- Start two large-bore IVs of Ringer's lactate or normal saline. For children, a large-bore IV is 22-gauge or larger.

- Obtain type and crossmatch and administer blood as ordered.
- Insert a nasogastric tube and urinary catheter.
- Prepare the patient for surgery.

Münchausen syndrome by proxy

Münchausen syndrome by proxy is a form of child abuse in which a parent or caregiver (usually the mother) fabricates or induces symptoms of an illness in a child. The mother involved is usually described as intelligent, knowledgeable, and genuinely concerned for the child.[9]

SYMPTOMS

- The fabricated illnesses typically include histories of fever, vomiting, diarrhea, seizures, rash, blackouts, apnea, hematemesis, and hematuria.
- The mother may actually induce symptoms in the child by suffocation, by administration of drugs or toxic substances, or by placing her own blood in the child's urine, vomitus, or stool specimens.

DIAGNOSIS

- Symptoms are observed only by the caregiver and disappear when the child is separated from the caregiver.
- There is a history of visits to the ED to treat illnesses for which no cause can be determined.
- The child has been treated in numerous medical facilities.
- There are unusual symptoms that make no clinical sense.
- There are discrepancies between the history and physical findings.[9]

TREATMENT

- The treatment will be based on the child's actual clinical presentation.
- Do not allow the mother to have access to any laboratory specimens, since she may attempt to alter the specimen.
- Document all physical findings and the history given by the mother.

NURSING ALERT

Document all findings thoroughly but in an objective manner. Body diagrams and photographs may be helpful in delineating the location and size of the injuries. This information may be very helpful later in court. Do not alienate the parents or caregivers. Keep them informed of the plan of care. Be non-

judgmental during your communication and interactions with
the parents or caregivers. *Remember:* it is the law in every
state to report suspected child abuse to the appropriate child
protection agency.

Sexual abuse in children

Explain to the child during the interview that you are there
to listen. Convey interest, sincerity, and respect. Never interview the child in front of the possible abuser. Determine
and use the child's own terminology for describing body
parts. The following questions may help when interviewing
the child:

"Sometimes kids are asked to keep secrets. These secrets
can be scary. You are safe with me. Has this happened
to you? Can you tell me about the secret?"[4]

"Sometimes grownups do things to kids that hurt and are
scary. Has someone hurt you?"[4]

Assessment of the genitals and rectum should only be
done once, if at all possible, to prevent unnecessary psychologic trauma to the child. Thus the nurse and physician
should do this together. To examine the genitals, place the
child supine in the frogleg position. For anal examination,
place the child in the lateral decubitus position. To help
the child relax, a trusted family member, social worker, or
nurse should be at the head of the examining table to comfort the child. The child should not be restrained for this
part of the examination. If the child is very uncooperative,
the examination should be stopped and the child sedated
if necessary.

SYMPTOMS

- Symptoms include inflammation, redness, drainage, discharge, or bleeding from the genitals; lacerations, abrasions, or ecchymosis of the genitals; and tears, abrasions,
edema, or discharge of the anus.

NURSING ALERT

Victims of child abuse will often need to be seen in a pediatric or gynecology clinic that is capable of performing a col-
poscopy. A colposcope allows an examination of the external
genitalia as well as the vagina and cervix. Vascular changes,

Continued

NURSING ALERT—cont'd

scars, and variations are best noted with a colposcope.
However, this instrument does not eliminate the need for a
gross examination in the ED.

DIAGNOSIS
- Diagnosis is based on an examination and history
  obtained during the interview with the child (and
  parent).

TREATMENT
- Unless life-threatening bleeding is present, definite treatment may not be needed in the ED.
- Document the child's statements from the interview and
  any abnormal physical findings.
- It may be necessary to refer the child to a play
  therapist.
- Follow-up of culture results and treatment will be
  necessary.
- Report the suspected abuse to the appropriate child protection agency.

Battered women

A battered woman is 16 years of age or older and is physically, emotionally, or psychologically abused by a husband
or significant other.[4] Some characteristics often associated
with battered victims include the following:

1. Denial of battering because of fear or shame
2. Self-blame for what has happened
3. Feelings of confusion, depression, and low self-esteem
4. Reluctance to take action because of emotional and financial dependence on batterer or lack of emotional
   and financial resources
5. Reluctance to take action because of fear of retaliation
   by the abuser
6. A tendency to rationalize the incident because the batterer was intoxicated

The batterer will often accompany and stay with the victim to prevent her from reporting the abuse. Ask the accompanying spouse, mate, or friend to wait in the lobby.
Interview the woman in a place that affords privacy. Some
women will admit that a boyfriend or spouse beat them,
whereas others will not. Questioning should be conducted
in a supportive, nonjudgmental, and nonassuming man-

ner. The following questions may be helpful in eliciting a history:

"It seems that the injuries you have could have been caused by someone hurting or abusing you. Did someone hurt you?"[4]

"Sometimes when people come to the ED with physical symptoms like yours, we find that they are having some sort of trouble at home. I am concerned that someone is hurting you. Is this happening to you?"

See the "Injuries Commonly Seen in Battered Women" box.

SYMPTOMS
- Symptoms will be based on the injuries.

DIAGNOSIS
- Diagnosis is based on an examination and on a history obtained from the patient.

TREATMENT
- Perform a primary survey to identify all life-threatening injuries.

INJURIES COMMONLY SEEN IN BATTERED WOMEN

Alterations in skin integrity

- Burns resulting from:
  Splashes
  Friction (being dragged on the ground)
  Chemicals
  Cigarettes or cigars
- Knife wounds
- Scalp, facial lacerations
- Oral mucosa lacerations

Alterations in musculoskeletal system

- Facial or nose contusions or fractures
- Skull fractures
- Patterned bruises
- Torso injuries
- Breast contusions
- Fractured ribs
- Abdominal contusions (especially during pregnancy)
- Back or spine injuries

Continued

INJURIES COMMONLY SEEN
IN BATTERED WOMEN—cont'd

Neurologic impairment

- Altered consciousness from strangulation attempts
- Intracranial hemorrhage
- Postconcussion symptoms
- Visual impairment resulting from corneal abrasion or retinal detachment

Obstetric complications

- Miscarriages
- Abruptio placentae
- Premature uterine contractions
- Intrauterine fetal demise
- Low-birth-weight infant

- After intervening for any life-threatening conditions, perform a secondary survey to identify any other injuries.
- Assess the potential for homicide (see Chapter 3).
- Battered women may stay in an abusive relationship for many understandable reasons. Notify the appropriate adult protection agency according to your hospital policy and state laws.
- Document all injuries. Body maps may be helpful in delineating the locations and sizes of the injuries.
- Instruct and assist the woman in developing an emergency safety plan if she needs to leave the home immediately.
- Provide the woman with the phone number of the closest women's shelter.

Elder abuse

Elder abuse can include any of the following:

1. Physical abuse: The willful infliction of bodily harm onto a person 60 years of age or older by a spouse, child, family member, or primary caregiver; examples include pushing, kicking, hitting, slapping, punching, rough handling, inappropriate use of physical or chemical restraints, or sexual assault or rape
2. Psychologic and emotional abuse: Infliction of mental

anguish caused by actions or verbal assaults against the victim's well-being; examples include name-calling, insults, attacks on the victim's self-esteem, treating the victim as a child, threats of violence against the victim, controlling the victim's activities

3. Neglect: Passive or active withholding of services necessary to maintain the health and welfare of the victim; includes food, clothing, medications, basic hygiene, and health-related services

4. Exploitation: Improper use of the victim or the victim's resources by the caregiver for purpose of financial or material gains

Elder abuse rarely occurs in isolation or as a single incident. It is usually a recurring problem that may increase in frequency and severity over time. It will be necessary to interview the caregiver and the elder patient separately. Provide a private, quiet place for the interview. Listen carefully and convey a nonjudgmental, empathetic attitude. Ask open-ended questions. The following questions may be used as a guideline:

"We sometimes see people with injuries like yours. Sometimes they are the result of an argument. Has this happened to you?"

"Can you describe what happens when you and your family member (caregiver) argue or have problems? Do these behaviors include hitting or threats to harm you?"

"Have there been threats to abandon or confine you, or to withhold medicine or food from you?"

"Could you describe your routine day to me (activities, bathing, hygiene)?"

The following questions may be helpful in interviewing the caregiver:

"Caring for someone who is impaired as [the patient] is can be a very difficult task. It must be frustrating at times. How do you handle it?"

"Is it difficult to obtain the medications your [patient] needs?"

"Who is available to help you at home? Do you ever get a break to relax?"

"How do you cope with having to care for [the patient] all the time?"

"During the interview we noticed bruises on [the patient's] face and arms. Do you know how he (she)
got them?"

SYMPTOMS
• Symptoms depend on the injuries.

DIAGNOSIS
• Diagnosis is based on an examination and information
obtained from the history.

TREATMENT
• The treatment will depend on the specific injuries.
• Notify a social worker if possible. The social worker
may go into the home to assess the interactions and
environment.
• Carefully document information obtained from the interview and any physical findings.
• Provide the caregiver with information regarding community resources and support groups.

EXPECTED PATIENT OUTCOMES

1. Patent airway
2. Bilateral equal breath sounds
3. Heart rate of 60 to 100 beats/min (or age appropriate)
4. Systolic BP of >90 mm Hg (or age appropriate) or at
level needed to maintain adequate perfusion (see
Reference Guide 22 for vital signs in children)
5. Improvement or no further deterioration in neurologic
status
6. Open and effective communication between the patient
and nurse
7. Understanding of abuse and neglect as a crime against
the patient
8. Understanding and verbalization of community resources and support systems

DISCHARGE IMPLICATIONS

Child Abuse
1. Instruct the parent on alternative coping mechanisms to
deal with stress (e.g., leave the room immediately if
ready to hit the child, or phone a friend or relative).
2. Provide the parent with phone numbers of support
groups. These may be listed in local telephone books or
under city, county, or state information.

Battered Women

If a battered woman decides to return to the home, there are some things she can do to protect herself. Include these with the discharge instructions:

1. Have a room in the house that has a strong lock.
2. Keep a bag or suitcase packed.
3. Hide extra money, car keys, and important documents, such as the marriage license, Social Security card, and family birth certificates, in a safe, secure place so they can be obtained quickly.
4. Teach the children or encourage the neighbors to call the police during an attack.
5. Plan for a place to go in an emergency—a woman's shelter, a social agency, or the home of a trusted friend or relative.
6. When possible, call the police and get names and badge numbers of police officers in case there is need of a record of the attack.
7. Leave the house and take the children if an attack is imminent.
8. Go to a hospital or ask for medical attention when in a safe place. Usually domestic violence shelter programs will provide a staff member to accompany the at-risk individual to the hospital or ED. Sometimes women are hurt more seriously than they think during a physical assault.
9. Obtain and keep a record of any injuries, including photographs, to have the strongest possible case to press charges.

Even if the woman will not admit to being battered or abused, provide her with written information of spouse abuse centers and shelters in the area (when you suspect battering).

Elder Abuse

1. Community referrals are important with elder abuse. These referrals may include the department for social services, senior citizen centers, community mental health centers, long-term care ombudsmen, agencies on aging, and national committees dealing with elder abuse.
2. Instruct caregivers on alternative methods to cope with stress.

References

1. Campbell JC, Sheridan DJ: Emergency nursing interventions with battered women, *J Emerg Nurs* 14(1):12-17, 1989.
2. U.S. Department of Health and Human Services: *Elder abuse,* Washington DC, 1980, U.S. Government Printing Office.
3. Pollick MF: Abuse of the elderly: a review, *Holistic Nursing Practice* 1(2):43-53, 1987.
4. Sheridan D: Family violence. In Kitt S, Kaiser J, editors: *Emergency nursing: a physiologic and clinical perspective,* ed 2, Philadelphia, 1995, WB Saunders.
5. Fox G: Victims of abuse, *Nurs Times* 87(33):30-31, 1991.
6. Emergency Nurses Association: *Emergency nursing pediatric course manual,* ed 2, 1998, Park Ridge, Ill, The Association.
7. Kessler DB, Hyden P: Physical, sexual, and emotional abuse of children, *Clin Symp* 43(1):1-32, 1991.
8. Hauber DJ, Stokes JL: *Evidence collection handbook,* Frankfort, Ky, 1994, Kentucky State Police Laboratory.
9. Kelley SJ: Physical abuse of children: recognizing and reporting, *J Emerg Nurs* 14(2), 1988.

Chapter 3

Behavioral Conditions

B

Celeste Shawler

CLINICAL CONDITIONS
Violent Behavior Toward Others
Violent Behavior Toward Self
Victims of Abuse
Anxiety
Individuals in Crisis

TRIAGE ASSESSMENT
Violent Behavior
Assessment of patients with the risk for violence toward self or others requires knowledge of the dynamics of crises and expert interventions that will provide for a safe and therapeutic environment in the emergency department (ED). Staff awareness and preventive practices must be incorporated into the ED nurse's daily routine.[1,2] The manner in which the triage assessment is conducted is critical to the eliciting of accurate data to identify the risk for violence toward self or others.
Manner of speech
Talk in a slow, calm voice, and avoid argument or direct confrontation. *Remember:* The patient is probably in emotional disequilibrium and very anxious.
Agitated patient
If the patient is agitated, quickly get him or her into a less stimulating section of the ED and do not make him or her wait for treatment. Waiting greatly increases frustration and the potential for loss of control.
Topic of conversation
Pay attention to what the patient says and to how it is said.
Staff attitude
Be receptive to the patient. Demonstrate care and concern. Let the patient know immediately that you are concerned, that you are here to help, and that the ED is a safe place.

This will help to establish trust and credibility, which are stabilizing factors when interacting with those in crisis.

Staff protection

Use common sense and caution when interacting with someone who is violent toward others.[3] Allow space between yourself and the patient and do not attempt to control violent behavior by yourself.

Victims of Abuse
Domestic violence

Domestic violence should be considered a possibility when women seek treatment for either trauma or mental health problems.[4] As many as 30% of women who are seen in the ED exhibit one or more symptoms of physical abuse.[5]

Children

Children are frequently victims of abuse (see Focused Nursing Assessment).

Rape

Rape is a criminal offense. It is important to understand that there is a stigma attached to rape, and because of this the nurse should be extremely sensitive to the victim. Look for evidence indicating that force or coercion was used and that the sexual contact occurred against the victim's will.[6]

Anxiety

Most patients admitted to the ED will have some degree of anxiety. An understanding of the continuum of anxiety, from mild to moderate, severe, and panic, and the interventions appropriate to each level will be outlined.

General Observations

Focus on the following assessment areas.

Violent behavior toward others

- *Acting out behaviors:* Assess acting out behaviors (present and past).
- *Signs of potential violence:* Does the patient exhibit signs of alcohol or other drug use? If so, the risk for violence increases. Signs include pacing, violent gestures, a demanding attitude, profane and threatening verbal language, and the making of direct threats.
- *Reaction of patient to others:* Are there individuals present who calm or agitate the patient? If so, ask the one who calms the patient to remain with the patient and ask the others to remain at a distance from the patient.

- *Lethal weapons:* Are there lethal weapons in the possession of the patient or visitors? If so, follow your institution's policy for obtaining the harmful item(s).

Violent behavior toward self
- Does the patient have a suicide plan now?
- What is the history of suicide attempts?
- Are physical or psychiatric illnesses present?
- Has the patient experienced recent losses?
- What is the level and involvement of social support?
- Are alcohol or other drugs present?

Victims of abuse
- Assess specific injuries.
- Ask how and when any injuries occurred.
- Assess all physical complaints.
- Ask about stressors in the patient's life.
- Listen for consistency or lack of consistency in the patient's history. Lack of consistency may be because of high levels of anxiety.
- The patient should be interviewed alone.
- Begin to collect evidence as appropriate according to policy and law.

Behavior indicating emotional crises
Any patient admitted to the ED has the potential to be in any of the various stages of emotional crises.
- What recent stressful events have occurred in the life of this patient or family?[7]
- What has been the meaning of these events to the patient?
- Is there an actual or perceived threat to life?
- What is the medical emergency (e.g., overdose, drug reaction, or high-risk medical condition)?[8]
- Is there a psychiatric emergency?[8] Does the patient need seclusion, restraints, a crisis team, or security personnel?
- Assess the patient's ability to care for himself or herself.

Disordered thought processes
Patients may experience the following conditions, which are all indicative of disordered thought processes:
- Some individuals may be experiencing delusions or hallucinations and may have a diagnosis of schizophrenia.
- Some individuals may be severely depressed.
- Some individuals may be psychotic (out of touch with current reality).

FOCUSED NURSING ASSESSMENT
Violent Behavior
Nursing assessment should center on behaviors, cognitive abilities, thought processes, and the level of disequilibrium and disorganization.
Behaviors
- Describe the patient's present behavior (verbal and nonverbal).
- What is the patient's level of motor activity (especially if the patient is pacing)?
- What is the patient's physical appearance?
- How is the patient attired (e.g., appropriate for weather, or disheveled)?
- How much eye contact does the patient make?
- What is the patient's verbal presentation? How does the patient communicate and what is the content of the patient's speech (quality, quantity, and organization)?
- Describe the mood and emotions of the patient.
- If the patient has a suicide plan, are the means present (e.g., a knife or pills)? Is it a well-defined or a vague plan?
Thought processes and cognitive abilities
- How well is the patient oriented?
- How are the patient's perceptual abilities (e.g., hallucinations or illusions)?
- How much judgment and insight does the patient have? Does the patient understand the need for care?
- How good is the patient's memory?
- What are the patient's thought processes like (clarity, organization, symptoms)?
Level of disequilibrium and disorganization
- How have life changes and stressful events affected the patient's equilibrium?
- What is the patient's perception of these events?
- What situational support (or lack of support) does the patient have?
- What, if any, coping mechanisms has the patient used in the past and present?
- What was the triggering event, the "last straw" for the patient?
- How great is the patient's need for immediate attention?

B

Victims of Abuse
Types of injuries in domestic violence
- Bleeding injuries, especially to the head, face, breasts, abdomen, and chest
- Internal injuries, concussions, perforated eardrums, abdominal injuries, severe bruising, eye injuries, and strangulation marks on the neck
- Back injuries
- Fractured jaw, arms, pelvis, ribs, clavicles, and legs
- Burns from cigarettes, appliances, scalding liquids, and acids
- Psychologic trauma, anxiety, attacks of hyperventilation, heart palpitations, severe crying spells, and suicidal tendencies
- Miscarriages

Observe children for signs of stress caused by family violence. For example, children may exhibit emotional, behavioral, school, or sleep problems, or increased aggressive behavior.[9]

Physical symptoms indicating possible spouse abuse[9]
Chief complaints (without physical cause):
- Headache
- Abdominal pain
- Choking sensation
- Chest pain
- Back pain
- Dizziness
- "Accidents"

Presenting problems
The following are signs of high anxiety and chronic stress:
- Agitation
- Hyperventilation
- Panic attacks
- Gastrointestinal disturbances
- Hypertension
- Physical injuries
- Eating disorders
- Insomnia

Anxiety
Mild or normal anxiety
- Provides the energy to get on with tasks
- Growth-producing
- Constructive
- Necessary for survival

Moderate anxiety

- Anxiety narrows perceptual field
- Can pay attention when directed to do so

Severe anxiety

- High level of acute anxiety that occurs when stress is pervasive
- Perceptual field diminished to point where person can attend to only one specific detail
- Ability to solve problems very limited
- Efforts to relieve anxiety likely to be random and ineffective

Panic level of anxiety

- Most intense and pervasive level of anxiety
- Perceptual field so limited by anxiety that person is no longer able to process any outside stimuli from environment
- Anxiety likely to disorganize or immobilize the patient
- Panic not extending over long periods of time[10]

Risk Factors
Violent behavior

1. Individuals in possession of alcohol or other drugs
2. Individuals with history of agitated or disruptive behavior, especially under stress or in stressful times
3. Individuals with unstable relationships or lack of supportive relationships
4. Altered thought processes; psychotic symptoms such as delusions, paranoia, and hallucinations.
5. Situational or maturational crises with an already fragile homeostasis
6. Patients with a low tolerance for frustration and with poor impulse control[11]
7. Patients with seizure disorders (especially during postictal states), organic brain syndromes such as dementia, confusional states resulting from metabolic disorders, head trauma, drug toxicities, and drug withdrawal[11]
8. Adolescents with previous suicide attempts, early sexual behavior, substance abuse, trouble at school and with the law, depression,[12] social isolation, and impulsivity[13]

Victims of abuse

1. There is a history of violence and abuse. Violence is a learned behavior.
2. Men who abuse believe in being in control and dominant in the family, and abusing bolsters their low self-esteem.

3. Men who have extreme jealousy of their spouse are more likely to abuse.
4. Violence is more likely to occur when alcohol or other drugs are used. However, alcohol and drugs are an excuse for the abuse, not a cause.

Life Span Issues

1. The Centers for Disease Control and Prevention estimates that 300,000 high school students make a serious suicide attempt each year, resulting in 4000 ED visits. Follow-up studies suggest that 6% to 50% of these adolescents make another attempt and as many as 11% eventually take their own lives.[12,14]
2. Adolescents undergoing humiliating life experiences or having family conflict characterized by disruption and violence are at increased risk of suicidal behavior.[13]
3. Geriatric patients may need alternate assessment methods because of changes in hearing, speech, and mobility. Assess these patients for organic mental disorders and contributing medical problems.[8]
4. Pediatric patients need attention to family issues and developmental difficulties.[8] Offer interventions to change and improve the family functioning. Commend the family on any strengths noted, offer information about parenting and community resources, and encourage respite, support, and education for the parents.

INITIAL INTERVENTIONS

Violent Behavior Toward Others

Table 3-1 and the Priority Nursing Diagnoses and Interventions sections provide preventive measures and initial interventions related to violent behavior toward others.

1. Staff intervention should provide for the safety of the patient and others, using the least restrictive options possible.
2. Realize that physical aggression is an attempt to achieve security and control; thus, staff efforts to convey comfort, safety, and control reduce the risk of violence.
3. Talk with the patient calmly and respectfully, using short, concise explanations.
4. Allow the patient a lot of space, beware of touching the patient, and avoid physical entrapment of staff members. Focus on wanting to "help" or work with the patient.

Text continued on p. 158

TABLE 3-1 Care of the Violent Patient

Symptoms	Diagnosis	Treatment
No history of violence Basically satisfactory support system Social drinker only and is not drinking now May be slightly agitated or impatient but is able to be redirected	No predictable risk of violence	Use verbal interventions: 1. Talk with patient in calm, reassuring manner 2. Ask patient to sit in less stimulating environment 3. Ask family, friends with stabilizing influence to stay with patient, those who provoke to stay away 4. Encourage expression of anger verbally vs. acting out; give positive feedback for appropriate verbal expressions of anger 5. Offer choices to patient when possible

Has occasional ideation of assault and violence (including paranoid ideas) No history of assault or impulsive acting out Occasional drinking bouts and angry verbal outbursts Basically satisfactory support system No alcohol or drugs are present May be slightly agitated and verbalizing feeling out of control but able to be redirected	Low risk of violence	Use verbal interventions 1-5 above

Data from Cahill CD, et al: *Iss Mental Health Nurs* 12(3):139-252, 1991; Carpenito LD: *Handbook of nursing diagnosis*, ed 4, Philadelphia, 1991, JB Lippincott; Green E: *J Emerg Nurs* 15(6):523-527, 1989; Hoff LA: *People in crisis: understanding and helping*, ed 3, Redwood City, 1989, Addison-Wesley; Kurlowicz L: *Am J Nurs* 90(9), 1990; Martin L et al: *J Emerg Nurs* 17(6):395-401, 1991.

Continued

TABLE 3-1 Care of the Violent Patient—cont'd

Symptoms	Diagnosis	Treatment
Has frequent ideation of assault and violence but no specific plan Has history of impulsive acting out and verbal outburst while drinking or using other drugs Stormy relationships with periodic high-tension arguments Increased agitation (e.g., pacing, fist clenching, intensified facial expressions, raised voice, shouting) Can be directed by an individual staff member or a group of staff	Moderate risk of violence	Use 1-5 above, plus the following as needed: 6. Search for, remove harmful objects from patient's room 7. PRN medication may be indicated to decrease agitation, potential for violence 8. Redirect patient with group of staff "verbal show of concern" if an individual cannot redirect the patient

Has plan for violence now

Has history of frequent acting out against others

Has used drugs or ETOH frequently and to excess

Has indicators of drugs or ETOH use on board

May have paranoia or hallucination

Stormy relationships with much verbal fighting and occasional assaults

Rule out organic etiology (e.g., basilar skull fracture)

Body: Pacing, violent gestures

Verbal: Demanding, abusive, profane, threatening violence

May or may not be able to be redirected by a group of staff

High risk of violence

Use 1-8 above.

9. Anticipate, have ready group of staff to provide verbal external control

10. Physical control if patient unable to be redirected and patient progresses to an extremely high risk of violence; proceed immediately with next level of treatment (see below)

Data from Cahill CD, et al: *Iss Mental Health Nurs* 12(3):139-252, 1991; Carpenito LD: *Handbook of nursing diagnosis*, ed 4, Philadelphia, 1991, JB Lippincott; Green E: *J Emerg Nurs* 15(6):523-527, 1989; Hoff LA: *People in crisis: understanding and helping*, ed 3, Redwood City, 1989, Addison-Wesley; Kurlowicz L: *Am J Nurs* 90(9), 1990; Martin L et al: *J Emerg Nurs* 17(6):395-401, 1991.

Continued

TABLE 3-1 Care of the Violent Patient—cont'd

Symptoms	Diagnosis	Treatment
Has current highly lethal plan	Extremely high risk of violence	1. Psychiatric emergency: Requires immediate physical control to prevent harm to self and others
Has history of homicide attempts or impulsive acting out and strong urge to control and "get even" with someone		2. Team effort to provide external physical control for patient
History of excessive and continual use of drugs and/or ETOH		3. "Assistance Please" code
Very likely intoxicated		4. Team leader tells patient what team is going to do
May have paranoia or hallucinations		5. Five staff (one for each limb and one to protect patient's head)
Rule out organic etiology (e.g., basilar skull fracture)		6. Four-point restraint (see institution's policy); patient very vulnerable and requires constant observation
May arrive to ED in four-point restraints or actively threatening with violent gestures and/or weapon		
Verbal: Demanding, abrasive, profane		

- Apply restraints securely but not tight enough to interfere with circulation or respiration
- Tie to bed frame, not rails
- Hourly respiration and circulation checks
- Elevate head of bed slightly (if not contraindicated) to prevent aspiration
- Constant observation

7. PRN medications for safety and patient's comfort
8. If patient threatening with weapon, notify security stat

Data from Cahill CD, et al: *Iss Mental Health Nurs* 12(3):139-252, 1991; Carpenito LD: *Handbook of nursing diagnosis*, ed 4, Philadelphia, 1991, JB Lippincott; Green E: *J Emerg Nurs* 15(6):523-527, 1989; Hoff LA: *People in crisis: understanding and helping*, ed 3, Redwood City, 1989, Addison-Wesley; Kurlowicz L: *Am J Nurs* 90(9), 1990; Martin L et al: *J Emerg Nurs* 17(6):395-401, 1991.

5. Do not wear loose or dangling jewelry or a stethoscope around your neck.
6. Do not have pockets full of scissors, clamps, or other items that are potential weapons against you.
7. Respect the personal space of the patient.
8. Position yourself with the patient so that no obstacles exist between you and an exit.
9. Stand at about a 45-degree angle to the patient and maintain good eye contact.[1]
10. Attempt to control the factors in the environment that encourage development of previolent aggression (e.g., long waits, delays, or a stimulating environment).[15]
11. Use verbal strategies to deescalate the aggressive patient (e.g., acknowledge the patient's anger). Say, "We are not going to let you hurt yourself or others."
12. Implement teamwork with verbal strategies. A "show of concern" is a group of staff together with just one person talking to the patient.
13. Implement teamwork with physical control.[16]
14. Initiate specific strategies (e.g., IV sedation or a neuromuscular blocking agents after restraining patient) when a patient is out of control and physical danger to the staff is imminent.
15. Know your institution's policies and procedures for crises, such as a panic button or notification of the security department, police, or the crisis team.

Violent Behavior Toward Self

See the Priority Nursing Diagnoses and Interventions sections.

1. Get an oral contract from the patient stipulating that the patient agrees not to leave the ED.
2. Try to get a "no harm contract" from the patient. The patient is asked to articulate intentions regarding harm to himself or herself. Whether a patient has the ability to make this agreement affects the assessment of acuity and interventions needed.
3. All safety measures are to be carried out in a respectful, informative manner to minimize patients' and visitors' potential discomfort.
4. Prepare the patient's room so that it is as free as possible of harmful objects. Arrange to have one or two rooms designated as "safe" or have a plan to make a room "safe" by rolling out carts, locking cabinets, etc.

5. Inform the patient of and explain the rationale for safety procedures.
6. Remove dangerous objects (e.g., pills or weapons) from the patient.
7. Put the patient in hospital clothing to assess potential harmful objects or drugs hidden in the patient's own clothing and to help ensure that the patient remains in the ED. Pay attention to the removal of clothes if the patient is paranoid or if self-esteem and privacy are threatened and the patient begins to decompensate even more than in the current state.

Victims of Abuse
See Chapter 2.
1. Provide a safe environment by allowing for privacy.
2. Acknowledge the patient's fears and reassure the patient about his or her present safety.
3. Establish yourself and the ED as reliable, caring, and concerned.
4. Assess your own responses to human abuse, so that your own values and perceptions do not impede you in caring for the victims.
5. Be aware of your institution's policies and procedures and of state laws regarding documentation of injuries and collection of evidence.
6. For rape victims or other victims in psychologic crises, you may need to call psychiatric staff.
7. Call the rape crisis center for volunteers and information for follow-up care.
8. Report abuse to the appropriate authorities in the institution and the state.

Anxiety
1. Maintain a calm, nonthreatening manner.
2. Reassure the patient of his or her safety and security.
3. Use simple, brief messages.
4. Try to get the patient into a low-stimulation environment.
5. Pay attention to anything that causes fear in the patient.

Individuals in Crisis
1. Reduce the sensory stimuli in the environment.
2. In acute crises the patient is often quite anxious, so di-

rect questions to help the patient define the sequence and significance of events.

3. Offer reflective, acknowledging statements such as, "I can imagine with all the confusion and stress you have described, you feel quite overwhelmed."

4. Work toward finding something that will give immediate relief in at least one aspect of the patient's crisis[17] (e.g., child care, specific resources to attend to patient and family needs, or a voucher for some medications).

Disordered Thought Processes

Psychosis, schizophrenia, and major depression are characterized by major disturbances in thought processes. The patient may have a variety of symptoms, from simple thinking to bizarre thinking. The individual is at increased risk for harm to self because of the inability to attend to self-needs.

1. Generally, a firm, consistent, gentle approach is most effective.

2. Give clear, brief directions.

3. Do not argue with the patient about hallucinations or delusions—refer to "the voices." For example, "I believe you when you tell me you hear. . . . The voices must be troubling you. . . . We are here in the ED to help you. You are safe here."

4. Offer food, fluids, and other comfort measures.

PRIORITY NURSING DIAGNOSES

Risk for violence directed at others
Risk for self-directed violence
Risk for self-care deficit
Risk for alteration in thought processes
Risk for ineffective individual coping
Risk for anxiety

◆ **Violence directed at others** related to self-concept, biochemical alterations, alterations in thought process, impairment of ability to control impulses, and uncontrolled anger:

INTERVENTIONS
- Maintain a low level of stimuli.
- Observe the patient's behavior frequently (q15min) so that interventions can be implemented as required.

- Place the patient in a safe area.
- Remove all dangerous objects from the environment.
- Respond matter-of-factly to verbal hostility and avoid arguing.
- Convey a calm attitude.
- Have sufficient staff to indicate a "show of concern," if necessary.
- Administer tranquilizing medications prn.
- Observe the effectiveness and side effects of medications.
- If the patient is in physical restraints, the patient is highly vulnerable and needs constant observation.
- As agitation decreases, assess the patient's readiness for restraint removal.

◆ **Self-directed violence** related to depression, hopelessness, misinterpretation of reality, feelings of worthlessness, and unresolved grief:

INTERVENTIONS

- Ask the patient directly, "Have you thought about killing yourself? Do you have a plan? Do you have the means to do this?"
- Ask for specifics of the plan.
- Initiate a "no harm" contract, a short-term oral contract with the patient that he or she will not harm himself or herself during a specific time frame.
- If the patient is unable to make a contract, increase the level of observation and increase protection in the environment.
- Initiate frequent speaking contact with the patient (q15min).
- Maintain the patient in view of the staff and in a safe environment.
- Remove any potentially harmful objects from the patient and environment.
- Therapeutic interactions indicate that the patient is learning ways to deal with problems other than harming himself or herself.

◆ **Self-care deficit** related to perceptual or cognitive impairment:

INTERVENTIONS

- Offer nutritious snacks and fluids.
- Assist the patient to the bathroom hourly or as needed.
- If the patient is paranoid about food, give the food in the unopened container and let the patient open it.

- Ensure that the patient has appropriate clothing for weather conditions.
- Assist the patient with personal hygiene if needed.

◆ **Alteration in thought processes** related to impaired cognition or biochemical alterations:

INTERVENTIONS
- Accept the content of the patient's altered thinking.
- Do not reinforce the altered thinking. Use "the voices" instead of words like "they."
- Orient the patient to reality (e.g., "Even though I realize the voices are real to you, I do not hear any voices speaking").
- Reassure the patient that he or she is safe.
- Try to recognize persons in the patient's network whom he or she knows and can call, and who may calm and reassure the patient. Sometimes a familiar voice, even on the phone, can calm the patient and help him or her reestablish some sense of control and balance.

◆ **Ineffective individual coping** related to a poor support system, poor problem solving, and a lack of prior experience in dealing with similar crises:

INTERVENTIONS
- Recognize that the behavior is purposeful and attempt to reduce the patient's anxiety and insecurity.
- Help the patient identify his or her own strengths and resources and those in the community.

◆ **Anxiety (panic)** related to situational and maturational crises, threats to self-concept, and the threat of death:

INTERVENTIONS
- Maintain a calm, nonthreatening manner.
- Reassure the patient of his or her safety and security.
- Use simple words and brief messages.
- Keep stimuli in immediate surroundings reduced.
- Administer tranquilizing medications as ordered.

PRIORITY DIAGNOSTIC TESTS

Serum toxicology screening
Electrolyte levels
Blood ethanol levels
Urinalysis and urine drug screen
CT scan (e.g., to rule out tumors, space-occupying lesions, and aneurysms).
ED protocol for physical injury and evidence should be followed.

COLLABORATIVE INTERVENTIONS

Overview

In general, a crisis may occur when there have been stressors (e.g., situational, maturational, or social) that exceed the coping abilities of the individual, family, or community. The coping strategies that are usually effective fail to maintain the balance for those involved. The resulting disorganization, anxiety, and preoccupation with the difficulty often overwhelm those involved, and many may seek the services of the ED.

Likewise, the ED is a place where a variety of crises are treated. Traumatic injuries, abuse, and suicide attempts after losses are some examples of crises treated in the ED. Any individual with a perceived life-altering or life-threatening occurrence may be in a high to a panic state of anxiety, and nursing interventions should reflect an understanding of this. Because anxiety is contagious, the nurse should try to maintain a calm, nonthreatening manner when working with a patient in crisis so that the patient's feeling of security will be enhanced.

Clinical Conditions
Violent behavior toward others

Prevention measures are critical in the ED. The symptoms, diagnoses, and treatment of violent behavior are listed in order of acuity. Interventions for the protection of the patient are listed from least restrictive to most restrictive.

A designated safe, quiet area or room for psychiatric emergencies is needed.[1,2] Staff must have education and practice in the use of verbal strategies to deescalate patients, the use of nonviolent physical control techniques, and the use of restraints. Available hospital staff and security should also be part of the ED resources. Teamwork is important.

The importance of teaching and coaching the staff to be respectful of the patient's dignity regardless of exhibited behavior cannot be emphasized enough. Hunt[18] emphasizes that it is important for the ED nurse to realize that the patient is in the midst of a psychiatric emergency and that the patient needs to be reassured and checked frequently. She also emphasizes the importance of using knowledgeable, sensitive nursing interventions and states, "I'd like to think if I or a friend or family member were in the ED, the nurse would . . . offer me a warm blanket, even though I am yelling and agitated, because you notice I am shivering."

The ED environment must be carefully monitored to prevent escalation of anxious, agitated persons. For example, long delays in treatment and an overstimulating environment, for someone who has low impulse control or who is anxious and agitated, automatically increase the person's acuity and increase the chance that a psychiatric emergency will occur.

Table 3-1 outlines the symptoms, diagnoses, and treatments of the patient with behavior that is violent toward others. The table goes from low acuity and least restricted environment to high acuity and most protective environment.

Violent behavior toward self

For specific drug overdoses, see Chapter 19. Table 3-2 outlines the symptoms, diagnoses, and treatment of the patient with violent behavior toward self. The symptoms, diagnoses, and treatment of suicidal behavior are listed in order of acuity from least restrictive to most protective. Interventions for the safety of the patient are listed in the following table.

Victims of abuse

(See Chapter 2.)

Rape

- Do not leave the person alone.
- Maintain nonjudgmental care.
- Maximize emotional support, stay with the victim, show concern for the victim's needs, and encourage problem solving whenever possible.
- Ensure confidentiality.
- Encourage the victim to talk.
- Engage a support system (family and friends) when appropriate.[19]
- Obtain proof of force, including the following:
  1. Written descriptions and pictures of physical injuries
  2. Documented direct quotes
- Obtain information for identifying the assailant, including the following:
  1. Sperm and seminal fluid specimens from which DNA markers can be drawn
  2. Head hair or pubic hair of the assailant, found on the victim
- Proof of sexual contact includes the following:

TABLE 3-2 Care of the Suicidal Patient

Symptoms	Diagnosis	Treatment
No notion of suicide No history of attempts Has satisfactory social supports Close contact with significant others Engages in appropriate conversation Vague feelings of depression and helplessness No alcohol or drug problems EMV: 15 on the Glasgow Coma Scale	No predictable risk of immediate suicide	Verbally contract with patient not to leave ED, record contract If patient leaves, give information for follow-up Assign patient to designated safe room where visible to staff Treat presenting complaint If possible, make follow-up appointment Discharge instructions to include resources for follow-up
Has considered low-lethality methods of suicide No history of attempts No recent or serious losses Has satisfactory support network No withdrawal from social contacts	Low risk of immediate suicide	Contract with patient not to leave ED and not to harm self; record contract Accompanied by family or friend who agrees not to let patient leave If patient leaves, give information for follow-up

From Bradley V, Shawler C: *J Emerg Nurs* 19(5):393-395, 1993.

Continued

B

TABLE 3-2 Care of the Suicidal Patient—cont'd

Symptoms	Diagnosis	Treatment
May be mildly depressed No alcohol or drug problems Basically wants to live EMS: 15 on Glasgow Coma Scale		Assign patient to room where visible to staff Check patient hourly in waiting room or in treatment area and record hourly check If discharged, make follow-up appointment
Has considered suicide with moderately to highly lethal method No specific plan or has plan with low-lethal method History of low-lethal methods Some changes or losses Few or only one significant other(s) Some feelings of helplessness, hopelessness, and withdrawal Moderate amount of depression Depends on ETOH or other drugs for stress relief Weighing the odds between life and death—may give no-harm contract None to some disorientation or disorganization, confusion, or anxiety	Moderate risk of immediate suicide	Contract that patient will not leave or harm self, record contract Accompanied by friend or family member who agrees not to let leave 30-min checks by hospital staff while patient in lobby or family room If unable to do 30-min checks, take patient to treatment area Assign patient to safe room Continue 30-min checks Offer something to eat or drink Anticipate laboratory studies: ETOH and toxicity Anticipate psychiatric consult If discharged, make follow-up appointment

	High risk of immediate suicide	Triage nurse takes patient to safe room
Has current high-lethality plan, obtainable means		Register in back
History of attempts with moderate to high lethality		One-to-one with hospital staff
Some losses recently		Contract with patient for no self-harm if possible
Only one or no significant other(s)		Offer something to eat or drink
Unable to communicate with significant other		Anticipate laboratory studies: ETOH and toxicology
Withdrawal		Anticipate psychiatric consult
Moderate to high level of depression		
Has used drugs or ETOH to excess		
Depressed and wants to die—may not give no-harm contract		
Some to moderate disorientation, disorganization, confusion, disturbed thought process, or appears anxious		

From Bradley V, Shawler C: *J Emerg Nurs* 19(5):393-395, 1993.

Continued

TABLE 3-2 Care of the Suicidal Patient—cont'd

Symptoms	Diagnosis	Treatment
Has current high-lethality plan with available means	Very high risk of immediate suicide	Triage nurse takes patient to treatment area or requests assistance as needed
History of attempts with high lethality		Register in back
Significant losses or changes		One-to-one with hospital staff
Cut off from resources or significant others		STAT call to psychiatric consult team
Psychosis with command hallucinations (e.g. "The voices tell me to hurt myself")		Offer something to eat or drink
Severe depression		Anticipate laboratory studies: ETOH and toxicology
Uses ETOH and other drugs continually and to excess		Psychiatric consult
Wants to die		
Probably will not give no self-harm contract		
Marked disorientation, disorganization, confusion, or appearance of anxiety		
Severely disturbed thought processes		

From Bradley V, Shawler C: *J Emerg Nurs* 19(5):393-395, 1993.

1. Presence of motile or nonmotile sperm on or in the victim
2. Presence of acid phosphatase in vaginal fluid (highly suggestive of recent sexual contact because it is in high concentrations in seminal fluid and all but absent in vaginal fluids)[15]

Domestic violence
Women

1. Reassure the victim of her present safety.
2. Allow an open, accepting interview so the patient feels more comfortable talking.
3. Reassure the victim that intrafamily violence is not OK, and encourage treatment.
4. Offer treatment possibilities (e.g., information about shelters, counseling for the victim, and community liaisons as supports to women).

Children

1. Collect and document data indicating abuse.
2. Report to the appropriate institutional and state authorities.
3. Discuss parenting challenges and suggest supports for the parents.
4. Seek ways to meet the needs of parents so that they may better parent.

Anxiety

1. Identify the severity of the anxiety.
2. Panic requires immediate intervention as follows:
   - Remain with the patient.
   - Maintain a calm manner.
   - Use short, simple sentences.
   - Minimize environmental stimuli.
   - Suggest an antianxiety medication to relieve the panic anxiety level.
3. Interventions for moderate to severe anxiety are as follows:
   - Walking or other use of large muscle groups
   - Relaxation exercise with deep breathing and tensing and relaxing muscle groups (with direction from nurse)
   - Reducing external stimuli (e.g., sound, color, and people) but not isolating patient[10]

Individuals in crisis

The patients with mental health disturbances who enter the ED are in various states of disequilibrium and dysfunction. Indeed, if one uses a holistic view of patients, any insult to the patient's system has the potential to cause psychologic disequilibrium and dysfunction. Thus all patients admitted to the ED need assessment of and intervention for psychologic and psychosocial stressors.

Recognition and prevention strategies for potential crises can greatly enhance the functioning of patients and families. A model that focuses on crisis intervention and the problem-solving approach is illustrated in Figure 3-1. This model views human beings as being in a state of equilibrium until a stressful event occurs. The stressful event causes disequilibrium. For the problem to be resolved, the balancing factors must be present. If one or more of the balancing factors are absent, disequilibrium increases and the likelihood of crisis increases.

The first step in the nursing process is an assessment of the problem using this model as a guide.

1. Assessing the meaning of the problem (sample questions):
   • How does this problem affect your life now?
   • How do you see this problem affecting your future?
   • Are others around you affected by this problem?
   • What does this problem mean to you and your life?
2. Assessing situational supports (sample questions):
   • With whom do you live?
   • Is there someone you are close to?
   • Do you have family or friends available to you?
   • Whom do you trust?
   • Are you involved with a church?
   • Are you involved in any community activities?
3. Assessing coping skills (sample questions):
   • How do you usually cope with stress?
   • Can you do that now?
   • Is it working or not?
   • Has anything like this ever happened before?
   • What else do you think might help you now?

REMEMBER: All questions may not be appropriate for every patient, and other questions may be helpful in assessing the balancing factors.

This assessment helps with 1) the prevention of potential crises and 2) interventions at various levels of disequilibrium.

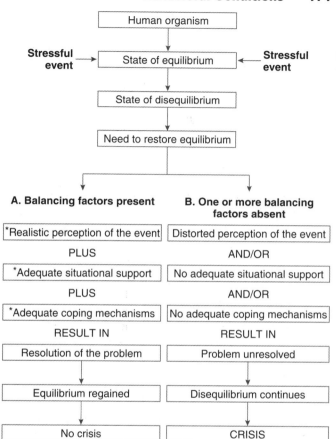

Figure 3-1 Paradigm: the effect of balancing factors in a stressful event. (From Aguilera D, Messick J: *Crisis intervention theory and intervention,* ed 6, St Louis, 1989, Mosby.)

Prevention of crises: maintaining balancing factors
SYMPTOMS
- The patient is experiencing situational stressor(s) such as chronic or acute physical illnesses, relocation, or others.
- The patient is experiencing maturational and developmental events such as pregnancy, divorce, the death of a family member or friend, a new marriage or relationship, or a change in job or economic status.

DIAGNOSIS
- The patient and family are in severe stress and are effectively coping, but a crisis may be imminent.
- Watch and listen for cues indicating that the ability to cope is waning, such as the following:
  "I'm hanging in there, but I'm not sure how much longer I can do this."
  "My friends are helping me with all that's going on in my life, but they are getting tired too."
  "Even the little things take a lot of my energy."

TREATMENT
- Assist the patient and family in recognizing their strengths.
- Look for ways to expand the support network.
- Find interventions that give immediate relief to one or more areas of the patient's life.
- Recommend education options (e.g., premarital counseling, prenatal classes, support groups, or community support).
- Help to normalize thoughts and feelings related to distress.
- Help patients to pace themselves and delegate or delete unnecessary activities and expectations.

Disequilibrium continues: restoring balancing factors
SYMPTOMS
- The patient feels anxious and helpless.
- Distress and crisis is perceived as overwhelming.
- The patient is disorganized and unable to plan, reason, or comprehend and engages in frenzied activity.
- The patient has acute somatic complaints (e.g., shortness of breath, GI disturbances, and fatigue).
- The patient's attempts to use the usual coping mechanisms fail.
- Coping mechanisms offer minimal and brief relief.

DIAGNOSIS
- The patient is at the beginning of crisis.
- Balancing factors are not maintained.
- Disequilibrium is evident.

TREATMENT
- Listen actively and with concern.
- Help the patient understand the crisis and that he or she is getting help and support now.
- Use the strategies listed in "Prevention" with consideration that anxiety is higher and cognitive functioning is decreased.
- Explore additional supports.
- Assist the patient with expanding his or her coping mechanisms.

Crisis apparent: emergency situation

SYMPTOMS
- The patient is feeling increasingly tense, anxious, helpless, and panicky.
- The patient may engage in "wishful thinking" and denial, hoping to get relief.
- The patient is using more unusual or primitive coping mechanisms in a hit or miss manner.
- The patient's behavior and problem solving are increasingly disorganized.
- The patient's thoughts are severely to completely disorganized.
- The patient's coping efforts continue to fail.

DIAGNOSIS
- This is an emergency: crisis is evident.

TREATMENT
- The patient needs immediate help and interventions to restore equilibrium.
- The interventions are short term and focus on solving the immediate problem.
- The patient may need a protective environment (e.g., hospitalization, a designated stable and safe environment with family or significant others, frequent follow-up with home care, or clinical appointments).

NURSING SURVEILLANCE

1. Monitor behaviors.
2. Monitor the trend of behaviors, environmental factors

affecting the patient's behavior, and various intervention strategies.
3. Assess biochemical imbalances and overdoses.
4. Recheck restraints:
    • Monitor the patient hourly.
    • Evaluate the range of motion to all extremities at least every 4 hours by releasing one restraint at a time.
    • Maintain skin care during every shift.
    • Maintain appropriate documentation (reason for restraint and restraint checks).
    • Attempt a trial release from the restraints if the patient's behavior indicates that this is safe.
5. Reevaluate the patient's risks of harm to himself or herself or others.
6. Evaluate the patient's response to medications and other interventions.
7. Assess the patient's level of consciousness.
8. Monitor the patient's vital signs as indicated.

EXPECTED PATIENT OUTCOMES

1. There is no evidence of violent behavior by the patient toward himself or herself or others.
2. The patient makes no further suicide attempts during the ED stay.
3. The patient is able to name resources outside the hospital to use if he or she is feeling suicidal.
4. The patient is able to control impulses to prevent acts of violence against himself or herself or others with assistance from caregivers (family if discharged home, hospital staff if hospitalized).[20]
5. The patient articulates feelings of increased self-worth.[21]
6. The patient can state some areas of his or her own strengths and weaknesses.
7. With assistance from caregivers, the patient can distinguish between reality-based and non–reality-based thinking.[20]
8. The patient is able to maintain anxiety at a level where he or she can problem solve and function in daily living.[20]
9. The patient is able to verbalize signs and symptoms of escalating anxiety and techniques for interrupting progression of the anxiety.

TABLE 3-3 Drug Summary

Drug	Dose/Route	Special considerations
Haloperidol	3-5 mg bid/tid PO (adults)	Management of acute and chronic psychoses, agitated behavior
	2-5 mg q4-8hr IM (adults)	More severe symptoms of agitated behavior; may be administered as often as every 60 min depending on response
	0.05-0.15 mg/kg/day PO (child)	—
Chlordiazepoxide (Librium)	25-50 mg initial dose then q1-2hr IM (adult)	Minor tranquilizer or antianxiety agent
Diazepam (Valium)	5-10 mg 1-2 hr up to 40 mg/day IM (adult)	Minor tranquilizer or antianxiety agent
Oxazepam (Serax)	10-30 mg up to 120 mg/day PO (adult)	Effective with anxiety, tension, agitation, irritability, anxiety associated with depression
Tricyclics		
Amitriptyline (Elavil, Endep)	75-200 mg/day; some patients may require as much as 300 mg/day PO (adult)	Major depression associated with organic disease, schizophrenia, or alcoholism Contraindicated with MAOIs and antiarrhythmics

Continued

B

TABLE 3-3 Drug Summary—cont'd

Drug	Dose/Route	Special considerations
Imipramine (Tofranil, Janimine)	100-150 mg/day; after 2 weeks and symptomatic relief not achieved, may increase to 250-300 mg/day PO (adult)	Major depression associated with organic disease, schizophrenia, or alcoholism Contraindicated with MAOIs and antiarrhythmics
	30-40 mg/day. Rarely exceed 100 mg/day PO (adolescent, geriatrics)	—
Monoamine oxidase inhibitors (MAOIs)		
Phenelzine (Nardil)	45-90 mg/day PO (adult)	Depression Contraindicated in hypersensitivity to MAOIs, geriatric, hypertension, severe hepatic, cardiac, or renal disease
Tranylcypromine (Parnate)	20-60 mg/day PO (adult)	—

Serotonin reuptake inhibitors (SSRIs)

Fluoxetine (Prozac)	10-40 mg PO (adult) Initial dose 20 mg/day in AM Dosage may be increased after several weeks if no clinical improvement Doses above 20 mg/day should be bid; maximum dose 80 mg/day	Major depression Contraindicated with MAOIs
Sertraline (Zoloft)	50-200 mg/day PO (adult)	Major depression Not to be used within 14 days of MAOI Use with caution with renal or hepatic impairment

10. Victims of abuse are able to make changes and take necessary actions to protect themselves and eliminate violence in their lives.[4]

DISCHARGE IMPLICATIONS

1. Teach the patient and family or significant others about the need for follow-up treatments.
2. Provide the patient with information about community resources.
3. Instruct the family or significant others in recognizing signs of increased anxiety and agitation, in strategies to decrease anxiety and agitation, and in when to seek treatment at the ED or other facilities.
4. Evaluate the need for psychiatric nursing-home care.
5. Make appointments for follow-up counseling.

References

1. Glasson L: The care of psychiatric patients in the emergency department: preparation, staff awareness, preventive practices, and the psychiatric patient, *J Emerg Nurs* 19(5):385-391, 1993.
2. Glasson L: RAP-DEE-responding to disruptive/violent behavior in the emergency department, *J Healthc Prot Manage* 1(2):112-114, 1992.
3. Kurlowicz L: Violence in the emergency department, *Am J Nurs* 90(9):35-40, 1990.
4. Hadley S: Clinical articles: working with battered women in the emergency department: a model program, *J Emerg Nurs* 18(1):18-23, 1992.
5. Henry SL, Roth M, Gleis LH: Domestic violence—the medical community's legal duty, *KMA Journal* 90(4):162-169, 1992.
6. Ledray LE: The sexual assault examination: overview and lessons learned in one program, *J Emerg Nurs* 18(3):223-230, 1992.
7. Hoff LA: *People in crisis: understanding and helping,* ed 3, Redwood City, Calif, 1989, Addison-Wesley.
8. Talley S, King MD: *Psychiatric emergencies: nursing assessment and intervention,* New York, 1984, Macmillan.
9. Swanson RW: Battered wife syndrome, *CMAJ* 130:709, 1984.
10. Haber J et al: *Comprehensive psychiatric nursing,* ed 2, New York, 1982, McGraw-Hill.
11. Cahill CD et al: Inpatient management of violent behavior: nursing prevention and intervention, *Issues Ment Health Nurs* 12(3):139-252, 1991.
12. Piacentini J: Pediatric update: evaluating adolescent suicide attempters: what emergency nurses need to know, *J Emerg Nurs* 19(5):465-466, 1993.

13. Srnec P: Children, violence, and intentional injuries, *Crit Care Nurs Clin North Am* 3(3):471-478, 1991.
14. Kalogerakis MG: Emergency evaluation of adolescents, *Hosp Community Psychiatry* 43(6):617-621, 1992.
15. Lavoie FW et al: Emergency department violence in United States teaching hospitals, *Ann Emerg Med* 17(11):12-27, 33, 1988.
16. Morton PG: Managing assault, *Am J Nurs* 86(10):1114-1116, 1986.
17. Kercher EE: Crisis intervention in the emergency department, *Psychiat Aspects Emerg Med* 9(1):219-232, 1991.
18. Hunt E: Guest editorial: on avoiding "psych" patients, *J Emerg Nurs* 19(5):375-376, 1993.
19. Burgess A, Holstrom L: *Rape: victims of crisis,* Bowie, Md, 1975, Prentice Hall.
20. Townsend MA: *Nursing diagnoses in psychiatric nursing,* Philadelphia, 1988, FA Davis.
21. Perrin KO, Williams-Burgess C: The suicidal patient in the CCU: nursing approaches, *Crit Care Nurse* 10(7):59-64, 1990.

B

Chapter 4

Burns

Julia Fultz
Marci Messer

CLINICAL CONDITIONS
Thermal Burns
Inhalation Injury
   Carbon Monoxide Poisoning
   Upper Airway Injury
   Lower Airway Injury
Electrical Burns
Chemical Burns

Patients with burn injuries are considered multiple trauma patients because of the physiologic effect of the burn on organ systems. In addition to the burn injury, patients often have traumatic injuries. The goals of burn management in the emergency department (ED) are to stop the burning process, maintain the airway, breathing, and circulation (ABCs), preserve viable tissue, and prevent infection.

TRIAGE ASSESSMENT

The first priority of care with the burn patient is to eliminate the source of the heat if it is still present. Clothing and jewelry that are producing heat must be removed, and any chemicals in the form of a dry powder should be brushed off the skin. Protective gear must be worn to protect the caregiver from the chemicals, and care must be taken to prevent contamination of the ED if the patient has been exposed to a hazardous material (e.g., phosphorus, ammonium, or hydrofluoric acid). Once the source of the burning has been eliminated, caregiver attention turns to ABCs.

NURSING ALERT

Protective gear (gloves, face shield, and clothing) must be donned to prevent the accidental contamination of the caregiver. Employer hazardous material policy and procedure must be followed. If the clothing is contaminated, it must be placed in an isolation bag.

The burned areas should be cooled with tepid water as soon as possible. Chemical burns must be flushed immediately with copious amounts of water for 20 to 30 minutes or until the burning sensation and pain subside. Chemical injuries to the eye require immediate eye irrigation with 1 to 2 liters of normal saline or Ringer's lactate. Tar, plastic, or asphalt should be left in place and flushed with water until it has solidified and cooled. Clothing adhered to the skin should be left in place. Trying to remove the substance or clothing may result in increased tissue damage.

General Observations

- Ensure that the burning process has been stopped.
- Ensure that ABCs are intact.
- Patients with the potential for ABCs problems and patients with anything other than minor superficial burns should be directly admitted to the treatment area. Patients with what appear to be "minor burns" may also be admitted to the treatment area for pain relief measures if necessary.
- Assuming that lifesaving interventions are not necessary, elicit the following data from the patient, family, friends, or emergency medical personnel:
  1. *"AMPLE"* history (*A*llergies, *M*edications, *P*ast medical history, *L*ast meal, *E*vents of the incident)
  2. Type of burning agent
  3. Length of time of exposure
  4. Whether the patient was in an enclosed area
  5. Concurrent trauma
  6. Any prior treatment
  7. History of alcohol or drug use before the event
  8. History of smoking
  9. Voltage, amperage, and current for electrical burns
  10. Advanced directives

11. Tetanus immunization status
12. Possibility that injury suggests maltreatment

FOCUSED NURSING ASSESSMENT

The first priority in caring for the burn patient is to stop the burning process. Once that goal has been achieved, the burn patient is treated as a trauma patient and the nursing assessment follows the primary and secondary assessment outlined in Chapter 20. In addition, the following assessment parameters should be applied. As with all trauma patients, a high index of suspicion must be maintained to anticipate and treat potentially life-threatening situations. Evaluation of the burn injury occurs after the initial assessment and interventions have taken place.

Airway

- Inspect the mouth and nose for soot, burns, blisters, and edema. Look for singed nasal and facial hairs. If such signs are present, maintain a high index of suspicion for an inhalation injury.
- Monitor the patient for abnormal inspiratory sounds (e.g., crowing, stridor, and hoarseness) that may be associated with partial occlusion of the pharynx or larynx from burn edema.
- Circumferential burns to the neck may compromise the airway as a result of the tourniquet-type effect of edema.

NURSING ALERT

An inhalation injury should be suspected in a patient who was in a burning environment in a confined space or in a patient who apparently has an altered level of consciousness. Inhalation injuries may not manifest themselves for several hours after the time of the injury. Prepare for prophylactic endotracheal intubation in any patient who exhibits questionable respiratory mechanics or has clinical indications for an inhalation injury.

Breathing

- Evaluate the respiratory rate, use of accessory muscles, chest wall symmetry, and excursion. Circumferential third-degree burns to the chest may impair chest expansion because of eschar formation. An escharotomy may need to be performed to allow the chest to expand with inspiration.

- Auscultate the lungs for bilateral air movement and adventitious sounds.
- Assess for agitation or change in the level of consciousness.
- In addition to the signs of potential inhalation injury stated in the airway assessment, hoarseness, stridor, wheezing, cough, carbonaceous sputum, tachypnea, dyspnea, and agitation may be found during the breathing assessment.

Perfusion

- Assess vital signs frequently. The patient's heart rate is the second most reliable indicator of adequate fluid resuscitation (urine output is the first).[1] Patients with a serious burn will experience a fall in cardiac output within the first few minutes of the injury.[1] The swelling of a burned limb invalidates the readings from a noninvasive blood pressure (BP) cuff placed on that limb.
- Assess pulses, especially those distal to the burn. Nonpalpable pulses should be evaluated with a Doppler. Circumferential third-degree burns on an extremity may require an escharotomy.
- Assess capillary refill, torso and extremity temperature, and skin color.
- Assess cerebral perfusion by evaluating the patient's LOC. The affinity of hemoglobin for carbon monoxide is over 200 times that for oxygen. Signs and symptoms of inadequate perfusion may indicate carbon monoxide poisoning (see section on Carbon Monoxide Poisoning).
- Remove rings and other constricting jewelry.

Extent of Burn

Once the primary survey, initial resuscitation interventions, and secondary survey are complete, the burn injury is evaluated. The extent of the burn is calculated as a percentage of the total body surface area (TBSA) with partial- or full-thickness burns. First-degree burns are not included in the estimates of TBSA because the skin does not lose its ability to function. The Rule of Nines (Figure 4-1) can be used to estimate the TBSA involved. It must be adapted for accurate assessment of infants and toddlers, because their body proportions are different from those of adults.

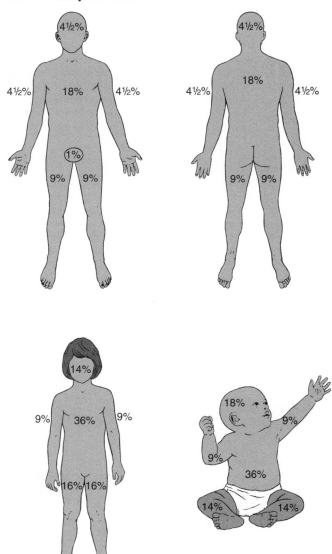

Figure 4-1 Rule of Nines.

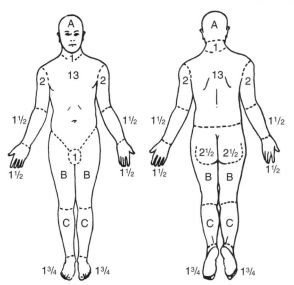

Relative percentage of areas affected by growth

	Age in years					
	0	1	5	10	15	Adult
A—½ of head	9½	8½	6½	5½	4½	3½
B—½ of one thigh	2¾	3¼	4	4¼	4½	4¾
C—½ of one leg	2½	2½	2¾	3	3¼	3½

Figure 4-2 Lund and Browder chart. (From Griglak, Martin: Thermal Injury, *Emerg Med Clin North Am* 10(2):374, 1992.)

- A modified Rule of Nines used for the child proposes that for each year of life after 2 years of age, 1% is subtracted from the head and 0.5% is added to each leg.
- For estimating the percent of patchy burns, use the size of the palmar surface of the patient's hand, which equals 1% of the body surface area.
- Age-related charts, such as the Lund and Browder chart (Figure 4-2), may provide a more accurate determination of the extent of the injury in children.

Risk Factors

The following risk factors are associated with a burn injury:

1. Children less than 5 years of age and adults more than 65 years of age
2. Hot water heaters set too high
3. Workplace exposure to chemicals or electricity
4. Complacency in the workplace
5. Use of alcohol
6. Carelessness with burning cigarettes
7. Inadequate or faulty electrical wiring
8. Wearing flammable clothing, especially flammable nightwear

Life Span Issues
Pediatric Patients

1. Since young children do not have the motor dexterity to quickly remove themselves from the heat source and since their skin is thinner, their burns are more severe than those an adult would sustain given the same exposure.
2. Airway compromise occurs more rapidly because of the smaller size of the airway.
3. Lack of bone ossification and increased bone pliability result in early exhaustion of a child with constrictive chest burns from the decreased chest wall compliance.[2]
4. Children are further compromised by a higher metabolic rate, which causes increased oxygen consumption.
5. Heart rate is a reliable indicator of the degree of shock because cardiac output is maintained in young children by increasing the heart rate rather than the stroke volume.
6. BP is not a reliable indicator of shock. Compensation from vasoconstriction will maintain the BP in an acceptable range until cardiovascular decompensation occurs.
7. Special attention should be given to preserving body heat. Children have a larger body surface area to weight ratio in comparison to adults and will have a greater degree of heat and evaporative water loss.
8. Children are predisposed to hypoglycemia because of low glycogen stores. Maintenance fluids (which must be calculated in addition to the burn resuscitation fluids) containing glucose should be used to supplement the Ringer's lactated resuscitation, to avoid hypoglycemia.[3]

Geriatric Patients

1. Geriatric patients have a diminished sensory capacity and are sometimes cognitively impaired. A reduced reaction time coupled with frequently impaired mobility and declining physical strength increases their risk for injury. As is the case with children, the skin is thinner, resulting in more severe burns.
2. Preexisting cardiopulmonary disease decreases the ability to tolerate pulmonary stressors such as inhalation burns.
3. Preexisting disease (e.g., chronic obstructive pulmonary disease, coronary artery disease, hypertension, renal compromise, or diabetes) results in a reduced reserve capacity of the body system affected by the disease. Thus, the elderly are predisposed to organ dysfunction with increased morbidity and mortality.
4. Fluid resuscitation necessitates close monitoring to prevent complications from underresuscitation or overresuscitation.

Pregnancy

1. A spontaneous termination of pregnancy usually occurs with TBSA burns of 60% or more.[2]
2. The fetus totally depends on stable maternal vital signs. Large amounts of supplemental oxygen are required to ensure adequate fetal oxygenation.
3. Patients beyond 20 weeks' gestation (uterus at the level of the umbilicus) may need to be placed on either their right or left side to prevent compression of the vena cava by the uterus, which causes hypotension.
4. Fetal monitoring is essential. Patients should be transferred to a burn center.

NURSING ALERT

Plasma volume increases in pregnancy. As a result of this volume increase, 1200 to 1500 mL of the blood volume may be displaced before signs of hypovolemia are seen.[4] The placenta is sensitive to catecholamine release and has little autoregulatory capability; thus it cannot compensate for the resulting vasoconstriction and hypoperfusion. Anticipation of shock in the pregnant patient is of the utmost importance in treatment of the fetus.

INITIAL INTERVENTIONS

1. Take precautions to prevent further contamination of the burns. Use sterile gloves for all burn wound contact, and use gowns, masks, and head covers for moderate or major burns.

2. Provide supplemental oxygen. Any patient with potential carbon monoxide poisoning should receive 100% oxygen per nonrebreather mask.

3. Inadequate respiratory effort must be assisted with a bag-valve device attached to a 100% oxygen source. Prepare for intubation in any patient with inadequate respiratory mechanics or noisy respiratory effort.

4. Take precautions to prevent aspiration in the unconscious patient by using the rescue position, if not contraindicated by concurrent trauma, and have functioning suction equipment at hand. Prepare for endotracheal intubation and nasogastric tube placement, which provide definitive protection.

5. Determine if chemical burns have been flushed adequately. The burns should have been flushed with copious amounts of water for at least 20 to 30 minutes and the patient should voice decreased pain and discomfort.

6. Attach a cardiac monitor, oxygen saturation monitor, and automatic BP cuff to the patient. Pulse rates of 110 to 125 beats/min after the initial resuscitation phase (a few hours following injury) can be a normal response in adults with large burn areas.[1,5] Heart rates in children will vary according to age. A tachycardia with rates of 120 to 170 beats/min may be present in children in the first 24 hours despite adequate urine output.[1,5,6] The patient's BP is not a reliable indicator of the adequacy of fluid resuscitation. However, a low mean pressure (i.e., ≤65 mm Hg in adults; ≤40 mm Hg in children)[1] can be indicative of the need for further evaluation of fluid status.

> **NURSING ALERT**
>
> Pulse oximetry may not be able to differentiate between hemoglobin saturated with carbon monoxide and hemoglobin saturated with oxygen. A high oxygen saturation reading may not indicate adequate oxygenation.

7. Burns may be cooled with tepid to cool moist compresses. Cooling of burns must be done with caution to prevent hypothermia. Ice and cold water are contraindicated for cooling burns. After the burns are cooled, wet bedding should be removed and patients should be covered with dry, clean sheets and blankets to maintain body temperature.
8. Eye care involves flushing with copious amounts of water or saline solution after inverting the eyelid and removing any particles (see Procedure 16).
9. Cover burns with clean, dry sheets until definitive wound care can be initiated.
10. Anticipate fluid resuscitation in adults with ≥20% TBSA burns, in young children with ≥10% to 15% TBSA burns, and in geriatric patients with ≥5% to 15% TBSA burns.[5]
11. Elevate the head of the bed 30 degrees to minimize edema of the face and to minimize cerebral edema if not contraindicated by concurrent trauma.
12. Obtain an accurate patient weight.
13. Initiate the transfer of patients requiring treatment in a burn center (see "American Burn Association Transfer Criteria" box).

AMERICAN BURN ASSOCIATION TRANSFER CRITERIA

Second- and third-degree burns greater than 10% BSA in patients less than 10 or more than 50 years of age
Second- and third-degree burns greater than 20% BSA in other age groups
Second- and third-degree burns with serious threat of functional or cosmetic impairment that involve the face, hands, feet, genitalia, perineum, and major joints
Third-degree burns greater than 5% BSA in any age group
Significant electrical burns, including lightning injury
Chemical burns with serious threat of functional or cosmetic impairment

---

BSA, Body surface area
From *Advanced Burn Life Support,* 1994 revision; National Burn Institute/American Burn Association. *Continued*

AMERICAN BURN ASSOCIATION TRANSFER CRITERIA—cont'd

Inhalation injury with burn injury

Circumferential burns of an extremity and chest

Burn injury in patients with preexisting medical disorders that could complicate management, prolong recovery, or affect mortality

Any burn patient with concomitant trauma in which the burn injury poses the greatest risk of morbidity or mortality

Burned children should be transferred to a hospital with qualified personnel and equipment

From National Burn Institute: *Advanced burn life support provider manual 1994*, 1994, Omaha, The Institute.

PRIORITY NURSING DIAGNOSES

Risk for fluid volume deficit

Risk for impaired gas exchange

Risk for altered peripheral tissue perfusion

Risk for pain

Risk for impaired skin integrity

Risk for infection

- ◆ **Fluid volume deficit** related to increased capillary permeability and loss of plasma volume from vascular space (fluid shift) as demonstrated by edema, decreased urine output, decreased central venous pressure, decreased pulmonary capillary wedge pressure, hypotension, or tachycardia:
  INTERVENTIONS
  - Monitor vital signs for tachycardia and hypotension.
  - Place two large-bore intravenous (IV) catheters for fluid resuscitation.
  - Place a urinary catheter to monitor output.
- ◆ **Impaired gas exchange** related to alveolar injury and decreased hemoglobin, as demonstrated by carbonaceous sputum, a hoarse voice, singed nasal hairs, burns to the face, a decreased Po_2, or an increased Pco_2:
  INTERVENTIONS
  - Provide 100% oxygen by nonrebreather mask.
  - Assist ventilations with a bag-valve device if inadequate respiratory effort exists.

- Prepare for intubation for patients with signs of potential airway obstruction.
- Elevate the head of the bed for patients with potential inhalation injuries unless concurrent trauma precludes doing so.
- Monitor oxygen saturation by pulse oximetry (pulse oximetry may not differentiate between carbon monoxide- and oxygen-saturated hemoglobin).
- Prepare for an escharotomy in the case of circumferential burns of the chest that compromise chest expansion and the patient's ability to breathe.
- Monitor hemoglobin.
- Monitor carboxyhemoglobin levels for patients with carbon monoxide poisoning.

◆ **Altered peripheral tissue perfusion** related to generalized edema, avascular tissue, decreased cardiac output, and hypovolemia as demonstrated by diminished peripheral pulses, loss of sensory function, and cool extremities:
INTERVENTIONS
- Evaluate peripheral pulses, sensory function, skin temperature, and capillary refill.
- Place a BP cuff on the unaffected limb if possible.
- Remove jewelry and constrictive clothing.
- Prepare to assist with an escharotomy for a patient with a circumferential burn of an extremity associated with perfusion deficits.

◆ **Pain** related to stimulation of exposed pain sensors as demonstrated by moaning, hostility, crying, clenched teeth, facial grimacing, complaints of pain, irritability, an increased heart rate and BP, or restlessness:
INTERVENTIONS
- Cool burns with tepid to cool moist compresses, taking care to avoid hypothermia.
- Cover cooled burns with a clean dry sheet to prevent irritation of exposed nerve endings from air currents.
- Administer pain medications as ordered.
- Advise the patient of all procedures to be performed and of what to expect during the procedure.

◆ **Impaired skin integrity** related to burns, edema, and impaired physical mobility as demonstrated by destruction of dermis, epidermis, and underlying structures, fluid-filled blisters, and mottled, waxy, white, cherry red, or blackened skin color:

INTERVENTIONS
- Eliminate the source of burning.
- Flush chemical burns with water for 20 to 30 minutes.
- If the ears are burned, secure endotracheal and gastric tubes away from the ears.
- Tar, asphalt, and plastic that adhere to the skin must be cooled with water.
- Turn the patient every 2 hours.

◆ **Infection** related to an altered integumentary system as demonstrated by destruction of the dermis and epidermis:
INTERVENTIONS
- Use sterile gloves for all wound contact.
- Use sterile gowns, masks, and shoe and head covers for moderate or major burns.
- Use strict aseptic technique.
- Use sterile linens for patients with moderate to severe burns.
- Administer antibiotics and tetanus toxoid as ordered.

PRIORITY DIAGNOSTIC TESTS

Laboratory

Serum electrolyte levels: Initially, levels may be normal, but they will change during the early course of treatment.

Serum BUN and creatinine: Blood urea nitrogen (BUN) and creatinine levels may be falsely elevated related to fluid deficits.

Blood glucose: The level may be elevated as a result of the stress response. Hypoglycemia in children may occur because of limited glycogen stores.

Arterial blood gas: The PO_2 may initially be normal with inhalation injuries. It is especially important to document a baseline pH with patients who sustain electrical burns, because acidosis is common. Patients with large burns will have a mild metabolic acidosis that will resolve with adequate resuscitation.

Complete blood count: Initially, the hemoglobin and hematocrit may be elevated as a result of the intracellular fluid shift.

Serum albumin: The level may be low because plasma proteins, principally albumin, are lost into injured tissue secondary to increased capillary permeability.

Serum drug and alcohol screens and urine drug screen: These are especially important if the patient is unconscious or obtunded.

B

Serum carboxyhemoglobin: Screening should be done with patients with suspected inhalation injuries. Signs and symptoms appear if the level is elevated >10% (see the "Indications" box).

Urine myoglobin: A urine myoglobin test should be done for patients with electrical burns. Myoglobin is released when muscle tissue breaks down. The urine will turn light red or tea colored, but there are no red blood cells present. Myoglobin can cause damage to renal tubules if the kidneys are not well flushed. Urine output needs to be 75 to 100 ml/hr until the color of the urine clears, then 50 ml/hr. Check cardiac enzymes if an electrical injury is involved.

Chest Radiograph
Chest radiographic changes are usually seen at approximately 48 hours after an inhalation injury. An admission chest x-ray examination will provide a baseline for comparison with later films.

Electrocardiogram
An electrocardiogram (ECG) is particularly indicated in electrical burns because cardiac dysrhythmias are common complications.

CT Scan
Rule out an intracranial hemorrhage in patients with a neurologic deterioration who have suffered an electrical injury.

INDICATIONS FOR ALTERED FLUID RESUSCITATION REQUIREMENTS

Inhalation injury
Delay in resuscitation
Associated trauma
Extensive depth and surface area burn
Circumferential burns requiring escharotomy release
High-voltage electrical injury
Extensive muscle damage
Preexisting medical conditions
Extreme age groups (infants and geriatric patients)

From Gordon MD, Winfree JH: Fluid resuscitation after a major burn. In Carrougher GJ: *Burn care and therapy,* St. Louis, 1998, Mosby.

COLLABORATIVE INTERVENTIONS

Overview

1. **Provision of oxygen:** Burn patients should receive 100% oxygen by nonrebreather mask. Patients with a possible inhalation injury should be positioned with the head of the bed elevated to decrease dependent edema of the upper airway unless a potential cervical injury precludes doing so. Prepare to intubate patients with signs of impending airway obstruction (stridor, hoarseness, dyspnea, or tachypnea). An endotracheal tube at least 7.5 mm in diameter is recommended for use with adult patients to facilitate pulmonary toilet or bronchoscopy. Nasal intubation is the preferred route for the burn patient if it is possible[2] (see Procedure 15). Avoid undue pressure against the burned skin and ears when securing an endotracheal tube, particularly during fluid resuscitation when edema formation is greatest. A well-secured endotracheal tube is of paramount importance in the initial resuscitation phase; a tube that is dislodged may be impossible to replace because of edema of the airway.

2. **Fluid replacement:** Fluid replacement can be expected in adults with ≥20% TBSA burns, in children with ≥10% to 15% TBSA burns, and in geriatric patients with burns ≥5% and ≤15% TBSA.[5] The goal of fluid replacement in the first 48 hours is to preserve vital organ perfusion, avoiding both overresuscitation and underresuscitation. Warmed Ringer's lactate is the replacement fluid of choice and should be infused through two large-bore IV catheters, preferably placed through unburned skin. Administer 2 to 4 ml/kg/% BSA burned in the first 24 hours following the time of the injury. Give one half of the total 24-hour volume in the first 8 hours (burned tissue is most permeable during the first 8 hours after injury), one fourth during the second 8 hours, and one fourth during the third 8 hours. (Parkland's formula recommends 4 ml/kg/% BSA in 24 hours, and the Modified Brooke Formula recommends 2 ml/kg/% BSA in 24 hours. The two formulas advocate consistent administration of the fluid over the first 24 hours post-injury.) Use of colloid solutions is controversial during the first

12 to 24 hours of resuscitation because increased capillary permeability causes a loss of plasma proteins interstitially, which traps water.[5] The "Indications for Altered Fluid Resuscitation Requirements" lists certain concurrent injuries that will alter the amount of fluid needed during resuscitation.

NURSING ALERT

Formulas for fluid resuscitation are only a guide. Fluid replacement should be sufficient to maintain an hourly urine output of 30 to 50 ml/hr in adults and 1 ml/kg/hr in children weighing <30 kg.[2,4]

---

3. **Nasogastric tube:** Adynamic ileus usually accompanies most burn injuries involving over 20% TBSA.[7] Patients with these burns should have gastric decompression until bowel function returns.
4. **Urinary catheter:** Use of a urinary catheter is essential because urine output serves as a guide for fluid resuscitation.
5. **Escharotomy:** An escharotomy is indicated for circumferential burns that constrict the chest or extremities and cause circulatory or respiratory compromise. The procedure is performed at the patient's bedside using sterile technique. The preferred sites on the extremities are midmedial or at the midlateral aspect, including the joints. The preferred incision and site on the chest are bilateral incisions in the anterior axillary lines from the clavicle to the costal margins. If the burn includes the abdominal wall, the incision should extend onto the abdomen along the costal margin.[4] Incisions must extend through the entire length and depth (to the subcutaneous fat) of the eschar. This allows separation of the tissue allowing for expansion from edema. Assess extremity pulses after the escharotomy. If pulses are not restored, a fasciotomy is required.[4]
6. **Tetanus toxoid:** Necrotic tissue is an ideal medium for *Clostridium tetani* to grow. Administer tetanus toxoid to previously immunized patients. Administer tetanus immunoglobulin for those not previously immunized or for whom the immunization status is unknown. (See Table 4-1)

TABLE 4-1 Drug Summary

Drug	Dose/route	Special considerations
Tetanus toxoid	0.5 ml IM	For tetanus-prone wounds and those not adequately immunized Give toxoid in unburned tissue
Tetanus immunoglobulin	250-500 U IM	Give if tetanus status is unknown and wound is tetanus prone Give in unburned tissue
Morphine	Adult 3-5 mg IV Children 0.05-0.1 mg/kg every 2-3 hr, as needed	Give by IV route; if it is given IM, poor tissue perfusion results in inadequate absorption Monitor blood pressure until pain controlled Monitor patient for respiratory depression if not intubated
Mannitol (Osmitrol)	25 g bolus followed by 12.5-25 g/L of Ringer's lactate IV	Administer through filter Monitor for hypotension Evaluate urine for color, amount, and pH

7. Administer pain medication. IV administration is preferred because intramuscular injections result in inconsistent absorption (see Table 4-1).
8. Administer antibiotics as ordered.
9. Initiate transfer to a burn center if the injury warrants. The American Burn Association has identified burns that

TABLE 4-1 Drug Summary—cont'd

Drug	Dose/route	Special considerations
Mafenide acetate (Sulfamylon)	Spread over burned area	Has good eschar penetration capabilities; choice agent topically in infected wounds
		Painful for 30-40 min when applied; penetrates cartilage
		Premedicate patient for pain
		Do not use in cases of sulfa drug allergy or respiratory or kidney disease
Silver sulfadiazine (Silvadene)	Spread over burned area using gloved hand or tongue blade topically	Use sterile technique to apply
		Is not painful when applied
		Do not apply to face as may stain skin

may benefit from the care provided at a burn center (see the "American Burn Association Transfer Criteria" box).

Clinical Conditions
Thermal burns

The extent of the injury is a result of the intensity of the heat (temperature) and the duration of exposure.

SYMPTOMS

Superficial (first degree)
- First-degree burns involve the epidermis and are characterized by pain, edema, and erythema that blanches. First-degree burns are not calculated in the estimation of burn injuries because the skin does not lose its protective function. A patient with extensive superficial burns may exhibit headache, chills, and nausea and vomiting as a result of mild systemic response.[8]

Superficial partial-thickness (second degree)
- Second-degree burns involve the epidermis and part of the dermis. The skin is hyperemic and moist with thin-walled, fluid-filled blisters. Nerve endings are intact and irritated, causing extreme pain. The burned areas will blanch when pressure is applied.

Deep partial-thickness (second degree)
- Second-degree burns also can involve the epidermis and deep layers of the dermis. The skin is pale to waxy-white in color with blisters like tissue paper that contain little if any fluid. The wound has a decreased pinprick sensation that can make differentiation from full-thickness burns difficult.

Full-Thickness (third degree)
- Third-degree burns involve the epidermis and the entire dermis and extend into the subcutaneous tissues (Figure 4-3). The surface is dry, hard, inelastic, and insensate. The burn may appear waxy, white, cherry red, yellow, brown, or black. Nerve endings have been destroyed, although some sensation may be intact at the edges of the burn and cause discomfort.

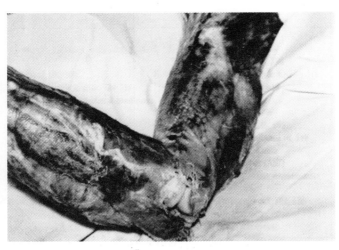

Figure 4-3 Full-thickness burn exposing elbow joint. (From Dressler DP, Hozid JL, Nathan P: *Thermal injuries,* St Louis, 1988, Mosby.)

DIAGNOSIS

- Diagnosis is based on history and on assessment of the skin.

TREATMENT

- Initial treatment is focused on stopping the burning process and on airway management, breathing, and fluid resuscitation.
- Cool burned areas with tepid to cool moist compresses. Once the burn is cooled, remove all wet bedding and dressings.
- Maintain the body temperature. Hypothermia results in vasoconstriction that will further compromise circulation to the injured area. Maintain a body temperature of 99° F to prevent further damage.[1] Cover the patient with a clean sheet and a blanket for comfort.
- Ensure adequate pain and anxiety control, especially before cleansing the injury.
- If the patient is to be transferred to a burn center, it is not necessary to debride the burn or dress it with topical ointments. Cover the patient with a clean, dry sheet and blanket.[2]
- If admission to the hospital or transfer to a burn center will be delayed beyond 12 hours, wound care should be initiated after consultation with the receiving physician. Topical ointments may need to be applied (see Table 4-1).
- Gently cleanse the wound with a mild soap and rinse with warm water.
- Pieces of clothing, foreign matter, and charred skin should be removed by soaking, rinsing, or gentle cleansing with wet gauze. Sloughed or necrotic skin will need to be debrided according to hospital protocol if the patient is not to be transferred. Controversy exists regarding the debridement of burn blisters; leave the blisters undisturbed, drain them and leave the injured epithelium in place, or remove the injured epithelium completely.[7] The physician treating the patient will determine the care. The wound should be cleansed before the dressing is applied regardless of which method of dealing with the blisters is chosen.
- Evaluate circumferential burns for circulatory compromise and prepare for an escharotomy if compromise occurs.

- Assess for vascular compromise from swelling or compartment syndrome (Chapter 10).
- Tar, asphalt, or plastic that remains on the skin should be cooled, and covered with a petroleum-based ointment (e.g., mineral oil or bacitracin) or commercially prepared solvent to dissolve it. Cover the area with a dressing. The tar will dissolve within 18 to 24 hours and then the burn can be assessed and treated.

Inhalation injury

An inhalation injury is caused by chemicals, gases, or heat being inhaled, and the severity is related to the amount and composition of the inhaled substances. Inhalation injuries significantly increase the morbidity and mortality of burn-injured patients.[2,9] There are three types of inhalation injuries: carbon monoxide inhalation, upper airway injury (above the glottis), and lower airway injury (below the glottis).[2]

Carbon monoxide inhalation

Carbon monoxide (CO) is a byproduct of the combustion of organic material. It is a colorless, odorless gas with an affinity for hemoglobin that is over 200 times that of oxygen. CO binds to hemoglobin, blocking the uptake and transport of oxygen with a resulting hypoxia. Patients who were in an enclosed area during a fire are predisposed to CO poisoning.

SYMPTOMS

- Symptoms are related to the amount of hemoglobin saturated with CO (carboxyhemoglobin) (see the "Signs and Symptoms of Carbon Monoxide Poisoning" box).

SIGNS AND SYMPTOMS OF CARBON MONOXIDE POISONING

0%-10%	Normal, smokers, and those living in urban areas
10%-20%	Headache, confusion, and dyspnea on exertion
20%-40%	Fatigue, severe headache, visual disturbances, dizziness, nausea and vomiting, and chest pains in individuals with coronary artery disease
40%-60%	Tachycardia, tachypnea, hallucinations, combativeness, respiratory failure, shock, convulsions, coma, cherry-red skin color, and death
>60%	Usually results in death

Data from Fitzgerald KA, McLaughlin EG: *ACCN Clin Issues Crit Care Nurs* 1(3):535-542, 1990; Ruth-Sahd L: *Nursing* 92:33, 1992.

- Mild symptoms include a headache and confusion.
- More severe symptoms include vomiting, tachycardia, tachypnea, hallucinations, and eventual coma and death.
- Symptoms result from tissue hypoxia, not from parenchymal injury.

DIAGNOSIS

- Note the history and duration of exposure to products of combustion, especially in an enclosed area.
- Record the carboxyhemoglobin level (clinical indicators are unreliable, as are blood gases).

TREATMENT

- Administer warmed and humidified 100% oxygen by nonrebreather mask if the patient can maintain his or her own airway or by intubation if indicated by a decreased LOC. The half-life of carboxyhemoglobin is 5 to 6 hours with room air, 30 to 90 minutes with 100% oxygen, and 20 to 25 minutes with hyperbaric treatment.[3,10]
- Monitor carboxyhemoglobin levels. Patients should remain on 100% oxygen until carboxyhemoglobin levels are <10%. In severe cases (elevated carboxyhemoglobin associated with a pH of less than 7.4) hyperbaric oxygen therapy may be suggested.[11] During hyperbaric oxygen therapy the CO molecule is removed from the hemoglobin.

Upper airway injury (supraglottic)

An upper airway injury may result from a thermal injury or inhaled chemicals or gases that have a high water solubility and are rapidly absorbed on the moist surfaces of the mouth, nose, and upper airway (e.g., chlorine, ammonia, and sulfur oxides and dioxides).[5,12,13]

SYMPTOMS

- Symptoms may be absent initially. Edema peaks at 24 to 48 hours after injury.[9]
- Symptoms include erythema, edema, hoarseness, blisters, or ulcerations of the oropharynx and larynx.
- Symptoms also may include a mechanical obstruction of the airway secondary to edema (e.g., stridor, tachypnea, dyspnea, and crowing respirations). Hypovolemia may initially delay the development of edema.

DIAGNOSIS

- There is a history of heat or hot liquids entering the airway.
- Direct visualization of damage to the larynx, pharynx, and vocal cords.

TREATMENT
- Elevate the head of the bed.
- Provide warm, humidified oxygen.
- Administer aerosolized epinephrine.
- Prepare for early intubation of patients who have the potential for airway obstruction.

Lower airway injury (infraglottic)

The ability of the supraglottic area to cool hot air usually prevents thermal injury to the infraglottic structures. Inhalation injuries to the infraglottic structures are usually a result of inhaled toxic fumes, gases, mists, and particles and affect primarily the upper and small airways. Exposure to a fine mist will affect the small airways and the lung parenchyma.[9]

SYMPTOMS
- The onset of symptoms is unpredictable, and frequently the patient is initially asymptomatic.
- Damage depends on the chemical content of the inhaled substance and on the length of exposure.
- The patient may have sooty sputum (generally reliable), burns to the face, singed nasal hairs, and inflammation of oropharyngeal mucosa. Inhalation injuries to the lower airway may occur without evidence of external signs.
- The onset of cough, hoarseness, dyspnea, wheezing, and stridor is delayed.

DIAGNOSIS
- The patient has a history of exposure to products of combustion, especially in a small area.
- A bronchoscopy will reveal tracheobronchial injuries such as mucosal inflammation, ulcerations, necrosis, soot, foreign particles, and edema.[9] These clinical findings often present before obvious respiratory compromise.
- A xenon ventilation perfusion scan identifies injury to small airways and parenchymal injury. The scan is usually performed within 24 to 48 hours after the injury. A delay in the clearance of xenon from the lungs is indicative of parenchymal injury.[9]

TREATMENT

Minimal to mild injury
- Provide warm humidified oxygen per nonrebreather mask.
- Implement incentive spirometry to prevent atelectasis.

- Use bronchodilators for bronchospasms and wheezing.
- Monitor arterial blood gases and pulse oximetry, and for changes in assessment indicating a delayed airway obstruction.
- Those who are asymptomatic but have a history of significant exposure need close observation for 24 hours because of the unpredictable course of inhalation injuries.[2]

More severe injury

- Provide humidification of inspired oxygen.
- Begin aggressive pulmonary toilet to mobilize and remove secretions.
- Use beta 2-agonist nebulizer treatments or IV bronchodilators for bronchospasms and wheezing.[9]
- Obtain an arterial blood gas analysis (nonspecific indicator of inhalation injury; however, with progression of pulmonary dysfunction, arterial oxygen desaturation and retention of carbon dioxide may occur).
- The patient may require greater fluid volume for resuscitation.
- Perform intubation and implement mechanical ventilation for respiratory failure.

Electrical burns

Electrical injuries are classified by the type and strength of current encountered.

- Types of current include "alternating current" (AC) found in households (voltage of 110 or 220) and "direct current" (DC) found in car batteries and electrosurgical devices. Contact with AC tends to cause muscle contraction, making it difficult for the victim to let go of the electrical source. Contact with DC tends to cause a single violent muscle contraction, often throwing the victim from the electrical source. Contact with AC tends to be more dangerous than contact with DC.
- The strength of current is divided into two categories: high voltage, 1000 volts or greater, and low voltage, below 1000 volts. High voltage usually causes more tissue destruction.

NURSING ALERT

Victims of an electrical injury who come to the ED in cardiopulmonary arrest should receive aggressive resuscitation.

NURSING ALERT

> As a result of the implosive and explosive effects of lightning, the victim can be thrown. Maintain a high index of suspicion for life-threatening blunt, traumatic injuries.

SYMPTOMS

- Electrical injuries produce a wide variety of injuries that initially may be difficult to determine. Careful observation and repeated assessment are necessary to treat the patient properly.

Cardiac

- Patients may be experiencing ventricular fibrillation (more common with AC exposure), asystole (more common with high voltage and lightning exposure), or respiratory arrest.
- Additional ECG changes may include sinus tachycardia, ST segment elevation, QT segment prolongation, ventricular ectopy, atrial fibrillation, and a bundle branch block.[14]
- Acute hypertension may occur, especially with lightning injuries.

Integument

- Externally, the thermal injuries range in depth from superficial to full thickness with the possible destruction and necrosis of underlying structures and organs.
- Contact points (often called entrance wounds) are usually dry and charred, whereas ground points (often called the exit wounds) are usually larger with irregular edges.[2,14] Identification of points of contact may help determine the path of the current.
- Oral burns may be seen in children who have been exposed by chewing on electrical cords.
- Lightning strikes frequently cause a flashover phenomenon in which the electrical current passes over the body instead of through it. This results either in superficial burns that are linear or punctate in form, or alterations in the skin (which are not actually thermal injuries) such as feathering, which produces a red-branching pattern on the skin, described as spidery or featherlike in appearance.[2,14]

Neurologic

- Neurologic injury may be immediate or delayed.
- The patient may have a history of a transient level of con-

sciousness or experience confusion, amnesia, and short-term memory loss.[14,15]

- The patient may have headaches, skull fractures, intracranial hemorrhage, and seizures, especially if the electricity entered through the head.
- The patient may have spinal cord injuries from high-voltage contact and may also have paraplegia.

Vascular
- Internally, nerves, blood vessels, and muscles have low resistance and are good conductors, and therefore they are more easily injured, whereas fat and bone have high resistance.
- The patient may experience thrombosis from heating of the blood vessels, more so in smaller vessels since they do not have the blood flow to help dissipate the heat.
- The patient may experience vascular spasms, especially with lightning injuries. Extremities will be cold, blue, mottled, and pulseless. This usually resolves within a few hours without treatment. If it does not, consider compartment syndrome or thrombosis of the vessels.

Pulmonary
- The patient may have contusions, especially in cases involving a lightning strike.

Musculoskeletal
- Fractures or dislocations from violent muscle contractions or falls may occur.
- Compartment syndrome may develop.
- The lack of an external burn does not rule out internal damage to an extremity.

Urine
- The urine may be discolored, red to reddish brown; this may be indicative of either hemoglobin or myoglobin.

Sensory
- The patient may experience visual disturbances from eye damage.
- The tympanic membrane may rupture.

DIAGNOSIS
- Diagnosis is based on history. The burn can be difficult to diagnose if adequate history is not available.
- Diagnosis is also based on an assessment of the wounds.

TREATMENT
- Manage any ABC problems first.
- Provide spinal immobilization if the potential for frac-

tures from falls is present. Many electrical injuries occur in those who work on elevated electrical wires, cut trees, or are in construction.

- Use electrocardiographic monitoring. Be prepared to treat dysrhythmias with standard advanced life support measures.

- The use of traditional burn formulas is not applicable in electrical injuries because of the inability to calculate the TBSA affected. Appropriate fluid resuscitation is essential to preventing renal failure from myoglobinuria. Fluids should be titrated to maintain a urine output of 0.5 to 1 ml/kg/hr for clear urine or 1 to 1.5 ml/kg/hr for pigmented urine.[14]

- An osmotic diuretic such as mannitol may be used initially to promote renal perfusion if myoglobinuria is present. If it is administered, urine output can no longer be used as the major determinant of adequate fluid resuscitation.

- Treat severe acidosis secondary to muscle necrosis by adding 50 mEq of sodium bicarbonate to each liter of IV fluids. Maintaining slight alkalinization of the blood (pH = 7.45) also ensures the urine pH is alkaline. An alkaline urine pH increases the solubility of myoglobin in the urine and improves the rate of clearance.[2,14]

- Perform frequent extremity vascular checks. If vascular compromise is present, an escharotomy or fasciotomy must be performed.

- Frequently orient those who are confused.

- Maintain pain and anxiety control.

Chemical burns

Chemical burns occur when a chemical compound reacts with the skin, causing a chemical reaction (see the "Treatment of Specific Chemical Burns" box). Some absorption may occur and cause systemic reactions. Outcome is related to four things: the type of chemical (acid, alkali, or organic compounds), the length of exposure, the concentration of the substance, and the amount of the substance. The chemical reaction and subsequent tissue injury continue until the chemical is removed from the skin. The earlier the treatment, the less the damage. Acid burns cause coagulation necrosis and protein precipitation, which limit the extent of the tissue damage. Alkali burns cause more damage than acid burns because they produce

TREATMENT OF SPECIFIC CHEMICAL BURNS

B

Hydrofluoric acid

Hydrofluoric acid is used in manufacturing and research, and in the home as a rust remover, in bathroom cleansers, and as an acidifier in swimming pools.

Action	Penetrates the skin and causes intense pain; pain onset may be delayed for hours Can cause systemic toxicity, including dysrhythmias and hypocalcemia Can cause damage to the bones
Treatment	1. Aggressively lavage with water or, if available, a solution of benzalkonium chloride for 15-30 min immediately after contact. 2. Treat topically with a calcium gluconate gel. Deeper burns may require subcutaneous infiltration or an intraarterial infusion of 10% calcium gluconate. 3. Eyes must be treated with copious irrigation of water or normal saline. 4. Inhalation injury should be treated with nebulizer treatment of calcium gluconate solution. 5. Blisters must be removed because they may harbor fluoride ions.

Phenols

Phenols are found in chemical disinfectants and commercially available germicidal solutions and are used in industrial, agricultural, cosmetic (face peels), and medical fields.

Action	Causes coagulation necrosis Absorbed phenol may cause profound CNS depression, coma, respiratory failure, hypotension, hypothermia, and a metabolic acidosis

Data from Edlich RF, Moghtader JC: Chemical injuries. In Rosen P et al, editors: *Emergency medicine concepts and clinical practice,* ed 4, St Louis, 1998, Mosby; National Burn Institute: *Advanced burn life support provider manual 1994,* 1994, Omaha, The Institute; Winfree R, Barillo DJ: *Nurs Clin North Am* 32(2):275-278, 1997.

Continued

TREATMENT OF SPECIFIC CHEMICAL BURNS—cont'd

Phenols—cont'd

Action —cont'd	May induce fatal systemic toxicity by affecting the liver and kidneys
	Dilute solutions more rapidly absorbed than concentrated ones

Treatment	1. Irrigate with large volumes of water under low pressure.
	2. Phenol is poorly soluble in water; removal and dilution are best accomplished by swabbing with undiluted polyethylene glycol, either 300, or 400 if available.
	3. Phenols may become trapped in hair; any contaminated hair should be removed as soon as possible.

Alkalis

Alkalis are commonly found in fertilizers and oven and drain cleaners and are formed when dry cement is mixed with water.

Action	Produces liquefaction necrosis
	Saponification of fats (converts fat into a soap)
	Dehydrates cells

Treatment	1. Begin copious irrigation with large volumes of water under low pressure.
	2. Strong alkalis require prolonged (may take up to 12 hours for the pH to return to normal) irrigation to limit the severity of the injury.
	3. Certain chemicals contacting water produce heat; however, the large volumes of water used to irrigate the injury tend to limit this exothermic reaction.

Data from Edlich RF, Moghtader JC: Chemical injuries. In Rosen P et al, editors: *Emergency medicine concepts and clinical practice,* ed 4, St Louis, 1998, Mosby; National Burn Institute: *Advanced burn life support provider manual 1994,* 1994, Omaha, The Institute; Winfree R, Barillo DJ: *Nurs Clin North Am* 32(2):275-278, 1997.

B

TREATMENT OF SPECIFIC CHEMICAL BURNS—cont'd

White phosphorus

White phosphorus is commonly found in fireworks and weaponry and is used in the manufacture of insecticides, rodent poisons, and fertilizers.

Action	Danger of spontaneous combustion when exposed to air; when ignites, is oxidized and forms acids with the addition of water
	Tissue injury caused by heat production
	Metabolic abnormalities (hypocalcemia and elevated phosphorus level)
	ECG changes—prolonged QT interval, bradycardia, ST-T wave changes
Treatment	1. Remove the patient's clothing and the chemical particles from the skin.
	2. Submerse the affected area in cool water to isolate the chemical from the air (white phosphorus becomes a liquid at warmer temperatures [$44°$ C]).
	3. Wash the patient with a suspension of 5% sodium bicarbonate and 3% copper sulfate in 1% hydroxyethyl cellulose as soon as available (made by hospital pharmacy). If absorbed systemically, copper sulfate is toxic; treatment with the suspension is limited to 30 minutes, then the suspension is thoroughly washed from the skin.
	4. Phosphorus can be seen under a fluorescent light (Wood lamp). This may be an alternative for removing the phosphorus.

Continued

TREATMENT OF SPECIFIC CHEMICAL BURNS—cont'd

Elemental metals (sodium and potassium)

Action Harmless until activated with water
Tissue damage because of thermal and chemical injury

Treatment 1. DO NOT USE WATER.
2. In a prehospital setting, a class "D" fire extinguisher or sand should be used to suppress flames; the patient is then transported, with metal covered with oil (mineral oil or cooking oil) to separate it from water.
3. ED treatment involves removing small pieces of metal from the skin, and then debridement and cleansing of the thermal injury.

Data from Edlich RF, Moghtader JC: Chemical injuries. In Rosen P et al, editors: *Emergency medicine concepts and clinical practice*, ed 4, St Louis, 1998, Mosby; National Burn Institute: *Advanced burn life support provider manual 1994*, 1994, Omaha, The Institute; Winfree R, Barillo DJ: *Nurs Clin North Am* 32(2):275-278, 1997.

a tissue liquefaction necrosis, denaturation of protein, and loosening of tissue planes, allowing a deeper spread of the chemical and thus a more severe burn. Organic compounds cause cutaneous damage and can be absorbed, leading to liver and kidney damage.[15] Certain chemicals such as hydrofluoric acid can penetrate into the subcutaneous tissues and cause damage for several days after exposure.

SYMPTOMS
- The patient has skin damage resembling that of a thermal injury, with erythema, blistering, or full-thickness loss.
- The patient may have a history of inhaling chemical fumes.

NURSING ALERT

The extent of the tissue injury may be deceptive. Extensive necrosis, fluid loss, and systemic toxicity may occur during the first 24 to 36 hours after the injury.

B

DIAGNOSIS

- Diagnosis is determined by a history and assessment of the skin.
- Identification of the chemical agent is appropriate but is secondary to the removal of contaminated clothing and immediate irrigation of the affected area.

TREATMENT

- Emergency caregivers should observe strict universal precautions to avoid contaminating their own eyes, skin, and lungs. The patients' contaminated clothing should be removed and disposed of according to hospital policy.
- Dry powder residue should be brushed off before irrigation.
- Irrigation of the area with water should be done immediately for a minimum of 20 to 30 minutes. With few exceptions, neutralizing solutions have no advantage over water. Irrigation should continue until the patient voices a significant decrease in pain or the pain stops.
- Irrigation of the eye should begin with at least 1 to 2 liters of normal saline or Ringer's lactate and should continue until the eye's pH is 7.4.[16] If only one eye is involved in the chemical exposure, make sure the irrigation fluid runoff does not contaminate the uninvolved eye.
- Treatment for a tissue injury is the same as for a thermal burn.
- Frequent assessment should be performed for pulmonary involvement, which may range from mild tracheal irritation to adult respiratory distress syndrome.
- The "Treatment of Specific Chemical Burns" box provides a list of some chemical burns that require special treatment modalities or antidotes.

Special precautions with burns

Ears: Rupture of the tympanic membrane is common with patients struck by lightning.[14] Cartilage has a poor blood supply, which means the healing process is slow. With thermal burns, pressure must be kept off the ears; therefore the use of pillows must be avoided. Cloth ties used to secure endotracheal tubes and nasogastric tubes must be kept away from the ears (Figure 4-4).

Lips: Position endotracheal tubes to prevent pressure on the lips. Use bacitracin to prevent drying and cracking.

Eyes: The single most important treatment is copious irrigation with normal saline within seconds of the injury.

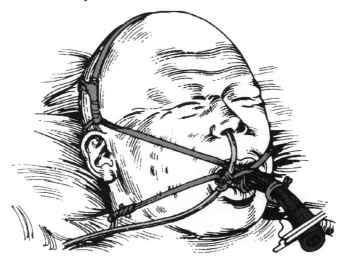

Figure 4-4 Cloth ties used to secure gastric and endotracheal tubes are kept away from the ears.

Invert the eyelid and remove any particles before irrigating. Irrigate for 30 minutes. Assess for eyelash inversion, which will cause corneal abrasions. The cornea must be kept moist (see Chapter 9). If only one eye is injured, prevent contamination of the unaffected eye from irrigation fluid runoff. Topical anesthetics may help decrease the pain and aid in irrigation.

Hands and feet: Preserving function is of the utmost importance. Elevate the extremity above the heart to prevent dependent edema that will delay healing. If fingers and toes are wrapped, they are wrapped individually; do not "mitten" them. If the patient cannot maintain the fingers in a position of function independently, the hand should be splinted.

Perineum: A urinary catheter must be placed until the edema resolves. Massive swelling occurs in the scrotum as a result of dependent edema. If the patient is on bed rest, the area must be cleansed thoroughly and ointment applied after voiding or defecation.

Joints: Exposed bones or tendons should be kept moist with saline-soaked sterile gauze.

NURSING ALERT

Burns of the hands, eyes, face, perineum, or joints require the special treatment available in a burn center.

NURSING SURVEILLANCE

1. Conduct repeated primary and secondary examinations of the affected body systems and injuries.
2. Monitor the urine for myoglobin (identified by reddish brown or tea-colored urine and urinalysis results negative for red cells).
3. Evaluate the effectiveness of pain and anxiety control.
4. Ensure infection control and aseptic techniques.
5. Obtain vital signs and an admission weight.
6. Monitor serum electrolyte levels.

EXPECTED PATIENT OUTCOMES

1. Urine output of 50 ml/hr for an adult, 1 ml/kg/hr for children under 30 kg, and 50 to 100 ml/hr for patients with electrical burns
2. Urine negative for myoglobin
3. Adequate pain control evaluated by self-scoring pain scale
4. Palpable pulses in all extremities
5. Capillary refill <2 seconds in all extremities
6. Heart rate <100 beats/min (<120 in patient with extensive burns as a result of hypermetabolic state); BP and cardiac rhythm within normal limits for patient's age
7. Core temperature remains 37° C (98.6° F) or higher
8. Maintained Glasgow Coma Scale score of 15
9. Decreasing carboxyhemoglobin level
10. Transfer to burn center within 4 hours of injury (see the "American Burn Association Transfer Criteria" box)

References

1. Gordon M, Goodwin CW: Initial assessment, management, and stabilization, *Nurs Clin North Am* 32(2):237-249, 1997.
2. National Burn Institute: *Advanced burn life support provider manual 1994*, Omaha, 1994, The Institute.
3. Lasear SE: Tissue integrity burns. In Neff JA, Kidd PS, editors: *Trauma nursing*, St Louis, 1993, Mosby.

4. American College of Surgeons: *Advanced trauma life support: student course manual,* ed 6, Chicago, 1997, The College.

5. Gordon MD, Winfree JH: Fluid resuscitation after a major burn. In Carrougher GJ: *Burn care and therapy,* St Louis, 1998, Mosby.

6. Cortiella J, Marvin JA: Management of the pediatric burn patient, *Nurs Clin North Am* 32(2):311-327, 1997.

7. Oman KS, Reilly EL: Initial assessment and care in the emergency department. In Carrougher GJ: *Burn care and therapy,* St Louis, 1998, Mosby.

8. Faldmo L, Kravitz M: Management of acute burns and burn shock resuscitation, *AACN Clin Issues Crit Care Nurs* 4(2):351-366, 1993.

9. Cioffe W Jr: Inhalation Injury. In Carrougher GJ: *Burn care and therapy,* St Louis, 1998, Mosby.

10. Jordon BS, Barillo DJ: Prehospital care and transport. In Carrougher GJ: *Burn care and therapy,* St Louis, 1998, Mosby.

11. Edlich RF, Moghtader JC: Thermal burns. In Rosen P et al, editors: *Emergency medicine concepts and clinical practice,* ed 4, St Louis, 1998, Mosby.

12. Carrougher GJ: Inhalation injury, *AACN Clin Issues Crit Care Nurs* 4(2):367-377, 1993.

13. Gough D, Young G: Airway burns and toxic gas inhalation. In Dailey RH et al: *The airway: emergency management,* St Louis, 1992, Mosby.

14. Cooper MA: Electrical and lightning injuries. In Rosen P et al, editors: *Emergency medicine concepts and clinical practice,* ed 4, St Louis, 1998, Mosby.

15. Winfree R, Barillo DJ: Nonthermal injuries, *Nurs Clin North Am* 32(2):275-278, 1997.

16. Edlich RF, Moghtader JC: Chemical injuries. In Rosen P et al, editors: *Emergency medicine concepts and clinical practice,* ed 4, St Louis, 1998, Mosby.

Chapter 5

Cardiovascular Conditions

Theresa M. Glessner

C

CLINICAL CONDITIONS
Myocardial Infarction
Angina
Congestive Heart Failure
Cardiogenic Shock
Sudden Death
Cardiac Arrest
Endocarditis
Pericarditis
Acute Aortic Dissection
Acute Arterial Occlusion
Venous Thrombosis

TRIAGE ASSESSMENT

The most common cardiac conditions encountered in the emergency department (ED) are myocardial infarctions (MIs), angina, congestive heart failure (CHF), pericarditis, endocarditis, cardiogenic shock, sudden death, and cardiac arrest. Common vascular conditions include acute aortic dissection, acute arterial occlusion, and venous thrombosis. At triage it is important initially to assess the patient's airway, breathing, and circulation (ABCs) and to take care of life-threatening conditions first and then determine the exact condition that has presented itself. Many cardio-vascular conditions have similar initial presentations, so it is important to do a carefully focused survey. If the cardiovascular system is involved, the patient will need to be closely monitored. Assuming that life-threatening conditions will be cared for per ACLS protocol, the fol-lowing must be obtained at triage based on the patient's chief complaint.

216   Chapter Five

Pain

Use the "PQRST" mnemonic as a systematic way to obtain information about pain:

   P (provoke): What provokes the pain? What makes it better or worse? What are positions of comfort and discomfort?

   Q (quality or character): What type of pain is it (burning, tight, crushing, tearing, pressure)?

   R (radiation): Where does the pain start? Where does it go? Have the patient point with one finger to where the pain is the most uncomfortable.

   S (severity): How severe is the pain on a scale of "0" to "10" ("0" representing no pain and "10" representing the worst pain)?

   T (time): When did the pain start? How long did it last? What time did the intensity change?

If the patient feels severe, crushing, left-sided chest pain radiating to the left shoulder, arm, or jaw, often accompanied by nausea, suspect an MI.[1]

Shortness of breath

Is the patient short of breath? Is this shortness of breath worse on exertion or with a position change? Does the patient experience orthopnea or paroxysmal nocturnal dyspnea (PND)? When did the shortness of breath begin and how long does it last? Is the patient able to function during periods of shortness of breath? If the patient is short of breath on exertion and has chest pain, suspect myocardial ischemia.

Cough

Does the patient have a cough? When did the cough begin? Does the cough produce any sputum and what does the sputum look like? Does pain or shortness of breath accompany the cough? If the patient has a dry, nonproductive cough accompanied by shortness of breath, especially on exertion, suspect fluid overload or CHF.

Nausea and vomiting

Has the patient experienced any nausea or vomiting? Was it accompanied by diaphoresis or chest pain? Patients frequently have some vague nausea accompanied by diaphoresis with their chest pain while having an MI or an episode of angina.

Extremity pain

If the complaint involves an extremity, is there pain? What are the color, temperature, and capillary refill of the extremity? Is there clubbing or edema? Are the pulses present above and below the involved area of the extremity? What is the size of the involved extremity compared to the uninvolved extremity? Do rest and elevation improve or worsen the pain? Can the patient walk? If so, how far can the patient walk before the onset of pain? What is the location of the pain when it occurs during ambulation? If the patient has pain, edema, and cyanosis of one extremity, suspect an arterial or venous occlusion. Patients with arterial occlusion have rest pain, a pain that starts when the patient is at rest or sleeping and wakes the patient up. Typically, rest pain starts over the top of the foot and is a severe, aching pain. Claudication can be caused by arterial or venous disease and can begin at any level, calf, thigh, or buttocks.

Injuries

Has the patient sustained any type of injury that would account for any of the symptoms? What is the location of the injury and the time and mechanism of the injury's occurrence? If the patient was involved in a motor vehicle crash, was the patient restrained? What type of restraint was used (e.g., lap and shoulder belts)? Was the vehicle equipped with airbags, and did they inflate? At what speed did the crash occur? Was there damage to the interior or exterior of the car or steering wheel? What was the extrication time? How many vehicles were involved? Was any object impacted? Were there any fatalities caused by the crash? If the patient has been involved in a motor vehicle crash without impact of the chest area and is having chest pain, suspect angina or an MI. If the chest was impacted, suspect a myocardial contusion and have a high index of suspicion for arrhythmia and tamponade.

Other symptoms

Other pertinent symptoms include a history of palpitations, syncope or near syncope, numbness, a headache, and activity intolerance. For patients with suspected arterial or venous disease, it is imperative to inspect the skin and note any alopecia, nail changes, or ulceration.

Medical history

It is important to determine if the patient has a history of cardiac disease (past MIs, angina, CHF, hypertension, congenital anomalies, angioplasties, or cardiac surgery). These patients are at increased risk for developing a recurrence of a problem or developing a related problem. For example, patients who have had an MI are at greater risk for recurrence or for developing angina or CHF. Also determine if the patient has a history of pulmonary disease (asthma, chronic bronchitis, emphysema, pulmonary hypertension, pleurisy, and congenital pulmonary anomalies or black lung), diabetes (type, how controlled, and a history of complications), renal disease (acute or chronic, type of dialysis, and access used), vascular disease, hepatic disease, smoking, or alcohol abuse. A history of any of the above puts the patient at increased risk for having cardiac or vascular insufficiency.

Medication history

Obtain a complete medication history from the patient, family, or pharmacist. The medication history should include not only prescription medications, but also over-the-counter (OTC) and recreational drug use.

FOCUSED NURSING ASSESSMENT

Nursing assessment centers mainly on perfusion.

Perfusion
Heart sounds

The presence of S_3 or S_4 may indicate heart failure. The presence of a murmur may indicate valvular or septal insufficiency.

Breath sounds

The presence of rales or crackles that do not clear with coughing may indicate CHF.

Color

Pale or cyanotic color may indicate poor cardiac output secondary to an MI or a great vessel problem. Pale or cyanotic extremities that are cool or pulseless indicate an arterial or venous occlusion.

Peripheral pulses

Weak or absent pulses may indicate an acute arterial or venous occlusion; weak pulses may also indicate low cardiac output secondary to an acute MI, CHF, or a great vessel problem.

Capillary refill

Delayed capillary refill indicates low cardiac output, a vessel occlusion, hypothermia, or shock.

Skin temperature

Cool extremities may indicate a vessel occlusion or low cardiac output; also assess skin for diaphoresis, which may indicate pain, anxiety, or low cardiac output.

Blood pressure and heart rate

Obtain blood pressure (BP) and heart rate. A rise in heart rate may indicate anxiety, fluid volume depletion, or low cardiac output. A fall in heart rate may indicate an SA nodal problem or cardiovascular insufficiency. A rise in BP may indicate anxiety, noncompliance with medications, pain, or vasoconstriction. A fall in BP indicates vasodilation, dehydration, or cardiovascular collapse. Prescribed medications such as beta-blockers and calcium channel blockers can adversely affect heart rate and BP.

Ventilation
Breathing patterns

Assess the patient's breathing pattern. Low cardiac output and CHF produce respiratory distress because of pulmonary congestion caused by fluid volume overload in the ventricle. The patient will appear short of breath, have rales on auscultation, or exhibit peripheral edema on examination.

Cardiovascular Risk Factors

1. *Medical history* (see Nursing Alert Box).

NURSING ALERT

Patients with past cardiac or vascular conditions, diabetes, or renal or hepatic disease are at increased risk for additional cardiac or vascular conditions because these patients already have some blood vessel compromise and are at risk for additional insult.

---

2. *Congenital conditions:* Cardiac or pulmonary anomalies can cause patients to be at risk for an MI or the development of CHF.
3. *Smoking history:* Patients who smoke or live with smokers have an increased risk for cardiac and vascular diseases because cigarette smokers and those inhaling second-hand smoke develop blood vessel changes.[2]
4. *Medication history:* Female patients who smoke and use contraceptives experience an increased incidence of vascular disease and have been shown to develop blood clots much more readily.[2] Cocaine users are at risk for developing tachyarrhythmias and myocardial ischemia leading to cardiovascular insufficiency and collapse.[3]

5. *Gender:* Research results suggest that men are at increased risk for heart disease. Hormonal and stress factors have a part in the development of heart disease in men and postmenopausal women.[4]

6. *Heredity:* Patients with a family history of cardiac or vascular disease are at increased risk for these conditions.[4]

7. *Stress and anxiety:* Research has shown that stress and anxiety, as well as a "type A" personality, can lead to an MI.[4]

8. *Age:* As the age of a patient increases beyond the third decade, the risk of cardiovascular disease increases because of blood vessel changes associated with aging.[5]

9. *Hypertension:* Those with uncontrolled or undercontrolled hypertension are at increased risk for an MI because of increased afterload and increased preload on the left side of the heart.[2]

10. *High cholesterol:* Hypercholesterolemia increases risk for an MI because of the increased risk for plaque formation leading to occlusions in the coronary arteries.[2]

11. *Sedentary life style:* Lack of exercise and activity increases the risk for an MI and for vascular occlusion that is related to the development of pooled blood leading to blood clots in the small vessels.[6,4]

12. *Obesity:* Because of the increased risk of a sedentary life style and an increased load on the heart, obese patients are more likely to have vascular occlusions and an MI.[2]

13. *Ethnic and racial origin:* Research demonstrates that nonwhites are more likely to develop cardiovascular disease than whites. Blacks are more likely to develop cardiovascular disease at an early age.[4]

Life Span Issues
Pediatric patients

Cardiovascular conditions in pediatric patients may be diagnosed or undiagnosed congenital anomalies and complications related to their treatment. Cardiovascular complications include CHF, acute MI, and conduction disturbances. CHF is a result of inadequate pumping and may be related to anomalies such as a ventricular septal defect. An MI is always an ischemic event, not an atherosclerotic event, and may be secondary to an anomaly. Bradycardia can be caused by hypoxemia or a conduction disturbance anomaly or may follow surgical correction of a congenital anomaly.[7,8]

Women

More women than men report loss of appetite, paroxysmal nocturnal dyspnea, and back pain as the first symptoms noted in relationship to the onset of an MI. Women are also less likely to report symptoms and less likely to seek or receive treatment for symptoms of an MI.[9]

NURSING ALERT

Always carefully evaluate chest pain during pregnancy.

Pregnancy

Pregnancy-induced cardiomyopathy and pulmonary embolism are life threatening to the mother and the fetus. Hemodynamic changes during pregnancy include a marked increase in blood volume and cardiac output. Peripheral vascular dilatation causes an increased heart rate and decreased BP. During the postpartum period, deep venous thrombosis and pulmonary emboli develop from amniotic emboli. Other conditions that may interfere with the cardiovascular system during pregnancy include pregnancy-induced hypertension, gestational diabetes, vaginal bleeding, spontaneous abortion, placenta previa, abruptio placentae, and postpartum hemorrhage (see Chapter 15).[1]

Geriatric patients

There is an increased incidence of cardiovascular disease in the geriatric patient because of the development of arteriosclerosis that causes increased peripheral vascular resistance. The heart loses elasticity with age and thus is less responsive to demands. It takes the geriatric patient's heart much longer to increase its rate in response to increased activity. There are an increased number of silent myocardial infarctions with increasing age because the nerve innervation to the heart is decreased. Symptoms are not always well described by the geriatric patient because of communication problems, neuropathies, and other physiologic changes associated with aging.[5]

INITIAL INTERVENTIONS

Regardless of the cardiovascular condition, the following interventions may be beneficial:

1. Assess breathing and implement measures to facilitate breathing such as elevating the head of the bed, decreasing sensory stimulation, and allowing the patient to assume a position of comfort. Prepare for endotracheal intubation if there is evidence of severe respiratory distress with airway compromise and no evidence of compensation. If the patient is not breathing, open the airway, ventilate the patient, administer oxygen at 100% per bag-valve mask, and prepare to intubate.

2. Administer oxygen to keep the patient's SpO_2 >90%. If the patient is in no apparent respiratory distress, administer oxygen at 2 L/min per nasal cannula. If the patient appears to be in respiratory distress, administer oxygen at 100% per nonrebreather mask.

3. Assess circulation. If no pulse is present, administer CPR. If there is a pulse present, assess pulses and capillary refill. Establish peripheral intravenous (IV) access, preferably an 18-gauge or larger, and administer D_5W or normal saline at a keep-vein-open rate. If the patient is hypotensive (SBP <90), establish two large-bore IVs and administer a bolus of Ringer's lactate or normal saline and then reassess. If hypotension continues, repeat the procedure.

4. Initiate ECG, blood pressure, and pulse oximetry monitoring as soon as possible.

5. Obtain a 12-lead ECG.

6. Obtain laboratory specimens as ordered by the physician. Anticipate drawing at least an electrolyte panel and a CBC, and possibly a PT/PTT level.

7. If the pain is determined to be possibly cardiac in origin, administer nitroglycerin 0.4 mg sublingual as ordered—approximately one every 3 to 5 min as tolerated by the patient's blood pressure (SBP >90 mm Hg) for three doses, then prepare to initiate a nitroglycerin drip as ordered (Table 5-1). The patient may also be started on nitropaste—1 to 2 inches to the chest wall—or may be given 1 to 3 metered doses of nitrospray to relieve the pain. Continuously monitor the patient's pain, BP, and ECG during nitroglycerin administration, and note any changes.

Text continued on p. 229

TABLE 5-1 Drug Summary

Drug	Dose/route	Special considerations
Abciximab	0.25 mg/kg bolus 10-60 min before starting PTCA	Administration associated with increased frequency of a major bleeding event; contraindicated in patients with a history of recent bleed or surgery Administer in a dedicated IV line, monitor coagulation profile, observe bleeding precautions Coadministered with ASA and heparin, followed by continuous infusion of 10 µg/min for 12 hr postangioplasty
Adenosine	Initial dose: 6 mg rapid IV push (over 1-3 sec); if SVT not resolved in 1-2 min, may administer 12 mg rapid IVP; may repeat × 1 followed by rapid saline flush	Half-life of adenosine is <5 sec Side effects are common but resolve quickly; include flushing, chest pain, and dyspnea Periods of bradycardia and ventricular ectopy may be seen after resolution of the SVT. Patients receiving theophylline, dipyridamole, and carbamazepine may not be candidates for adenosine therapy
Bretylium	Load: 5 mg/kg IV push, then increase to 10 mg/kg IV push every 15-30 min, up to 30 mg/kg Maintenance: 1-2 mg/min IV infusion	Initial bolus may cause hypotension Continuous infusion causes orthostatic hypotension, nausea, and vomiting Use with caution in patients receiving digoxin; this drug increases possibility of toxicity

Continued

C

TABLE 5-1 Drug Summary—cont'd

Drug	Dose/route	Special considerations
Digoxin	Load: 0.5-1 mg orally or IV in divided doses over 24 hr	Observe for toxicity (nausea, vomiting, anorexia, irregular pulse); monitor pulse, serum potassium, and renal function closely
Diltiazem	Bolus: 0.25-0.35 mg/kg IV Maintenance: initiate infusion at 5 mg/hr, titrate to effect	Monitor for hypotension and bradycardia; regulate infusion accordingly Use in patients with atrial fibrillation or flutter with rapid ventricular rates Do not use in patients with AV blocks, WPW, severe hypotension, or shock
Dobutamine	2-20 μg/kg/min IV infusion	Monitor blood pressure and ECG closely; these patients are prone to PVCs and tachycardia
Dopamine	2-20 μg/kg/min IV infusion	Monitor urine output, heart rate, and blood pressure closely DO NOT mix with sodium bicarbonate Extravasation causes tissue necrosis; can be treated with local Regitine
Epinephrine	0.1-1 mg IV bolus; if no effect, may increase to 3-5 mg IV bolus every 5 min Maintenance: IV infusion 1-4 μg/min	DO NOT mix with sodium bicarbonate Adverse effects include hypertension, tachycardia, and ventricular tachycardia

Continued

c

Drug	Dosing	Monitoring
Furosemide	20-200 mg at 20 mg/min IV push	Monitor for alkalosis, nausea, vomiting, diarrhea, hypocalcemia, hyperglycemia, and digoxin toxicity
Heparin	Bolus: 5000 U IV push Maintenance: 800-1200 U/hr IV infusion	Monitor PTT Initiate bleeding precautions Anticoagulant activity of heparin can be reversed with protamine
Hydralazine	10-40 mg IV at 1 mg/min or IM	Monitor for anginal symptoms, tachycardia, hypotension, and palpitations
Enalaprilat	1.25-5 mg q6hr IV over 5 min	Decrease dose with concurrent diuretic therapy; do not use in patients with known renal artery stenosis, monitor creatinine in patients receiving ACE inhibitor for the first time Delayed absorption with hepatic failure; monitor BP closely while administering this medication
Lidocaine	Bolus: 1-1.5 mg/kg IV; may repeat in 3-5 min at half the initial dose to a total of 3 mg/kg bolus, infuse at 3 mg/min, and for a 2.5-3 mg/kg bolus, infuse at 4 mg/min Maintenance: for a 1 mg/kg bolus, infusion rate is 2 mg/min; for a 1.5-2 mg/kg bolus, infuse at 3 mg/min; for a 2.5-3 mg/kg bolus, infuse at 4 mg/min	Maintenance dose may be decreased for geriatric patients or those with poor hepatic function, CNS depression, drowsiness, confusion, or tinnitus

TABLE 5-1 Drug Summary—cont'd

Drug	Dose/route	Special considerations
Metoprolol	5 mg rapid IV push every 2 min for 3 doses	Monitor heart rate and blood pressure; may precipitate heart failure and angina; give with caution in patients with COPD; treat over-dose with atropine
Morphine	1-10 mg every hr IV push or drip; 1-10 mg q2-4hr IM	Titrate dose to effect May cause respiratory depression and pupil constriction Use with caution in patients with hypotension or increased intracra-nial pressure Give Narcan for overdose
Nifedipine	10-20 mg PO or SL (may be avail-able IV in the future)	Main side effect is hypotension; dosage may have to be altered if the patient is receiving concurrent carbamazepine therapy
Nitroglycerin	Begin IV infusion at 5 µg/min and titrate to effect; 0.4 mg SL every 3-5 min as tolerated by blood pressure or pain relief	Closely monitor heart rate and blood pressure Mix IV nitroglycerin in glass bottle and administer through non-PVC tubing to prevent absorption into plastic
Nitroprusside	0.5-10 µg/kg/min IV infusion	Rapid vasodilator; monitor blood pressure closely Drug may be titrated up every 5 min for effect; mix in 5% dextrose in water and protect from light; monitor for toxicity by drawing thio-cyanate levels

Procainamide	Load: 1 g at 20 mg/min IV; infusion: 2-5 mg/min	Stop loading dose for widened QRS or hypotension Monitor drug levels daily Signs of toxicity include fever and torsades de pointes
Streptokinase	1.5 million U IV over 1 hr	Side effects include bleeding, hypotension, arrhythmias, and allergic reactions The patient must not have a repeat dose for 6 months because anaphylaxis may develop Patients who receive streptokinase may be started on low-molecular-weight heparin therapy after their streptokinase dose
TPA	100 mg IV over 3 hr (but protocols may vary)	Administer within 6 hr of onset of chest pain Half-life is 3-5 min Side effects include bleeding and arrhythmias; screen patient for any history of bleeding before drug administration Patients who receive tPA will also receive heparin therapy following tPA administration
Urokinase	6000 IU/min for up to 2 hr IA IV: 4400 U/kg over 10 min followed by 4400 U/kg/hr for 12 hr[16]	Hypotension, bleeding, and arrhythmias are the main side effects Usually given in conjunction with heparin

IA, Intraarterially.

Continued

TABLE 5-1 Drug Summary—cont'd

Drug	Dose/route	Special considerations
Verapamil	5-10 mg IV bolus over 2 min, then repeat doses of 10 mg after 30 min	Hypotension and bradycardia followed by asystole are significant adverse effects; bradycardia and asystole usually result from pushing drug too fast
		May depress myocardial contractility, so give with caution to patients receiving concurrent beta-blocker therapy; also, some patients develop reflex tachycardia as result of accessory pathways; if this occurs, administer calcium and choose another drug to slow the heart rate
		Dosage may have to be adjusted if patient is receiving carbamazepine therapy

8. If the pain is localized to an extremity and possibly related to vascular insufficiency, monitor the color, pulses, pain, movement, and edema in the affected extremity. If an arterial occlusion is suspected, prepare the patient for an angiogram. If a venous injury or occlusion is suspected, anticipate that noninvasive venous studies will be needed.

9. If the pain is caused by a large vessel problem, the patient's BP should be monitored closely and IV sodium nitroprusside or IV labetalol initiated if hypertension develops (IV nifedipine is also being used experimentally for control of hypertension). Anticipate an aortogram or CT scan of the abdomen if aortic disruption is suspected. Hypotension is considered an ominous sign and should be treated with volume resuscitation (Ringer's lactate or normal saline), dopamine, Levophed, or epinephrine drips (Table 5-1).

PRIORITY NURSING DIAGNOSES[6,10]

Risk for decreased cardiac output
Risk for altered tissue perfusion
Risk for pain
Risk for anxiety
Risk for impaired gas exchange
Risk for activity intolerance
Risk for fluid volume excess
Risk for impaired skin integrity
Risk for noncompliance

♦ **Decreased cardiac output** related to inability of the damaged myocardial tissue to pump effectively, as demonstrated by decreased peripheral perfusion, decreased mentation, and poor urinary output:

INTERVENTIONS

• Focus on increasing contractility with medications and decreasing myocardial oxygen demand by decreasing afterload and preload with diuretics, vasodilators, and pain management.

♦ **Altered tissue perfusion** related to decreased cardiac contractility, obstruction of blood flow to vital tissues, or decreased blood volume, as demonstrated by peripheral cyanosis, diminished peripheral pulses, altered mentation, decreased urinary output, chest pain, shortness of breath, decreased cardiac output, cardiac dysrhythmias, increased afterload, increased pulmonary artery pressure, and in-

creased central venous and pulmonary capillary wedge
pressure:

INTERVENTIONS

- Focus on increasing contractility with medications and
  increasing circulating blood volume with fluid.
- Vessel obstruction should be relieved with vasodilators,
  anticoagulants, thrombolytic therapy, or percutaneous
  angioplasty.

♦ **Pain** related to poor tissue perfusion because of obstruction in blood flow, as demonstrated by verbal complaints of
crushing chest pain and extremity pain:

INTERVENTIONS

- Focus on pain relief with medications or positioning.

♦ **Anxiety** related to pain and poor mentation, as demonstrated by behavior, restlessness, and repetitive questioning
about condition:

INTERVENTIONS

- Focus on relieving anxiety with medication or by offering
  reassurance.

♦ **Impaired gas exchange** related to diminished cardiac
contractility and increased afterload, as demonstrated by
poor arterial blood gases, increasing shortness of breath, and
decreased pulse oximetry readings:

INTERVENTIONS

- Administer oxygen to the patient.
- Possibly begin diuresis to relieve some of the volume
  overload.

♦ **Activity intolerance** related to decreased functional
capacity of the heart, as demonstrated by shortness of
breath, fatigue, chest pain, and vital sign changes with
activity:

INTERVENTIONS

- Maintain the patient on strict bed rest during the acute
  phase of the illness.

♦ **Fluid volume excess** related to decreased contractility,
increased afterload, and decreased renal perfusion, as
demonstrated by decreased urinary output, increased peripheral edema, increased pulmonary secretions, decreased cardiac output, and increased pulmonary capillary
wedge pressure:

INTERVENTIONS

- Relieve the fluid overload with diuretics and afterload
  reduction.

♦ **Impaired skin integrity** related to decreased peripheral perfusion, as demonstrated by skin breakdown in the affected areas:

INTERVENTIONS

- Turn the patient frequently.
- Provide pressure relief with pillows and pressure-reduction mattresses.
- Change wound dressings as ordered and note further areas of skin breakdown.

♦ **Noncompliance** related to denial of the severity of the condition, as demonstrated by repeated admissions, low blood levels of measurable medications, and articulation that medication and activity regimen are not being followed:

INTERVENTIONS

- Provide good discharge teaching for the patient and family.
- Provide adequate support for frequent dressing changes and laboratory specimen acquisition, such as home health or local hospital or MD office.
- Provide adequate support for smoking cessation.

PRIORITY DIAGNOSTIC TESTS

Cardiac Conditions

ECG: An electrocardiogram (ECG) determines areas of cardiac injury, myocardial infarction, or conduction disturbance (see Table 5-2).

TABLE 5-2 Location of Infarct and ECG Changes

Location	Changes
Anterior MI	ST elevation in V_1-V_4
Septal infarct	ST elevation in V_1 and V_2
Inferior MI	ST elevation in lead 2, 3, and aV_F
Lateral MI	ST elevation in lead 1, aV_L, V_5, and V_6
Posterior MI	Reciprocal changes in V_1 and V_2—tall R wave, ST depression, and upright T wave
Right ventricular MI	Significant ST elevation in a V_R in patients with an inferior wall MI
Apical infarct	ST elevation in V_5 and V_6

Data from Dubin D: *Rapid interpretation of EKG's*, ed 3, Tampa, 1978, Cover Publishing; Lewis V: *Nurs Clin North Am* 22(1):15-32, 1987; Marriott HJ: *Practical electrocardiography*, ed 7, Baltimore, 1983, Williams & Wilkins.

Laboratory tests

Cardiac isoenzymes: CK and CKMB elevate after an MI. CK first appears in the blood 4 to 6 hours after the onset of pain and peaks at 16 to 36 hours. CKMB is cardiac specific. Also, there is an inversion of LDH_1 and LDH_2 isoenzymes that occurs approximately 24 hours after the onset of pain.[11]

Troponin-1: The test for troponin-1 has a high specificity and sensitivity for cardiac injury. Levels of troponin-1 are elevated very early after a myocardial injury has occurred.

Complete blood count: The white blood cell (WBC) count is elevated with any type of infectious process, and this can be a cause for chest or cardiac pain. Decreased hematocrit would indicate bleeding.

Serum electrolytes: Electrolyte abnormalities can cause a variety of symptoms that are similar to those caused by decreased cardiac output. If diuretics are administered to decrease preload, potassium, sodium, and chloride levels could be altered.

Serum magnesium, phosphorus, and calcium: Low levels of serum magnesium, phosphorus, and calcium could diminish the ability of the heart to pump even further.

PT/PTT: Initially a baseline is helpful. It is nice to know if the patient has an underlying clotting problem, especially if thrombolytic therapy is needed.

Liver function tests: The liver metabolizes many of the cardiac drugs administered.

Arterial blood gases: Deterioration in the respiratory status can be monitored, and an initial baseline is helpful.

Serum creatinine and BUN: Serum creatinine and blood urea nitrogen (BUN) provide an indication of renal function. One or both of these values will be elevated in renal failure and will continue to increase in the presence of renal insufficiency or hypoperfusion.

Radiographic tests

Chest x-ray: A chest x-ray examination rules out any radiographic cause of chest pain and gives an indication of the presence of pulmonary disease and edema.

Other tests

Echocardiogram: An echocardiogram gives an indication of myocardial damage by looking at wall motion and giving an indication of ejection fraction. Echocardiography is

helpful for assessing valve function using the transthoracic approach.[4]

Pericardiocentesis: A pericardiocentesis is done in the event
of ventricular asystole or pulseless electrical activity. If fluid
is present and can be evacuated, cardiac function will increase because the heart will be able to contract better.

Diagnostic cardiac catheterization: A diagnostic cardiac
catheterization visualizes patency of the coronary arteries and valves and measures ventricular ejection fraction. Coronary angioplasty and stent placement can
be done at the same time as the catheterization if the
lesions are such that the patient will benefit from the
procedure.

Exercise tolerance test: A dramatic increase in the heart
rate with little work is indicative of the heart's inability to
pump effectively. ST depression (>1 mm) during exercise indicates ischemia. This is a test that may be ordered
on an outpatient basis and may be part of the discharge
instructions.[4]

Vascular Conditions

Angiography: An angiography directly images an artery
through a percutaneously inserted sheath to visualize any
narrowing, occlusion, or rupture.[12] Percutaneous angioplasty and stent placement can be done at the time of
this procedure to relieve any occlusion or stenosis that
may be causing poor perfusion.

Duplex examination: A duplex examination is a combination of both Doppler flow through a blood vessel and direct ultrasound color-flow imaging of an occlusion. This
may be done to image an artery or vein.[13]

Laboratory tests

Serum electrolytes: Assess for any electrolyte imbalance
and obtain a baseline before any drug administration.

Serum creatinine and BUN: These tests provides an indication of renal function.

Complete blood count: The result of a CBC indicates any
blood loss or infectious process.

Liver function tests: The result of a liver function test indicates any liver damage that could interfere with drug administration or blood clotting.

Type and crossmatch: Obtaining a type and crossmatch allows for blood and blood products to be available if

bleeding starts or if operative management of the condition occurs.

Arterial blood gases: Baseline acid-base status is important and oxygenation to poorly perfused areas should be optimal. This also gives an indication of pulmonary function that would be important if operative management were necessary.

PT/PTT: A baseline and continuous monitoring are necessary, especially if anticoagulants are administered.

Radiographic tests

Chest x-ray: A chest x-ray examination will detect any widening of the mediastinum indicating aortic dissection. This is also done for preoperative evaluation if surgical intervention is necessary.

Acute abdominal series: An acute abdominal series rules out any problem or disruption of the abdominal aorta—aneurysms will occasionally be seen on x-ray films.[12]

CT scan of the abdomen: A CT scan of the abdomen will give a transverse view that will show an abdominal aortic aneurysm and give a measurement of the aneurysm.[12] This also rules out other processes that may be present in the abdomen.

Other tests

Electrocardiogram: Obtaining a baseline is necessary preoperatively. Repeat ECGs may be ordered to monitor for changes in response to treatment.

Doppler flow studies: These studies are noninvasive and they give an indication of arterial and venous flow in the extremities. They also measure pressures in the extremities. When a systolic wave is prolonged, there is a probable occlusion.[12]

Venogram: A venogram provides direct visualization through injected contrast of the vein, and any occlusion can be visualized.[12]

COLLABORATIVE INTERVENTIONS

1. Oxygen should be provided to all patients with cardiovascular insufficiency in order to optimize oxygenation to all cells.
2. Initiate IV access in order to administer any medications that may be needed and as a precaution if the patient should arrest.

3. Allow the patient to assume a comfortable position in bed in order to allow for adequate oxygenation and minimal anxiety.
4. An ECG allows for diagnosis of any cardiac problem and gives a basis for treatment.

Clinical Conditions
Myocardial infarction
SYMPTOMS

- The patient experiences chest pain with or without radiation to the left arm, neck, or jaw. The pain is sometimes accompanied by nausea, diaphoresis, pallor, or shortness of breath.
- Pain may be described as sharp, heaviness, tightness, crushing, burning, or squeezing; it may be severe or vague and may occur at rest or during activity.

DIAGNOSIS

- A 12-lead ECG will show changes (Table 5-2), but changes may not be evident on the initial ECG; therefore history and risk factors should be considered.
- Changes in cardiac isoenzymes will occur; the CPK increases 4 to 6 hours after the onset of the infarct and peaks 16 to 36 hours after the infarct.[11]
- The troponin-1 level begins rising within 1 hour of the injury; it is the most sensitive and reliable test to indicate an MI.[11]
- The LDH level also increases within 24 hours of an infarct and peaks 48 to 72 hours after the infarct.[11]
- Abnormality in the LDH isoenzymes (LDH_1 and LDH_2) also indicates myocardial necrosis.[11]
- Other positive indicators of myocardial damage include an echocardiogram, which assesses cardiac wall motion and valvular function, and a diagnostic cardiac catheterization. A cardiac catheterization provides direct visualization of the coronary arteries in order to detect spasm or blockage and measures cardiac pressures as well as LV function.

TREATMENT

- Provide continuous cardiac monitoring.
- Administer oxygen therapy (2 L/min per nasal cannula if not in respiratory distress).
- Administer nitroglycerin titrated to pain relief and BP.

- Begin thrombolytic therapy (tPA or streptokinase) in conjunction with heparin, aspirin, beta-blockers such as Lopressor IV, and calcium channel blockers such as diltiazem IV.[14] The earlier that thrombolytic therapy is initiated, the greater is the survival benefit.[15]
- If pain continues after thrombolytic therapy, morphine sulfate IV should be administered. Morphine is the drug of choice for relief of pain associated with an acute MI.[15]
- Later interventions include percutaneous transluminal coronary angioplasty (PTCA) for blocked coronary arteries, coronary artery bypass grafting, and intraaortic balloon pumping to increase coronary artery perfusion, decrease afterload, and relieve continuing pain.

Angina
SYMPTOMS
- The patient experiences substernal or epigastric pain that occurs with activity or emotional stress.
- Pain usually lasts 3 to 5 minutes but may last up to 20 minutes.
- Pain varies in severity and presents as a heaviness, tightness, fullness, squeezing, or crushing.
- Pain is intermittent in origin and usually develops in those patients who have a history of angina, a previous MI, hypertension, or diabetes.

DIAGNOSIS
- If the patient is having pain at the time that the ECG is done, ischemia will be evident on the ECG and will show ST segment depression.
- There will be no elevation in cardiac enzymes.

TREATMENT
- Provide oxygen, nitroglycerin for pain relief, beta-blockers, and calcium channel blockers.
- Decreasing stress, finding a position of comfort, decreasing environmental stimuli, and maintaining a calm manner while caring for the patient may also alleviate anginal symptoms.

Congestive heart failure
SYMPTOMS
- CHF is associated with fluid overload.
- Symptoms of CHF include peripheral edema, cough, crackles, tachypnea, orthopnea, shortness of breath, fa-

tigue, weight gain, and S_3 gallop; later symptoms include pink, frothy sputum, tachycardia, and cyanosis.

DIAGNOSIS

- A chest x-ray examination will show infiltrates and an enlarged heart.
- Arterial blood gases will show hypoxemia and acidosis.
- The ECG will show ventricular enlargement.

TREATMENT

- Provide oxygen (may require higher concentration of oxygen to keep saturation >95%).
- Assist the patient in maintaining a position of comfort.
- Obtain IV access for administration of furosemide and administration of inotropic agents such as digoxin, dobutamine, or morphine to decrease anxiety and decrease the work of breathing.
- Anticipate the use of vasodilators such as nitroglycerin, nitroprusside, or hydralazine to decrease BP as well as afterload.
- Maintain an anxiety-free environment to ensure a better outcome for the patient.

Cardiogenic shock

SYMPTOMS

- The most common cause is an MI, so symptoms are similar but much more severe.
- Cardiogenic shock can also be caused by chest trauma or end-stage cardiomyopathy.
- All symptoms center on decreased cardiac output: confusion; decreased urine output; poor peripheral perfusion; signs of pulmonary congestion, including crackles, tachypnea, and orthopnea; tachycardia; and usually a feeling of impending doom ("I'm going to die").

DIAGNOSIS

- An ECG may show cardiac arrhythmias and usually an MI. Arterial blood gas studies show hypoxia and metabolic acidosis.

TREATMENT

- Provide oxygen and prepare for endotracheal intubation.
- Establish IV access to provide a combination of medications, such as furosemide and nitrates, to decrease preload; medication such as dopamine and dobutamine to

increase contractility; and medications such as nitroprus-side to decrease afterload.

- If cardiac output and tissue perfusion continue to be in-adequate, consider intraaortic balloon pump therapy.[16] Also, be prepared to initiate ACLS protocol; mortality from this state of shock is 80% to 90%.

Sudden cardiac death

SYMPTOMS

- Sudden cardiac death is sometimes accompanied by pal-pitations, dizziness, chest pain, or shortness of breath, but some patients have no warning.
- If the patient has lived through multiple episodes of sud-den death, there may be an aura that the patient can relay.
- There is a loss of consciousness with a period of loss of pulse and blood pressure.

DIAGNOSIS

- The electrocardiogram shows ventricular fibrillation or ventricular tachycardia.

TREATMENT

- Per ACLS protocol, establish an airway, begin ventilation, and administer oxygen (see Reference Guide 1).
- Administer CPR.
- Defibrillate.
- Establish IV access and administer antidysrhythmics such as lidocaine, bretylium, and procainamide.
- If the patient survives sudden death, evaluation for an automatic implantable cardioverter-defibrillator (AICD) should be initiated.
- If the patient has an AICD in place, ACLS protocol should be followed. The rescuer will not be shocked by the AICD as long as rubber gloves are worn while doing chest compressions, and the defibrillator will not damage the AICD.[7]

Cardiac arrest

SYMPTOMS

- There is an absence of respiration and an absence of pulse and blood pressure.
- The patient is unresponsive and cyanotic, and pupils do not react to light.

DIAGNOSIS

- An ECG shows ventricular fibrillation or tachycardia or pulseless electrical activity or asystole in two leads.

- ABGs show metabolic and respiratory acidosis, especially if the patient has been in cardiac arrest for a prolonged period.

TREATMENT

- After taking care of the ABCs, try to determine the underlying cause, such as cardiac tamponade, hypovolemia, hypoxemia, a tension pneumothorax, or acidosis, and treat if possible.
- Use ACLS protocol to treat cardiac arrest.
- Epinephrine will be the first and most frequently used drug before and after IV access has been established; epinephrine may be given through the endotracheal tube if IV access has not been obtained.
- Always ensure that the ECG leads are properly applied before deciding that the patient is in asystole and ALWAYS check asystole in two leads.

Endocarditis

SYMPTOMS

- Symptoms include fever, chills, fatigue, weight loss, anorexia, and night sweats.
- The patient usually has a history of cardiac surgery or some other invasive procedure, such as IV drug use, or of congenital heart disease or rheumatic heart disease.
- The patient is often tachycardic, has a new cardiac murmur or petechiae, and has signs of cardiac failure such as peripheral edema.

DIAGNOSIS

- The WBC count is increased.
- Blood cultures are positive.
- The serum glucose level is increased secondary to the infectious process.
- A chest x-ray examination shows a heart enlargement.
- The erythrocyte sedimentation rate is elevated secondary to the ongoing inflammatory process.
- Definitive diagnosis is made by an echocardiogram that shows valvular incompetence or valvular vegetation.

TREATMENT

- Administer antibiotics that are specific to the infectious agent.
- Provide palliative treatment for fever, such as Tylenol.
- Provide symptomatic treatment of heart failure.

Pericarditis

SYMPTOMS

- The patient experiences sudden, severe, sharp chest pain that may radiate to the back or shoulders and increases with movement or inspiration; the pain usually occurs after open-heart surgery or radiation therapy.
- A pericardial friction rub is audible along the left lower sternal border.
- The patient may experience tachycardia and hypotension that may be the result of decreasing cardiac output associated with cardiac compression from the accumulated fluid in the pericardial sac.

DIAGNOSIS

- A chest x-ray examination will show cardiomegaly with clear lung fields.
- An ECG will show ST elevation in the limb leads and in the precordial leads, but there are no QRS changes.
- An echocardiogram will be definitive in showing an accumulation of fluid in the pericardial sac.

TREATMENT

- Pericardiocentesis may need to be performed for a large effusion to prevent cardiac tamponade and cardiac failure.
- Antiinflammatory drugs or analgesics will help relieve the associated pain.
- Treatment of any underlying condition such as an MI, infection, or rheumatic fever is paramount.
- Surgical interventions such as a pericardial window or pericardiectomy will decrease discomfort and accumulation of fluid.

Acute aortic dissection

SYMPTOMS

- Back pain and pain between the shoulder blades are the most common presenting symptoms.
- Late symptoms include decreasing hematocrit and hypovolemic shock associated with profound blood loss.
- If the dissection involves the thoracic aorta, chest pain may be the presenting symptom. The pain is knife-like and radiates down the back and into the lower extremities.
- There is a BP difference in the right and left extremities or in the upper and lower extremities.
- Peripheral pulses will be diminished or absent.

DIAGNOSIS

- A chest x-ray examination will show a widening of the aorta in the area of the dissection.
- A definitive diagnosis is an aortogram that rules out acute dissection.

TREATMENT

- Controlling the arterial BP to maintain mean arterial pressures between 60 and 80 mm Hg is paramount; use of sodium nitroprusside is indicated acutely.
- If the patient is in shock associated with leaking or rupture, vigorous fluid resuscitation is indicated.
- Replacement of blood loss with packed red blood cells may be necessary.
- If symptoms progress, surgical intervention is necessary.

Acute arterial occlusion

SYMPTOMS

- The patient may experience a sudden onset of extremity pain and numbness; this usually occurs in the patient with a history of peripheral atherosclerotic disease.
- A pale, cool, cyanotic extremity with the absence of peripheral pulses associated with paresthesia is a common presentation.

DIAGNOSIS

- Doppler flow studies will clearly show arterial occlusion.
- Invasive studies such as arteriograms also show arterial occlusion.[2]

TREATMENT

- Initiation of heparin therapy is common, along with intraarterial urokinase infusions.
- If the occlusion is severe, the patient may require an embolectomy or angioplasty.

Venous thrombosis

SYMPTOMS

- The patient experiences pain, tenderness, swelling, and warmth of the affected extremity, along with a positive Homans' sign.
- The patient usually has had a period of bed rest for some reason, including acute or chronic illness, or is receiving IV injections.

DIAGNOSIS

- A venogram is a definitive indicator of a deep venous thrombosis.[2]

- Other diagnostic indicators include a venous duplex examination and measurements of the extremities to show a difference right to left.

TREATMENT
- Heparinization is the definitive treatment for DVT.
- Follow-up treatment includes warfarin sodium (Coumadin) therapy, usually for 1 year after deep venous thrombosis.

NURSING SURVEILLANCE

1. Monitor vital signs, including oxygen saturation.
2. Monitor for relief of pain.
3. Monitor for level of pain.
4. Monitor I/O and continually assess fluid balance.
5. Monitor the ECG for any changes or dysrhythmias.
6. Monitor mentation, an indicator of perfusion.
7. Monitor peripheral perfusion and peripheral pulses.

EXPECTED PATIENT OUTCOMES

1. Pain decreases in severity as documented on the "1 to 10" pain scale.
2. Systolic BP is maintained above 90 mm Hg.
3. Heart rate is maintained above 60 beats/min and below 100 beats/min.
4. Urine output is >30 ml/hr.
5. Mental status is at baseline; the patient is awake and alert.
6. Oxygen saturations are >95%.
7. Peripheral perfusion is restored or maintained.

DISCHARGE IMPLICATIONS
Cardiac

1. Teach the patient and family the signs of an MI and when medical assistance is needed for symptoms. Teach the patient and family to use 911.
2. Teach the patient how to use sublingual nitroglycerin or nitropaste.
3. Instruct the patient and family about the use of discharge medications and give medication information sheets to the patient or family for reference.
4. Instruct the family on the importance of CPR training in the event of a cardiac arrest.

5. Instruct the patient and family on the importance of follow-up care.

Vascular

1. Instruct the patient and family on the importance of getting coagulation studies checked frequently.
2. Instruct the patient on what to look for in the event of reocclusion.
3. For patients with suspected or documented aortic aneurysms, teach signs of rupture and impending rupture. Stress the importance of follow-up care.
4. For patients with peripheral vascular disease, teach palliative measures for their pain, such as the use of support hose and elevation of the extremity.

References

1. Rea R et al, editors: *Emergency nursing core curriculum,* ed 4, Philadelphia, 1994, WB Saunders.
2. Doyle J: Treatment modalities in peripheral vascular disease, *Nurs Clin North Am* 21(2):241-253, 1986.
3. Vazquez M, Lazear S, Larson E: *Critical care nursing,* ed 2, Philadelphia, 1992, WB Saunders.
4. Rossi L, Leary E: Evaluating the patient with coronary artery disease, *Nurs Clin North Am* 27(1):171-188, 1992.
5. Ebersole P, Hess P: *Toward healthy aging: human needs and nursing response,* ed 3, St Louis, 1990, Mosby.
6. Herman J: Nursing assessment and nursing diagnosis in patients with peripheral vascular disease, *Nurs Clin North Am* 21(2):219-231, 1986.
7. Lundberg GD, editor: Guidelines for cardiopulmonary resuscitation and emergency cardiac care: recommendations of the 1992 national conference of the American Heart Association, *JAMA* 268(16):2135-2302, 1992.
8. Majoros K: Comparisons and controversies in clot busting drugs, *Crit Care Nurs Q* 16(2):46-69, 1993.
9. Penque S et al: Women and coronary disease: relationship between descriptors of signs and symptoms and diagnostic and treatment course, *Am J Crit Care* 7(3):175-182, 1998.
10. Gordon M: *Manual of nursing diagnosis,* New York, 1987, McGraw-Hill.
11. Lewis V: Monitoring the patient with an acute myocardial infarction, *Nurs Clin North Am* 22(1):15-32, 1987.
12. Massey J: Diagnostic testing for peripheral vascular disease, *Nurs Clin North Am* 21(2):207-218, 1986.

13. Faust G, Cohen J: *Vascular surgery,* ed 3, Baltimore, 1998, Williams & Wilkins.
14. Leach R: A tPA ninety minute protocol, *J Emerg Nurs* 19:338-339, 1993.
15. Marino PM: *The ICU book,* ed 2, Baltimore, 1998, Williams & Wilkins.
16. Horvath P, editor: *Care of the adult cardiac surgery patient,* New York, 1984, John Wiley & Sons.

Chapter 6

Communicable Diseases

Pamela S. Kidd

C

CLINICAL CONDITIONS
Acute Rheumatic Fever
Acute Streptococcal Infection
Cellulitis and Skin and Soft Tissue Infection
Diphtheria
Food Poisoning
Hepatitis
Human Immunodeficiency Virus
Lyme Disease
Measles
Meningococcal Infection
Mononucleosis
Mumps Parotitis
Pertussis
Rubella (German measles)
Tetanus
Tuberculosis
Varicella (chickenpox)

TRIAGE ASSESSMENT

Many patients will come to the triage area with symptoms of a communicable or infectious disease. This chapter provides an overview of the communicable and infectious diseases most frequently encountered in the emergency department (ED). It is not meant to be a comprehensive review. The reader may need to refer to a communicable disease text for more information. A thorough history at triage is necessary, since many of these patients will need to wait for treatment. The triage nurse must determine if isolation of the patient is necessary before determining if a treatment bed is available.

Start with questions about the following topics to help determine if isolation or mask protection may be necessary. In general, most communicable diseases are spread by droplet routes through coughing and sneezing. A patient who is unable to use hygiene measures (e.g., turning head or covering mouth) during coughing and sneezing because of cognition level or physical status should be masked. If symptoms suggest the possibility of tuberculosis, masking the patient is appropriate until diagnosis is made and treatment is initiated. A patient with a visible rash or vesicles (those not covered with clothing) should be taken to a separate, private waiting area (such as the grief or quiet room).

Exposure
Ask if another member of the family or work and school contacts have been ill. If so, have the patient describe their symptoms. Table 6-1 includes incubation periods for common communicable diseases.

Travel
Travel to other countries may be associated with a higher incidence of drug-resistant tuberculosis (DR-TB), hepatitis A and E, *Escherichia coli* food poisoning, and Lyme disease (e.g., travel to Asia is associated with an increased risk for DR-TB).

Malaise
If the patient complains of malaise, lethargy, anorexia, and frequent colds and cough, ask about the patient's sexual history, history of injection drug use, and hemophilia. Primary human immunodeficiency virus (HIV) infection produces symptoms of fever, myalgia, fatigue, and sore throat.

Communicable disease history
Determine if the patient has or has had a communicable disease. HIV-positive individuals should be considered tuberculosis positive until proven otherwise.[1,2] Determine the date of diagnosis of HIV, since progression to acquired immunodeficiency syndrome (AIDS) usually occurs within 10 years after initial infection. Complications such as subacute sclerosing panencephalitis (progressive neurologic deficit) occur later in childhood after either a measles infection or inoculation with the live measles virus vaccine. A patient may have had other episodes of shingles (herpes zoster).

Treatment for previous or current communicable disease
If the patient has had a communicable disease, determine the course of treatment. DR-TB generally occurs in people

Text continued on p. 254

TABLE 6-1 Comparison of Communicable Disease

Disease	Adult symptoms	Pediatric symptoms	High-risk group	Diagnosis	Treatment	Incubation period	Transmission route	Peak period	Complications
Pertussis	Persistent cough lasting >7 days	Paroxysmal cough Whoop Cough-induced vomiting Leukocytosis	Infants 1-2 mo old Females >males <3 doses of DTP vaccine	Antipertussis toxin 1 g G antibody measured by enzyme-linked immunosorbent assay Culture of nasopharyngeal secretions	Erythromycin	7-13 days	Respiratory secretions	Every 3-4 yr	Pneumonia Seizures Cranial nerve abnormalities
Rubeola (typical)	Fever Macular rash progressing head to toe Koplik's spots Photophobia	Fever Macular rash progressing head to toe Koplik's spots Photophobia	Persons in late teens and early 20s	Hemoagglutination inhibition and complement-fixation tests	Symptomatic Antipyretics Fluids Dark room Measles vaccine within 72 hours of exposure	10-12 days	Droplets from nasopharyngeal tract	Winter and spring	Encephalitis
Rubeola (atypical)	Headache Arthralgia Abdominal pain Macular rash starting with extremities and moving central	Headache Arthralgia Abdominal pain Macular rash starting with extremities and moving central	Adults born between 1957 and 1967	Hemoagglutination inhibition and complement-fixation tests	Symptomatic	10-14 days	Droplets from nasopharyngeal tract	Winter and spring	Rare

Continued

C

TABLE 6-1 Comparison of Communicable Disease—cont'd

Disease	Adult symptoms	Pediatric symptoms	High-risk group	Diagnosis	Treatment	Incubation period	Transmission route	Peak period	Complications
Mumps	Epididymo-orchitis Testicular atrophy Meningitis	Low-grade fever Headache Vomiting Sore throat Unilateral or bilateral paroid swelling	15-19-yr-olds (not vaccinated or infected)	Clinical presentation	Symptomatic Adult males are placed on bed rest Analgesics	2-3 weeks	Droplet, oral contact Contact with articles recently contaminated with saliva	Winter and early spring	Sterility Meningitis
Rubella	Rash Low-grade fever Malaise Conjunctivitis Sore throat	Pink papular rash on face and neck that spreads to extremities	7 mo to 40 yr	Rubella antibody assay tests	Symptomatic Antipyretics (no aspirin)	14-21 days	Droplets from nasopharyngeal tract	Winter and early spring	Arthralgia Arthritis, congenital rubella syndrome for infants born to females who acquire rubella in first trimester of pregnancy

Varicella (chickenpox)	Low-grade fever Lesions in several stages (macules, papules, vesicles, crusted lesions) Rash appears on trunk, then face and scalp Lesions in mouth, throat, and conjunctiva	Low-grade fever Lesions in several stages (macules, papules, vesicles, crusted lesions) Rash appears on trunk, then face and scalp Lesions in mouth, throat, and conjunctiva	Immuno-compromised individuals	By clinical presentation	Antihistamines 125-625 U of Varicella immunoglobulin in within 96 hours of exposure, use in pregnant women, immunocompromised	10-21 days	Direct contact with vesicle discharge or mucous membranes	Winter and spring	Encephalitis Pneumonia May precede Reye's syndrome
Tetanus	Pain Stiffness in the jaw, abdomen, or back Dysphagia Reflex spasms	Pain Stiffness in the jaw, abdomen, or back Dysphagia Reflex spasms	Occupational groups (wounds obtained in farming, forestry activities) Persons over age 50	By clinical presentation and absence of serum antibody level	500-6000 U IM of human tetanus immunoglobulin Benzodiazepines to treat spasms Neuromuscular blocking agents (e.g., pancuronium)	2 hours to 7 days	Contact between an open wound and spores in the soil	Variable, based on contact with soil, especially where horses are present	Respiratory failure

C

Continued

TABLE 6-1 Comparison of Communicable Disease—cont'd

Disease	Adult symptoms	Pediatric symptoms	High-risk group	Diagnosis	Treatment	Incubation period	Transmission route	Peak period	Complications
Multidrug-resistant tuberculosis	Weight loss Fever Night sweats Cough Hemoptysis Chest pain (treatment for adults is 6 months)	Children may have more extrapulmonary symptoms (e.g., abdominal pain) (treatment for children is 9 months)	Foreign-born persons from India, China, Philippines Alcoholics, IV drug abusers Institutionalized individuals (prisons, nursing homes)	Presence of acid-fast bacilli on sputum smear Lesions on chest x-ray Positive tuberculin skin test	Respiratory isolation for 2 weeks Usually treated with isoniazid and rifampin	2-10 weeks, although can be latent for over 50 years (immuno-suppressed individuals will usually develop active TB within 4-8 weeks)	By droplets from nasopharyngeal tract through coughing, talking, sneezing, singing	Variable	Meningitis Hematologic abnormalities Pleural effusion
Tuberculosis	Cough Weight loss Diarrhea Abdominal pain Changes in mental status	Cough Weight loss Diarrhea Abdominal pain Changes in mental status	Immuno-compromised individuals (HIV positive)	Anergy testing comparing reaction to purified protein derivative with other antigen reactions	Treatment should last for at least 12 months Treatment requires use of at least 3 drugs not used previously (INH, rifampin, ethambutol, pyrazinamide, streptomycin)	2-10 weeks, although can be latent for over 50 years (immuno-suppressed individuals will usually develop active TB within 4-8 weeks)	By droplets from nasopharyngeal tract through coughing, talking, sneezing, singing	Variable	Meningitis Hematologic abnormalities Pleural effusion

	Symptoms (Adult)	Symptoms (Children)	Risk Groups	Diagnostic Tests	Treatment/Prophylaxis	Incubation	Transmission	Course	Complications
Hepatitis A	Anorexia Nausea and vomiting, aversion to cigarettes Right upper quadrant abdominal pain	Same symptoms as adult but less severe	Contact with family member who is infected Day care centers, foreign travel	Anti-HAV IgM antibody confirm active hepatitis A, or previous	Immunoglobulin given for anticipated exposure (0.02 ml/kg IM)	15-50 days	Fecal-oral transmission spread by saliva, contaminated food and water	Variable	No chronic implications; confers lifelong immunity
Hepatitis B	Jaundice Anorexia Nausea and vomiting Right upper quadrant abdominal pain Jaundice Rash and arthralgias Jaundice is less severe	Same symptoms as adult but less severe	Health care workers Sexually promiscuous IV drug abusers	HBsAg—presence of hepatitis B surface antigen HBeAg—"e" antigen indicates high infectivity	Hepatitis B immune globulin (0.06 ml/kg IM) and hepatitis B vaccine given after exposure (0, 1, 6 mo)	45-160 days	Parenteral or sexual transmission via blood, saliva, semen, and vaginal secretions	Variable	Chronic hepatitis Liver cancer
Non-A, non-B hepatitis (hepatitis C)	Blood dyscrasia Arthritis Hepatomegaly Malaise	Same symptoms as adult but less severe	Health care workers IV drug abusers Hemophiliacs Renal patients	Elevation of alanine aminotransferase Anti-hepatitis C antibodies in serum	Symptomatic treatment Corticosteroids may be used Acyclovir Immunoglobulin (0.06 ml/kg ×2 within firs 2 weeks of exposure)	2-26 weeks	Percutaneous transmission through blood transfusions, pooled plasma products, IV drug abuse, hemodialysis	Variable	Chronic hepatitis Cirrhosis Liver cancer

Continued

TABLE 6-1 Comparison of Communicable Disease—cont'd

Disease	Adult symptoms	Pediatric symptoms	High-risk group	Diagnosis	Treatment	Incubation period	Transmission route	Peak period	Complications
Hepatitis D (coinfection with hepatitis B)	Hepatomegaly Jaundice (more severe symptoms than seen with hepatitis B alone)	—	IV drug abusers Hemophiliacs	Anti-hepatitis D antibodies in serum	Hepatitis B immune globulin and hepatitis B vaccine given after exposure	15-64 days	Parenteral or sexual transmission	Variable	Chronic hepatitis
Hepatitis E	Anorexia Nausea and vomiting Right upper quadrant abdominal pain Jaundice	Occurs rarely in children	Visitors to developing countries Rare in U.S.	No diagnostic test available	Symptomatic	15-50 days	Fecal-oral; spread by contaminated water	Variable	High mortality rate in pregnant women
Human immuno-deficiency virus	Vaginal candidiasis Recurrent shingles Oral candidiasis Skin condition Fatigue Visual changes Fever Sore throat	Vaginal candidiasis Recurrent shingles Oral candidiasis Skin condition Fatigue Visual changes Fever Sore throat	Homosexuals, predominantly male IV drug abusers Hispanics Blacks Sex workers (prostitutes) Hemophiliacs	Western blot positive for antibodies against HIV	Zidovudine Acyclovir Treatment of opportunistic infections (e.g., Pneumocystis, Candida)	Unknown	Parenteral or sexual transmission	Variable	May present first with hepatitis B, syphilis, and tuberculosis

Lyme disease	Bull's eye rash Fever Headache Neck pain Myalgia	Bull's eye rash Fever Headache Neck pain Myalgia	Children between 5 and 14 years old Hikers in New England, mid-Atlantic, north central U.S. regions	Punch biopsy of rash shows spirochetes with antibodies to *Borrelia burgdorferi*	Doxycycline, ampicillin, or azithromycin	3-30 days	Bite of tick infected with *B. burgdorferi*	Summer and early fall	Carditis Encephalitis Arthritis
Acute rheumatic fever	Appears rarely as primary disease in adults	Fever Malaise Weight loss Arthralgia Carditis Chorea Subcutaneous nodules	Ethnic groups Children (less likely after puberty)	Presence of streptococcal antibodies Positive throat culture for group A *Streptococcus*	Salicylates Supportive treatment Steroids may be given for carditis	2-3 weeks	Initial infection with group A *Streptococcus* (usually strep throat or fever)	Variable	Carditis/valve disease Polyarthritis Chorea

who have had incomplete treatment for TB or in natives of a country or region with a high rate of DR-TB (e.g., Haiti, Latin America, or Southeast Asia). Several factors may activate dormant TB lesions, including diabetes, steroid therapy, malnutrition, and alcohol abuse.

Living conditions

A large family, bedroom overcrowding, inadequate access to clean water, and poor ventilation have been associated with streptococcal infections (e.g., acute rheumatic fever), tuberculosis, and hepatitis A.

Cough

Pertussis should be considered in all people who have had a cough lasting more than 7 days.[3] A paroxysmal cough is associated with pertussis in all age groups. Persistent, unrelieved coughing that interrupts sleep is associated with tuberculosis. When a cough persists for 3 weeks or more after a cold, TB should be considered.[4] Hemoptysis is also associated with tuberculosis.

Genetic factors

Ask if another member of the family has a history of communicable diseases. Acute rheumatic fever has been linked with genetic factors.

Medical history

Acute rheumatic fever may have developed in patients with an earlier diagnosis of streptococcal infection. Persons with impaired venous drainage (as a result of peripheral vascular disease or coronary bypass graft surgery using the saphenous vein) are at increased risk for cellulitis. Diabetes associated with hypertension causes a greater number of skin and soft tissue infections. Latin and Native American diabetic patients have diabetic complications earlier. Hemophilic patients and those receiving hemodialysis have a higher incidence of hepatitis B, C, and D. An altered immune system increases the likelihood of a herpes zoster infection.

Speech

Numbness around the mouth and slurred speech with muscle weakness and malaise are associated with botulism.

Mood and memory changes

Ask about mood and memory changes, headaches, and neck stiffness, since encephalitis and meningitis are complications from several communicable diseases (e.g., measles, acute rheumatic fever, Lyme disease, and chickenpox). Patients may exhibit complications and not the initial

illness. These symptoms also suggest the possibility of an
opportunistic infection for an HIV-infected individual.

Injection drug use

Hepatitis B, C, and D and HIV infection are more common
among injection drug users.

Nausea, vomiting, and diarrhea

Gastrointestinal complaints occur in several varieties of
food poisoning. If the patient complains of nausea, vomiting, diarrhea, and abdominal cramping, obtain a diet history for the preceding 24 hours (Table 6-2). Ask about the
number of stools and their character in the past 24 hours.
Determine the number of times the patient vomited in the
past 24 hours.

Immunizations

Ask if the patient has had prior immunizations and, if so,
what vaccines were used, the number of doses that were
given, and when the immunizations were received.
Underimmunized children are at increased risk for complications from most communicable diseases (Table 6-1). If
the patient has received the varicella vaccine, the likelihood of a varicella or herpes zoster infection is minimal.

Over-the-counter drug use

Ask if over-the-counter (OTC) medications have relieved
the patient's symptoms. The arthritis associated with acute
rheumatic fever responds dramatically to aspirin.

Pain

In some communicable diseases the pain is more severe
than associated physical findings would indicate. Arthritis
pain caused by acute rheumatic fever is severe, but joint inflammation signs may be minimal. The pain associated with
a herpes zoster infection is confined to a specific location
and may involve burning or tingling.

Insect bite

Ask if the patient was bitten by an insect and, if so, by what
type. Did the patient bring the insect with him or her? In
the case of Lyme disease, the likelihood of an infection increases with the duration of the tick's feeding.

NURSING ALERT

Do not attempt to remove a feeding tick by using a lighted
match, chemicals, or petroleum jelly. These substances may
cause the tick to release more organisms (spirochetes) into

Continued

NURSING ALERT—cont'd

the patient's skin. Ticks should be removed using tweezers and gentle traction pulling at the mouth. Squeezing the abdomen may release a greater number of spirochetes. Attach the tick to an index card using clear tape. Label the date of the bite, the part of the body bitten, and the locale from which the tick came. The tick can be checked for the presence of spirochetes.

Vital Signs

- *Tachycardia:* Tachycardia out of proportion with fever is a sign of carditis. Carditis is a symptom of acute rheumatic fever. Many times, the patient will seek health care for complications from a strep infection but not for the initial infection because the initial infection was mild. Tachycardia

TABLE 6-2 Varieties of Food Poisoning

Organism	Susceptible foods	Symptoms	Incubation period
Staphylococcus aureus	Cream pastries Mayonnaise Mayonnaise-based salads	Vomiting Headache	1-8 hr
Clostridium botulinum	Canned low-acid vegetables Canned fruits Canned fish	Descending weakness Paralysis Ptosis Pupillary abnormalities Dysphagia Dyspnea	18-24 hr
Bacillus cereus	Fried rice	Vomiting Abdominal cramps	1-6 hr
Escherichia coli	Contaminated water Unpeeled vegetables and fruits	Watery diarrhea Green slimy stools, positive for leukocytes Abdominal cramps Low-grade fever	24-72 hr

with hypotension may be present if the patient is in hypovolemic shock from fluid volume deficit caused by the vomiting and diarrhea associated with food poisoning.
* *Fever:* Temperature elevation is common with communicable diseases. Low-grade fever is present in chickenpox,
measles, and mumps. High-grade fever is associated with
atypical measles and a *Streptococcus* infection. Very high
fever may occur in tetanus because of the overactivity of
the autonomic nervous system.

General Observations
Skin rash
* Although it is not possible to have the patient undress at
triage, all visible skin should be examined for the presence of a rash or lesion(s). Figure 6-1 illustrates the rash
distribution of commonly encountered conditions in the

TABLE 6-2 Varieties of Food Poisoning—cont'd

Organism	Susceptible foods	Symptoms	Incubation period
Vibrio cholerae	Contaminated water Unpeeled vegetables and fruits	Severe diarrhea and vomiting Hypovolemic shock	1-3 days
Salmonella	Raw or undercooked poultry, eggs, ground beef	Nausea and vomiting Fever Abdominal pain Watery diarrhea, Loose, slimy, green stool with rotten egg odor	8-48 hr
Trichinosis	Undercooked pork or wild game	Abdominal pain Nausea Fever Diarrhea	24-48 hr
Ciguatoxin	Barracuda, red snapper, grouper, sea bass	Diarrhea Ataxia, dizziness	1-6 hr

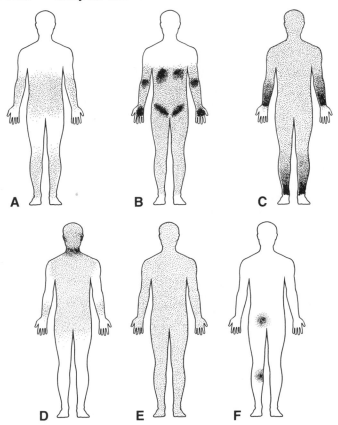

Figure 6-1 A, Meningococcemia. Meningococcemica begins as macules, progresses to petechiae, then forms purpura. It is located on extremities and trunk. **B,** Atypical measles. This type of measles is manifested as a maculopapular rash along skin creases. **C,** Rocky Mountain spotted fever. The fever produces a diffuse rash with heavier concentration at distal extremities. **D,** Typical measles. Typical measles starts behind ears and moves first to the face and neck, then downward over the rest of the body; the measles appear as discrete spots on the patient's extremities. **E,** Rubella. Rubella begins on the face and progresses to the neck, trunk, and extremities, respectively. **F,** Lyme disease. Lyme disease produces a centrifugal rash that varies in diameter with a red outer border and a clearer center. The rash is seen in higher frequency in the popliteal and groin regions. The patient with Lyme disease may have multiple or singular lesions.

ED. Subcutaneous nodules over bony prominences are associated with acute rheumatic fever. Petechiae or purpura (an indirect indicator of thrombocytopenia) is common in meningococcemia and indicates a very ill patient who needs to be treated immediately.

C

NURSING ALERT

Do not be fooled by skin and soft tissue infections. A streptococcal skin infection can be life threatening and advances systematically and rapidly. When in doubt about the origin of a skin infection, triage immediately to the treatment area.

Skin lesions
- Skin and mucous membrane lesions may appear in histoplasmosis, an opportunistic infection associated with HIV infection. Multiple discrete papules may appear on the extremities, trunk, and face. The lesions will be associated with fever and anorexia.

Wounds
- Examine wounds and lacerations thoroughly. Tetanus-prone wounds include those contaminated with dirt or saliva, puncture wounds, avulsions, gunshot wounds, burns, and frostbite. Closed-fist injuries sustained by hitting knuckles against teeth as well as animal and human bites are particularly prone to cellulitis.
- Examine drainage, if present, from the wounds. Creamy, yellow pus suggests the presence of staphylococci. Group A beta-hemolytic streptococci produce erythema without drainage. Brownish, foul-smelling drainage suggests anaerobic bacteria.

Gland enlargement
- Swelling of the parotid glands may be apparent in cases of mumps.

Pharynx
- It is helpful to perform a quick inspection of the patient's mouth and throat at triage, using a penlight and tongue depressor. A red, irritated pharynx with or without pustules may be present in *Streptococcus* infections. The patient may be given a mask or asked not to cough without covering his or her mouth while awaiting treatment. A patient with Koplik's spots (bright red macules with a bluish white spot in the center) on the buccal mu-

cosa of the inner lip may have measles, and this patient is highly contagious and must be isolated immediately. Koplik's spots precede the measles rash by 48 hours.

Tongue and mouth

- Swelling of the tongue, drooling, dysphagia, and pain in the floor of the mouth are associated with Ludwig's angina. Because of the potential for respiratory compromise resulting from edema, patients exhibiting these symptoms should be triaged immediately to the treatment area.
- Oral mouth lesions may be present in thrush, an opportunistic infection associated with HIV infection.

Height and weight

- Assess height and weight in relation to stature. Weight loss is common in patients with tuberculosis and HIV infection. Anorexia is a common complaint of these patients.

Dehydration

- Assess skin turgor and look for sunken fontanels and orbits. Assess lethargy and any change in mentation. Dehydration occurs rapidly in food poisoning (e.g., *Escherichia coli, Salmonella,* and *Staphylococcus*).

Hygiene

- Impetigo, folliculitis, furuncles, and carbuncles are associated with poor hygiene. Poor dental hygiene is associated with Ludwig's angina.

FOCUSED NURSING ASSESSEMENT

Nursing assessment should focus on ventilation, perfusion, mobility, mental status, and neurovascular status.

Ventilation
Airway

Maintain patency of the airway. Patients with a stiff jaw and dysphagia are at risk of aspiration and laryngospasm. Suction equipment should be at the bedside, and the staff should be prepared to assist with intubation and to administer a neuromuscular blocking agent.

Breath sounds

Consolidation may be present in pneumonia associated with HIV infection and in TB. Wheezing may be present in pertussis.

Perfusion
Apical heart rate
The auscultation of a murmur may indicate acute rheumatic fever. A systolic mitral regurgitation murmur is best auscultated at the apex, using the diaphragm of the stethoscope while the patient holds his or her breath after exhaling. A diastolic aortic regurgitation murmur is best auscultated in the third, left intercostal space. Diminished heart sounds may indicate pericardial effusion (associated with carditis induced by acute rheumatic fever). Palpitations and fainting may occur because of conduction defects associated with disseminated Lyme disease.

Neck veins
Congestive heart failure (CHF) may be a complication of acute rheumatic fever. Patients exhibit jugular venous distention and facial edema. Neck veins may be flat and urine output decreased in cases of hypovolemia as a result of fluid loss from vomiting and diarrhea that are caused by food poisoning.

Mobility
Ataxia is present in some cases of food poisoning. Red, swollen joints that are warm to the touch may be present in cases of acute rheumatic fever.

Mental Status
Assess the patient's level of responsiveness and record a Glasgow Coma Scale score. Some infections may present with central nervous system changes (e.g., cytomegalovirus, meningitis, or encephalitis).

Neurovascular Integrity
Assess the neurovascular status of all extremities. Several skin and soft tissue diseases have vascular implications (e.g., necrotizing fasciitis, cellulitis, and Kaposi's sarcoma). The vascular status of extremities can be assessed by noting the level at which the skin loses its hair and becomes shiny. On palpation, the transition zone from warm to cold should be noted. Crepitus will be present on palpation in cases of necrotizing fasciitis. Because of the rapidity with which this disease progresses, patients with crepitus should be triaged immediately to the treatment area. Sensation

should be assessed using a pinprick or pinwheel. The point at which the patient begins to feel the prick and the point where the sensation turns to pain should be noted.

Risk Factors

1. Lyme disease affects mainly hikers or those involved in outdoor occupations such as farming and forestry. New England and mid-Atlantic states have a higher incidence of the disease.
2. Certain diseases are seasonal. Lyme disease has a higher incidence in the summer and early fall.
3. Determine the proximity of pets and livestock to the patient. Tetanus occurs more frequently from wounds contaminated with soil where horses have resided. Lyme disease may occur in domestic animals, with a higher incidence in cats.
4. Crowded living conditions, malnutrition, and alcoholism and other drug addiction are associated with TB infection.
5. Certain eating situations pose increased risks for food poisoning. These include the following:
   - Picnics during warm weather with mayonnaise-based salads
   - The eating of home-canned vegetables
   - Undercooked pork
   - Egg-based sauces
   - Fish
   - Fried rice
   - The eating of ice and unpeeled fruits and vegetables when traveling in another country
6. Bisexual and homosexual men still have the highest rates of HIV infection, and their rate of TB and DR-TB is rapidly increasing. Having received a blood transfusion before 1985 increases a person's risk for HIV.

Life Span Issues
Children

1. Children have fewer pulmonary symptoms with TB. They have fever, malaise, and weight loss. They have a higher incidence of extrapulmonary TB involving the brain (meningitis), hematologic system (miliary TB), and bones (arthritis).
2. Infants between 1 and 2 months of age are at the great-

est risk for pertussis and its complications (seizures, encephalopathy, and pneumonia). There is a higher rate among females than among males.

3. Acute rheumatic fever rarely occurs initially with adults. School-age children are at greatest risk.

4. The older the child is when developing acute rheumatic fever, the less likelihood there is of carditis developing as a complication.

5. Children with HIV infections may exhibit enlarged lymph glands, low platelet counts, and a history of recurrent otitis media or pneumonia.

6. Hepatitis A and E are usually milder with children and have a shorter course of disease. Fever may be absent. Hepatitis B, C, and D progress to chronic liver disease more frequently with infants than with adults.

7. Children from 5 to 14 years of age have the highest incidence of Lyme disease.

Women and pregnancy

1. Most vaccines are contraindicated during pregnancy because they contain live virus or organism. Several communicable diseases (e.g., rubella), when contracted during the first trimester, result in a high incidence of fetal anomalies and death. Amniocentesis counseling may be appropriate.

2. Hepatitis E that is transmitted by a fecal-oral route, mainly in developing countries, has a high mortality rate in pregnant women.

3. Women with cervical cancer, abnormal Pap smears, genital warts, recurrent pelvic inflammatory disease, and vaginal candidiasis have a higher rate of HIV infection.

Adulthood

1. Mumps is more serious for an adult because complications of meningitis and epididymoorchitis (infection of the epididymis and testicles) are more common.

Geriatric patients

1. The geriatric population is at the greatest risk of contracting tetanus. They may not be adequately immunized.

2. The geriatric population is at risk for TB because most were exposed to TB early in the century when prevalence was high (reactivation of previously acquired disease). They may have outlived their initial infecting organism and are now susceptible to reinfection. TB

may present as a pleural effusion in the geriatric population and initially be misdiagnosed as CHF.

INITIAL INTERVENTIONS

1. Measure and document the rash using a total body drawing, or photograph the rash (with the patient's permission).
2. Initiate intravenous (IV) access in anticipation of fluid and medication administration for cases of suspected food poisoning or severe infection.
3. Initiate cardiac monitoring when extra heart sounds are auscultated or hypotension, hypertension, or tachycardia is present.
4. Initiate pulse oximetry in cases of dysphagia, dyspnea, persistent coughing, or sputum production.

PRIORITY NURSING DIAGNOSES

Risk for fluid volume deficit
Risk for ineffective airway clearance
Risk for injury
Risk for decreased cardiac output

◆ **Fluid volume deficit** related to dehydration:
   INTERVENTIONS
   • Initiate IV access and administer crystalloids as ordered.
◆ **Ineffective airway clearance** related to excessive sputum production, inability to control secretions, laryngospasm, or nasopharyngeal edema:
   INTERVENTIONS
   • Insert a nasopharyngeal or oral airway as the condition indicates.
   • Suction the airway.
◆ **Injury** related to infection and seizure activity:
   INTERVENTIONS
   • Administer antibiotics and an anticonvulsant as ordered.
   • Anticipate the administration of neuromuscular blocking agents.
   • Initiate masking or isolation of the patient if the patient may be immunocompromised or infectious.
◆ **Decreased cardiac output** related to pericardial effusion or valve disease:
   INTERVENTIONS
   • Decrease oxygen demands by administering oxygen and minimizing activity.

- Administer diuretics as ordered.
- Anticipate surgical intervention.

PRIORITY DIAGNOSTIC TESTS

Laboratory Tests

Aspartate transaminase (SGOT): This level may be elevated in hepatitis.

Alanine transaminase (SGPT): This level may be elevated in hepatitis.

Anergy testing: Anergy testing may be initiated in the ED for geriatric and immunocompromised patients. These individuals may have a fading immune response to organisms to which they have been previously exposed. The person may react positively to inoculation with an organism, but the reaction may be so slight as to be misdiagnosed as negative. A battery of "control" antigens that all individuals are exposed to as part of life (e.g., *Candida*) are administered along with the organism of concern (e.g., TB). Reactions to all inoculations are compared with one another to determine severity of reaction and, subsequently, infection. If the test result is negative, a second dose is administered to elicit a booster or recall effect. A positive second test result is as significant as an initially positive test. A negative result from a TB test does not rule out TB. Immunocompromised individuals (e.g., those with HIV) may not be able to mount a reaction.

NURSING ALERT

Occasionally a patient wants his or her TB test read in the ED. Reactions should be read within 72 hours after administration. Induration (the degree to which the tissue is hard on palpation), not erythema, is significant. The following parameters should be used:

- 5 mm of induration is positive in a person with recent TB exposure, an HIV-positive individual, and a person with a chest film indicative of TB lesions.
- 10 mm of induration is positive in increased-risk groups.
- 15 mm of induration is positive in all groups.

Rapid antigen tests: These tests detect cell wall antigen of dead or viable bacteria and viruses by means of latex ag-

glutination or enzyme-linked immunosorbent assay
(ELISA). A positive test result indicates a current or previous infection.

Antibody tests: These tests can detect exposure to a particular organism if the patient is able to mobilize an immune response to the organism. The development of antibodies against a particular organism is a positive test
result. Antibody tests are used to detect exposure to hepatitis, *Streptococcus,* mumps, and several other diseases.

Bilirubin: Serum bilirubin levels are elevated in hepatitis.

CD4 count: This is a measurement of the number of
helper-T lymphocytes in the blood that bear the CD4 surface molecule, which is the cellular receptor for HIV.

CD8 count: This is a measurement of the number of sup-
pressor lymphocytes. People who are not infected with
HIV tend to have more CD4 than CD8 lymphocytes.

Complete blood count (CBC): Leukocytosis may be present, with an increased lymphocyte count for children
who have pertussis or measles.

C-reactive protein: This value may be elevated in Lyme
disease.

Culture and sensitivity testing: Wounds may be cultured for
the presence of spirochetes (Lyme disease) and tetanus.
Vesicles may be aspirated after cleansing with povidone-
iodine solution and rinsing with alcohol, using a small-
gauge needle attached to a tuberculin syringe. Sputum
cultures may be performed to test for acid-fast bacilli (tuberculosis). Nasopharyngeal cultures may be performed
to detect *Streptococcus* and pertussis infections. Stool cultures may be obtained to identify the causative organism
in suspected cases of food poisoning.

Erythrocyte sedimentation rate: This value may be elevated
in Lyme disease.

Monospot: This heterophil agglutination test detects antibodies to the Epstein-Barr virus (the usual causal agent
for mononucleosis).

Western Blot test: This test is used to confirm the presence
of certain antibodies as a follow-up to enzyme-linked immunosorbent assay testing. Viral proteins (e.g., HIV) are
readily visualized.

Radiographic Tests

Chest films: A chest film may be ordered to detect lesions
in tuberculosis. Cardiac enlargement and pericardial ef-

fusion may be detected in cases of carditis with acute rheumatic fever.

Extremity films: These may be ordered in cases of skin and soft tissue infection to rule out osteomyelitis or the presence of a foreign body or pathologic fracture.

Radionuclide scans: These may be used to confirm osteomyelitis. Increased radionuclide uptake in any area is a positive result for that area.

Other Tests

Electrocardiogram: The P-R interval may be prolonged in carditis (associated with acute rheumatic fever), producing a first- or second-degree heart block.

Echocardiogram: An echocardiogram may be obtained to document pericardial effusion and valve disease associated with acute rheumatic fever.

Lumbar puncture with cerebrospinal fluid (CSF) analysis: Certain communicable diseases may result in encephalopathy and meningitis. CSF is examined for antibodies to specific organisms, to confirm that neurologic complications are related to progression of a specific disease.

COLLABORATIVE INTERVENTIONS

Overview

1. Obtain a wound or rash culture (sometimes a punch biopsy may need to be performed by the physician) before cleansing the wound or rash site.
2. Administer the appropriate vaccine to provide active or passive immunity. Table 6-1 lists treatments for communicable and infectious diseases. Table 6-3 lists precautions with selective vaccines. The "Vaccination Pearls of Wisdom" box discusses misperceptions about vaccination to provide a resource for answering patient and parent questions.

Clinical Conditions
Acute rheumatic fever

Acute rheumatic fever only occurs after an upper respiratory infection of group A streptococci.

SYMPTOMS

- Arthritis and fever usually occur first.
- Cardiac involvement can range from minor dysrhythmias to severe CHF.

TABLE 6-3 Vaccine Precautions

Vaccine	Side effects	Dose	Special considerations
Measles, mumps, and rubella (MMR)	Rash, low-grade fever, seizures, arthritis	0.5 ml SC Peds: 1st dose at 15-18 mo, 2nd dose at 4-6 yr	Contraindicated in pregnancy, persons allergic to eggs or who have hypersensitivity reaction to neomycin
Diphtheria, tetanus, pertussis (DTP)	Fever, crying, irritability, seizures	0.5 ml IM	Persons with known seizure history at greater risk of experiencing seizure after administration Persons with 105° F temperature or greater or persistent crying after previous administration should not receive another dose
Tetanus toxoid (Td) diphtheria	Local redness and tenderness, headache, malaise	0.5 ml IM or SC	Contraindicated in persons with a known allergy to gamma globulin or thimerosal
Tuberculin skin test	Local redness at injection site	0.1 ml of 5 tuberculin units of purified protein derivative IC	Induration (degree to which tissue is hard or firm), not erythema, is significant Test should be read within 72 hr

TABLE 6-3 Vaccine Precautions—cont'd

Vaccine	Side effects	Dose	Special considerations
Varicella vaccine	Rash, low-grade fever, malaise	Adults: 0.5 ml SC × 2 doses, 4-8 wk between doses Peds: give at age 12 mo or older, 0.5 ml SC × 1 dose	Contraindicated Wait 5 wk if immune globulin has been given Do not give to immuno-compromised or pregnant patient, active TB or febrile illness[8]

C

VACCINATION PEARLS OF WISDOM

1. Acellular pertussis vaccines have been developed that provide protective immunity with fewer side effects (fever, crying, irritability, seizures, and encephalopathy).
2. The combination antigen vaccine DTP (diphtheria, tetanus, and pertussis) is used for children less than 7 years of age. Tetanus and diphtheria (Td) is recommended for individuals 7 years of age and older because side effects from the pertussis vaccine are more severe in this age group.
3. If a series of immunizations is started but is interrupted, it is not necessary to restart the series or to give extra doses.
4. Patients who served in the Armed Forces since 1941 can be assumed to have received at least one dose of tetanus vaccine.
5. An episode of tetanus does not provide immunity, so a complete series of immunizations is indicated.
6. Persons who received the measles vaccine from 1957 to 1967 should receive additional vaccination or have a measles antibody titer drawn to confirm immunity.

- Mitral and aortic valve disease may be present.
- A nonpruritic pink-red rash with a sharp outer edge (erythema marginatum) may appear on the trunk.
- Chorea (involuntary purposeless movements of the extremities and face) may occur in conjunction with heart problems.

DIAGNOSIS
- Diagnosis is based on the revised Jones' criteria.[5]
- The patient must have evidence of a previous group A streptococcal infection, the presence of two major criteria, or the presence of one major criterion and two minor criteria (see "Revised Jones' Criteria" box).

TREATMENT
- Acute rheumatic fever can be prevented by adequately treating the initial streptococcal infection. Once acute rheumatic fever occurs, it can reappear, and secondary prophylaxis is then indicated. Recurrences are less likely after puberty.
- Controversy exists over the length of time antibiotics should be administered. Suggestions range from until the individual reaches 18 years of age to lifetime administration.
- Patients with valve disease will require additional antibiotic preparation before dental and surgical procedures.

REVISED JONES' CRITERIA FOR ACUTE RHEUMATIC FEVER

Major criteria

Carditis
Polyarthritis
Chorea
Erythema marginatum (skin rash)
Subcutaneous nodules

Minor criteria

Arthralgia
Fever
Prolonged P-R interval on electrocardiograph
Elevated erythrocyte sedimentation rate
Elevated C-reactive protein

- Intramuscular antibiotic injections may be given monthly, or daily oral medication may be used.
- In acute cases of carditis induced by acute rheumatic fever, diuretics and digoxin may be given in the ED.

Acute streptococcal infection

Acute streptococcal infection usually presents as a sore throat. However, children may have only fever and rash.

SYMPTOMS

- The patient may have a high fever (>38.5° C or 101.5° F), headache, nausea, and vomiting.
- Pharyngeal edema, exudative tonsillitis, and enlarged and tender cervical lymph glands may be present.
- The rash of scarlet fever (red, diffuse macules) may be present.

DIAGNOSIS

- Diagnosis is determined by a positive result on a throat culture for group A beta-hemolytic *Streptococcus* or by an increased serum level of antistreptolysin O or other antibodies to *Streptococcus*.

TREATMENT

- Antibiotic therapy is indicated for at least 10 days to prevent complications from strep infection, such as acute rheumatic fever.
- Cephalosporin or erythromycin is recommended for penicillin-allergic individuals. Beware of potential for cross-sensitivity in patients who are allergic to penicillin.

Cellulitis and skin and soft tissue infection

SYMPTOMS

- Erythema, tenderness, and hot, red, edematous skin with enlargement of regional lymph nodes are characteristic of cellulitis.
- Blisters may be present.
- In children, facial cellulitis may result from *Haemophilus influenzae* infection.
- The skin becomes dusky and purplish with facial edema.
- Ludwig's angina is a type of cellulitis that results from infection of the second and third lower molar. It is a rare but life-threatening illness characterized by tongue swelling, dysphagia, and drooling.

DIAGNOSIS

- A skin biopsy may be performed, but diagnosis in the ED setting is frequently based on clinical presentation.

TREATMENT
- Antibiotics are initiated.
- Surgical drainage may be used for abscesses.
- Analgesics will be administered before drainage.
- Assess the tetanus status and administer Td or Hyper-Tet as indicated.
- Cultures of the drainage should be obtained before starting antibiotic therapy.
- Heat application may facilitate drainage and earlier healing.
- Elevation of the affected part decreases edema and pain.
- Bleeding wounds should be dressed in dry gauze until the bleeding stops.
- A wet-to-dry saline dressing can be applied to draining wounds.
- In Ludwig's angina, treatment focuses on airway maintenance, IV antibiotic therapy, pain control, and nutritional support.

Diphtheria
Diphtheria is an acute infection of the skin or upper respiratory tract. It is a rare disease in the United States. For more information, please refer to a communicable disease textbook, call the Centers for Disease Control and Prevention (CDC), or visit the CDC web site at www.cdc.gov.

SYMPTOMS
- Diphtheria toxin destroys epithelium. A gray pseudomembrane forms over the tonsils and pharynx. The toxin may spread to other organs (e.g., lungs, heart, and kidney) where it damages organ structure and function.

DIAGNOSIS
- Diagnosis is determined by clinical presentation.

TREATMENT
- Treatment is supportive, by artificially maintaining organ function until the toxin clears.

Food poisoning
Food poisoning can occur from a variety of organisms (see Table 6-2 for more information regarding incubation periods and symptoms). Food poisoning can be classified as having either gastrointestinal- or neurologic-based symptoms. Both kinds of poisoning can be life threatening.

SYMPTOMS
- Food poisoning with neurologic effects will manifest itself by descending paralysis, ataxia, dizziness, pupillary

changes, and, ultimately, respiratory compromise (e.g., botulism and ciguatoxin).
- Gastrointestinal effects are nausea, vomiting, watery diarrhea, abdominal pain, and fever (e.g., *Staphylococcus, Bacillus, E. coli,* cholera, *Salmonella,* and trichinosis).

DIAGNOSIS
- Diagnosis is based on clinical and diet history.
- The history of other individuals with similar symptoms who ate at the same function or restaurant is a significant factor.
- Stool cultures may be performed in cases where confirmation of an organism is needed.

TREATMENT
- Oral glucose or electrolyte solutions may be used for patients who are not severely dehydrated. Oral rehydration therapy should consist of a solution with 75 to 90 mEq/L of sodium. The dose varies according to degree of dehydration (10 to 100 ml/kg over 4 hours).[6]
- IV fluids may be administered.
- Antiemetics and antimotility agents may be ordered.
- Antibiotics may be used if the patient is immunocompromised or in a toxic condition.
- Botulinum-trivalent antitoxin must be administered early before toxin confirmation in cases of suspected botulism.
- Endotracheal intubation and mechanical ventilation may be initiated.

Hepatitis
Hepatitis is an acute inflammation of the liver. It may be produced by a virus, a chemical or drug reaction, or alcohol abuse. Viral hepatitis infection is either transmitted by a fecal-oral route (hepatitis A and E) or by a blood or sexual transmission route (hepatitis B, C, and D). See Table 6-1 for comparisons of the various forms of hepatitis.

SYMPTOMS
- Regardless of the origin, symptoms are similar and include fever, malaise, anorexia, arthralgia, vomiting, diarrhea, right upper quadrant pain, and color changes in the stool (clay), urine (dark), and skin (jaundice).

DIAGNOSIS
- Diagnosis is based on an elevation of the level of liver enzymes, antibody testing (except in hepatitis E, where no test is available), and a liver biopsy. HIV and syphilis testing should be initiated.

TREATMENT

- Treatment of hepatitis A is supportive, consisting of rest and fluids. Immune globulin is administered to all patient contacts and to the patient. Hepatitis B is experimentally treated with interferon, but there is no cure. Hepatitis C is treated with 3 million units of interferon subcutaneously, three times a week for 24 weeks. Acyclovir may be used. A hepatitis D infection can occur only if the patient has a hepatitis B infection; therefore prevention of hepatitis B is the best prevention for hepatitis D. No treatment is available for hepatitis D or E. Fulminant hepatitis is treated with bed rest, a low-protein diet, and neomycin or lactulose (orally or rectally as indicated) to decrease blood ammonia levels.

Human immunodeficiency virus

Patients may arrive at the ED with a known HIV infection or with symptoms and an unconfirmed suspicion of the disease. The goals of the ED visit should be to improve the immune status and to prevent or treat opportunistic infections.

SYMPTOMS

- Weight loss, fever, malaise, oral and skin lesions, visual changes, persistent coughing, and a sore throat may be present, depending on whether it is an initial HIV infection or an opportunistic infection with an earlier diagnosed HIV infection. A specific discussion of all opportunistic infections is beyond the scope of this book.

DIAGNOSIS

- HIV is confirmed by a positive result on the ELISA and Western Blot tests.
- Syphilis, hepatitis B, and TB testing may be performed because these diseases often occur in tandem.
- WBC and T-helper cell counts are predictive of opportunistic infections (see the "T Helper Cell Counts" box). Patients with suspected *Pneumocystis carinii* pneumonia (PCP) who have an oxygen saturation <90% or a Po_2 <60 mm Hg usually require hospital admission.

TREATMENT

- Zidovudine is used to treat an HIV infection (Table 6-1). This drug may produce anemia and thrombocytopenia. Other retroviral agents, nucleoside analogs, and protease inhibitors may be used.
- Immunizations may be administered prophylactically.
- If PCP is diagnosed, steroids and pentamidine may be initiated in the ED.

T HELPER CELL COUNTS AND OPPORTUNISTIC INFECTION SUSCEPTIBILITY

- T helper cell count 200-500/mm^3 = Tuberculosis, Kaposi's sarcoma, thrush, and oral hairy leukoplakia
- T helper cell count 200-250/mm^3 = *Pneumocystis carinii* pneumonia, toxoplasmosis
- T helper cell count below 50/mm^3 = cytomegalovirus, lymphoma, meningitis

---

Lyme disease

Lyme disease is caused by a spirochete that is transmitted by a tick bite. The spirochete may travel by the vascular or lymph system to any organ in the body.

SYMPTOMS

- There are three stages. Early localized infection is characterized by erythema migrans (an expanding circular lesion usually occurring at the site of the tick bite).
- In cases of an early disseminated infection, patients may have joint and tendon pain.
- Patients complain of fatigue and malaise.
- Palpitations and fainting may occur because of atrioventricular conduction blocks.
- Chronic infection may take a year or longer to occur.
- Chronic arthritis may develop.
- Encephalopathy may result in mood changes and memory and sleep disturbances.

DIAGNOSIS

- Testing for Lyme disease is most frequently conducted using antigen tests.
- The spirochete may be cultured from skin lesions.

TREATMENT

- Treatment includes antibiotics, PO or IV depending on the severity of the symptoms noted.
- Penicillin or tetracycline derivatives are prescribed.

Measles

SYMPTOMS

- A dry cough, headache, low-grade fever, sore throat, Koplik's spots, and a nonblanching, diffuse rash are characteristic of measles.
- A hacking cough, conjunctival irritation, and photophobia may occur before the appearance of Koplik's spots.

- Atypical measles is a form of the disease that strikes individuals who received measles vaccine containing the killed measles virus instead of live attenuated virus. Persons immunized between 1957 and 1967 are at risk for atypical measles.
- Symptoms of atypical measles include a high-grade fever, edema of the feet and lips, and a rash that begins on the extremities and migrates to the head.

DIAGNOSIS

- Diagnosis is usually based on clinical presentation, exposure, and vaccination history.
- The WBC may be low, with lymphocytosis present.

TREATMENT

- Treatment is symptomatic.
- Antipyretics and fluids are given.
- Rest in a darkened room may be suggested if photophobia is present.
- All exposed, susceptible persons such as other members of the household should receive postexposure prophylaxis with immune globulin (0.25 mg/kg, maximum dose 15 ml; immunocompromised patients should receive 0.5 mg/kg), preferably within 72 hours but up to 6 days after exposure.

Meningococcal infection

Meningococcal disease is transmitted by nasopharyngeal droplets. In most individuals, disease does not develop from infection. The disease can occur as acute meningitis or as fulminant meningococcemia characterized by disseminated intravascular coagulation (DIC) and septic shock.

SYMPTOMS

- If the organism produces meningitis, symptoms are fever, nuchal rigidity, and a decreased level of consciousness.
- Petechiae and purpura are common with both the meningitis and meningococcemia forms.
- The rash produces lesions on the extremities and trunk (Figure 6-1).
- Lesions may be macules before becoming petechiae.
- Malaise, hypotension, and pulmonary edema with CHF may occur in sepsis.

DIAGNOSIS

- Diagnosis is determined by clinical presentation and a history of viral upper respiratory infection.

- Cultures of blood, lesions, and cerebrospinal fluid will reveal meningococci.

TREATMENT

- Penicillin (300,000 U/kg/day IV) is the treatment of choice.
- Volume replacement and vasopressors may be required.
- Heparin may be used in cases of DIC.

Mononucleosis

Adolescents, college students, and military recruits are most susceptible to this disease. Transmission of the virus is by nasopharyngeal droplets.

SYMPTOMS

- A fever, swollen glands, a sore throat, and lethargy are common.
- The spleen is enlarged in some cases.

DIAGNOSIS

- A positive monospot test result confirms the diagnosis.
- Liver enzymes may be elevated.
- Lymphocytosis may be present in the WBCs.

TREATMENT

- Supportive treatment with fluids and rest is recommended.
- Contact sports and aspirin products should be avoided for up to 8 weeks to help prevent splenic rupture and bleeding.

Mumps parotitis

SYMPTOMS

- The major symptom of mumps is nonsuppurative swelling and tenderness of the salivary glands.
- A fever is often present.
- Males may have unilateral swelling of the genitalia.

DIAGNOSIS

- Diagnosis is based on clinical presentation and antigen testing.
- A mumps infection confers lifelong immunity.

TREATMENT

- Treatment is supportive, since there is no cure.
- Antipyretics and analgesics may be ordered.
- Topical warm or cold compresses may relieve discomfort.
- Patients should be placed on bed rest until their temperatures return to normal. This appears to limit the severity of the disease.

- Scrotal support should be used in cases of orchitis and epididymitis.
- Avoid sour foods, since these cause pain secondary to stimulation of salivary flow.

Pertussis

SYMPTOMS

- Pertussis begins with a low-grade fever, nasal congestion, and a mild cough. After 2 weeks the cough worsens.
- In adults, leukocytosis and lymphocytosis may be absent, whereas it is frequently present in children with pertussis.
- Children have a greater incidence of protracted paroxysmal coughing that is worse at night.

DIAGNOSIS

- Diagnosis is confirmed by the antipertussis' toxin antibody production.

TREATMENT

- Treatment is supportive, using fluids and antipyretics.
- Antibiotics may be ordered to prevent a bacterial respiratory infection and pneumonia.

Rubella (German measles)

Rubella can be difficult to distinguish because it presents similarly to measles and scarlet fever.

SYMPTOMS

- A low-grade fever, a sore throat, and a pink papular rash on the face and neck that spreads to the trunk and extremities are characteristic.
- Postauricular and suboccipital lymph nodes are enlarged and usually tender.
- The WBC count is normal.

DIAGNOSIS

- Diagnosis is determined by rubella antibody assay tests.

TREATMENT

- Antipyretics and antipruritic medications may be ordered.

Tetanus

Tetanus is caused by a spore-forming rod found in contaminated soil. It most commonly follows an acute injury, but it can also infect chronic wounds (e.g., decubiti and skin abscesses). The spores can live in the body for months or years, producing disease at a time removed from the initial injury.

SYMPTOMS

- Tetanus produces rigidity and spasms of skeletal muscle.
- The toxin spreads by way of the circulation.

- Nerves with the shortest axons are affected first.
- Symptoms begin in the facial muscles and jaw, progressing to the neck and trunk.
- Dyspnea and dysphagia are common.
- If the spasms are controlled by medication, overactivity of the sympathetic nervous system may result in dysrhythmias, tachycardia, peripheral vasoconstriction, and cardiac arrest.
- Urinary retention may occur.

DIAGNOSIS
- Diagnosis is usually based on clinical presentation.

TREATMENT
- Rapid deterioration is expected; therefore the patient is intubated and given neuromuscular blocking agents (e.g., pancuronium).
- Tetanus immune globulin is administered to prevent further absorption of the toxin.
- Wounds should be debrided, and antibiotics may be initiated.
- Patients will require immunization because the amount of toxin causing the disease is inadequate to confer immunity.

Tuberculosis

SYMPTOMS
- For persons younger than 60 years of age, nightsweats, anorexia, and weight loss are the predominant symptoms.
- In individuals 60 years of age and older, cough, sputum production, and weight loss are frequent symptoms.
- It is possible to have active disease without symptoms.

DIAGNOSIS
- Diagnosis is usually based on a positive tuberculin skin test result and lesions appearing on a chest film.
- For immunocompromised individuals, diagnosis may be based on clinical presentation.

TREATMENT
- Isoniazid and rifampin are initially used to treat TB. For DR-TB, simultaneous administration of several drugs may be needed.
- Generally, isoniazid, rifampin, pyrazinamide, and ethambutol or streptomycin are given (Table 6-1).
- Steroids may be used in severe cases.
- Baseline liver function should be assessed before any TB medication is started because of the side effects of these medications.

- Visual acuity must be examined before and during ethambutol therapy.
- Since it is difficult to measure visual acuity in children, ethambutol is not recommended for pediatric use.
- High-efficiency particulate (HEPA) respirators have been recommended by the CDC for use in health care facilities to prevent the transmission of tuberculosis; however, they are expensive and their efficacy is not clear. Masking the patient while the patient is in the ED is a good precaution. When it is available, use a HEPA respirator.

Varicella (chickenpox)

SYMPTOMS

- The rash associated with chickenpox is extremely pruritic and ranges from macules to papules, to vesicles, and to crusted lesions simultaneously.
- A low-grade fever may be present.
- Reactivation of the varicella virus may occur in the form of herpes zoster (shingles).
- Vesicles are gray in appearance and are located along a dermatome (nerve fiber). They arise from an erythematous base and contain clear fluid. Common sites include the thoracic area (50%), lumbosacral and cervical region (10% to 20%), and the trigeminal nerve (10% to 20%).[7]

NURSING ALERT

Beware of vesicles on the side or tip of the nose. This is highly associated with trigeminal nerve involvement. An immediate ophthalmic consultation is warranted because of the high incidence of complications, including, but not limited to, optic neuritis and glaucoma. Perform a visual acuity check.[8]

DIAGNOSIS

- Diagnosis is usually determined by clinical presentation, although antibody testing may be done.

TREATMENT

- For immunocompromised individuals, varicella immunoglobulin (125 units/10 kg up to 625 units) can be administered within 96 hours of exposure to prevent or modify illness.
- The immunoglobulin will protect the person for 3 weeks. Wait 5 weeks after administration before administering the varicella vaccine.

- Analgesics, antihistamines, and steroids may be given to provide relief from symptoms.

NURSING ALERT

Remember to warn patients and parents not to use aspirin or aspirin products if the patient is younger than 21 years of age because of the association between Reye's syndrome and aspirin use.

NURSING SURVEILLANCE

1. Monitor the cardiac pattern and treat potentially lethal dysrhythmias (second- and third-degree heart block may occur in acute rheumatic fever).
2. Monitor the trend of the patient's temperature. An elevated temperature may further dehydrate a patient with fluid volume deficit.
3. Monitor urine output and color to assess core perfusion and liver dysfunction.
4. Trend oxygen saturation. Desaturation may occur in a patient who is not responding to drug therapy or who requires artificial ventilation because of respiratory paralysis or spasm.
5. Monitor the patient's level of consciousness.

EXPECTED PATIENT OUTCOMES

1. The fever decreases or is absent.
2. The airway remains patent.
3. The breathing pattern is adequate (whether maintained by patient or artificially) as demonstrated by SpO_2 >94% and arterial blood gases normal for condition.

DISCHARGE IMPLICATIONS

Discharge instructions should be based on the clinical diagnosis of the patient. Refer to Table 6-1 for specific information regarding transmission routes, incubation periods, and complications associated with diseases. Some diseases require greater detail in discharge instruction and are discussed below.

1. *Acute rheumatic fever:* Patients should be examined daily for the first weeks of the disease to detect carditis early, before valve damage. The seriousness of this disease and

the need for long-term antibiotic therapy must be explained to the patient.

2. *Hepatitis:* Patients discharged with hepatitis should be instructed to rest and to anticipate low energy levels for up to 6 months. Alcoholic beverages should be avoided for 6 to 12 months. Instruct the patient that immunity to one type of hepatitis does not confer immunity to another type.

3. *HIV:* If HIV testing has been performed (with written informed consent of the patient), certain counseling must be provided. Patients must be informed about the medical significance of the test, whether the test result is negative or positive; test limitations; how HIV is spread; the availability of medical and psychosocial care; and social consequences of testing.[9] HIV-infected individuals should be referred to support groups and instructed on the prevention of disease transmission to others.

4. *Lyme disease:* Patients should be instructed to wear light-colored clothes and long sleeves and pants with wrist and ankle bands before entering tick-infested areas. Insect repellent may be used.

5. *Mumps:* The patient is contagious until the swelling subsides. The patient should remain home from work and school.

6. *Rubella:* The patient should remain home from work and school for 7 days after the onset of the rash. After receiving the MMR vaccine, the female, postpubertal patient should be warned not to become pregnant for at least 3 months. All pregnant first-trimester patients should be referred to an obstetrician.

7. *Skin conditions:* Encourage all family members to wash with antibacterial soap and not to share razors or towels and washcloths.

8. *Tuberculosis:* Patients should be taught to report early signs of hepatitis because of the toxic liver effects of TB medications. Anorexia, nausea, weakness, jaundice, clay-colored stools, and dark urine should be reported quickly to their primary health care provider.

9. *Varicella and herpes zoster:* Active lesions are potentially infectious. Inform the patient to avoid neonates, pregnant women, and immunosuppressed patients.

NURSING ALERT

Both ED and prehospital personnel should receive tuberculin skin testing every 3 to 6 months because of their high potential for exposure. Personnel should wear respiratory protection when suctioning the airway of high-risk individuals. Personnel should have a TB skin test immediately after a known exposure. Hepatitis B testing is recommended yearly to determine the antibody level for personnel repeatedly exposed to blood. A booster vaccine should be administered if the antibody levels fall below 10 IU.[10]

References

1. Elpern E, Girzadas A: Tuberculosis update: new challenges of an old disease, *Medsurg Nurs* 2:176-183, 1992.
2. Franckhauser M: Tuberculosis in the 1990s, *Nurse Pract Forum* 4:30-36, 1993.
3. Centers for Disease Control and Prevention: Resurgence of pertussis—United States, *MMWR* 42:952-960, 1993.
4. Dutt A, Stead W: Tuberculosis in the elderly, *Med Clin North Am* 77:1353-1368, 1993.
5. American Heart Association: Special writing group of the committee on rheumatic fever, endocarditis, and Kawasaki disease of the council on cardiovascular disease in the young: guidelines for the diagnosis of rheumatic fever, *JAMA* 268:2069-2073, 1992.
6. Straughn A, English B: Oral rehydration therapy: a neglected treatment for pediatric diarrhea, *Matern Child Nurs* 6:144-147, 1996.
7. Bjorgen S: Clinical snapshot: herpes zoster, *Am J Nurs* 98(2):46-47, 1998.
8. Reifsnider E: Common infectious adult skin infections, *Nurse Pract* 22(11):17-20, 23-24, 26-27, 1997.
9. Gold J: HIV-1 infection, *Med Clin North Am* 76:1-18, 1992.
10. Schiff E: Viral hepatitis today, *Emerg Med* 24:115-116, 119, 122-124, 126, 129-130, 132, 1992.

Chapter 7

Ear, Nose, Throat, and Facial and Dental Conditions

Mark Parshall

CLINICAL CONDITIONS
Epiglottitis
Croup (Laryngotracheobronchitis)
LeFort Fractures
Airway Foreign Bodies
Ludwig's Angina
Parapharyngeal Abscess and Peritonsillar Abscess
Epistaxis
Facial Fractures
    Mandibular Fractures
    Nasal Fractures
Dental Avulsions
Auricular and Nasal Septal Hematomas
Facial Lacerations
Ménière's Disease and Acute Labyrinthitis (Vestibular Dysfunction)
Esophageal Foreign Body
Nasal and Ear Foreign Bodies
Otitis Media
Otitis Externa
Sinusitis
Odontalgia
Acute Necrotizing Ulcerative Gingivitis
Cerumen Impaction

TRIAGE ASSESSMENT

Dental, facial, and ear, nose, and throat (ENT) emergencies range from life threatening to relatively minor. Emergency priority is given to upper airway injuries or obstructions (as a result of bleeding, swelling, infection, burns, or foreign bodies), to uncontrolled bleeding or hemodynamic instability, and to mixed presentations involving alterations in consciousness. In less pressing situations, attention is directed toward preservation or restoration of structural and functional integrity, to pain reduction, and to addressing psychosocial responses to potential disfigurement or disability.

NURSING ALERT

Any patient demonstrating airway symptoms or a high-energy injury to the face or neck with significant facial or neck swelling should be triaged directly to a resuscitation area.

Patients with high-impact blunt or penetrating injuries above the level of the clavicles require emergent initiation of spinal precautions.

Airway and Breathing
Impaired ability to speak or swallow
Cardinal signs of acute airway compromise include an impaired ability to speak or swallow, stridor, crowing, retractions, cyanosis, and, generally, obvious distress. Not all of these signs will be present in every instance.
Lethargy
A child who looks acutely ill but is lethargic, "too quiet," or apathetic should be triaged for emergency examination.
Position
If the patient assumes a "tripod" position or is deliberately quiet in an effort to improve air movement, suspect epiglottitis.[1,2]
Dysphagia, drooling, dysphonia, and distress
Classic signs of epiglottitis have been termed the "four D's"—dysphagia, drooling, dysphonia (muffled voice), and distress.[2] Drooling is not always present. Genuine difficulty swallowing (dysphagia) is accorded a higher triage priority than pain with swallowing (odynophagia).[3] The complaint of "difficulty swallowing" is often used by patients to describe painful swallowing.
Muffled speech, tongue protrusion, trismus, or torticollis
A pharyngeal wall abscess or cellulitis of the floor of the mouth or soft tissues of the neck should be triaged as a potential airway emergency if it is associated with muffled speech, tongue protrusion, trismus, or torticollis.

Mechanism of injury

High-energy blunt facial or soft tissue neck injuries that are considered at high risk for airway compromise or cervical spine injury include vehicular collisions (especially if victims were not restrained), motorcycle ejection, "clothesline" injuries, and being struck in the face or neck with a blunt instrument.

Breathing patterns

Abnormalities in rate, depth, or symmetry of breathing in conjunction with facial, oral, or pharyngeal swelling, infection, or a high-energy mechanism of injury may indicate an incomplete airway obstruction. An altered breathing pattern when the airway is clear may be a sign of a concomitant central nervous system (CNS) problem (e.g., a head or spinal cord injury).

Circulation

Bleeding (epistaxis, facial wounds)

Bleeding from epistaxis or facial wounds may be profuse. In most cases, bleeding can be readily controlled with direct pressure.

Tachycardia and narrowed pulse pressure

Although epistaxis is relatively common in patients with hypertension, at triage the blood pressure (BP) is rarely so elevated as to have actually caused the bleeding episode.[4] It is more common at triage to find the patient's vital signs consistent with mild or moderate blood loss (e.g., tachycardia and, initially, a narrowed pulse pressure).

Tachycardia and hypotension

In otherwise healthy patients, bleeding from anterior epistaxis or isolated facial trauma is rarely severe enough to cause significant hemodynamic compromise. Therefore a finding of tachycardia and moderate to severe hypotension in triage should heighten the examiner's index of suspicion for posterior bleeding in epistaxis or for some other source of concealed hemorrhage among patients with facial injuries.

Syncope

The patient may respond to the sight of blood or the presence of pain with a vasovagal syncopal episode. Accordingly, triage judgment with respect to bleeding involves more than vital signs and estimation of blood loss.

Other Triage Considerations
Symptom description
Obtain information related to the rapidity of symptom onset and associated symptoms or complaints; medications, allergies, and tetanus status should be obtained in triage or as soon as possible.

Ice
Ice should be applied to areas of traumatic facial swelling while the patient is waiting to be seen.

Domestic violence
Victims of domestic violence often have facial injuries and may need to be triaged as emergency status for their safety and to initiate crisis intervention, even when there is no threat to the airway or hemodynamic status.

Corrosive ingestions
Corrosive ingestions (e.g., battery acid or lye) require immediate triage to a resuscitation area.

Avulsed teeth
Avulsed teeth are accorded a higher triage priority than most other dental complaints (e.g., odontalgia) because of the limited window for replantation (see Collaborative Interventions).[5-7]

FOCUSED NURSING ASSESSMENT
Risk Factors
Injury
1. Soft tissue facial trauma is most commonly related to falls. Facial fractures are most commonly related to vehicular collisions and interpersonal violence.[8]
2. Midfacial fractures (e.g., orbital blowout and LeFort II and III fractures) increase the risk of permanent eye injury.[9]
3. Facial trauma resulting from interpersonal violence is often associated with alcohol or drugs and possible ongoing belligerence.[8] It may be necessary to triage a patient to a secure area and have security personnel immediately on hand, even in cases where the injuries themselves may not be emergent.

Life Span Issues
Infants and children
1. Airway structures are less rigid in children than in adults, and hence more likely to be compromised by swelling, infection, or trauma.

2. Infants less than 3 months of age are obligate nose breathers, so even nasal congestion can lead to significant respiratory embarrassment for this age group. Nasal flaring with infants is often a sign of significant respiratory compromise or distress.
3. Retractions in any age group are a potentially serious sign; for children, supraclavicular retractions are usually most indicative of severe effort.
4. Epiglottitis can occur in any age group but is most prevalent among children between 3 and 6 years of age.[1-4]
5. Croup is most common from 3 months to 3 years of age[3,4] with a peak incidence around 2 years of age.[10]
6. The possibility of aspiration of a foreign body should be considered in the case of a child with a sudden onset of wheezing or stridor and retractions, or in the case of a child with chronic wheezing that is unrelieved by aerosolized bronchodilators.
7. Falls are the most common cause of facial injuries to children.[8] The nurse should be alert to injuries that appear inconsistent with the mechanism reported or allegedly resulting from activities beyond the developmental abilities of the child.
8. Midfacial fractures are relatively uncommon among school age and younger children. When present, they suggest a high-energy mechanism of injury with an increased risk of intracranial injury.
9. Nasal foreign bodies occur most commonly in childhood, especially with toddlers. Foreign bodies of the ear are also common in childhood but are found in individuals of any age, often related to using various small objects to "clean" the ear canals.

Adults

1. The most common cause of facial fractures to young adults is interpersonal violence. With males, this tends to arise from altercations with strangers in settings where alcohol has been ingested. In cases involving females, assailants are more frequently known to the victim—often domestic partners.[8]
2. The initial onset of Ménière's disease generally occurs between 30 and 50 years of age.

Geriatric patients

1. Falls are the most common cause of facial and head injuries for the geriatric population.[8] The nurse must be

alert to an alleged mechanism of injury inconsistent
with the injuries seen.

2. It is important in cases of geriatric patients who have
sustained falls to determine if there was a loss of consciousness either before or after the fall. Of particular
concern is a history of several falls or increasing confusion over a span of several weeks because this could indicate a subacute or chronic subdural hematoma.

3. Older adults are also more prone to posterior epistaxis[11,12] and profuse bleeding from facial and scalp
wounds.

4. Ludwig's angina, a severe cellulitis of the oral cavity, is
most common among geriatric patients who have some
degree of immune compromise.[7]

E

INITIAL INTERVENTIONS

1. A patient with actual or potential airway compromise
should be triaged directly to a treatment area where suction and intubation equipment is immediately at hand.

2. Cardiac and continuous pulse oximetry monitoring
should be initiated if signs of airway compromise are
present. (Epiglottitis in children may be an exception—
see Collaborative Interventions.)

3. When possible, elevate the head of the bed to facilitate
air movement.

4. Bleeding should be controlled with direct pressure.

5. Large-bore IV access should be established if the patient
is hemodynamically unstable.

6. A patient with epistaxis should be triaged to an examination chair unless he or she is hypotensive or syncopal.

PRIORITY NURSING DIAGNOSES*

Risk for ineffective airway clearance
Risk for aspiration
Risk for cervical spine injury
Risk for impaired gas exchange
Risk for fluid volume deficit
Risk for brain injury
Risk for pain

---

*Because of the heterogeneous nature of clinical conditions, nursing
diagnoses in this chapter are stated in terms of related factors or risk
factors. Interventions are discussed under Clinical Conditions.

Risk for sensory-perceptual alteration: auditory, visual, or proprioceptive

Risk for impaired skin or mucous membrane integrity

Risk for infection

Risk for body image disturbance

- ◆ **Ineffective airway clearance:**
  RISK FACTORS
  - Upper airway swelling related to infection or trauma
  - Foreign body aspiration
  - Diminished level of responsiveness
  - Bleeding
- ◆ **Aspiration:**
  RISK FACTORS
  - Positioning (e.g., spinal precautions)
  - Diminished level of responsiveness
  - Gastric distention (e.g., traumatic ileus)
  - Foreign body in upper airway
- ◆ **Cervical spine injury:**
  RISK FACTORS
  - High-energy blunt or penetrating mechanism of injury
  - Vehicular ejection
  - Injury above clavicles
  - "Clothesline" injury
- ◆ **Impaired gas exchange:**
  RISK FACTORS
  - Upper airway swelling related to infection or trauma
  - Aspiration of foreign body
  - Posterior nasal packing[4,11-13]
- ◆ **Fluid volume deficit** related to bleeding, vomiting, or impaired swallowing
- ◆ **Brain injury:**
  RISK FACTORS
  - High-energy blunt or penetrating mechanism of injury above clavicles
  - Known or suspected period of airway compromise or hypoxia
  - Orbital cellulitis or severe sinusitis
- ◆ **Pain** related to trauma, infection, or inflammation
- ◆ **Sensory-perceptual alteration: auditory, visual, or proprioceptive** related to trauma, infection, or vestibular dysfunction
- ◆ **Impaired skin or mucous membrane integrity** related to trauma

♦ **Infection:**
RISK FACTORS
- Foreign body in ear or nose
- Open facial fractures
- Odontalgia or dental abscess
- Open mandibular fractures
- Nasal septal or auricular hematoma

♦ **Body image disturbance:**
RISK FACTORS
- Facial trauma
- Preoccupation with cosmetic consequences of injury

E

PRIORITY DIAGNOSTIC TESTS
Laboratory Tests
Arterial blood gas: An ABG is useful in cases of partial airway obstruction or trauma. Avoid the test in cases of suspected pediatric epiglottitis (see "ABG" in Collaborative Interventions).

Blood studies as indicated or by trauma protocol: Perform a CBC, ethanol, chemistry panel, and blood bank (type and screen or crossmatch and coagulation studies).*

Cultures: Obtain blood cultures in cases of orbital or pharyngeal cellulitis or peritonsillar abscess. Obtain a pharyngeal culture. Rapid strep cultures (i.e., 24 hours) have a lower false negative rate than latex agglutination (strep antibody) screens (never swab throat if epiglottitis is suspected).

Radiographic Tests
Plain radiographs: Obtain a cervical spine series (according to mechanism of injury and trauma protocols); a lateral soft tissue neck film (foreign bodies and often in epiglottitis); facial films (choice of views depends on what should be visualized and whether the cervical spine has been cleared); a chest x-ray film; a KUB; a soft tissue neck film; or a "babygram" (to localize a radiopaque foreign body).

CT scans: CT scans are useful in cases of facial injuries in multiple trauma or head injury, in cases of penetrating

---

*In posterior epistaxis, a baseline CBC, PT and PTT, and type and screen are often ordered in the ED. They are rarely necessary in cases of anterior epistaxis.

trauma or impalement, or in cases of orbital cellulitis or severe sinusitis.

Panorex:* Panorex films may be obtained for mandible injuries, multiple dental avulsions, and periodontal abscess.

Barium (Ba^{++}) swallow: Use a barium swallow for an esophageal foreign body, particularly food.†

Other Tests

Fiberoptic endoscopic procedures (laryngoscopy, bronchoscopy, and esophagoscopy): These are diagnostic, as well as definitive, treatments for some foreign bodies.

Continuous pulse oximetry: Continuous pulse oximetry is useful in cases of suspected airway compromise and to monitor response to oxygen therapy. A patient may have a "normal" SpO_2 and still require oxygen (e.g., if hemoglobin is low); therefore SpO_2 is more useful for establishing a trend. It should not be the sole criterion on which a decision to initiate oxygen therapy is made.

COLLABORATIVE INTERVENTIONS

Overview

Collaborative interventions are grouped by human response patterns to acute alterations in structure and function (e.g., risk of airway compromise or bleeding).

Clinical Conditions
Epiglottitis (supraglottitis)

Risk for airway compromise

SIGNS AND SYMPTOMS

- Epiglottitis is bacterial (usually *Haemophilus influenzae*) and is characterized by rapid onset of high fever (>39° C) and a toxic appearance.
- In addition to the classic signs previously discussed (see Triage), open-mouth breathing with tongue protrusion, a "sniffing" position, or a tripod position may be seen.[3]
- Cyanosis or pallor may be present.[1,2]

---

*A patient must be able to sit up in a special chair for a Panorex. If the patient cannot tolerate sitting up, or if the cervical spine has not been cleared, other studies, such as an AP face, reverse Waters' view, and plain mandible films, may be ordered.

†Alternatively, a cotton pledget soaked in contrast may be swallowed.[3]

- With adults, epiglottitis may have a more indolent onset and may not be characterized by high fever.
- Often the chief complaint is of the worst sore throat of the patient's life.[3]

DIAGNOSIS

- With children, epiglottitis is diagnosed primarily by clinical presentation and rapidity of onset.
- Lateral soft tissue neck films may be helpful in ambiguous presentations but are not always necessary.
- If a child is sent to the x-ray department, a parent should be allowed to remain with the child, a crash cart should be immediately available, and the child should be attended by an emergency nurse or physician.
- With adults, indirect laryngoscopy (e.g., with a mirror) can be performed[4] and lateral soft tissue neck films may be more helpful.

TREATMENT

- Children: The child and parent should be triaged immediately to a resuscitation area, and the child should be allowed to remain in whatever position facilitates breathing.[2]
- As soon as epiglottitis is suspected, an emergency nurse or physician should continuously observe the child.[2]
- The child will not tolerate lying down and should not be made to do so.[2,4]
- Because of the child's tenuous airway, the nurse should avoid performing, and protect the child from, intrusive procedures.
- Blow-by oxygen and a cardiac monitor may be used if the child will tolerate them without increased distress, but no attempt should be made to secure a mask or nasal cannula to the child's face.[1]
- Usually the airway will be secured under direct visualization by an otolaryngologist or anesthesiologist in the operating room, in case an emergency tracheostomy is required.[2-4]
- In crash situations in the field or ED, a cricothyrotomy may be necessary.[2,4]
- Once the airway has been secured, attention can then be directed toward obtaining laboratory studies, initiating IV fluids, and administering antibiotics—usually second- or third-generation cephalosporin or ampicillin/sulbactam (Unasyn).[14]

- Adults with epiglottitis are often treated with high-dose steroids in addition to antibiotics.[3] Adults are less likely than children to need emergency intubation; development of stridor is a strong predictor of the need for intubation or tracheostomy for the adult.[15]

Croup (laryngotracheobronchitis)

SIGNS AND SYMPTOMS

- Croup can be a cause of severe airway compromise.
- The child will have frequent paroxysms of the characteristic barking cough, inspiratory stridor, and retractions.
- Fever is often present in laryngotracheobronchitis (LTB), but usually is not as high as in epiglottitis.
- Often the symptoms of LTB worsen at night, and the parents frequently report that the child sounded worse at home than on arrival in the ED (because of the soothing effect of cooler, moister air outside).
- Depending on the degree of distress, it is acceptable to attempt to measure vital signs and oxygen saturation in triage.
- In cases of severe distress, triage is immediate. In older children, the coughing may be intermittent with relatively normal breathing in between.
- Depending on department volume and waiting times, it may be prudent to categorize even milder cases of LTB as emergencies.

DIAGNOSIS

- Diagnosis of LTB is based on clinical presentation and progression of symptoms. Most croup is viral.
- The croupy cough is pathognomonic.
- In contrast to epiglottitis, the typical history is a respiratory infection of more insidious onset that has worsened, often over several days.
- Membranous croup (MLTB) is a rare but potentially life-threatening condition. Symptoms are similar to viral LTB, but MLTB tends to occur with a slightly older age group (around 5 years of age) and the child appears to be in a more toxic condition than the child with viral croup. MLTB is probably a bacterial superinfection of a viral upper respiratory tract infection. The child with MLTB requires admission to an intensive care unit and may require endotracheal intubation. Unlike viral LTB, MLTB necessitates parenteral antibiotics.[10]

TREATMENT

- Triage acuity and the rapidity with which treatment is instituted depend on the vital signs and on the degree of respiratory distress.
- If triage is immediate, oxygen should be started by whatever means the child will tolerate (e.g., blow-by) while vital signs are being assessed.
- Continuous oxygen saturation monitoring should be initiated.
- Treatment is with cool mist. In more severe cases, aerosolized racemic epinephrine may be used alone or in conjunction with a parenteral steroid, most commonly dexamethasone sodium phosphate.[10] Steroids have a much slower onset but much longer duration of action than racemic epinephrine. Therefore they may decrease the total number of doses of racemic epinephrine but are not a substitute for it.[10]
- Traditionally, patients who require racemic epinephrine have been admitted or at least placed on holding or observation status for several hours because of the short duration of action.[10]
- Some authorities suggest that it may be appropriate to discharge patients who have received steroids in addition to racemic epinephrine, provided that: (1) they have been observed closely for several hours, during which time they have remained free of signs of respiratory distress (e.g., retractions and stridor), and (2) the parent or caregiver is responsible, understands signs and symptoms of a worsening condition, and can easily return or access appropriate follow-up.[16]
- Antibiotics are generally reserved for cases serious enough to warrant admission and are not a mainstay of emergency treatment.

LeFort II and III fractures
SIGNS AND SYMPTOMS

- LeFort II and III fractures are high-energy injuries from direct blows to the midface, and they should be considered based on mechanism of injury.
- Patients generally have nasal and pharyngeal bleeding and massive swelling and ecchymosis around the eyes, nose, maxilla, and upper oral cavity.
- Abnormal approximation of the teeth is common.

- The patient may be obtunded because of a concomitant head injury.
- Cerebrospinal fluid (CSF) rhinorrhea may be present but may be obscured by bleeding.
- A "halo" test on a piece of filter paper is helpful.
- LeFort I fractures are less serious, but loose or avulsed teeth may still represent an airway hazard.

DIAGNOSIS
- The face may look elongated in cases of a LeFort II or III fracture.
- Instability of the facial architecture is present.
- A definitive diagnosis is radiographic; a computed tomography (CT) scan is usually necessary.
- The fractures are often complex and may be mixed (e.g., a LeFort II pattern on one side with a III pattern on the other).
- A LeFort III fracture is a craniofacial separation. The fracture extends across the upper maxilla and nasal bones through the orbit and zygoma.
- A LeFort II fracture is pyramidal and involves the maxilla, nasal bones, palate, and inferior or medial orbit.
- A LeFort I fracture is a linear maxillary alveolar fracture.

TREATMENT
- LeFort fractures require surgical repair, often on a delayed basis.
- From a nursing standpoint, the anatomic distinctions are less important than the recognition of a high-impact injury that may communicate with intracranial structures.
- Based on the mechanism of injury, the patient initially will require spinal precautions that increase the risk of aspiration.
- Yankauer or larger-bore suction should be immediately at hand, and the patient may require intubation.
- Prophylactic intravenous (IV) antibiotics may be ordered.
- If a CSF leak is present, the patient will require neurosurgical consultation.

Airway foreign bodies
SIGNS AND SYMPTOMS
- Acute foreign body aspiration generally presents as moderate to severe respiratory distress with stridor, wheezing, or impaired phonation.
- Breath sounds may be diminished unilaterally or diffusely.

- An occult foreign body (e.g., one that was aspirated at some previous time and not recognized) may present with signs and symptoms of chronic cough, unequal breath sounds, and localized wheezing on forced expiration.[17]

DIAGNOSIS
- Foreign bodies of the airway may be diagnosed by means of a history of sudden onset of distress, by radiograph (lateral neck or chest x-ray), or by fiberoptic laryngoscopy or bronchoscopy.
- An occult foreign body may be suspected with an individual who has suffered recurrent bouts of pneumonia.[17]

TREATMENT
- Patients should be triaged to a resuscitation area and allowed to remain in whatever position in which breathing is most comfortable and least fatiguing—usually sitting up.
- A baseline O_2 saturation should be checked and high-flow cool mist oxygen per mask or blow-by should be initiated.
- The most common foreign body in adults is a food bolus.
- In cases involving children, small toys, buttons, coins, and nuts are common.
- Removal is generally performed with a fiberoptic laryngoscope and forceps or via bronchoscopy.

Ludwig's angina
SIGNS AND SYMPTOMS
- Ludwig's angina is a diffuse cellulitis of the sublingual, submental, and submandibular tissues characterized by high fever, tense brawny edema of the submandibular area, and tongue protrusion.[7]
- Ludwig's angina can cause airway compromise and can extend to the mediastinum, resulting in mediastinitis.

DIAGNOSIS
- This condition is usually seen with older adults, often with some degree of immune compromise.[7]
- Diagnosis is based on the location and appearance of cellulitis.
- A complete blood count (CBC) and blood cultures are generally ordered as a baseline septic workup.
- Lateral soft tissue neck and chest x-rays may also be needed.

TREATMENT
- The patient should be admitted and given IV antibiotics, usually high-dose penicillin G and cefoxitin or metroni-

dazole. Ampicillin and sulbactam or ticarcillin and clavulanate may also be used.[14]

Parapharyngeal, retropharyngeal, and peritonsillar abscess

SIGNS AND SYMPTOMS

- Most patients with these conditions are febrile and complain of moderate to severe neck or pharyngeal pain, odynophagia (painful swallowing), and dysphagia (difficulty swallowing).
- Patients may also exhibit dysphonia (muffled, "hot potato" voice) or signs of airway compromise (e.g., stridor).
- Peritonsillar and parapharyngeal abscesses are unilateral and cause uvular displacement. Trismus also may be present.[3]
- A parapharyngeal abscess often presents with torticollis.[3]

DIAGNOSIS

- Diagnosis is determined by clinical symptoms.
- A peritonsillar abscess is more localized. The patient is usually symptomatic for 48 hours before the abscess becomes apparent.[4]
- A parapharyngeal abscess usually extends down into the tissue planes of the neck and is more serious, though less common than a peritonsillar abscess.
- A retropharyngeal abscess may be a sequel to a puncture of the posterior pharyngeal wall by a foreign body (e.g., a bone shard) or iatrogenic instrumentation (e.g., endotracheal intubation or endoscopy). It may also occur as a complication of diabetes or a compromised immune response (e.g., alcoholism, malignancy, or an HIV-related disease).[18]
- In cases of retropharyngeal abscess, swelling of the posterior pharyngeal wall may not be visible on physical examination.[18]
- Lateral soft tissue neck radiographs or a CT scan may be necessary to confirm or differentiate among diagnoses.[4,18]
- Leukocytosis is a common clinical finding in these conditions. A baseline septic work up may be ordered.

TREATMENT

- Patients with a parapharyngeal abscess are admitted, and high-dose parenteral antibiotic therapy is initiated.
- Peritonsillar abscesses are generally aspirated, or incised and drained in the ED; on occasion the patient may be

discharged from the ED, but often patients are admitted for a short stay and IV antibiotics.

- Patients with a retropharyngeal abscess may require emergency examination in an operating room under general anesthesia, operative incision and drainage, and admission for high-dose parenteral antibiotic therapy.

Epistaxis

SIGNS AND SYMPTOMS

- Active epistaxis is obvious. Even in cases where the patient appears to be bleeding from both nares, epistaxis is almost always unilateral.
- It is helpful at triage to have the patient identify on which side bleeding was first evident and whether the direction in which bleeding was first noted was from the naris or in the pharynx.[11,12]
- Unless syncopal, the patient should be triaged to an ENT examination room.

DIAGNOSIS

- The basic diagnostic question in epistaxis is the location of bleeding.
- The vast majority of epistaxis is anterior, most commonly from the mucosa of the anterior (cartilaginous) nasal septum (known as Kiesselbach's area or Little's area).[13,19]
- Identification of an anterior bleeding site is diagnostic. Anterior bleeds rarely require hematologic and coagulation studies unless the patient is receiving anticoagulants or is uremic.[4]
- Posterior epistaxis is more profuse and more difficult to control.
- Epistaxis unresponsive to pressure over Little's area suggests a posterior site, as does bleeding around or behind a preexisting anterior nasal pack.

TREATMENT

Anterior epistaxis

- The patient should sit upright and apply firm, continuous bilateral pressure between thumb and forefinger to the septal cartilage just above the alae for about 10 minutes.
- Often it is helpful for the nurse to apply the pressure initially so the patient can acquire the "feel" for the location and amount of pressure.
- If the patient is unable to maintain the pressure, the nurse should maintain it.

- The patient should be supplied with a basin or suction for oral secretions but should be instructed not to expectorate forcefully or blow the nose until immediately before the nasal examination.
- Typical supplies for a nasal examination include a head lamp, nasal speculum, bayonet forceps, a Frazier suction tip, silver nitrate applicators, and bacitracin ointment.
- Cocaine diluted to a 4% or 5% solution is commonly used as a topical anesthetic and vasoconstrictor. Alternatively, a mixture of tetracaine (Pontocaine) or 4% lidocaine with phenylephrine or epinephrine can be used.[4,11,12]
- At the beginning of the examination, the patient is instructed to blow out any clots from nares. Suction with a Frazier tip should be set up and ready beforehand.
- The physician uses bayonet forceps to place cotton pledgets moistened with anesthetic in the nasal vestibule. The pledgets should be left in place for 5 to 10 minutes, after which any localized bleeding sources can be cauterized.[11,12]
- Silver nitrate cautery is preferred over electrocautery because it is less likely to damage the septum.[12]
- Once hemostasis has been achieved, an anterior pack with a long ribbon of petrolatum gauze or a cellulose (Merocel) tampon or Oxycel packing can be placed.[4,11-13]
- Petrolatum gauze or Merocel packing should be removed in 1 to 2 days in the ED or by the patient's private physician.
- Oxycel does not have to be removed; it desiccates and can be blown out by the patient in a few days.
- Patients should be counseled to avoid drinking beverages that are either very hot or very cold while packing is in place.
- Patients should also avoid aspirin and nonsteroidal anti-inflammatory drugs for at least several days.
- Patients should be instructed not to lift heavy objects or engage in straining while a pack is in place.
- Patients may be more comfortable at home resting in an orthopneic position (e.g., with enough pillows to elevate the head and upper torso to the equivalent of a semi-Fowler's position).

Posterior epistaxis
- If an anterior site cannot be identified, or if bleeding continues in spite of packing or resumes after an anterior pack is in place, a posterior bleed is suspected.[11,12]

Posterior bleeds are usually from a branch of the ethmoid artery and can be profuse or intermittent.[11] Generally, a posterior bleed necessitates an ENT consultation. If a posterior pack is placed, the patient should be admitted. Geriatric patients or those with chronic obstructive pulmonary disease may require ICU admission because of a risk of hypoxemia or hypercapnia with a posterior pack in place.[4,12] Ultimately, the patient may require surgical ligation. The most common means of tamponading a posterior bleed is a double balloon catheter (Naso-Stat or Epi-Stat).[11-13] The proximal balloon fills up the nasal cavity and the distal balloon is inflated in the nasopharynx to block retrograde bleeding and keep the larger, nasal balloon in place. The balloons may be inflated with sterile water or normal saline. A combination of petrolatum gauze or Oxycel anterior packing may be used in conjunction with balloon tamponade.[13]

- Posterior gauze packs are rarely used anymore because they are extremely uncomfortable; however, they are occasionally needed if balloon tamponade is ineffective. A posterior gauze pack consists of a wad of tightly folded gauze sponges that are firmly tied together by a minimum of three ties that are at least 6 inches long. A Robinson catheter is passed through to the nasopharynx and brought out through the mouth. Two of the ties are tied through the eyelet of the catheter, and the third is taped to the cheek. The catheter is pulled back out the nose, and traction is applied to the two ties until the pack lodges firmly in the nasopharynx. The two nasal ties are taped to the outside of the nose or the cheek. Systemic analgesics are usually needed for pain; some physicians may order a sedative as well. On occasion, patients will have a vasovagal episode resulting from the pain and stimulation of the pack.

Facial fractures (altered structural integrity)
The treatment of facial bone fractures varies with the location and the amount of bony displacement. Nasal and mandibular fractures are the most common. Ice should be applied acutely to any areas of facial swelling as soon as the patient has been triaged. Because most of the facial bones are not mobile and it is difficult to assess the degree of deformity while acute swelling is present, many patients with facial fractures may be discharged with instructions to fol-

low up with a plastic surgeon or ENT specialist after the swelling has gone down. Surgical intervention, if indicated, is often elective.

Mandibular fractures

SIGNS AND SYMPTOMS

- Classic signs of a mandibular fracture are malocclusion and an inability to open the mouth completely.
- Forcible displacement of two or more adjacent lower teeth toward the tongue is another sign of a probable mandibular fracture.[7]

DIAGNOSIS

- Because of its shape, the mandible is frequently fractured in more than one location; hence the desirability of a Panorex film, because this shows the entire mandible in the same plane.[7,20]
- The most common fracture sites are the mandibular angle, body, and symphysis.[7,20]
- If clinical signs of a mandibular fracture are evident, it should be assumed that any intraoral laceration in the mandibular region is an open fracture.[7]

TREATMENT

- Patients with mandibular fractures frequently need suction to help with the removal of blood and oral secretions that can be especially problematic if spinal precautions are in place.
- Often, the patient or a family member can be given a Yankauer suction and shown how to use it; if the patient is too obtunded or uncooperative, the nurse should anticipate that frequent suctioning may be necessary.
- Recent literature suggests that open reduction and internal fixation is gaining favor over intermaxillary fixation.[20]

Nasal fractures

SIGNS AND SYMPTOMS

- Nasal fractures are the most common facial bone fracture and are characterized by pain, swelling, possible deformity, and epistaxis or clotted blood in the nares.

DIAGNOSIS

- Diagnosis of nasal fractures is generally made on clinical grounds.
- The patient will need a nasal speculum examination to rule out a septal hematoma.
- Radiographs are generally unnecessary, and even when positive they rarely influence treatment.[21,22]

TREATMENT

- A fractured nose is generally not urgent unless the fracture is open or a septal hematoma is present.
- Ice should be applied while the patient is awaiting treatment.
- As with facial bone fractures, the necessity of surgical repair for nasal fractures is generally evaluated after swelling has gone down, 1 to 2 weeks after the injury.

Dental avulsions

SIGNS AND SYMPTOMS

- A completely avulsed tooth is generally obvious.
- Often, intraoral bleeding or a bloody socket is present.
- A luxation is a displacement of a tooth.

DIAGNOSIS

- A luxation can be identified by manual examination.
- In cases of complete avulsion, the tooth may be replantable, particularly if replantation occurs within 2 hours of the injury.
- The best salvage rate for replantation occurs when extraoral time is <30 minutes.[5,6] Therefore it is important to establish the time of injury and how the tooth has been handled.

TREATMENT

- While awaiting replantation or while en route to the hospital, it is best to keep the tooth in a container with milk or saline as a transport medium.
- Plain water should not be used because of its hypotonicity.[5,6]
- Alternatively, the patient may carry the tooth in the sublingual or buccal sulcus, but only if the patient is alert and a suitable transport medium is unavailable.[5] (Saliva is hypotonic and highly contaminated with bacteria.) There are commercially available tooth preservation sets that use Hank's solution, a buffered solution that contains glucose, Mg^{++}, and Ca^{++} in a small jar with a basket inside for holding the tooth.[6]
- The root of the tooth should not be handled. Before replantation the root of the tooth should be gently flushed with sterile saline.
- Early dental consultation is indicated.
- Dental fractures are less urgent and have variable prognoses, depending on what part of the tooth is involved.
- Higher priority should be accorded broken teeth that have exposed pulp. This may appear as a vascular core or

at times as a pink-tinged pulsation visible through a
dentinal surface.[5]

Auricular and nasal septal hematomas

SIGNS AND SYMPTOMS

- An auricular hematoma is caused by a blunt blow to the
  external ear.
- The hematoma is an obvious injury, characterized by
  swelling and ecchymosis.
- A nasal septal hematoma is not obvious to gross inspection but is a risk when the patient has a fractured nose.

DIAGNOSIS

- An auricular hematoma is diagnosed by direct observation.
- A nasal septal hematoma is diagnosed by direct inspection of the septum, using a nasal speculum.

TREATMENT

- Cartilage is avascular and receives its blood supply from
  the perichondrium.
- A hematoma of the auricle or nasal septum threatens the
  viability of the underlying cartilage because the extravasated blood is between the cartilage and the perichondrium. This can cause avascular necrosis of the cartilage that leads to either a "cauliflower ear" or a
  saddle-nose deformity.[12,21]
- The treatment for either an auricular or a nasal septal
  hematoma is an incision and drainage (I & D) of the
  hematoma.[12,21]
- Following the I & D, in the case of the auricle, the convo-
  lutions of the auricle are packed with petrolatum gauze.
  Several gauze sponges are laced between the auricle and
  the scalp to hold it in a neutral position, then the entire
  area is padded with fluff gauze and secured with a roll
  gauze bandage that covers the dressed ear.[12]
- In the case of the septal hematoma, following the I & D,
  a small drain (e.g., a sterile rubber band) is placed and
  an anterior pack is inserted as with anterior epistaxis.[12]
  In either case the packing and dressing must be changed
  daily and the respective structures inspected for evidence
  of reaccumulation or infection.

Facial lacerations

Open facial wounds should be dressed with moist saline
dressings or cleansed with saline or Shur-Clens. Betadine
should not be applied directly to open facial wounds unless

it is diluted because it is toxic to subcutaneous tissue and can increase scarring. Ice packs should be applied to areas of swelling. If the cervical spine is clear, elevation of the head is helpful in reducing swelling.

Ménière's disease and acute labyrinthitis (vestibular dysfunction)

SIGNS AND SYMPTOMS

- Symptoms of Ménière's disease include tinnitus, rotational vertigo, and unilateral, progressive sensorineural hearing loss.[23]
- During recurrent, acute episodes, the vertigo and tinnitus become profound and may be associated with severe nausea and vomiting that can be sufficiently severe to cause dehydration and prostration.
- Acute labyrinthitis has a similar presentation but is not characterized by chronic tinnitus or a progressive hearing loss.

DIAGNOSIS

- Definitive diagnosis for Ménière's disease requires tests that are not performed on an emergency basis (e.g., audiometry and electronystagmography).
- Patients who give a history of multiple episodes of severe vertigo should be referred for a workup.

TREATMENT

- Treatment of an exacerbation of Ménière's disease is aimed at correcting fluid and electrolyte imbalances and relieving vertigo, nausea, and vomiting.
- Antiemetic drugs such as promethazine or droperidol may be necessary.
- Treatment for acute labyrinthitis is supportive and aimed at relieving symptoms.
- Oral meclizine is commonly prescribed to relieve vertigo, frequently in conjunction with a benzodiazepine such as diazepam that helps stabilize vestibular function.[24]
- Patients need to be counseled to change positions gradually and to avoid sudden head movements.

Esophageal foreign body

SIGNS AND SYMPTOMS

- Esophageal foreign bodies, although less serious than airway foreign bodies, are extremely uncomfortable, and often it is difficult at triage to be certain that a foreign body "in the throat" is in fact esophageal.

- If there is any doubt regarding the location of the foreign body (i.e., trachea versus esophagus), it is safest to triage immediately to a treatment area.
- At times the patient can describe the sensation clearly enough that the diagnosis is reasonably certain.
- Phonation is generally not impaired, and stridor should not be present.
- The patient may be retching without nausea.
- Esophageal foreign bodies commonly occur while eating and may be associated with stricture, especially in older adults.

DIAGNOSIS

- Esophageal foreign bodies may be diagnosed by plain radiographs if the object is radiopaque.
- Food and radiolucent objects may be diagnosed by a barium swallow.

TREATMENT

- Often, an esophageal foreign body will gradually pass.
- IV glucagon is occasionally helpful in relaxing the distal (smooth muscle) segment of the esophagus.
- Esophagoscopy is occasionally necessary.
- Depending on the size, nature, and location of the foreign body, it may be removed or pushed into the stomach by means of the endoscope.

Nasal and ear foreign bodies

SIGNS AND SYMPTOMS

- In cases involving children, foreign bodies frequently have delayed presentations that mimic infections such as sinusitis or suppurative otitis.
- Foreign bodies of the ear often present as a conductive hearing loss.
- Occasionally an insect crawls into the ear canal and can be extremely painful and distressing at any age.

DIAGNOSIS

- Foreign bodies of the nose may be visible on direct examination, but an index of suspicion must be maintained in cases of foul, purulent drainage.
- A foreign body of the ear can be seen via otoscopy, but if some time has elapsed since its introduction into the ear canal, cerumen or purulent drainage may obscure it.

TREATMENT

- In the cases of nasal foreign bodies there is some degree of risk that the foreign body might be converted to an airway foreign body if pushed during a removal attempt.

- With ear foreign bodies there is a risk of a tympanic membrane rupture or laceration of the external auditory canal during removal.[25]
- Because of these risks, foreign body removals in the ED are generally performed by or under the supervision of a physician. It is best to set a time limit before undertaking a removal because more harm can be caused by determined removal attempts than has been caused by the foreign body itself. If the time limit has been reached without success, it is best to involve an ENT specialist.[12,25,26]
- Vegetable matter, such as a bean or wood, is difficult to remove because it swells up and becomes too soft to be grasped with a forceps. Hard, spherical foreign bodies, such as beads, are also difficult to grasp.
- Foreign bodies of the ear may be removed by means of alligator forceps, suction tip, or passing an ear curette or Fogarty catheter beyond the foreign body and gently pulling it out. Nursing responsibilities during removal consist primarily of assisting with the examination and removal. Small children will be frightened and will often need to be secured with a sheet or on a papoose board. On occasion, conscious sedation may be ordered for a child before removal.
- Insects in the ear canal can be killed by means of filling the ear canal with microscope immersion oil (highly refined mineral oil),[27] vegetable oil,[27] or 4% topical lidocaine solution.[12] Microscope immersion oil has recently been found to be the most rapid and effective in immobilizing and killing cockroaches in vitro.[27] The killed insect can be removed by irrigation or suction or with forceps.[12,27]
- Nasal foreign-body removal can be performed with alligator forceps, with a suction tip, or by passing a Fogarty catheter past the foreign body, in much the same manner and with the same nursing responsibilities as with ear foreign bodies (see preceding entry). It is helpful to instill a topical vasoconstrictor before any removal attempts.
- Alternatively, a "positive pressure" removal technique has been described for nasal foreign bodies in children.[28,29] A topical vasoconstrictor is instilled into the naris. While waiting for the vasoconstrictor to take effect, the parent or caregiver is instructed to occlude the noninvolved naris manually and "give a puff of 'mouth to mouth'" to the child by making an airtight seal and blowing briefly

(but sharply) into the child's mouth.[28] The child is positioned supine and asked to open his or her mouth so the parent or caregiver can bestow "a big kiss."[28] Compared with instrumentation, the procedure is relatively atraumatic and less stressful to the parent and child, and theoretically it poses less risk of conversion to an airway foreign body.[28] If it is unsuccessful, more-invasive techniques can be used.

Otitis media

Signs and Symptoms

- Acute otitis media is most common among children below school age because of their short, relatively flat eustachian canals.
- Typically, there is a history of several days of a upper respiratory infection followed by increasing fussiness, fever, pain, and emotional distress of the child and parent alike. Symptoms may be unilateral or bilateral.

Diagnosis

- Diagnosis is made by otoscopic examination. The tympanic membrane is red and does not move normally with air insufflation.
- Small children are often discomfited or frightened by ear examinations and may need to be held securely.
- Initially, the parent should hold the child seated in his or her lap with the parent's arms crossed over the child's arms.
- If the child is too restless or uncooperative, the child can be positioned supine, with the arms extended upward.
- The nurse should hold the child's upper arms at either side of the head, and a second person (staff or parent) should hold the child's thighs just above the knees. This permits the examiner to gently hold the head still with one hand while using the otoscope with the other.
- If the tympanic membrane cannot be visualized because of cerumen, the ear canal is generally curetted by the physician.

Treatment

- Although it is not without controversy, ED treatment typically involves oral antibiotics. Amoxicillin is generally appropriate as a first-line agent for children or adults; trimethoprim-sulfamethoxazole and erythromycin-sulfisoxazole are acceptable alternatives if the patient is allergic to penicillin.[14,16,24,30] If adherence is doubtful, a single IM injection of ceftriaxone (50 mg/kg) may be ordered.[16]

- Acetaminophen or ibuprofen may be ordered for pain relief.
- In general, a child with otitis media should be reexamined 1 to 2 weeks after completing a course of antibiotics to make sure the infection has been adequately treated. This is especially important for younger children (<2 years of age) or those with persistent symptoms or a history of recurrent otitis media.[16] If the child is not improving within a few days of starting treatment, a reexamination is in order and a change in antibiotics may be necessary.

Otitis externa

SIGNS AND SYMPTOMS

- An infection of the external auditory canal can be quite painful. It is often related to swimming or diving and is most common in adults and older children.

DIAGNOSIS

- Diagnosis is made by otoscopy. The external auditory canal may be inflamed or contain exudative debris.

TREATMENT

- Treatment consists of gentle debridement of the ear canal with a curette or calcium alginate swab and instillation of polymyxin B–neomycin–hydrocortisone drops.[12,26]
- On occasion, a "wick" (an antibiotic-soaked strip of packing gauze) may be placed in the ear canal to help distribute the medication more evenly and prevent it from coming out of the canal.
- The patient should be instructed to avoid swimming or getting the ear canals wet for a period of about 2 weeks.
- At times, analgesic drops may be helpful.
- Older diabetics may develop malignant *(Pseudomonas)* otitis externa and may need to be hospitalized and given parenteral antibiotics.[14,26]

Sinusitis

SIGNS AND SYMPTOMS

- Complaints of "sinus" congestion or headaches are extremely common, and it is essential to clarify more precisely what the patient's symptoms are.
- Sinusitis generally is accompanied by a sensation of pressure in the affected region and a purulent nasal discharge.
- The patient may be febrile.

DIAGNOSIS

- Definitive diagnosis can be made by an x-ray examination or a CT scan but often is presumptive and based on clinical presentation.
- Transillumination may be used as a diagnostic adjunct.

TREATMENT

- Untreated sinusitis can progress and, as with orbital cellulitis, lead to cavernous sinus thrombosis or other intracranial infections.[31]
- Treatment usually consists of a broad-spectrum antibiotic and a decongestant.
- To avoid inspissation of mucus, antihistamines should be avoided unless allergy is deemed a significant etiologic factor.[12]
- Rarely, irrigation of the sinuses by an ENT specialist may be required.

Odontalgia

SIGNS AND SYMPTOMS

- Patients complaining of severe dental pain commonly come to the ED at night or on weekends when they may have difficulty accessing a dentist. If an abscess is the cause, the patient's jaw or cheek may be swollen on the affected side.
- The patient may be febrile.
- Patients frequently arrive believing they must be seen by a dentist immediately to have an emergency extraction. This is rarely necessary.
- It is helpful in triage to reorient the patient's expectations for the visit: diagnosis of the problem, pain relief, determination of whether an antibiotic is indicated, and facilitation of prompt follow-up care.

DIAGNOSIS

- Odontalgia is a symptom. Diagnosis is directed toward establishing the underlying cause and initiating appropriate treatment.
- Dental or Panorex radiographs may be needed.
- Common causes of odontalgia are abscesses and broken teeth with exposed dentin or pulp.[5]

TREATMENT

- An I & D of an abscess by the physician may be necessary.
- Nursing care is directed toward pain relief.
- The patient will generally be sent home with antibiotics and systemic analgesics.

- Patients with chipped or broken teeth may have them temporarily sealed with calcium hydroxide paste by the emergency physician if there is exposure of dentin or pulp.[5]
- In facilities that do not have dentists on staff, it is helpful for the ED to have some arrangement with area dentists for follow-up of ED visits.

Acute necrotizing ulcerative gingivitis

SIGNS AND SYMPTOMS

- Acute necrotizing ulcerative gingivitis (ANUG) is a mixed anaerobic gingival infection often referred to as trench mouth or Vincent's angina.
- Painful gingivostomatitis, headache, sore throat, anorexia, and halitosis characterize ANUG.

DIAGNOSIS

- Diagnosis is determined by the characteristic appearance of the oral cavity.

TREATMENT

- Treatment is with oral penicillin and with bicarbonate or peroxide mouth rinses.[3,5]
- Follow-up dental referral is recommended.
- Recurrences are common and, on occasion, gingival debridement by a dentist may be necessary.[5]

Cerumen impaction

SIGNS AND SYMPTOMS

- The typical presentation is a complaint of one ear, or occasionally both, feeling plugged or of a sensation of fullness, or some degree of diminished auditory acuity.[26,32]

DIAGNOSIS

- Impaction is easily noted on an otoscopic examination.

TREATMENT

- Removal may be by curette or more commonly by irrigation[26,32] (see Procedure 13).
- Irrigation should be avoided if there is suspicion of tympanic membrane rupture. A ruptured tympanic membrane will not ordinarily lead to hearing loss, but it may be associated with vertigo.[26]
- Patients often have mild discomfort during irrigation but should not experience vertigo, nausea, or severe pain.
- If a patient becomes increasingly symptomatic during irrigation, it should be discontinued and the physician should be notified.
- Removal may be attempted by curette, or the patient may be referred to a specialist.

- For all age groups, impacted cerumen is generally related to attempts to remove cerumen, usually with cotton swabs that tend to tamp it further into the ear canal. At times, patients hold a mistaken belief that cerumen is a pathologic secretion, a belief that may contribute to inappropriately zealous removal attempts. Patients should be instructed not to attempt to remove wax with swabs, match sticks, paper clips, or other small objects.
- Ceruminolytic agents may be recommended to prevent recurrence. Anecdotally, over-the-counter (OTC) liquid docusate sodium (Colace liquid, 1% solution, 10 mg/ml)* instilled once a month is reported to be more effective than either OTC or prescription ceruminolytics (Debrox or Cerumenex, respectively).[33] ENT follow-up is generally not indicated unless a tympanic membrane rupture has been found.

NURSING SURVEILLANCE

1. Airway maintenance
2. Oxygen saturation monitoring and administration as indicated
3. Control of bleeding and monitoring of fluid and blood replacement as indicated
4. Vital signs as appropriate to condition and departmental policy
5. Fever control and seizure prevention
6. Adequacy of pain relief and evaluation of responses to other interventions

EXPECTED PATIENT OUTCOMES

1. The airway shall be spontaneously maintainable, or an artificial airway shall be in place.
2. Oxygen saturation should have remained above 91% throughout stabilization, and vital signs should not have deteriorated.
3. In cases of epistaxis, bleeding should be controlled and vital signs should be within the normal range at the time of admission or discharge. For the patient with a posterior pack, oxygen saturation monitoring and adequate

---

*This product comes in a 30-ml bottle with a calibrated dropper. Docusate sodium syrup should never be used for this purpose.

IV access to permit administration of blood products, if needed, should be instituted.

4. For febrile children, a reduction in fever should be documented before discharge.

5. Nausea and vertigo should be improved at the time of discharge. The patient should be tolerating clear liquids PO.

6. Certain types of pain, particularly resulting from otitis media and odontalgia, may not be completely controllable in the course of a brief visit but should at least be reduced.

7. After disimpaction of cerumen, auditory acuity should be improved.

E

DISCHARGE IMPLICATIONS

1. The patient and family must understand the plan of care, expected self-care, medications, and expected time frames for symptom resolution and follow-up.

2. Means of providing humidified air (e.g., a bedside humidifier or using the shower to steam up the bathroom) should be discussed with parents of children with croup if they are well enough to be discharged. Clear criteria that would warrant a return to the ED should be discussed as well.

3. Patients with anterior nasal packs should understand what to do if bleeding recurs and when to follow-up for packing removal.

4. Parents of children with otitis media or other febrile conditions must know how to measure a child's temperature, how to administer antipyretics and antibiotics, and how to recognize signs and symptoms of deterioration.

5. A patient with a nasal fracture should be instructed to follow up with an ENT or plastic surgeon after the swelling has gone down (1 to 2 weeks) if it is difficult to breathe out of one naris or if the patient is not satisfied with the appearance of the nose.

6. Patients who have had an auricular or nasal septal hematoma incised and drained need to know when to return (or follow-up with a specialist) for dressing or packing changes and drain removal.

7. Patients with dental complaints should be helped to understand the importance of expeditious follow-up with a dentist or oral surgeon. The extent to which fear of den-

tal procedures or financial constraints may have put the patient at risk for a given problem should be explored with the patient in a nonjudgmental fashion.

References

1. Neff JA: Epiglottitis, *J Emerg Nurs* 13:184, 1987.
2. Nemes J, Schmidt E, Kelly L: Epiglottitis: ED nursing management, *J Emerg Nurs* 14:70, 1988.
3. Kimmitz TP, Defries HO: Pharyngeal emergencies, *Top Emerg Med* 6(3):66, 1984.
4. Weimert TA: Common ENT emergencies part 2: the acute nose and throat, *Emerg Med* 24(6):26, 1992.
5. Klokkevold P: Common dental emergencies: evaluation and management for emergency physicians, *Emerg Med Clin North Am* 7:29, 1989.
6. Krasner PR: Treatment of tooth avulsion by nurses, *J Emerg Nurs* 16:29-35, 1990.
7. Shesser R, Smith M: Oral emergencies, *Top Emerg Med* 6(3):48, 1984.
8. Hussain K et al: A comprehensive analysis of craniofacial trauma, *J Trauma* 36:34, 1994.
9. Joseph E et al: Predictors of blinding or serious eye injury in blunt trauma, *J Trauma* 33:19, 1992.
10. Cressman WR, Myer CM III: Diagnosis and management of croup and epiglottitis, *Pediatr Clin North Am* 41:265, 1994.
11. Josephson GD, Godley FA, Stierna P: Practical management of epistaxis, *Med Clin North Am* 75:1311, 1991.
12. Votey S, Dudley JP: Emergency ear nose and throat procedures, *Emerg Med Clin North Am* 7:117, 1989.
13. Jacobs EE, Ota HG, Turner PA: Control of epistaxis. In May HL et al, editors: *Emergency medicine*, ed 2, Boston, 1992, Little, Brown.
14. Sanford JP: *Guide to antimicrobial therapy*, Dallas, 1993, Antimicrobial Therapy.
15. Kass EG et al: Acute epiglottitis in the adult: experience with a seasonal presentation, *Laryngoscope* 103:841, 1993.
16. Pfaff JA, Moore GP: Eye, ear, nose, and throat, *Emerg Clin North Am* 15:327, 1997.
17. Wolkove N et al: Occult foreign-body aspiration in adults, *JAMA* 248:1350, 1982.
18. Tannebaum RD: Adult retropharyngeal abscess: a case report and review of the literature, *J Emerg Med* 14:147, 1996.
19. McGarry GW, Moulton C: The first aid management of epistaxis by accident and emergency medicine staff, *Arch Emerg Med* 10(4):298, 1993.
20. Chu L, Gussack GS, Muller T: A treatment protocol for mandible fractures, *J Trauma* 36:48, 1994.

Ear, Nose, Throat, Facial/Dental Conditions   315

21. Sharp JF, Denholm S: Routine x-rays in nasal trauma: the influence of audit on clinical practice, *J R Soc Med* 87(3):153, March 1994.
22. Nigam A et al: The value of radiographs in the management of the fractured nose, *Arch Emerg Med* 10(4):293, 1993.
23. Emergency Nurses' Association: *Emergency nursing core curriculum*, ed 4, Philadelphia, 1994, WB Saunders.
24. Weimert TA: Common ENT emergencies part 1: the acute ear, *Emerg Med* 24(5):134, 1992.
25. Bressler K, Shelton C: Ear foreign-body removal: a review of 98 consecutive cases, *Laryngoscope* 103(4):367, 1993.
26. Reich JJ, Turbiak TW: Otic emergencies, *Top Emerg Med* 6(3):19, 1984.
27. Leffler S, Cheney P, Tandberg D: Chemical immobilization and killing of intra-aural roaches: an in vitro comparative study, *Ann Emerg Med* 22:1795, 1993.
28. Backlin SA: Positive pressure technique for nasal foreign body removal in children, *Ann Emerg Med* 25:554, 1995.
29. Shapiro RS: Foreign bodies of the nose. In Bluestone CD, Stool SE, Scheetz, MD, editors: *Pediatric otolaryngology*, ed 2, Philadelphia, 1990, WB Saunders.
30. Celin SE et al: Bacteriology of acute otitis media in adults, *JAMA* 266:2249, 1991.
31. Clayman GL et al: Intracranial complications of paranasal sinusitis: a combined institutional review, *Laryngoscope* 101:234, 1991.
32. Zivic RC, King S: Cerumen impaction management for clients of all ages, *Nurs Pract* 18(3):33, 1993.
33. Chen DA, Caparosa RJ: A nonprescription ceruminolytic, *Am J Otol* 12:475, 1991.

Endocrine Conditions

Pamela S. Kidd

TRIAGE ASSESSMENT

Other than diabetes, endocrine conditions are extremely rare. Acute endocrine crises are life threatening and require rapid interventions. Patients may not realize they have an endocrine disorder, and the diagnosis may be made or suspected for the first time in the emergency department (ED). Because hormones affect several target organs, symptoms are multiple and diverse. The goal of triage is to accurately detect a pattern of symptoms related to an endocrine disorder. Specific diagnosis and treatment of the problem will occur in the treatment area. Questions in the following areas should help to detect endocrine disorders.

Existing health problems

Asking about existing health problems will alert you to whether the patient is aware that he or she has an endocrine problem. It also helps to rule out other etiologies of symptoms. For example, if the patient denies a heart problem but has tachycardia and palpitations, hypoglycemia or overproduction of thyroid hormone may be the cause. Tuberculosis has been associated with Addison's disease.[1]

Medication history

If the patient is taking medication, ask about the dosage. Insulin-dependent diabetic patients are at increased risk for ketoacidosis. Thiazide diuretics decrease serum potassium levels and induce hyperglycemia. A steroid-dependent person who stops taking steroid medications can precipitate Addison's disease. Table 8-1 highlights commonly prescribed drugs that may precipitate endocrine problems.

Gestational history

A gestational history is important for females if diabetes is suspected. Previous episodes of gestational diabetes are linked to postpartum diabetes.

Family history

A family history of autoimmune diseases (Hashimoto's thyroiditis, Graves' disease, Addison's disease, and diabetes) is significant.

TABLE 8-1 Drugs That May Precipitate
Endocrine Problems

Drug	Effect	Condition
Hydrochlorothiazide	Decreases insulin secretion and increases insulin resistance	DKA, HHNC
Beta-blocking agents (e.g., propanol)	Decreases insulin secretion	DKA
Dilantin	Decreases insulin secretion	DKA
Alcohol	Decreases insulin secretion	DKA
Calcium channel blockers (e.g., nifedipine)	Decreases insulin secretion	DKA
Cortisol	Increases insulin resistance	DKA, HHNC
Terbutaline	Increases insulin resistance	DKA
Sedatives	Decreases oxygen consumption	Hypothyroidism
Tranquilizers	Decreases oxygen consumption	Hypothyroidism
Diuretics	Decreases circulating blood volume	Hypothyroidism
Ketoconazole	Decreases steroid synthesis	Addison's disease
Rifampin	Decreases steroid synthesis	Addison's disease

DKA, Diabetic ketoacidosis; *HHNC*, hyperosmolar, nonketotic coma.

Stress

Several endocrine disorders (e.g., ketoacidosis and Cushing's disease) are precipitated or exacerbated by stress caused by cortisol secretion.

Dehydration

Determine if the patient has been vomiting, having diarrhea, urinating excessively, or not drinking fluids in a hot, humid environment. Vomiting is associated with diabetic ketoacidosis (DKA). All of these factors promote dehydration, which can precipitate DKA and hyperosmolar, nonketotic coma (HHNC). Vomiting and diarrhea are associated with hyperthyroidism.

Thirst

Thirst is associated with diabetes.

Energy

Fatigue is associated with myxedema, Addison's disease, and diabetes.

Pain

Elicit a description of the pain. Headaches are associated with hypoglycemia. Abdominal pain is associated with DKA and acute adrenal insufficiency.

Mood changes and insomnia

Mood changes and insomnia are characteristic of hyperthyroidism.

Weight

Weight loss is common in hyperthyroidism and Addison's disease.

Vital signs

- *Breathing pattern:* Kussmaul breathing (deep, accelerated, sighing respirations) indicates a pH below 7.2 and acidosis.
- *Blood pressure:* Hypotension is associated with dehydration and decreased circulating blood volume. Orthostatic changes in both blood pressure and pulse may be present. Diastolic hypertension is present in patients with chronic hypothyroidism (myxedema) caused by peripheral vasoconstriction as an effort to maintain body core temperature. Systolic hypertension is associated with Cushing's disease related to fluid retention and oversecretion of catecholamines.
- *Heart rate:* Bradycardia is present in hypothyroidism. Tachycardia and palpitations occur in hyperthyroidism.
- *Fever:* Note any temperature elevation. Infection may be subtle and still increase insulin requirements beyond

what the patient is capable of delivering, precipitating hyperglycemia and hyperosmolarity. A temperature >104° F may be present in hyperthyroidism.

General Observations
Skin
- Assess the patient's hydration status by examining skin turgor, mucous membranes, and orbits. Dry, hot skin is associated with an addisonian crisis. Flushed, dry skin indicates dehydration. Dehydration is associated with Addison's disease, HHNC, and ketoacidosis. Flushed, wet skin is associated with hyperthyroidism.
- Cool, pale skin is associated with hypothyroidism.
- Darkly colored (hyperpigmented) skin in white patients suggests Addison's disease. Hyperpigmentation may be most visible on the back of the hands, elbows, and knees.

Goiter
- A goiter may be present in hyperthyroidism.

Exophthalmos
- Exophthalmos (bulging eyeballs) may be present in hyperthyroidism.

Diaphoresis
- Excessive diaphoresis may occur in hyperthyroidism.

Edema
- Generalized edema may be present in hypothyroidism and syndrome of inappropriate secretion of antidiuretic hormone (SIADH). People with Cushing's disease tend to have round, plump faces with fat pads on the shoulders.

Obesity
- Obesity is a symptom of Cushing's disease.

FOCUSED NURSING ASSESSMENT

The areas of ventilation, perfusion, cognition, and sexuality should be assessed in greater detail.

Ventilation

Auscultate breath sounds. Pulmonary edema, characterized by crackles, may occur in hypothyroidism. Diminished breath sounds may indicate infiltrates and possible infection as a precipitating cause of DKA, HHNC, and thyroid disorders.

Undress the patient and assess the breathing pattern for symmetry and depth of excursion. As noted earlier, deep, rapid respirations indicate acidosis.

E

Perfusion
Auscultate heart sounds. A murmur may be present in high-flow (e.g., Cushing's disease and hypothyroidism) or hyperdynamic (e.g., hyperthyroidism) states.

Assess peripheral pulses. Vasoconstriction is present in Cushing's disease. Diminished pulses may be present in instances of dehydration.

Cognition
Perform a neurologic assessment and document a Glasgow Coma Scale (GCS) score for the patient (see Reference Guide 10). A person who is not oriented may be manifesting symptoms of cerebral edema from hyperosmolality or may be at risk for becoming dehydrated and precipitating hyperosmolarity. Cognition is almost always impaired in HHNC.

Assess the patient for tremors. Tremors and hyperreflexia occur frequently in hyperthyroidism.

Sexuality
Impotence and abnormal menses are associated with Cushing's disease.

Secondary sexual characteristics may be overpronounced (e.g., gynecomastia, and breast development with males) in Cushing's disease.

There is a decrease in body and pubic hair among females with Addison's disease.

Risk Factors
1. A history of diabetes predisposes the patient to hypoglycemia and hyperosmolar coma whether related to ketoacidosis or HHNC.
2. Black males and Native Americans from the Pima tribe have the highest incidence of diabetes in the United States.
3. Obesity is a risk factor for non–insulin-dependent diabetes mellitus (NIDDM).
4. Lung cancer is frequently associated with SIADH (oat cell).

Life Span Issues
Pregnancy
1. Pregnancy may potentiate DKA.
2. Pregnancy may stimulate hyperthyroidism. Failure to gain weight in pregnancy is an indicator of hyperthy-

roidism. Thyrotoxicosis or hypothyroidism may occur in
the postpartum period.
3. Gestational diabetes may occur. This diabetes is more
common among nonwhite and older women.

Children
1. The peak onset of insulin-dependent diabetes mellitus (IDDM) is 11 to 13 years of age. The onset of puberty and the increase of growth hormone may lead
to ketoacidosis.

Adults
1. The risk of NIDDM increases after the age of 40.
2. Thyroid crisis or storm occurs more among females in
the 30- to 50-year-old age range.
3. Addison's disease is more common among 30- to 50-
year-old adults.

Geriatric Patients
1. HHNC is more common in older individuals with
NIDDM.
2. Hypothyroidism causes decreased oxygen consumption
and heat generation. In the geriatric population, oxygen
consumption and heat generation decline as part of aging. Myxedema is diagnosed more frequently in the
geriatric population because symptoms are more pro-
nounced because of less compensatory reserve.

INITIAL INTERVENTIONS

1. Administer low-flow oxygen as needed until laboratory
tests return. Endocrine disorders affect metabolism,
and oxygen administration promotes oxygen availability in both overproduction and underproduction of
hormones.
2. Initiate pulse oximetry monitoring. Oxygen saturation
readings can provide clues regarding acidosis, phosphate levels, and core body temperature. An increased
affinity of oxygen to hemoglobin occurs in these states.
3. Initiate cardiac monitoring. Endocrine disorders may
produce dysrhythmias, conduction defects, and congestive heart failure (CHF).
4. Initiate continuous BP monitoring. Cardiovascular decompensation may occur as a result of the endocrine
problem or in response to rapid treatment. Changes
from baseline should be conveyed immediately.
5. Insert an IV catheter and obtain blood for potential tests
(CBC, electrolyte levels, glucose level, and hormone

function). An intermittent infusion device may be attached until further assessment is completed or laboratory data are returned, since overhydration may be a problem in some endocrine disorders. If dehydration is suspected, administer IV fluid.

PRIORITY NURSING DIAGNOSES

Risk for ineffective breathing patterns
Risk for decreased cardiac output
Risk for injury
   The following nursing diagnoses apply to patients with endocrine disorders.

♦ **Ineffective breathing patterns** related to fatigue, acidosis, and electrolyte abnormality:
   INTERVENTIONS
   • Administer oxygen per physician order.
   • Monitor oxygen saturation.
   • Prepare for endotracheal intubation, neuromuscular blockade, and mechanical ventilation.

♦ **Decreased cardiac output** related to dehydration or decreased contractility resulting from chronic left ventricle overdistention:
   INTERVENTIONS
   • Administer volume or diuretics as case dictates per physician order.
   • Decrease metabolic needs by treating fever, pain, and infection.
   • Monitor intake and output.

♦ **Injury** related to electrolyte disturbances (usually hyponatremia, hypokalemia [except in Addison's disease], or hypophosphatemia):
   INTERVENTIONS
   • Administer electrolyte replacement as laboratory values and the patient's condition indicate.
   • Monitor intake and output.
   • Perform frequent neurologic assessments.

PRIORITY DIAGNOSTIC TESTS

Laboratory Tests

A quick bedside calculation of laboratory tests used in DKA and HHNC is located in Table 8-2.

Adrenocorticotropic (ACTH) test: ACTH will be elevated in Cushing's disease.

TABLE 8-2 Bedside Calculation of Laboratory Tests in Diabetic Ketoacidosis and Hyperosmolar, Nonketotic Coma

Type	Rationale	Formula
Sodium correction	Serum sodium levels appear lower than they actually are as hyperglycemia is corrected	Add 2.8 mmol to the patient's reported sodium level for every 100 mg/dl increase in blood sugar above normal; normal considered 100 mg/dl (example: if blood glucose is 500 mg/dl, multiply $4 \times 2.8 = 11.2$; add 11.2 mmol to actual reported serum sodium value)
Serum osmolality	Measured osmolality by laboratory includes all molecules	$2 \times$ (serum Na + serum K) + blood glucose / 18 = calculated serum osmolality
	Calculated osmolality allows you to examine only molecules that contribute to dehydration; if calculated osmolality is less than measured and patient is comatose, there is another cause other than dehydration for coma	
Anion gap	Indicates an acidotic state but does not tell you what kinds of acids have produced the state (e.g., lactic acid vs. ketones)	Sodium − (chloride + bicarbonate) Normal range = 8-16 or Na + K − (chloride + bicarbonate) Normal range = 12-20

Aldosterone level: This will be decreased in Addison's disease.

Anion gap: An elevated anion gap indicates acidosis. An anion gap >20 mmol/L indicates DKA.

Arterial blood gases: The pH values will be low in both ketoacidosis and HHNC. They will be below 7.2 in ketoacidosis. Bicarbonate levels will be below 15 mEq/L in DKA.

Cortisol (serum): This will be at a decreased level in Addison's disease.

Cultures: Blood, urine, and sputum cultures may be needed to determine if an infection is present in HHNC and DKA, since the WBC count is normally elevated in these states.

Glucose: Glucose levels will be low in hypoglycemia, acute adrenal insufficiency, Addison's disease, and hypothyroidism. They will be elevated in ketoacidosis, HHNC, and Cushing's disease. A level >300 mg/dl suggests dehydration or impaired renal function. The highest levels (average = 1100 mg/dl) are found in HHNC.

Potassium: The level of potassium will be high in Addison's disease and untreated hyperosmolar states. As the patient is rehydrated, potassium moves back into the cell and levels may fall below normal.

Rapid synthetic corticotropin stimulation test: This test is used to determine if adrenal dysfunction is causing Addison's disease. Synthetic ACTH is administered IV and cortisol levels are measured at baseline and 30- and 60-minute intervals after administration. Failure of cortisol levels to increase indicates a primary adrenal problem.

Serum osmolality: This value will be elevated in both ketoacidosis and HHNC. A value >340 mOsm/L produces a comatose state.

Sodium: Hyponatremia may be present in Addison's disease and myxedema.

Thyroid Stimulating Hormone: This level will be low in secondary hypothyroidism (pituitary tumor) and in hyperthyroidism. It will be elevated in primary hypothyroidism (loss of functioning thyroid tissue).

Triiodothyronine (T_3) level: The level of T_3 is elevated in hyperthyroidism.

Thyroxine (T_4) level: The level of T_4 is elevated in hyperthyroidism.

Urine-free cortisol test: This 24-hour test detects cortisol excretion in the urine, commonly seen in Cushing's disease. If the test result is positive for cortisol, ACTH tests are conducted to determine the etiology of the disease.

Urine ketones: Ketones will be present in DKA but absent in HHNC.

WBCs: The WBC count is normally elevated without infection in diabetic patients. Levels of 40,000 cells/mm^3 have been noted in DKA without infection. An increased neutrophil count indicates infection in diabetic patients. Hypothyroid patients may be unable to elevate the WBC count in infection because of depressed bone marrow activity. An elevated band count on the differential indicates infection in these patients.

Radiographic Tests

CT scan: Scans of the adrenal, pituitary, and thyroid glands may be performed to identify gland enlargement, atrophy, and tumors.

Other Tests

ECG: T-wave changes during fluid resuscitation for dehydration may indicate impending CHF. Sinus bradycardia, a prolonged QT interval, and low voltage are seen on the ECG in hypothyroidism.

COLLABORATIVE INTERVENTIONS

Overview

1. Anticipate drug administration before the return of laboratory data because of serious consequences from many endocrine disorders (Table 8-3).
2. Draw blood for diagnostic testing before initiating medication in order to provide accurate baseline hormonal levels.[2]
3. Invasive hemodynamic monitoring may be initiated because of a need for monitoring vascular response to treatment. Assist with insertion and obtain measurements.
4. A urinary catheter is frequently inserted to monitor renal response to treatment.

TABLE 8-3 Drug Summary

Drug	Dose/Route	Use	Special considerations
Aminoglutethimide	1-2 g PO in divided doses	Cushing's disease	Causes rash, somnolence
Bromocriptine	2.5-15 mg PO	Cushing's disease	Causes nausea, headache, fatigue
Cyproheptadine	Up to 24 mg/day PO	Cushing's disease	Causes weight gain, somnolence
Demeclocycline	600-1200 mg/day PO	SIADH	Causes fever, headache, paresthesia
Dexamethasone	2 mg IV q6h	Thyroid storm	Stops peripheral conversion of T_4 to T_3
Fludrocortisone	50 µg q D; 200 µg/day PO	Addison's disease	Causes flushing, hypertension, headache
Hydrocortisone	In thyroid storm: 300 mg IVP followed by 100 mg q8h IV In Addison's disease: 100 mg IV push followed by 100 mg q4-6h IV	Thyroid storm, Addison's disease May also be given in myxedema to prevent acute adrenal insufficiency precipitated by levothyroxine administration	Causes rash, itching
Ketoconazole	600-1200 µg IV 200 mg PO qd; increase to 400 mg if needed	Cushing's disease	Causes hepatotoxicity, nausea, and vomiting

E

Drug	Dose	Indication	Comments
Levothyroxine	500 µg IV	Myxedema coma	Causes tachycardia, hypertension
Methimazole (MMI)	20 mg q4h PO	Thyrotoxicosis	Causes nephrotoxicity and rash
Metyrapone	2-6 g PO	Cushing's disease	Causes nausea, headache, and rash
Mitotane	9-10 g PO	Cushing's disease	Causes vomiting
Potassium iodide	1 g PO or NG or 5 drops q6h	Thyroid storm	Do not give until new thyroid hormone synthesis has been blocked with MMI or PTU
Propranolol	1 mg q5min IV prn	Thyroid storm	Blocks beta-adrenergic effects of thyroid hormone synthesis and inhibits conversion of T_3 to T_4
Propylthiouracil (PTU)	In thyrotoxicosis: 300-450 mg PO; In thyroid storm: 1 g PO or NG tube	Thyrotoxicosis; Thyroid storm	Inhibits thyroid hormone synthesis and inhibits conversion of T_3 to T_4
Sodium iodide	1-2 g IV over 24 hr	Thyroid storm	Do not give until new hormone synthesis has been blocked with MMI or PTU

Clinical Conditions
Diabetic ketoacidosis

Diabetic ketoacidosis (DKA) can be present with or without hyperosmolar coma. The use of free fatty acids for energy vs. glucose produces ketoacids. The most frequent cause of DKA is an undetected infection.

SYMPTOMS

- Hyperglycemia induces diuresis, so the patient complains of polyuria, thirst, and fatigue.
- In order to differentiate DKA from HHNC, note that patients with DKA may complain of abdominal pain related to gastric dilatation, that their respiratory rate may be rapid with deep breaths (Kussmaul's), and that CNS changes may not be present.

DIAGNOSIS

- Ketones will be present in the urine.
- Arterial blood gases will reveal a pH below 7.35.
- Blood glucose levels will be elevated (>250 mg/dl).[3]
- The serum osmolarity level will be high in some cases.
- The serum bicarbonate level may be low (<15 mEq/L).

TREATMENT

- If the patient is hypotensive, 0.9% normal saline (NS) is administered; otherwise 0.45% NS is given.
- Insulin is administered at a higher rate in DKA than HHNC (4 to 8 U/hr). The goal is to decrease the serum glucose level by 75 to 100 mg/dl per hour.[3] A more rapid reduction may precipitate cerebral edema.
- Potassium replacement may be necessary. When the potassium level reaches 5.5 mEq/L, 10 to 15 mEq/hr by may be initiated. As diuresis proceeds, potassium losses are great.
- Phosphate levels are typically lower with rehydration in DKA; thus phosphate may be given. Table 8-4 compares the treatment of DKA and HHNC.

Hyperosmolar, nonketotic coma

Patients who have HHNC may not have had diabetes diagnosed. Frequently, HHNC is the first indicator of a chronic problem. Almost all cases are precipitated by infection.

SYMPTOMS

- Massive diuresis occurs. Patients complain of polyuria, thirst, and fatigue related to calcium, potassium, and magnesium losses.
- CNS symptoms are common as a result of a high serum osmolality level.

TABLE 8-4 Comparison of Treatment for Diabetic Ketoacidosis and Hyperosmolar, Nonketotic Coma

Rehydration	Correction of Hyperglycemia
In both DKA and HHNC	**In DKA**
If serum sodium level is >165, administer 2.5% dextrose solution	Administer regular insulin IV bolus of 0.1-0.2 U/kg
If serum sodium level is 145-165, administer 0.45% normal saline (NS)	Follow with 0.1-0.2 U/kg/hr IV drip until glucose level reaches 300 mg/dl
If serum sodium level is <145, administer 0.9% NS	**In HHNC**
	Administer insulin 1-2 U/hr (not based on weight—takes much less insulin to correct problem)
Rate	
Administer 2 L within first 2 hours followed by 1 L q2h	
Give ½ of fluid deficit within first 12 hr	
Give last ½ of deficit over next 24 hr	
Start D_5NSS when glucose level reaches 300 mg/dl	
If potassium level is 4.5 or less, give 20-40 mEq of K^+/L of fluid/hr of treatment	
If pH is <7.0, give 1 ampule (44 mEq) of bicarbonate unless patient is comatose Bicarbonate may be administered 2 mEq/kg IV over 1-2 hr	

DKA, Diabetic ketoacidosis; *HHNC,* hyperosmolar, nonketotic coma.

- Patients complain of visual changes.
- Patients may be aphasic, stuporous, and actively seizing and hallucinating.

DIAGNOSIS
- Serum glucose (>400 mg/dl) and osmolarity (>315 mOsm/kg) levels will be high.
- Urine ketones will be negative.
- The arterial pH will be <7.25.

- The result of a urine test may be positive for a urinary tract infection.
- A chest film may indicate pneumonia.

TREATMENT
- Rehydration is accomplished through administration of 0.45% NS.
- IV insulin is administered in dosages of 1 to 2 U/hr.
- Insulin is decreased once the glucose level drops to 300 mg/dl.
- Potassium and phosphate replacement may be necessary.

> **NURSING ALERT**
>
> When treating both DKA and HHNC, it is crucial for the nurse to reassess the patient's breath sounds and neurologic status frequently to detect impending fluid overload; overaggressive rehydration will cause cerebral and pulmonary edema.

Hypoglycemia

Hypoglycemia may occur with a diabetic patient because of inadequate food intake in relation to insulin dosage. Exercise, infection, and emotional stress may also alter blood glucose levels. Nondiabetic patients are also susceptible to hypoglycemia.

SYMPTOMS
- Symptoms are sudden in onset.
- The patient may complain of a headache and dizziness and may appear confused.
- Diaphoresis, tachycardia, and palpitations may be present.

DIAGNOSIS
- The blood glucose level will usually be below 50 to 60 mg/dl.

TREATMENT
- Hypoglycemia is rapidly reversed with administration of IV glucose (50 ml of dextrose 50% solution) or oral glucose if the patient is alert enough to prevent aspiration. Glucagon 1 ml IM may be given as an alternative.

Thyrotoxicosis and thyroid storm

Thyroid storm is a life-threatening illness caused by the excessive release of thyroid hormones, usually precipitated by infection, injury, or the beginning of treatment for hyperthyroidism.

Symptoms
- Symptoms include elevated metabolism, tachycardia, diaphoresis, tremors, and hyperthermia.

Diagnosis
- T_3 and T_4 levels are elevated.
- Hyperglycemia is present.
- Levels of liver enzymes may also be elevated.
- There is debate concerning when thyrotoxicosis becomes thyroid storm. The presence of mental status changes usually signals progression of the hyperthyroid state.
- Tachycardia (>140 beats/min), atrial fibrillation, systolic flow murmurs, and fever (>106° F) indicate thyroid storm.

E

Treatment
- Antithyroid medication is administered (e.g., propylthiouracil or methimazole, see Table 8-3).
- Steroids may be given.
- Acetaminophen is administered and hypothermia measures are initiated.
- Beta-blocking agents (e.g., propranolol) may be given to decrease the cardiac response to thyroid hormone.

Myxedema

Myxedema coma is an acute manifestation of hypothyroidism.

Symptoms
- Altered mental status is present and may range from disorientation to psychosis.
- Hypothermia is another classic symptom.
- A precipitating illness or event usually stimulates a hypothyroid crisis.
- Common associated conditions are stroke, infection, and traumatic injury.

Diagnosis
- Diagnosis is based on the triad of symptoms discussed above.

Treatment
- IV levothyroxine is administered on suspicion of hypothyroidism, since it does not harm a euthyroid patient.
- Respiratory assistance may be needed because of the tendency to retain carbon dioxide. Intubation and mechanical ventilation may be initiated prophylactically because cardiovascular collapse occurs quickly with respiratory depression.

- CHF is a common complication. Diuretics and digoxin are used to treat this problem.
- Hypothermia is treated using core rewarming (e.g., warmed IV fluid, nasogastric fluids, and dialysis).

NURSING ALERT

External warming is avoided in the hypothyroid patient because peripheral vasodilation may produce cardiovascular collapse. Hypotension is a grave sign in hypothyroid patients.

Acute adrenal insufficiency and Addison's disease
Adrenal insufficiency is a devastating disease related to the effects of decreased glucocorticoids (energy availability), decreased mineralocorticoids (e.g., aldosterone) (dehydration), decreased androgens, and increased melanocyte-stimulating activity (hyperpigmentation). Rifampin, used to treat tuberculosis, may cause adrenal insufficiency.

SYMPTOMS
- General symptoms are fatigue, weight loss, dehydration related to nausea and vomiting, hypotension, abdominal pain, increased skin pigmentation, and depression. Females may have decreased body hair.

DIAGNOSIS
- Addison's disease may be caused by a primary adrenal problem or induced secondary to a hypothalamic or pituitary problem.
- ACTH levels will be low if a hypothalamic or pituitary problem exists.
- If cortisol production does not increase after administration of ACTH, an adrenal problem exists.

TREATMENT
- Hypovolemia and sodium depletion are treated with D_5NSS IV infusion. IV hydrocortisone is administered.
- Fludrocortisone is also administered to replace mineralocorticoids.

Cushing's disease
Cushing's disease is the overproduction of cortisol as a result of overactivity of ACTH. Immune suppression caused by cortisol overproduction increases the patient's risk for early death and masks signs of existing infection.

SYMPTOMS
- Obesity, hypertension, fatigue, abdominal pain, and osteoporosis are common symptoms.

DIAGNOSIS
- A urine-free cortisol test and measurement of the ACTH level are used to diagnose the disease.

TREATMENT
- Multiple medications are used in treating Cushing's disease (see Table 8-3). These medications have undesirable side effects and interfere with compliance.
- Surgery and pituitary irradiation may be used in some cases.

Syndrome of inappropriate secretion of ADH

SIADH is associated with lung cancer, CNS disorders, and chemotherapy.

SYMPTOMS
- Generalized edema and decreased urine output are frequent symptoms.
- CHF and changes in the level of consciousness (LOC) are later signs.

DIAGNOSIS
- Thyroid and adrenal function are normal, but the serum osmolarity level is decreased.
- Hyponatremia is present.

TREATMENT
- Fluid restriction is initiated (500-750 ml/24 hr).
- Demeclocycline is administered.
- Chemotherapy aimed at obliterating tumors may be indicated.
- Furosemide 1 mg/kg IV and NS infusion to replace urine losses of sodium are administered.

NURSING SURVEILLANCE

1. Monitor the cardiac pattern and treat potentially lethal dysrhythmias (e.g., tall peak T-waves indicating hyperkalemia, severe bradycardia, and severe tachycardia).
2. Monitor the patient's temperature. Administer antipyretics to decrease oxygen demands. Provide supportive warming in hypothyroidism. Beware of rapid rewarming and subsequent hypotension.
3. Monitor intake and output to determine renal response to volume replacement or diuresis.

4. Monitor the patient's LOC because of increased susceptibility for cerebral edema from a rapid reversal of hyperosmolar state.

EXPECTED PATIENT OUTCOMES

1. The patient's temperature returns to normal.
2. Blood pressure and heart rate stabilize.
3. Urine output is at least 30 ml/hr.
4. The patient's GCS score remains the same or improves.

DISCHARGE IMPLICATIONS

1. Patients on hormone replacement should be instructed
   to pay attention to signs of infection. Drug doses may
   need to be increased in fever and diarrhea.
2. Dramatic changes in weight, the addition of other medications for other problems, and advancing age can alter
   the required dosage and should be reported to the primary care provider.
3. In many cases of hormone replacement, dosage routines
   can be modified to fit patient response and comfort
   (e.g., twice daily vs. three times daily dosage).
   Encourage the patient to discuss dosage routines with
   the primary care provider.
4. Patients taking steroids should be told to inform other
   physicians, dentists, and other appropriate health care
   workers of steroid use before undergoing a procedure.
5. Patients with an endocrine disorder should wear a
   "Medic Alert" bracelet because changes in the LOC occur frequently; some endocrine disorders are rare and
   may not be diagnosed by the care provider available during the acute crisis.

Addison's Disease
The patient should be furnished with a needle, syringe,
and soluble corticosteroid preparation to use during an
acute crisis when traveling to areas without easy health care
access.

Diabetes
Diabetic patients generally will be discharged home after 4
hours of treatment if their pH is >7.35 and their bicarbonate level is >20 mEq/L.[4] Ensure that the patient understands how to prevent dehydration. Have the patient

demonstrate correct measurement of blood glucose and urine ketones using an appropriate device. Instruct the patient to either notify his or her primary provider or return to the ED if any of the following occur[5]:

- The blood glucose level is ≥250 mg/dl, instruct the patient to check for urine ketones when the blood glucose level reaches this figure.[3]
- Urine ketones are positive.
- The patient experiences illness that lasts longer than 24 hours.

Instruct the patient on signs of hypoglycemia and hyperglycemia.

References

1. Davis-Martin S: Disorders of the adrenal glands, *J Am Acad Nurs Prac* 8:323-326, 1996.
2. Bresler MJ, Sternbach GL: *Manual of emergency medicine,* St Louis, 1998, Mosby.
3. American Diabetes Association: *Clinical practice recommendations: diabetes care 20* (suppl 1), city, Alexandria, Va, 1997, The Association
4. Fleckman A: Diabetic ketoacidosis, *Endocrinol Metab Clin North Am* 22(2):181-207, 1993.
5. Suave D, Kessler C: Hyperglycemic emergencies, *AACN Clin Iss* 3:350-360, 1992.

E

ENVIRONMENTAL CONDITIONS

Patty Sturt

TRIAGE ASSESSMENT

Common environmental conditions encountered in emergency department (ED) patients include heat-related, cold-related, and near-drowning emergencies. Depending on geographic location, other environmental emergencies can include high-altitude illnesses, diving emergencies, venomous snake bites, arachnid envenomation, and bee, wasp, and fire ant stings. The patient demonstrates mild symptoms at triage that progress quickly to life-threatening conditions. The following data can help to identify the type of environmental emergency and its severity:

• Ask about events and activities preceding and at the time of the onset of symptoms.
• Record the patient's age, weight, medical history, use of alcohol, and current medications. Infants and geri-

atric patients are highly susceptible to cold- and heat-related emergencies. Alcohol and certain medications increase the risk of weather-related environmental emergencies.
- Note the weather conditions near or at the time of the onset of symptoms. This information may help in identifying cold- or heat-related emergencies.
- Note any recent animal bite or sting (suspect exposure to poisonous venom).

E

Vital Signs
- *Tachycardia and hypotension:* Tachycardia and hypotension may be related to a decreased circulating volume secondary to diaphoresis from a heat illness, to cold diuresis from hypothermia, vasodilation from snake bite venom or anaphylaxis, or to coagulation defects from pit viper envenomation.
- *Bradycardia:* Bradycardia may be related to myocardial depression secondary to hypothermia.
- *Fever:* Fever may be related to a failure of the temperature regulatory mechanism in heat stroke.
- *Tachypnea:* Tachypnea is often related to acidosis and hypoxia, which may occur in heat stroke, animal envenomation, anaphylaxis, altitude illness, and diving emergencies.

General Observations
Respiratory distress
- Stridor, wheezing, and respiratory distress (suspect laryngeal edema and bronchospasm) may occur from anaphylaxis secondary to envenomation or from pulmonary edema secondary to near-drowning.
Local skin changes
- Note the presence of localized erythema, ecchymosis, pain, and swelling (suspect bite or sting).
- Assess for the presence of red, painful skin areas (superficial reaction to an insect sting or bite).
- Note the presence of yellow, waxy skin areas (suspect frostbite).
Diaphoresis
- Observe for the presence of diaphoresis (suspect heat exhaustion or sympathetic nervous system [SNS] stimulation secondary to anaphylaxis).

Seizures

- Seizure activity may occur from brain hypoxia secondary to pulmonary changes from near drowning, diving, or high-altitude emergencies.

FOCUSED NURSING ASSESSMENT

Nursing assessment should focus on oxygenation and ventilation, perfusion, and cognition.

Oxygenation and Ventilation
Airway

Stridor and wheezing may be present in anaphylaxis from animal envenomations and in near-drowning. The patient with a decreased level of consciousness (LOC) is at risk for airway compromise.

Breath sounds

Wheezing and crackles frequently occur in near-drowning victims from alveolar capillary membrane damage, decreased surfactant, and atelectasis. Crackles are present in high-altitude pulmonary edema (HAPE), pulmonary edema from heat stroke, and air embolism in divers. Breath sounds will decrease, because of respiratory muscle weakness and paralysis, in moderate to severe coral snake envenomation.

Heart rate and rhythm

Obtain an apical pulse, and initiate cardiac monitoring. Tachycardia is a common and early response to hypovolemia. Bradycardia, atrial fibrillation, ventricular fibrillation, and asystole are possible with hypothermic patients.

Blood pressure

Hypotension can become severe in anaphylaxis, heat stroke, and hypothermia. A Doppler may be needed to obtain a blood pressure (BP) reading. Scorpion envenomation can produce hypertension from stimulation of the adrenergic system with a massive outpouring of catecholamines.

Peripheral circulation

Assess skin color, temperature, capillary refill, and peripheral pulses. Many environmental emergencies impair cardiac output from hypovolemia or vasodilation. Perfusion to the skin will be decreased, as exhibited by pale and cool skin, delayed capillary refill, and weak peripheral pulses. In cases of heat stroke, the skin may be warm and dry. Assess perfusion of the skin distal to areas with frostbite or edema from a venomous animal bite or sting.

Cognition
Level of consciousness
Increased intracranial pressure (ICP) from cerebral edema can occur in heat stroke, in high-altitude cerebral edema (HACE), and in arterial gas embolism from diving, near-drowning cases, and hypoxic events. Increased ICP will be manifested by changes in the LOC and possibly by seizures.

Pupil size and reaction
Vasodilation and hypovolemia may impair perfusion to the brain. Assess pupil size and reactivity. Pupils are often fixed and dilated in severe hypothermia.

Risk Factors
Heat-related illnesses
1. **Age:** The geriatric population may have decreased functioning of the sweat glands and diminished cardiac reserves. Infants are unable to increase sweat gland activity for evaporation and heat loss.
2. **Activity:** Amateur athletes, military recruits, and laborers are prone to heat-related illnesses and often are not acclimated to the environmental conditions.[1]
3. **Environmental conditions:** High heat, high humidity (decreases air evaporation so effective cooling is not maintained), a closed work space, and occlusive clothing contribute to heat-related emergencies.
4. **Medications:** Phenothiazines (e.g., Sparine) impair hypothalamic function. Antihistamines and tricyclic antidepressants dull the sweating response. Beta-blockers decrease cardiac response to the increased body temperature. Cocaine and amphetamines stimulate the SNS and further elevate body temperature. Lithium, diuretics, and anticholinergic drugs have also been identified as risk factors associated with heat-related illnesses.
5. **Medical history and current illness:** Status epilepticus generates a large quantity of heat from the intense muscle tension and activity. Alcoholism, obesity, and hyperthyroidism are other risk factors in heat-related illnesses.

Hypothermia
1. **Age:** Infants have a greater body surface area (BSA) for their weight, a smaller amount of fat stores for insula-

tion, and poor temperature-regulating mechanisms. The geriatric population may be less mobile and have chronic medical conditions. Geriatric individuals may not be able to sense cold well because of neuropathy and a decreased vasoconstriction response. Once stressed, geriatric individuals are unable to increase heat production.

2. **Activity:** Campers, hikers, and homeless individuals have greater exposure to environmental conditions associated with hypothermia and frostbite. Because of the high thermal conductivity of water, immersion can produce rapid hypothermia.

3. **Environmental conditions:** A wind speed above 5 MPH and exposure to an environment colder than one's body temperature are a basic requirement for hypothermia to occur.[2]

4. **Medications:** Phenothiazines impair the ability to shiver. Barbiturates and other depressants decrease the victim's awareness of cold environments and may have vasodilatory effects. Ethanol is a major risk factor because of its central nervous system (CNS) depressant and vasodilatory effects. The vasodilation increases heat loss from radiation.

5. **Medical history and current illness:** Hypothyroidism can depress the core temperature and heat production. Hypoglycemia decreases the ability to generate heat as a result of an inadequate supply of glucose to the CNS. Hypopituitarism and hypoadrenalism impair the body's ability to respond to a hypothermic state. Wernicke's encephalopathy and alcohol abuse cause decreased peripheral sensation and poor judgment that increase potential exposure times. Burn victims have greater evaporative loss.

6. **Multiple injury:** Victims of major trauma are at increased risk for hypothermia from open wounds, cold intravenous (IV) fluids and blood products, unwarmed oxygen, and being exposed in an open treatment area.

Near-drowning

Suicidal gestures, alcohol and other drug use that impairs judgment, exhaustion, unsupervised children, and reckless boating or water activities are risk factors for near drowning.

High-altitude illness

High altitude begins at elevations above 8000 feet. Ski enthusiasts and mountain climbers may be at risk for this illness. In pressurized cabins in planes, passengers with preexisting hypoxia or cardiac or pulmonary problems may have difficulty tolerating very high altitudes.

Diving illnesses

Inexperienced or exhausted divers, the use of alcohol and other drugs that impair judgment, and diving at depths of >33 feet are risk factors for diving illnesses.

Risk factors for various venomous animal bites and stings will be briefly discussed under Collaborative Interventions.

Life Span Issues
Children
1. Children younger than 4 years of age account for 40% of drownings.[3]
2. Mortality from hypothermia is greatest in neonates.

Adults
1. Drowning is the fourth-leading cause of accidental death and is second only to motor vehicle crash fatalities among males between the ages of 1 and 34 and females between the ages of 15 and 19.[4]
2. Hypothyroidism (a risk factor for hypothermia) is more common in women than in men.

INITIAL INTERVENTIONS

Regardless of the environmental condition, the following interventions should be considered:

1. Implement measures to maintain and protect the airway. These measures can include a chin lift–head tilt (if spinal trauma is not suspected), jaw thrust, nasopharyngeal airway, oropharyngeal airway if the patient is unresponsive or has no gag reflex, and preparing to assist with intubation. Have suction available to prevent aspiration.
2. Place the patient on a pulse oximeter to monitor oxygen saturation.
3. Initiate oxygen administration immediately if hypotension, tachycardia, or respiratory distress is present.
4. Initiate cardiac and BP monitoring.
5. Seizures may occur with conditions that result in hypoxia. Use seizure precautions by padding side rails,

keeping side rails up at all times, and having suction equipment at the bedside.

6. Inform the patient of the plan of care. Patients with environmental conditions are often anxious and fearful.
7. Support edematous extremities for comfort.
8. Determine the tetanus and diphtheria immunization status on any patient with altered skin integrity.

PRIORITY NURSING DIAGNOSES

Risk for ineffective airway clearance
Risk for impaired gas exchange
Risk for altered tissue perfusion
Risk for fluid volume deficit
Risk for knowledge deficit

♦ **Ineffective airway clearance** related to seizure activity:
  INTERVENTIONS
  • Techniques that can be used to maintain a patent airway include turning the head to the side to facilitate drainage, jaw thrust, suction, and insertion of a nasopharyngeal or oropharyngeal airway.

♦ **Impaired gas exchange** related to pulmonary edema or bronchospasms in near-drowning, arterial gas embolism from diving emergencies, respiratory muscle paralysis from severe coral snake envenomation, or pulmonary edema from heat stroke:
  INTERVENTIONS
  • Assist with intubation as needed.
  • Administer 100% oxygen (see Chapter 16).
  • Anticipate the need for arterial blood gases (ABGs).
  • Monitor ABG results.

♦ **Altered tissue perfusion** related to severe edema with compression of neurovascular structures (from venomous bites), vasodilation, or coagulation abnormalities:
  INTERVENTIONS
  • Monitor the amount of edema. Frequently assess pulses, capillary refill, color, sensation, movement, and pain distal to the edema.
  • Elevate the extremity.
  • Administer IV fluids and antivenin as ordered.

♦ **Fluid volume deficit** related to excessive diaphoresis, heat load, or inadequate fluid intake in hot and humid weather conditions:

INTERVENTIONS
- Oral balanced salt solutions can be administered if the patient is awake and alert.
- IV fluids should be given if the patient has a decreased LOC or is hypotensive.

◆ **Knowledge deficit** related to treatment of an environmental condition and prevention of future occurrences:
INTERVENTIONS
- Keep the patient and family and friends informed of the treatment plan.
- Include information on prevention in discharge instructions.

PRIORITY DIAGNOSTIC TESTS

Arterial blood gases (ABGs): An ABG detects hypoxia and acidosis from hypothermia, heat stroke, near-drowning, and arterial gas embolus.

Coagulation profile: A coagulation profile is necessary in heat stroke and pit viper envenomation. Disseminated intravascular coagulation may occur with these conditions.

Electrolytes and glucose level: Hyperkalemia and hypoglycemia occur in heat stroke. Baseline electrolyte levels are usually obtained on all patients with environmental emergencies.

Complete blood count (CBC): A CBC is obtained to assess white blood cell (WBC) count and hemoglobin and hematocrit levels. Hematocrit levels may elevate in heat-related emergencies. The WBC count may be elevated in reaction to a pulmonary inflammatory response.

Liver enzymes: The level of these enzymes will be elevated in heat stroke.

Radiograph: A chest film may be ordered to assess lung fields for pulmonary edema. Pulmonary edema can occur in near-drowning, heat stroke, and HAPE.

COLLABORATIVE INTERVENTIONS

Clinical Conditions
Heat-related illnesses
There are a variety of clinical conditions that occur in heat illness. The symptoms appear as a result of the body's attempt to dissipate heat.

Heat cramps
SYMPTOMS
- Painful muscle spasms occur in heavily exerted muscle, most often the calves.[5]
- Nausea occurs as a result of the loss of sodium from sweating and salt-poor fluid intake.

DIAGNOSIS
- Diagnosis is based on history.
- The serum sodium level is often within normal range.

TREATMENT
- The patient should rest in a cool environment. An oral balanced salt solution such as Gatorade is administered if serum sodium levels are decreased.
- Salt tablets are not recommended and may be dangerous for some patients.

Heat syncope
Fluid and electrolyte losses occur via sweating, and blood is shunted to dilated peripheral vessels.

SYMPTOMS
- Headache, light-headedness, postural hypotension, and a brief loss of consciousness may occur.

DIAGNOSIS
- Diagnosis is based on history and orthostatic vital signs.

TREATMENT
- The patient should rest in a cool environment.
- An electrolyte solution is administered if the patient is not hypotensive.
- Modified Trendelenburg position (legs elevated) is the position of choice.
- Teach the patient to avoid sudden or prolonged standing in a warm environment.

Heat exhaustion
There is ineffective circulating blood volume caused by the excess loss of body water and electrolytes from diaphoresis and inadequate fluid intake.

SYMPTOMS
- Headache, nausea, vomiting, malaise, thirst, tachycardia, anorexia, syncope, anxiety, a slightly elevated temperature, cool or pale skin, hypotension, and diaphoresis may be present.

DIAGNOSIS
- Diagnosis is based on history.

TREATMENT

- The patient should rest in a cool environment. Oral hydration and IV fluids (NS, D_5NS, or $D_5 \frac{1}{2} NS$) are frequently used.

Heat stroke

Heat stroke is a rare but life-threatening emergency. Overexposure to high environmental temperatures, especially when accompanied with high humidity and low-wind conditions, can impair the release of body heat and lead to an abnormal rise in body temperature. Temperature regulatory centers in the hypothalamus fail, which further increases body heat. Cellular breakdown begins, and all organs can be affected.

SYMPTOMS

- Neurologic dysfunction is a hallmark of heat stroke. Symptoms may include confusion, a decreased LOC, visual disturbances, and seizures.
- Heat stress creates tremendous demands on the cardiovascular system. Tachycardia and dysrhythmias may be present.
- The patient may exhibit tachypnea and pulmonary edema.
- The patient may have hypotension.
- The patient's core temperature is $>105°$ F.
- The patient has decreased urinary output.
- The patient's skin may be warm and dry or clammy and diaphoretic.

DIAGNOSIS

- Diagnosis is based on history and a physical examination.

TREATMENT

- Support the airway, breathing, and circulation (ABCs). Intubation may be necessary.
- Administer 100% oxygen.
- Place the patient on a cardiac monitor.
- Use a large-bore IV.
- Administer a fluid bolus of 200 to 300 ml if the patient is hypotensive. Repeat as necessary.
- Check the glucose level and administer 50% dextrose if hypoglycemia is present.
- Begin rapid cooling—ice packs to the groin, neck, and axillae. Spray cold water over the body. Place fans close to the patient to facilitate evaporative heat loss. Place hy-

pothermia (cooling) blankets over and under the patient. Cold saline peritoneal lavage may be used in refractory cases. Consider cold saline gastric lavage.
- Ice water immersion is an effective method of rapidly lowering body temperature.[6]

NURSING ALERT

Rapidly cool the patient to 101° F. Once the temperature is 101° F, slow the cooling measures to prevent rebound hypothermia. Acetaminophen is not effective initially, since its use depends on a normally functioning hypothalamus. Shivering should be avoided, because it generates heat. Diazepam or lorazepam can be used to prevent or stop shivering. Thorazine is not recommended, since it is known to lower the seizure threshold and BP. Continuously monitor the patient's temperature with a temperature-sensing urinary catheter or rectal probe.

Cold-related illnesses
Frostbite
Frostbite is tissue damage from cold. It can be superficial or deep.
SYMPTOMS
- Superficial frostbite produces redness followed by blister formation in 24 to 36 hours. The face, hands, and feet are commonly involved areas. The skin remains soft. Burning, tingling, and numbness may be present.
- In deep frostbite the skin may appear yellow and waxy. It may feel hard on palpation. The patient will complain of a loss of sensation and a feeling of heaviness in the area. Edema may be present.
DIAGNOSIS
- Diagnosis is based on history and a physical examination.
TREATMENT
- Rapidly rewarm the affected area in warm water at 104° to 108° F, usually for 15 to 30 minutes or until thawing is complete.[6]
- Narcotic analgesics may be administered, since rewarming is usually painful.
- The area is gently dried after rewarming.
- A sterile dressing is applied to protect tissue.

- Blisters may be debrided.
- The area is elevated to prevent further swelling.
- Immunization status should be assessed.
- The tissue is handled gently because the frostbitten area will be fragile.

Hypothermia

SYMPTOMS

- See Table 9-1.

DIAGNOSIS

- Diagnosis is based on history, core temperature, and an examination.

TREATMENT

- If intubation is necessary, it must be done gently to prevent unnecessary stimulation and the onset of ventricular fibrillation. A good rule of thumb is to intubate the hypothermic patient as you would a patient with a possible cervical spine injury.
- The patient's temperature is continuously monitored by a rectal probe.
- IV access (two large-bore) is initiated.
- Moderate to severe hypothermic patients should be protected from inadvertent rough handling. Aggressive handling may shunt acidotic, cold blood in the periphery to the core of the body.

TABLE 9-1 Hypothermia

Stage	Core temperature	Symptoms
Mild	90°-95° F (32°-35° C)	Tachypnea, tachycardia, ataxia, shivering, lethargy, confusion, and occasional atrial fibrillation
Moderate	86°-90° F (30°-32.2° C)	Rigidity, hypoventilation, decreased level of consciousness, increased myocardial irritability, hypovolemia, blood sludging with metabolic acidosis, and Osborne or J-wave (positive deflection in the RT segment)
Severe	<86° F (30° C)	Loss of reflexes, coma, hypotension, acidosis, apnea, cyanosis, ventricular fibrillation, and asystole

- The patient is rewarmed by one or a combination of the following measures:
1. *Passive rewarming*
   - Passive rewarming results in spontaneous warming of the patient without the use of additional heat beyond the patient's intrinsic heat production.
   - This measure includes placing the patient in a warm room with blankets and preventing drafts.
   - This method is used for mild hypothermia.
2. *Active external rewarming*
   - Active external rewarming involves adding heat directly to the surface of the body.
   - This measure includes heat packs, warming blankets, and overhead radiant warmers.
   - This method is used in mild and moderate hypothermia and in conjunction with active internal rewarming in severe hypothermia.

NURSING ALERT

Apply heat to the trunk of the body and not to the extremities. This will prevent vasodilation in the extremities that would result in hypotension and movement of acidotic, cold blood from the periphery to the core.[7]

3. *Active internal rewarming*
   - This is the most invasive method of treating hypothermia and provides the quickest rewarming times.
   - It includes the following modalities: application of warmed humidified oxygen, warmed gastric lavage, peritoneal lavage with dialysate warmed between 40.5° and 42.5° C, closed pleural irrigation with warmed saline, and warmed IV fluids. Warmed IV fluids do not significantly raise core temperature but will prevent further heat loss. IV fluids can be warmed in a microwave oven. Heating times should be determined for each microwave oven and should average 2 minutes at high power for a 1-L bag of crystalloid. The fluids should be thoroughly mixed before administration, since "hot spots" are common.[6]
   - Active internal rewarming is used in moderate to severe hypothermia.

Near-Drowning

Near-drowning is defined as survival, at least temporarily, from submersion. Secondary drowning is death occurring minutes to days after the recovery. Near-drowning can be categorized as wet or dry. Wet drowning indicates aspiration of fluid and occurs in 80% to 90% of submersions. Dry drowning accounts for 10% to 20% of cases. Dry drowning is defined as asphyxia secondary to laryngospasm.[8] Near-drowning from either fresh or salt water produces intra-pulmonary shunting, decreased compliance, decreased functional capacity, pulmonary edema, and hypoxia.

SYMPTOMS

- Symptoms include shortness of breath, wheezing, crackles, an altered LOC, cardiac arrhythmias, chest pain, hypotension, and oliguria.
- Significant electrolyte imbalances do not occur in near-drowning survivors.

NURSING ALERT

Cerebral edema can develop up to 24 hours after the insult. Frequent neurologic checks are necessary. Initially, the chest film may be normal. Pulmonary insufficiency related to pulmonary edema may not develop for up to 24 hours following the submersion. Frequent pulmonary assessments are a "must."[9]

DIAGNOSIS

- Diagnosis is based on history, symptoms, and chest films.

TREATMENT

- Maintain a patent airway.
- Administer 100% oxygen by nonrebreather mask.
- Assist with intubation if respirations are absent or minimal, if the patient is comatose, or if the patient is unable to maintain a PaO_2 of 60 to 90 mm Hg with high-flow oxygen by nonrebreather mask.
- Positive-end expiratory pressure (PEEP) may increase the functional capacity of the alveoli.
- Bronchodilators are given to decrease wheezing.
- Prophylactic antibiotics (to prevent pulmonary infections) are not routinely used in near-drowning victims.

E

- Insert a urinary catheter to monitor the urinary output.
- Anticipate the need for osmotic diuretics if cerebral edema is suspected secondary to hypoxia.

NURSING ALERT

Always suspect the possibility of a cervical spine injury in a near-drowning victim. Cervical spine injuries are a possibility with falls, diving, or skiing events.

High-altitude illness
For most purposes, high altitude begins at elevations above 8000 feet, the height at which most people's arterial oxygen saturation falls below 90%.[10] In an unacclimated person, hyperventilation and increased erythropoietin secretion are insufficient to relieve the hypoxemia.

Acute mountain sickness
Acute mountain sickness (AMS) is a collection of symptoms brought on by acute exposure to high altitude.

SYMPTOMS
- Symptoms include a headache, insomnia, anorexia, nausea, vomiting, dizziness, dyspnea, weakness, oliguria, cough, chest pain, difficulty sleeping, and peripheral edema.
- Symptoms peak 24 to 36 hours after onset and resolve over 1 to 4 days.
- Most cases are benign and transient.

High-altitude pulmonary edema
High-altitude pulmonary edema is a life-threatening form of high-altitude illness.

SYMPTOMS
- Symptoms include cough, dyspnea, wheezing, orthopnea, hemoptysis, tachycardia, tachypnea, and fever.
- Neck veins are usually flat, and there is no hepatic engorgement.

High-altitude cerebral edema
High-altitude cerebral edema is a life-threatening form of high-altitude illness that usually occurs at elevations above 12,000 feet. However, cases have been reported at altitudes of 8000 to 10,000 feet.

SYMPTOMS
- Symptoms include a severe headache, ataxia, altered mental status, vomiting, aphasia, seizures, and weakness of the extremities.

DIAGNOSIS
- Diagnosis is based on history, an examination, and symptoms.

TREATMENT
- Descent remains the definitive and most successful treatment for all forms of high-altitude illness. Even a 1000-foot descent can result in the reversal of mild to moderate symptoms.
- Mild AMS can be treated symptomatically with rest and supplemental oxygen.
- Other treatment measures include continuous positive airway pressure (CPAP), acetazolamide (controversial), dexamethasone, diuretics, pulmonary vasodilators such as nifedipine, and analgesics to relieve the headache.

Diving emergencies
Decompression sickness
As the depth and pressure increase during scuba diving, larger and larger amounts of nitrogen and oxygen dissolve in blood and tissue. Unlike oxygen, nitrogen is not metabolized by tissue and tends to accumulate. If ascent occurs too rapidly, nitrogen quickly escapes from the tissues as gas bubbles. It is the release of the gas bubbles and the site of release that determine the symptoms. Symptoms usually present on breaking the surface or within 4 hours of surfacing.[11]

SYMPTOMS
- Symptoms include severe pain in or near joints, pruritus, rash, cough, dyspnea, chest discomfort, visual disturbances, weakness, vertigo, headache, aphasia, and coma.

DIAGNOSIS
- Diagnosis is based on a history of diving and on symptoms.

TREATMENT
- Place the patient in the left lateral decubitus position or supine with the head in the neutral position.
- Administer 100% oxygen by nonrebreather mask.
- Follow adult and child life support protocols for dysrhythmias.
- Start one large-bore IV with crystalloid infusion.
- Recompression is needed as soon as possible. Recompression is accomplished by the use of hyperbaric (high-pressure) facilities or chambers.[11]
- Patients with persistent symptoms may be treated with hyperbaric oxygen up to 7 days after the onset of symptoms.

Arterial gas embolism

If the breath is held on ascent or if air is trapped in the lung by bronchospasms during ascent, the volume of gas in the lung expands. When a pressure differential of 80 mm Hg is reached, air is forced from the alveoli through the pulmonary alveolar capillary membrane. This will result in air entering the interstitial space or arterial circulation. Embolized air bubbles transported by the arterial system may lodge in the heart, brain, or blood vessels.[8]

SYMPTOMS
- Symptoms occur very rapidly and include a decreased LOC, seizure activity, blindness, confusion, a headache, and paralysis.
- Symptoms of a pneumothorax are shortness of breath, decreased breath sounds on the affected side, and subcutaneous crepitus in the chest and neck.

DIAGNOSIS
- Diagnosis is based on history and symptoms.

TREATMENT
- Administer 100% oxygen by nonrebreather mask.
- Assist with intubation if there is a decreased LOC or severe respiratory compromise.
- Start one large-bore IV.
- Immediate recompression is a priority. Facilitate patient transfer to a facility with a hyperbaric chamber.

Venomous snake bites

SYMPTOMS
- See Box 9-1.

DIAGNOSIS
- Diagnosis is based on the history and symptoms and on a description of the snake.

TREATMENT
- Measure the circumference of the bitten extremity.
- Immobilize the extremity at or below the level of the heart.
- Remove any rings or constricting items from the involved extremity.
- Apply a compression dressing over the bitten area with an elastic wrap. The wrap should be tight enough (but with fingers still able to fit and slide under the dressing) to reduce lymphatic flow.
- Insert two large-bore IVs.
- Anticipate the need for antivenin (Table 9-2) for those who experience moderate to severe envenomation.
- Administer oxygen by nasal cannula or mask.

VENOMOUS SNAKE BITES

Pit vipers

(rattlesnakes, cottonmouths, copperheads)

Characteristics: Pit vipers have a pit midway between the eye and nostril on each side of the head; a triangular head; elliptic pupils; long, sharp, retractable fangs; and a single row of subcaudal plates.

Venom: The venom is primarily hematotoxic.

Location: Pit vipers are found in every state but Maine, Alaska, and Hawaii; they are the most common venomous snakes in the United States.

Symptoms

• The patient has fang punctures, edema, sharp, burning pain, and erythema of the site and adjacent tissues within 1 to 30 min of the bite. Edema may spread for 12 to 24 hr.[12]
• Minimal envenomation may cause regional lymphadenopathy and tenderness.
• Severe envenomation may be accompanied by hypotension and shock, paresthesias, anemia, and disseminated intravascular coagulation.

Coral snakes

Characteristics: Coral snakes lack facial pits. They have black snouts, round pupils, broad bands of red and black separated by yellow rings, and short, fixed fangs.

Venom: The venom is primarily neurotoxic.

Location: The Arizona coral snake is found primarily in Arizona and New Mexico. The eastern coral snake is found in North Carolina, south to Florida, and west through the gulf states to Texas.[12]

Symptoms

• There may be little or no swelling or pain immediately after the bite. There can be a delay of 1-5 hr before the onset of systemic symptoms.
• Moderate envenomation: The patient has fang punctures and minimal swelling. There is no complete respiratory paralysis.
• Severe envenomation: The patient experiences complete paralysis within 36 hr after the bite.

From Gold BS, Barish RA: Venomous snakebites, *Emerg Med Clin North Am* 10(2):249-266, 1992.

TABLE 9-2 Arachnid Envenomations

Type	Location and description	Symptoms	Treatment
Scorpion	Found mostly in the southwest United States (Arizona, New Mexico, and Texas)*	Intense pain with little or no erythema or swelling One species (*Centruroides sculpturatus*) injects lethal neurotoxic venom Symptoms may include wheezing, stridor, profuse salivation, diaphoresis, confusion, seizures, hypertension, tachypnea, tachycardia	Immobilize affected part Do not apply tourniquet Antihypertensives Ensure tetanus and diphtheria prophylaxis Analgesic Support ABCs
Black widow spider	Common in California and other parts of the U.S. Usually found in outdoor buildings such as barns and under rocks Black with red hourglass marking on abdomen*	Venom is neurotoxic Pain at bite site may be sharp and stinging or resemble light pinprick Limb pain, local redness and swelling Two tiny red marks may be present Muscle spasms, headache, nausea, vomiting, hyperactive reflexes, ptosis, hypertension, diaphoresis, fever, seizures, shock	100% oxygen by mask, IV access, diazepam and calcium gluconate (see Table 9-3) for muscle spasms Antivenin (see Table 9-3) in seriously ill patient† Immobilization of the limb and cool compresses

| Brown recluse | Found in wood piles, attics, closets, and dark places
Found in southeastern, south central, and southwestern states
Light brown with dark brown violin shape on back | Mild or no pain with bite, local edema, erythema, bleb formation, local ischemia
Severe ulcerative necrosis appears on third to fourth day
Fever, chills, malaise | Avoid further trauma to area
Determine tetanus and diphtheria immunization status
Antibiotics
Debridement of necrotic areas and sterile dressings
Dapsone may be administered to inhibit neutrophil function, a major cause of skin necrosis |

*Allen C: Arachnid envenomations, *Emerg Med Clin North Am* 10(2):269-297, 1992.
†Data from Auerbach PS: Disorders due to physical and environmental agents. In Saunder CE, Ho MT, editors: *Current emergency diagnosis and treatment*, Norwalk, Conn, 1992, Appleton & Lange, pp 703-729.

- The performance of a fasciotomy is controversial in extremities with elevated compartment pressures. Many authorities are now becoming more conservative with the use of fasciotomy.[12]
- Do not use ice.
- Incision and suction is not recommended in the ED.

Arachnid envenomations

For symptoms and treatment, see Table 9-2.

DIAGNOSIS

- Diagnosis is based on history, on a description of physical characteristics of the animal, and on the patient's symptoms.

Bee, wasp, and fire ant (Hymenoptera) stings

These insects inject venom through a stinger connected to a venom reservoir (sac). Stings are common in summer months and usually involve the head, neck, and extremities.

SYMPTOMS

- Local reaction: The patient has immediate pain at the site of the sting. Erythema, edema, and itching may be present.
- Systemic reaction: The patient has hives, nausea, vomiting, conjunctivitis, rhinitis, facial swelling, abdominal pain, laryngeal edema (stridor), bronchospasms (wheezes), and anaphylactic shock. Hypotension and tachycardia may also be seen in systemic reactions.

DIAGNOSIS

- Diagnosis is based on the history of insect stings and on symptoms.

TREATMENT

- Administer 100% oxygen by nonrebreather mask.
- Anticipate and prepare for a cricothyrotomy if severe stridor is present.
- Aerosolized albuterol or metaproterenol may be used for bronchospasms.
- Establish large-bore IV access.
- Infuse normal saline or Ringer's lactate and administer fluid boluses as needed to maintain a systolic BP of >90 mm Hg.
- Remove the stinger by scraping.
- Do not use forceps to grasp or pull the stinger out, since this may contract the venom sac and release more toxin.[13]
- IV diphenhydramine (Table 9-3) is often used in mild envenomations.

TABLE 9-3 Drug Summary

Drug	Dose and route	Special considerations
Antivenin (*Latrodectus mactans*—black widow species)	Single dose of 6000 U Entire vial of antivenin (2.5 ml) recommended for adults and children IV—each dose must be diluted with 2.5 ml sterile water for injection; shake vial to dissolve contents completely; further dilute in 50 ml of normal saline for injection; administer over 15 min Can be given IM	Test for sensitivity to horse serum before using; can test with skin or conjunctival test Skin test: inject into skin not more than 0.02 ml of test material (1:10 dilution of normal horse serum in physiologic saline)*; similar injection of normal saline can be used as a control; evaluate results in 10-20 min; urticarial wheal surrounded by zone of erythema is positive reaction Conjunctival test: for adults, instill into conjunctival sac one drop of 1:10 dilution of normal horse serum; for children, instill into conjunctival sac one drop of 1:100 dilution; itching, redness, and tearing of eye, usually within 10-30 min, is positive reaction Monitor vital signs closely, since acute anaphylaxis possible

Tankin, G.W. (1996) Emergency Management of Brown Recluse Spider Bites: A Review, Gema.library.UCSF.edu.
*Data from *Physician's desk reference*, Montvale, NJ, Medical Economics Publishing, pp 2643-2644, 1995.

Continued

TABLE 9-3 Drug Summary—cont'd

Drug	Dose and route	Special considerations
Antivenin (Crotalidae) polyvalent (for treatment of enveno-mation caused by bites of pit vipers)	Moderate to severe envenomation may require 30-150 ml (3-15 vials), depending on severity and toxicity of bite or bites Infuse 5-10 ml IV over 5 min; if no reaction, the rest should be given over approximately 30 min to 2 hr	Most effective within 4 hr of bite and less effective after 8 hr; however, should be given even after 24 hr have elapsed Should have negative skin or conjunctival test (see previous antivenin drug) before giving drug IV Monitor closely, since acute anaphylaxis possible
Calcium gluconate (for muscle spasms associated with black widow envenomation)	Adult: 10% calcium gluconate, 1-2 ml/kg IV up to 10 ml per dose† Do not exceed 2 ml/min‡	For IV use only Monitor for hypotension
Dapsone	50-100 mg BID	Administer until necrosis subsides in brown recluse spider bites
Dexamethasone (Decadron—used for AMS and HACE)	4-6 mg PO every 6 hr§	

E

Diphenhydramine (Benadryl)—used for symptoms associated with stings)	25-50 mg IV or IM; IV—25 mg over 1 min or deep IM; Children—1 mg/kg	Drowsiness a common side effect; patient should not drive until effects wear off
Epinephrine (1:1000) (distress from anaphylaxis associated with stings)	Subcutaneously—adult: 0.3-0.5 ml; pediatric: 0.01 mg/kg; IV—adult: 0.1 mg (1:1000), 0.1 ml diluted in 10 ml of normal saline§ IV; administer over 10 min	Administer with caution to geriatric patient, those with cardiovascular disease or hypertension; cardiac arrhythmias more likely to occur with these groups. Monitor patient for cardiac arrhythmias, chest pain, and hypertension
Hydrocortisone (for severe reactions to Hymenoptera stings)	100-250 mg or 2 mg/kg; IV—25 mg over 1 min	Incompatible with aminophylline and Benadryl

Tankin, G.W. (1996) Emergency Management of Brown Recluse Spider Bites: A Review, Gema.library.UCSF.edu.
†Data from Allen C: Arachnid envenomations, *Emerg Med Clin North Am* 10(2):269-297, 1992.
‡Data from Gahart BL: *Intravenous medications*, St Louis 1994, Mosby.
§Data from Auerbach PS: Disorders due to physical and environmental agents. In Saunders CE, Ho MT, editors: *Current emergency diagnosis and treatment*, Norwalk, Conn, 1992, Appleton & Lange, pp 703-729.

- For severe reactions, administer epinephrine (1:1000) subcutaneously, 0.3 ml in adults and 0.01 ml/kg in children (see Table 9-3).
- Hydrocortisone should be administered in severe cases (see Table 9-3).

NURSING SURVEILLANCE

1. Frequently assess airway patency, breath sounds, respiratory rate and pattern, skin perfusion, heart rate and rhythm, BP, LOC, and the amount of edema in extremities.

EXPECTED PATIENT OUTCOMES

1. Patent airway
2. Bilateral equal breath sounds with absence of stridor, wheezing, and shortness of breath
3. Core body temperature between 97° and 99° F
4. Heart rate of 60 to 100 beats/min
5. Absence of life-threatening dysrhythmias
6. Systolic BP of >90 mm Hg or at level needed to maintain adequate peripheral perfusion
7. Normal mentation
8. Urine output >30 ml/hr
9. Decrease or no further progression of edema in extremities

DISCHARGE IMPLICATIONS

Heat-Related Illnesses

1. Teach the need to increase the intake of oral balanced salt solutions during hot, humid weather conditions.
2. Stress the need for frequent rest periods when participating in outdoor activities.

Cold-Related Illnesses

Frostbitten areas are very susceptible to further injury. Stress the importance of protecting the area from cold exposure and trauma. These patients may need to return to the ED or physician's office for dressing changes and reevaluation.

High-Altitude Illnesses

Teach the need to increase altitude gradually. This is particularly important at elevations above 8000 feet.

Diving Emergencies
Encourage divers to participate in certified diving programs and courses.

Near-Drowning Emergencies
Teach parents the importance of constant and continuous monitoring of children near pools, ponds, lakes, and other areas with water or fluid.

Venomous Snake Bites
Stress the need to wear boots and pants during hiking or mountain-climbing activities.

References

1. Merchandani H, Hameli AZ, Pressler R, et al: Heat related deaths—United States, 1993, *JAMA* 270(7):810, 1993.
2. Jolly BT, Ghezzi KT: Accidental hypothermia, *Emerg Med Clin North Am* 10(2):329-337, 1992.
3. Olshaker JS: Near drowning, *Emerg Med Clin North Am* 10(2):339-349, 1992.
4. Neal JM: Near drowning, *J Emerg Med* 3:41-52, 1985.
5. Tek D, Olshaker JS: Heat illness, *Emerg Med Clin North Am* 10(2):299-309, 1992.
6. Danzel D, Pozos R, Hamlet M: Accidental hypothermia. In Auerbach P, editor: *Wilderness medicine,* ed 3, St Louis, 1995, Mosby.
7. Michal DM: Nursing management of hypothermia in the multiple-trauma patient, *J Emerg Nurs* 15(5):416-421, 1989.
8. Shinnick MA: Recognition of scuba diving accidents and the importance of oxygen first aid, *J Emerg Nurs* 20(2):105-110, 1994.
9. Glankler DM: Caring for the victim of near drowning, *Crit Care Nurse* 13(4):25-32, 1993.
10. Tso E: High altitude illness, *Emerg Med Clin North Am* 10(2):231-245, 1992.
11. Jerrard DA: Diving medicine, *Emerg Med Clin North Am* 10(2):329-340, 1992.
12. Gold BS, Barish RA: Venomous snake bites, *Emerg Med Clin North Am* 10(2):249-266, 1992.
13. Sollars G: Thermoregulatory emergencies. In Kitt S, Kaiser J, editors: *Emergency nursing,* Philadelphia, 1990, WB Saunders.

Extremity Trauma

Julia Fultz

Gregg Bayer

TRIAGE ASSESSMENT

Musculoskeletal injuries are evaluated after the airway, breathing, and circulation (ABCs) have been assessed. Hemorrhage is the only life-threatening injury associated with extremity trauma. It may be conspicuous or concealed internally and is most frequently associated with pelvic, femur, and multiple fractures. Once ABC problems have been addressed, a secondary assessment is performed and injuries involving the limbs and joints can be evaluated.

- Elicit a history from the patient. Family, friends, police, and emergency medical personnel may be able to provide valuable information.
  1. Obtain an *"AMPLE"* history (*A*llergies, *M*edications, *P*ast medical history, *L*ast meal, *E*vents preceding the injury).
  2. Determine the mechanism of injury to help predict injuries sustained.
  3. Ask about the treatment the patient received before arrival at the hospital.
  4. Assess any immediate or delayed dysfunction or pain experienced.
  5. Note any history of musculoskeletal injury.
  6. Has the patient used drugs or alcohol that may alter an assessment such as judgment of pain?
  7. Note the patient's tetanus toxoid history.
- Determine the patient's respiratory status. Evaluate the rate and quality of respiratory effort.

E

NURSING ALERT

In patients with lower extremity, pelvic, or multiple fractures, a fat embolism may cause a sudden onset of shortness of breath. Fat globules released from the fractured marrow enter into the vascular system and become trapped in the vascular bed of the lungs. In addition to dyspnea and tachypnea, symptoms include a petechial rash, unexplained restlessness, pulmonary edema, or fever. Symptoms usually appear within 12 to 24 hours of the injury. Immediate immobilization of a fracture and limited movement of fractured bones help prevent fat embolism syndrome.[1] The occurrence of a fat embolism is rare; however, the mortality rate associated with it is high.[2]

- Remove anything potentially constrictive from the injured extremity, such as clothing, jewelry, or circumferential dressings.
- Expose the extremities.
- Evaluate the extremity for open wounds. Determine wound length and depth. A laceration over a suspected fracture site is treated as an open fracture until further

assessment proves otherwise. Place a clean, sterile dressing over open wounds. If the wound is actively bleeding, provide a pressure dressing. If the bleeding is pulsatile (indicative of arterial bleeding), apply manual pressure and triage the patient directly to the treatment area. Pressure applied over the artery proximal to the wound can also be applied to stop the bleeding (Figure 10-1). If the extremity cannot be exposed at triage for adequate assessment, the patient should be given priority for a treatment bed so the assessment can be completed.

- Note hematomas and document their size.
- Evaluate bone stability—bony crepitus is indicative of a fracture.
- Inspect for swelling, deformities, abnormal rotation, or shortening of the limb in comparison to the contralateral limb.
- Evaluate the extremity for the "Ps"—pain, pallor, pulses, paresthesia, and paralysis. Compare the injured extremity with the uninjured extremity if possible.

Pain

The most common complaint with musculoskeletal injuries is pain. Point tenderness may indicate an underlying fracture. Pain that is inconsistent with the extent of the injury may indicate the development of compartment syndrome. Pain distal to the level of the injury is uncommon unless there is neurovascular damage.

Pallor

Ischemia produces color and temperature changes.

Pulses

Palpate pulses in all extremities. If possible, compare the pulses distal to the injury to the pulses in the unaffected limb. Pulses must be checked by palpation, or by Doppler if not palpable. One of the most important indicators of vascular injury is the quality or absence of pulses.[3] However, the presence of pulses does not rule out vascular injury with some residual flow or compartment syndrome.

Paresthesia

Tingling or numbness is indicative of vascular or neurologic damage.

Paralysis

Paralysis is indicative of neurologic injury.

NURSING ALERT

Compartment syndrome is a limb-threatening condition in which pressures in a muscle compartment rise high enough to interrupt the microvascular circulation, causing ischemia and eventual irreversible tissue damage. Symptoms include severe, progressive pain that does not parallel the injury sustained, pain on passive stretching of the muscle involved, tenseness, and a diminished sensation to touch.[4-6] It must be identified and treated swiftly (see Compartment Syndrome under Clinical Conditions). Patients must be triaged to the treatment area immediately.

NURSING ALERT

A vascular injury associated with circulatory compromise can pose a threat to limb viability. Patients should be triaged to the treatment area immediately.

- Ensure appropriate packaging of an amputated part (wrap in saline-moistened, sterile gauze, place in a plastic bag, and then place in a larger bag or container on top of crushed ice).[2,7]
- Angulated fractures and joints should be splinted as found. Patients with these injuries should be given high triage priority.

FOCUSED NURSING ASSESSMENT

Examination of an extremity for injury involves exposure, inspection, and palpation. Nursing assessment focuses on neurovascular integrity, mobility, and comfort.

Neurovascular Integrity

A neurovascular examination should be performed before and after any intervention involving the injured extremity and every hour otherwise. The examination should include an evaluation of pulses, capillary refill, color, temperature, movement, sensation, and pain.

- Pulses must be reassessed at hourly intervals. An alert patient can be asked to report the development of numbness or tingling in an extremity, which may be indicative of vascular compromise.

- Capillary refill in all extremities should be <2 seconds for pediatric patients and adult males. Adult female patients should have a capillary refill of <2.9 seconds and the geriatric patient <4.5 seconds.[8]

NURSING ALERT

Capillary refill varies under certain circumstances. Environmental factors such as cold cause a delay in capillary refill, as do certain medical conditions such as arterial insufficiency.

- Inspect each extremity for uniform color, mottling, cyanosis, and pallor. Compare the injured extremity to the contralateral extremities for each of these.
- Evaluate the extremity skin temperature. Note the temperature by touch and compare extremities. Note temperature variances within the same limb.
- Note extremity movement and any motion limitations.
- Evaluate sensory function distal to the injury site.
  Touch: Evaluate hypoesthesia (decreased sensitivity) and hyperesthesia (increased sensitivity) by touching the skin lightly with a fine wisp of cotton, and differentiate between sharp and dull (use a sterile needle) or two-point discrimination.
  Proprioception: Receptors respond to stretch, pressure, or position. Grasp the big toe or a finger and ask the patient to determine if you are moving it up or down. If the patient is unable to determine this, repeat with the ankle or wrist.
  Paresthesia (numbness and tingling): Nerve involvement as a result of ischemia begins distally and travels proximally. Identify the area of paresthesia and perform serial examinations.
- Note the patient's pain.
- Inspect hematomas, measure their size, and evaluate them for expansion.
- Inspect for edema and note any increase in size.
- Evaluate the wound for active bleeding. Note blood around the wound or soaked into clothing or temporary dressings. Lacerations in proximity to arterial pathways must be monitored for arterial bleeding (Figure 10-1). Evaluate dressings for effectiveness in stopping the bleeding.

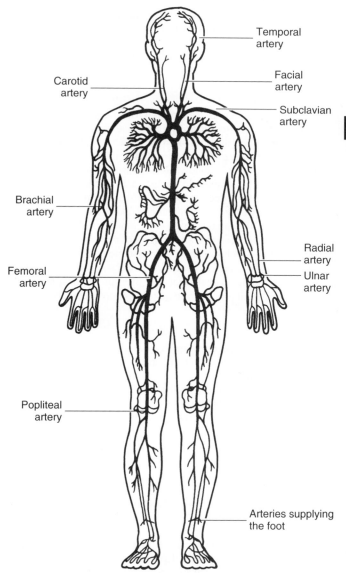

Figure 10-1 Pressure points for bleeding control.

- Immobilize potential fractures if this has not already been done. Immobilization helps prevent further tissue damage from the movement of fractured bone ends. Suspected joint dislocations should also be immobilized (see Procedure 28).

NURSING ALERT

The angulated joint with a suspected fracture should be splinted in the position in which it is found. A practical approach to splinting the angulated joint fracture is to use a conforming splint such as a vacuum splint or to splint and support the extremity with pillows. Neurovascular compromise in the presence of an angulated fracture or joint dislocation often necessitates the knowledge and skill of an orthopedist. In the acute setting, there is a thin line between the decision to straighten an angulated fracture with neurovascular compromise and the decision to wait for more definitive care. Joint fractures often involve associated dislocations. Attempts to straighten an angulated fracture involving a joint without the benefits of radiologic evaluation and orthopedic consultation may worsen the injury beyond its original presentation.

Mobility

Loss of mobility can result from neurovascular damage as a consequence of trauma to tendons, ligaments, bone, or muscles or from pain.

1. Inspect the exposed limb for the following:
   - Abnormal angulations
   - Shortening of one extremity in comparison to the other
   - External or internal rotation of an extremity
   - Discoloration (erythema, ecchymosis, paleness, or abrasions)
   - Edema
   - Exposed bone, tendons, ligaments, or muscle
2. Evaluate for a limitation in the range of motion of the injured extremity.
3. Evaluate the extremity muscle strength. Compare it with the unaffected extremity if possible. Note any atrophy.
   - Can the patient raise the extremity without assistance?
   - Can the patient raise the extremity against gravity (dangle the leg over the bed or have the arm hang by the patient's side)?

- Can the patient raise the extremity against resistance, such as the examiner's hand?
- Test flexion and extension by having the patient pull and push against the examiner's hand.
4. Gently palpate the extremity, moving proximal to distal for tenderness, crepitus, and increased heat. If a fracture is known to be present, crepitus does not need to be purposefully elicited. Further movement of the bone ends can cause additional injury.

Comfort
1. The most reliable indicator of pain is the patient's own interpretation of what is being experienced.
2. Evaluate the following characteristics of pain:
   - Location: Does the patient feel pain in a generalized large area, a localized small area, or a single point?
   - Intensity: The intensity of the pain should be evaluated on a standardized scale that can be repeated to evaluate changes in the level of pain, such as a scale of "0 = no pain" to "10 = the worst pain possible," in which the patient assigns the pain a number.
   - Quality: Is the pain prickling, burning, throbbing, aching, or radiating?
   - Onset: Did the patient feel the pain immediately after the event, or was there a delayed onset?
   - Duration: Is the pain continuous, steady, periodic, or momentary?
   - Variations: What makes the pain worse? What makes it better?
3. Immobilization of the extremity frequently diminishes the amount of pain experienced by preventing bone ends from grating together during muscle spasms.

Risk Factors
1. Repeated low-intensity activity (jogging or dancing) is a risk factor. Stress from repetitive activity is initially absorbed by muscles and soft tissue. As muscles begin to tire, the skeletal system absorbs more stress, which can lead to stress fractures and injured ligaments and joints.
2. Preexisting diseases that cause structural weakness of bones, joints, or muscles, such as osteoporosis, tumors, and Paget's disease, are also risk factors.
3. Other risk factors include high-risk sports activities such as skiing, rock climbing, motorcycle riding, or hockey.

4. Industrial and occupational work such as heavy machinery operation or construction work is another risk factor.
5. People of any age group in an abusive environment are at risk. Look for any injury to a limb that is incompatible with the explanation given for the injury, such as bruises at various stages of healing, inadequate care of a prior injury, bite marks, bilateral upper extremity bruising (from being held and shaken), or evidence of unset fractures.

Life Span Issues
Pediatric patients

1. Children who do not have completely developed motor skills are at an increased risk for injury.
2. A child's bones are more porous and more flexible than an adult's bones, so children may sustain incomplete fractures (greenstick and buckle fractures).
3. The epiphyses are cartilaginous growth zones in children that can often be mistaken on radiographs for fractures. Because of the relative weakness of this area, it separates before other structures are torn or broken.[4] Fractures through the epiphysis with disruption of the growth plate can cause growth disturbances.
4. Fractures of the clavicles are the most prevalent of all pediatric fractures.[9]

Geriatric patients

1. Geriatric patients who have decreased reaction times, a decreased range of motion, decreased muscle strength, and problems with balance have an increased potential for injury.
2. Increased frequency of degenerative bone disease with advancing age increases the incidence of fractures.
3. Fractures may occur spontaneously in osteoporotic bone.
4. Geriatric patients are at an increased risk for pressure sores as a result of decreased mobility if bed rest is needed.

Pregnancy

The hormone relaxin causes the pelvic ligaments to loosen. This, along with a change in the center of gravity caused by the enlarged abdomen, predisposes the woman to a loss of balance and to falls, causing musculoskeletal injuries.

INITIAL INTERVENTIONS

The goals of extremity injury management in the emergency department (ED) include the following:
- Hemorrhage control
- Identification of vascular injuries before irreversible ischemia develops
- Prevention of further tissue damage
- Ensuring peripheral perfusion
- Reduction of pain

1. Attend to any ABC problems.
2. Treat hemorrhage by direct pressure and pressure over the corresponding artery proximal to the injury (Figure 10-1).
3. Cover all open wounds with sterile gauze.
4. Elevate injured extremities above the level of the heart to decrease edema unless compartment syndrome is suspected; in this case, keep the extremity at the level of the heart to maximize tissue oxygenation.
5. Apply ice packs using a barrier between the ice pack and the skin.
6. Immobilize suspected fractures. Include the joint above and the joint below the suspected fracture. Assess neurovascular function before, during, and after immobilization (see Procedure 28 for specific fracture immobilization techniques).
7. Perform serial neurovascular checks (evaluation of pulses, capillary refill, color, temperature, movement, sensation, and pain).

PRIORITY NURSING DIAGNOSES

Risk for fluid volume deficit
Risk for altered peripheral tissue perfusion
Risk for pain
Risk for impaired physical mobility
Risk for infection

♦ **Fluid volume deficit** related to fluid loss from fracture sites or amputations, as demonstrated by decreased capillary refill, elevated heart rate, hypotension, diaphoresis, tachypnea, and altered mental status:

INTERVENTIONS
- Apply pressure dressings to active bleeding and use arterial pressure points if needed (Figure 10-1).

- Immobilize fractures to decrease blood loss from additional tissue damage.
- Insert two large-bore IV catheters (14- to 16-gauge), attach the catheters to large-bore trauma tubing with a maxi-drip chamber, and infuse crystalloid solution as ordered.

♦ **Altered peripheral tissue perfusion** related to neurovascular compromise, as demonstrated by decreased pulses, cool or pale skin, decreased motor or sensory function, and pain inconsistent with the extent of injury:

INTERVENTIONS
- Immobilize the injured extremity.
- Splint joint injuries and angulated fractures as found.
- Assess proximal and distal pulses every 30 to 60 minutes.
- Elevate the extremity to promote venous return, if not contraindicated as with compartment syndrome.

♦ **Pain** related to noxious stimuli from injury, tissue destruction, and invasive diagnostic procedures, as demonstrated by voiced complaints of pain, facial grimacing, skeletal muscle tension, irritability, restlessness, moaning, crying, anger, hostility, and withdrawal:

INTERVENTIONS
- Immobilize fractures.
- Administer pain medication as ordered.
- Advise the patient of what to expect with all procedures to be performed.
- Apply ice packs using a barrier between the skin and the ice pack.
- Elevate the extremity if not contraindicated as with compartment syndrome.

♦ **Impaired physical mobility** related to amputation, acute extremity pain, and extremity dysfunction, as demonstrated by difficulty walking, loss of manual dexterity, altered range of motion, paralysis or paresthesia of extremities, and verbalization of pain:

INTERVENTIONS
- Immobilize fractures and splint joint injuries and angulated fractures as found.
- Administer pain medication as ordered.
- Perform serial evaluations for neurovascular compromise.
- Train the patient in the use of a mobility aid (crutches, walker, or a cane).

◆ **Infection** related to altered skin integrity, as demon-
strated by exposed underlying structures, gross debris, and
lacerations:
INTERVENTIONS
- Remove any gross debris gently; if resistance is met,
  discontinue.
- Cover any opening in the skin with a sterile dressing.
- Administer antibiotics as ordered.

PRIORITY DIAGNOSTIC TESTS

E

Hemoglobin and hematocrit: For those patients with fractures of the pelvis, femurs, or multiple fractures, measure
hemoglobin and hematocrit because of the potential
blood loss (Table 10-1).

Type and crossmatch: Type and crossmatch should be obtained for potential blood transfusion if significant blood
loss from the fractures has occurred or is anticipated, or
for surgery to repair fractures.

Urine myoglobin: Myoglobin is a muscle protein that is released from the cell when the cell is severely damaged,
such as in crush injuries or compartment syndrome.
Myoglobin is excreted in the urine and will turn the
urine a reddish brown color.

TABLE 10-1 Potential Local Blood Loss in Fractures

Injured area	Amount (L)
Humerus	1.0-2.0
Elbow	0.5-1.5
Forearm	0.5-1.0
Pelvis	1.5-4.5
Hip	1.5-2.5
Femur	1.0-2.0
Knee	1.0-1.5
Tibia	0.5-1.5
Ankle	0.5-1.5
Spine or ribs	1.0-3.0

Data from Shires G: *Care of the trauma patient,* ed 2, New York, 1979,
McGraw-Hill; Walt AJ, editor: *Early care of the injured patient,* ed 3,
Philadelphia, 1982, WB Saunders.

Radiographs: Radiographs are a most useful tool in diagnosing fractures. Anteroposterior and lateral views should be included to view the entire bone and both proximal and distal joints.

Arteriogram: Perform an arteriogram to confirm or rule out a suspected vascular injury in the face of diminished or absent pulses.

CT scan: A CT scan is frequently used to identify acetabulum fractures and to evaluate the integrity of articulating surfaces such as the knee, hand, wrist, and ankle. It is also used to rule out cervical spine injuries when radiographs are inconclusive and to better define the characteristics of a known fracture. such as fragment placement and bony alignment.[6]

Magnetic resonance imaging: Magnetic resonance imaging identifies damage to bones, ligaments, cartilage, and menisci. This test is expensive and reserved for cases in which the diagnosis is in doubt and the treatment plan differs according to the test results.[6]

COLLABORATIVE INTERVENTIONS

Overview

1. Airway and breathing: Be prepared to assist with the management of airway and breathing problems should they develop. Airway adjuncts and intubation equipment should be readily available.
   - **Oxygen:** Supply supplemental oxygen to avoid local tissue hypoxia in patients who are hypotensive, in any multiple trauma patient who has fractures or any patient with multiple fractures, or to maximize tissue oxygenation in patients who have diminished or absent pulses. Monitor SpO_2.
   - **Hypovolemia:** Initiate crystalloid infusion via two large-bore IV catheters (14- or 16 gauge, 1¼ inches long) attached to large-bore tubing with a maxi-drip chamber. Pressure bags may be applied to increase the speed of fluid administration. Be sure to eliminate air from the bag to prevent an air embolus. Do not use extension sets or stopcocks because both diminish fluid flow.
2. Tetanus toxoid: Administer PRN.
3. Antibiotics: Administer as ordered.
4. Pain medication: Administer as ordered.

Clinical Conditions
Fractures
The most significant skeletal injury that can occur is termed a fracture. In addition to the insult to the bone tissue, injury may occur to surrounding soft tissue, blood vessels, and nerves. Significant risks of complications such as infection are often associated with fractures involving major soft tissue injury. A fracture that is explained by "minimal trauma" may indicate a predisposing structural weakness (e.g., Paget's disease, tumors, osteomalacia, rickets, or scurvy) or an abusive or violent situation.[6]

Fractures can be classified into two broad categories:
Closed fracture
A closed fracture is any fracture without an associated open soft tissue injury. The prognosis is generally better for closed fractures because of the limited risk of an infection. Closed fractures are also classified according to their specific type: comminuted, compression impacted, greenstick, oblique, spiral, and transverse (Figure 10-2).
Open fracture
An open fracture is any fracture with an associated open soft tissue injury. It is sometimes difficult to determine if a wound in proximity to a fracture actually communicates with the fracture. The general rule of thumb is to assume the wound is an open fracture until proven otherwise. Open fractures are treated as orthopedic emergencies because of the risk of infection and the potential complication of osteomyelitis.[6] Open fractures can further be defined according to severity (see the "Open Fracture Classification" box).
SYMPTOMS
Obtaining a mechanism of injury will help in identifying potential orthopedic injuries. The following symptoms are generally suggestive of a fracture. All need not be present to suspect a fracture:
- Pain at or around the site of injury
- Swelling at or around the site of injury
- Deformity of the extremity
- Instability of the extremity
- Crepitus (grating sound heard or felt when the ends of broken bones move together) on movement of the extremity
- Limited mobility and or limited range of motion of the extremity

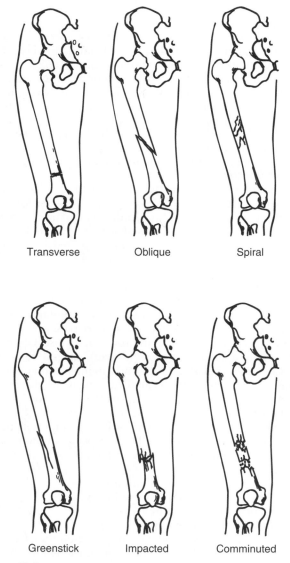

Transverse   Oblique   Spiral

Greenstick   Impacted   Comminuted

Figure 10-2 Classification of fractures.

OPEN FRACTURE CLASSIFICATION

Grade I   Small wound <1 cm long that has been punctured
             from below

Grade II   Well-circumscribed wound up to 5 cm long with
             little or no contamination and no excessive soft
             tissue damage or periosteal stripping

Grade III   Wound >5 cm and is associated with contamina-
             tion or significant soft tissue injury (tissue loss,
             avulsion, crushing injury) and frequently in-
             cludes a segmental fracture; soft tissue stripping
             of bone, major vascular injury, or periosteal
             stripping may be present

Data from American College of Surgeons: *Advanced trauma life support,* stu-
dent manual, ed 2, Chicago, 1993, The College; Geiderman JM:
Orthopedic injuries: management principles. In Rosen P et al, editors:
Emergency medicine concepts and clinical practice, ed 4, St Louis, 1998, Mosby.

- Muscle spasms
- Numbness or tingling

NURSING ALERT

Signs and symptoms of extremity fractures are often
grotesque in appearance. The site of a severely angulated
fracture may lead to "tunnel vision." It is paramount to realize that, in general, fractures do not cause life-threatening situations, and that even though the injury may be "limb threatening," proper perspective, diagnosis, and treatment of
life-threatening injuries must take priority.

DIAGNOSIS
- The diagnosis of a fracture is based on the mechanism of
  injury, clinical presentation, and radiographic studies.
  Generally, most orthopedic injuries involving the extremities are not life threatening, but the resulting trauma to
  body systems may be.

TREATMENT
Basic treatment of the fractured extremity involves the following steps:
- Establish control of the hemorrhage with sterile pressure
  dressings.

- Establish IV access for patients who have fractures that create the potential for fluid volume deficit.
- Cover open fracture wounds and exposed bone ends with saline-moistened sterile gauze.
- Splint the injured extremity, including the joint above and the joint below the injury.
- Apply ice packs to the injured site, placing a barrier between the skin and the ice pack.
- Elevate the extremity above the level of the heart.
- Evaluate pulses frequently.
- Avoid excessive movement or manipulation of the fractured site.

In addition to the general symptoms and treatment for fractures, specific extremity fractures may have distinct symptoms and treatment methods. Specific fractures are discussed in the following section. Splinting techniques for specific fractures can be found in Procedure 28.

Lower extremity fractures
Pelvic fracture

A pelvic fracture may be stable or unstable. Unstable fractures are a result of a great deal of force. They can result in hypovolemia from the potential loss of up to 4 L of blood that may occur because of torn arteries, damage to the venous plexus, and fractured cancellous bone surfaces.[10]

SYMPTOMS

- Little external deformity may be present, as a result of extensive overlying soft tissue.
- Blood may be seen at the meatus and on rectal examination (rectal, urethral, and bladder injuries are complications of pelvic fractures).
- Perineal ecchymosis or a scrotal hematoma may be observed.
- Abnormal rotation of the hips or legs may be present.
- External bleeding may be observed if the fracture is open.
- Distal circulation may be potentially impaired.
- The patient feels pain when pressure is applied to the anterosuperior iliac crests and the symphysis pubis.

TREATMENT

- Treatment requires a multispecialty team intervention to increase the chance of survival.[10]
- If the pelvic fracture is an open-book type of fracture, internally rotate the lower legs to reduce pelvic volume. Secure the legs together.[2]

- Splint the pelvis. Movement of the fractured bone ends can cause continued bleeding from the fracture site, so stabilization of the pelvis is of paramount importance. The pelvis may be stabilized using pillows, straps, and a backboard or vacuum splint. Military antishock trousers (MAST) can be used with low pressure (30 psi) to stabilize the pelvis. MAST are useful if a delay in definitive care is anticipated (such as a long transport), especially if hemodynamic instability is present. Some trousers have no air bladder in the posterior pelvis area. This may cause excessive pressure from the anterior compartment of the MAST and displace an otherwise stable fracture. MAST are often used in conjunction with a long spine board.
- Avoid unnecessary movement of the patient.
- Do not insert a urinary catheter if there is blood at the urinary meatus. A urethral injury will need to be ruled out.
- Bleeding from open fracture sites must be controlled by packing the wound.

Femur fracture

Bilateral femur fractures may represent a life-threatening injury secondary to hypovolemia (blood loss in each femur may be as much as 2 L). It takes a great deal of force to fracture the femur.

SYMPTOMS

- The patient will experience severe pain with midshaft femur fractures.
- Spasms of the quadriceps muscle as the result of bone ends overriding each other may cause extensive soft tissue injury. Deformity and tightening of the thigh may be noted with the spasm.
- The affected extremity may shorten in comparison to the unaffected extremity when they are parallel to each other.
- Distal femur fractures may involve the femoral or popliteal vessels, causing diminished pulses.

TREATMENT

- Immobilize the bone temporarily with a traction splint. Various types of traction splints are currently available, such as the Thomas, Hare traction, and Sager traction, each having its own unique application (see Procedure 28).

NURSING ALERT

Avoid the use of a traction splint if joint injuries are present on the ipsilateral side of the femur injury because further damage to the joint may result. The femur still needs to be immobilized using a nontraction splinting method such as a wire ladder splint or by securing the patient to a long board with necessary padding to stabilize the femur.

Knee fracture

Patellar fractures commonly occur with dislocations resulting from high energy transmission, and these fractures may be associated with a popliteal vessel injury.

TREATMENT

- Do not attempt to straighten angulation of the knee. These fractures may coexist with dislocations.
- Immobilize knee fractures as found, because of the proximity of joints both proximal and distal and the potential neurovascular compromise.
- When a leg that is straight is being immobilized, the knee should be flexed 10 degrees to take pressure off neurovascular structures.[2]

Tibia and fibula fractures

Tibial and fibular fractures may occur together or independent of each other and are generally the result of a direct blow (e.g., a pedestrian struck by an automobile). The tibia commonly fractures during falls because of its weight-bearing property.

SYMPTOMS

- Tibial fractures may remain "in line" if there is no insult to the fibula; however, bearing weight on the injured extremity is not possible.
- Tibial fractures may be associated with the development of compartment syndrome.[8] Evaluate for progressive pain that seems excessive in light of the injury sustained, pain on passive stretching of the muscle involved, tenseness of the area involved, diminished sensation, and weakness of the lower leg.
- Patients with a fibular fracture and a stable tibia may be able to place weight on the extremity. Posterior examination of the lower leg may reveal symptoms consistent with a fracture.

TREATMENT

- Splinting goals are aimed at providing stability while maintaining neurovascular function. Any splint that immobilizes the lower leg can be employed.

Ankle fracture

Ankle fractures commonly occur with connective tissue (e.g., ligament) injuries.

TREATMENT

- Dislocations may accompany fractures of the ankle and a specialist should undertake attempts at reduction.
- Immobilization of the ankle must be inclusive of the foot and the distal half of the lower leg.
- Pad bony prominences.

Foot fracture

Foot fractures are usually associated with dislocations and sprains, and it may be virtually impossible to differentiate the fractured foot from the sprained foot without the use of radiographs. Injuries secondary to axial loading may result in calcaneal (heel) fractures, and the energy may be transferred upward, causing spinal compression or burst fractures.

TREATMENT

- Conforming splints such as the pillow splint or commercially designed splints specifically for application to the foot should be employed. Toes should be exposed as a means for continuous reassessment.

Upper extremity fractures

Scapula fracture

Suspect scapular fractures with significant soft tissue injuries to the shoulder and when the mechanism of injury suggests a high level of kinetic energy transmission. Scapular fractures mandate a careful evaluation for damage to surrounding structures because they are frequently associated with shoulder dislocations, pulmonary contusions, rib fractures with the potential for an underlying pneumothorax, vertebral compression fractures, and upper extremity fractures.[11]

SYMPTOMS

- Patients frequently demonstrate a limited range of motion in the ipsilateral extremity.

NURSING ALERT

Life-threatening and limb-threatening injuries (such as a hemothorax, pneumothorax, or pulmonary contusion) or the

Continued

NURSING ALERT—cont'd

absence of ipsilateral extremity pulses may occur with scapular fractures as a result of the blunt forces commonly associated with them.

TREATMENT

- Rule out or treat potentially life-threatening injuries.
- Apply a sling and swathe to immobilize the arm and shoulder, thereby decreasing movement of the scapula. The sling cradles the arm so the elbow is bent just under a 90-degree angle, thus preventing extension and, to a certain extent, flexion. The swathe prevents abduction and adduction.
- Frequently assess neurovascular status.

Clavicle fracture

Clavicular fractures often cause damage to underlying structures such as the lung (pneumothorax, hemothorax), the subclavian vein, or the airway.

SYMPTOMS

- Patients often demonstrate shoulder instability as a result of a loss of support to the shoulder girdle.
- Evaluate the neurovascular status of the extremity, since these fractures are frequently associated with neurovascular compromise.
- This fracture may be associated with a pneumothorax, hemothorax, or brachial plexus compression.

TREATMENT

- Rule out underlying structure damage.
- Treatment of clavicular fractures may include a figure-eight splint that takes the pressure from the rest of the shoulder girdle off the clavicle and maintains proper clavicular alignment.

Humerus fracture

Humerus fractures may be associated with damage to the brachial artery and damage to the radial, ulnar, and median nerves. Because of the anatomic location of the neurovascular bundles, suspected fractures of the distal humerus should have a thorough and documented neurovascular examination. Direct force to the olecranon process can result in indirect fractures to the distal humerus.

TREATMENT
- Splint with a sling and swathe.
- Splint proximal shaft fractures by applying the swathe.

Radius and ulna fractures

SYMPTOMS
- Concern for fractures near the elbow and wrist relate to neurovascular compromise; therefore these require meticulous neurovascular evaluation and documentation.
- Colles' fracture is one of the more common fractures of the radius and ulna. It is commonly characterized as taking on a "silver fork" type of appearance, with the wrist turned up in relation to the radius and ulna.

TREATMENT
- Apply a rigid splint.
- When splinting for a Colles' or "silver fork" fracture, use a conforming splint such as a ladder splint and pad the spaces with rolled gauze (Kling or Kerlex) to provide more stability.

Hand fracture

The position of the hand during the injury is essential, since this information may yield valuable insight into potential fracture sites, damage to tendons, and damage to the neurovascular system of the hand.

SYMPTOMS
- Assess for rotational alignment. Normal rotational alignment occurs when the patient gently flexes the fingers in a loose fist and imaginary lines drawn down through the middle of the fingernail beds all meet in the area of the scaphoid. Digits may overlap if phalangeal or metacarpal fractures are present. Comparing the injured hand to the uninjured hand in this position also aids in this assessment.[12]
- Hand fractures are frequently associated with soft tissue injuries. Figure 10-3 shows anatomic landmarks useful in describing injury locations.

TREATMENT
- Remove rings promptly.
- Dress the soft tissue injury appropriately.
- Place the hand in a position of function (fingers slightly flexed with the thumb abducted away from the palm), and place rolled gauze (Kling or Kerlex) in the patient's palm.

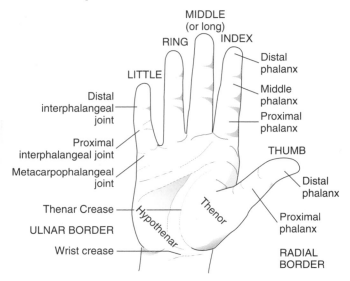

Figure 10-3 Volar view. Anatomic terminology useful in describing the hand.

- Wrap the hand, ensuring the fingertips are exposed for reassessment.
- Apply a rigid splint or conforming splint, taking care to place the splint distal to the wrist in order to provide complete immobilization of the hand and prevent further injury.

Compartment syndrome

Compartment syndrome is an emergency condition that occurs when the pressure within a muscle compartment rises to a level that interferes with microvascular circulation and impairs the neurovascular integrity. Over a period of hours, the interstitial tissue pressures rise above that of the capillary bed, resulting in ischemia of nerve and muscle tissue. It is most commonly caused by edema or bleeding into the compartment space from a crushing injury, fracture, prolonged compression of an extremity, burn (electrical or thermal), or bite (animal, human, snake, or spider).[2,4] Iatrogenic causes of compartment syndrome include MAST, an automatic BP cuff, a cast or dressing that is too tight, intraosseous line placement (occurs within 20 min-

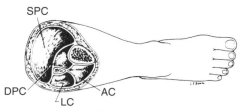

Four compartments of the leg: the anterior compartment *(AC)*, the lateral compartment *(LC)*, the superficial posterior compartment *(SPC)*, and the deep posterior compartment *(DPC)*.

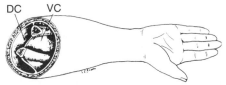

Two compartments of the forearm: the volar compartment *(VC)* and the dorsal compartment *(DC)*.

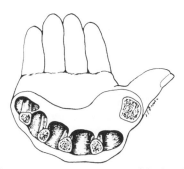

Five interosseous compartments of the hand.

Figure 10-4 Extremity compartments.

utes of line placement), thrombolytic therapy following radial artery cannulation, and anticoagulant use.[2,13]

The most common sites include the four compartments of the lower leg, the interosseous compartments of the hands, and the volar and dorsal compartments of the forearm (Figure 10-4).

The onset of ischemia depends on the amount of pressure and its duration.[6,14] The most frequently affected compartment is the anterior compartment of the lower leg, which is located lateral to the tibia.

SYMPTOMS

- Progressive and severe pain that is out of proportion with the underlying injury; pain aggravated by passive movement of the involved muscles
- Diminished sensation to touch
- Weakness of the involved extremity
- Tense swelling, asymmetry
- Paresthesias
- Pallor of the extremity (late sign)
- Loss of pulses (the cause of compartment syndrome occurs at the cellular level in the capillaries, so loss of pulses is a late sign if it is seen at all) [10,14]
- Delayed capillary refill (late sign)

DIAGNOSIS

- Diagnosis is based on clinical findings by examination.
- Confirmation of the diagnosis is made by direct compartment pressure measurement. Normal compartment pressure is <20 mm Hg. At 30 mm Hg, blood flow to the microcirculation is impaired.[6] Tissue pressures >35 to 45 mm Hg are critical because of the probable impairment of capillary blood flow.[2]

TREATMENT

- Place the limb at the level of the heart.

NURSING ALERT

Do not raise the limb above the level of the heart because arterial and venous pressure, and therefore oxygenation of the tissue, could decrease further.[5,6,15]

- Remove anything constricting the extremity (e.g., clothing, jewelry, cast material, or circumferential dressings).
- Continue to monitor pulses, capillary refill, sensation, range of motion, skin temperature, and pain.
- Evaluate the patient for rhabdomyolysis, myoglobinuria, and hyperkalemia.[6]
- An emergency fasciotomy of the affected compartment may be necessary.

Amputations—complete and incomplete

A complete amputation entails complete separation of some portion of the limb. An incomplete amputation involves partial separation of the limb without evidence of neurovascular activity distal to the partial separation.

The only life-threatening complication of an amputation is hemorrhage. In the complete amputation, constriction and retraction of the arteries in conjunction with a pressure dressing will usually control bleeding. In the incomplete amputation, partial laceration of an artery prevents retraction and the extremity may continue to bleed. Control of bleeding can be achieved through local pressure or pressure dressings and elevation of the extremity. If control of the hemorrhage cannot be obtained, a proximal tourniquet can be placed only as a temporary measure so the patient can be resuscitated.[7]

SYMPTOMS

• There is an obvious complete separation of the extremity or partial separation of the extremity associated with no capillary refill, no sensation, no pulses (by palpation or by Doppler), and no movement distal to the injury.

DIAGNOSIS

• Diagnosis is based on visualization of complete separation of the extremity at any level or a partial separation of the extremity without any neurovascular activity.

TREATMENT

Treatment for the patient involves the following:

• Place two large-bore IV catheters (14- or 16-gauge) $1\frac{1}{4}$ inches.
• Begin volume replacement with Ringer's lactate or normal saline (NS) as indicated.
• Implement pain management.
• Infection management includes antibiotics and tetanus toxoid. Wounds are usually tetanus prone, especially if degloving and crush injuries are involved.
• If the patient has a complete amputation or partial amputation with neurovascular compromise, prepare to transport him or her to a reimplantation center.

Treatment for the stump involves the following:

• Apply direct pressure to control the hemorrhage if needed.
• Remove gross dirt or debris by irrigation with Ringer's lactate or NS solution.
• Apply a sterile, moist dressing to the stump.
• Apply splint fractures.
• Elevate the extremity above the level of the heart.
• Monitor dressings for hemorrhage because active bleeding can be concealed.

Treatment for the amputated part involves the following:
- Collect and keep all amputated parts.
- Rinse with Ringer's lactate or NS to remove gross contamination.
- Wrap the part in sterile, saline-soaked gauze and place it in a dry plastic bag.
- Place the plastic bag with the amputated part on top of ice in another plastic bag or larger container. The plastic bag with the part should rest on top of the ice. The amputated part and ice should not come into direct contact. Cooling slows the chemical processes, and thereby increases viability and survival. Tissue tolerance of ischemia differs. Bone, tendon, and skin tolerate 8 to 12 hours of warm ischemia and 24 hours of cold ischemia. Muscle tolerates 6 hours of warm ischemia and 12 hours of cold ischemia.[7]

NURSING ALERT

It is up to the surgeon who provides definitive care to decide if any, all, or part of the amputation can be reimplanted. All amputated pieces and parts should accompany the patient to a reimplantation center.

NURSING ALERT

Determining if a partially amputated extremity should be cooled can sometimes be difficult. An incomplete amputation should be cooled if there is no evidence of circulation in the extremity distal to the injury, as determined by palpation and Doppler. Cooling can be done with ice packs. Ice must not come into contact with tissue. The goal is to slow the chemical processes to increase the viability of the tissue. The extremity should not be cooled if there is any active bleeding from the cut edge of the partially amputated part.[7] If neurologic or vascular activity is present distal to the injury, splint the extremity after applying dressings to the open wound.

Dislocations

Dislocation occurs when bone ends are displaced from the joints. (If the bone ends are only partially displaced, the injury is termed a subluxation.) The most frequent major dislocation seen in the ED is dislocation of the anterior shoulder.[6]

SYMPTOMS
- Severe pain to the joint area involved
- Deformity of the joint
- Extremity "locked" in an abnormal position
- Swelling of the joint
- Loss of range of motion
- Instability of limb if dislocation is accompanied by a fracture
- Numbness, loss of sensation, and loss of pulses distal to the injury (a dislocation can compromise the function of arteries and nerves in proximity)

E

DIAGNOSIS
- Diagnosis is based on the mechanism of injury.
- Diagnosis is also based on clinical presentation.
- Radiographs are used in diagnosis.

TREATMENT
- Do not attempt to straighten any dislocated joint without radiographs or orthopedic consultation because straightening the joint may worsen the original injury.
- Assess neurovascular integrity.
- Immobilize the potential dislocation in the position found.
- Splint the affected extremity in the position found.
- Provide padding to fill void spots, and then take the weight off the joint.
- Consider ice to reduce swelling in the joint area.
- Consider medication for pain control if it is not contraindicated by other injuries.

Sprains (ligament injury)

A sprain is a complete or partial tear of a ligament caused by sudden stretching of the joint beyond the normal range of motion.

SYMPTOMS
There are three grades of strains[6]:
Grade I
- Stretching or a small tear of the ligament
- Minimal swelling and hemorrhage, local tenderness
- No abnormal joint motion
Grade II
- Partial tearing of the ligament
- Tenderness, edema, and moderate hemorrhage, pain associated with motion and weight bearing
- Abnormal joint motion

Grade III
- Complete disruption of a ligament
- Joint may be obviously deformed
- Marked tenderness and swelling
- Joint may be unable to bear weight
- Grossly abnormal joint motion

DIAGNOSIS
- Diagnosis is determined by history and assessment.
- Perform radiograph examinations to rule out a fracture; avulsion fractures may occur with sprains.

TREATMENT
Grade I
- Apply ice, elevate for 12 hours, apply a compression dressing, and direct the patient to maintain light weight bearing with crutches.

Grade II
- Apply ice for 24 hours, immobilize the joint if necessary, apply compression bandages, and direct the patient to maintain light weight bearing with crutches.

Grade III
- Apply ice for 48 hours.
- Elevate the joint and apply a compression dressing or cast for immobilization.
- Surgical repair may be necessary.
- Avoid weight bearing.

Strains (injury to a muscle or tendon attachment)

A strain is the weakening or overstretching of a muscle where it attaches to a tendon. A strain is also referred to as a pulled muscle.

There are three grades of strains[6]:

SYMPTOMS
Grade 1
- Mild strains—minor tearing
- Local pain, point tenderness, swelling, slight muscle spasm

Grade 2
- Moderate strains—increased number of fibers torn
- Local pain, point tenderness, swelling, discoloration, and inability to use limb for prolonged periods

Grade 3
- Severe strains—complete separation of the muscle from muscle, muscle from tendon, or tendon from bone
- Localized pain, point tenderness, swelling, discoloration, and "heard a snapping noise"

DIAGNOSIS
- Diagnosis is determined by history and assessment.
- Perform a radiographic examination to rule out a fracture. Avulsion fractures may occur with second- and third-degree strains.

TREATMENT
Mild strain
- Apply an intermittent cold pack, elevate the extremity above the heart, and apply a compression bandage.
- Direct the patient to maintain light weight bearing on the extremity.
- Administer analgesics.

Moderate strain
- Apply cold packs for 24 hours, elevate the extremity above the heart, and apply a compression bandage.
- Direct the patient to maintain light weight bearing only on the extremity.
- Administer analgesics.

Severe strain
- Apply cold packs for 24 to 48 hours, elevate the extremity above the heart, and apply a compression bandage.
- Direct the patient not to bear weight on the affected extremity for 48 hours.
- Administer analgesics.
- Obtain an orthopedic consultation.

NURSING SURVEILLANCE

1. Monitor for airway and breathing problems with patients who have fractures of long bones or the pelvis or multiple fractures.
2. Monitor for continued hemorrhage and hypovolemia.
3. Evaluate hematomas for expansion.
4. Evaluate pulses.
5. Monitor skin color, temperature, and capillary refill.
6. Monitor sensory function distal to the injury.
7. Evaluate the effectiveness of pain control.
8. Evaluate the effects of splint and traction splint application.
9. Monitor for a fat embolism in patients with fractures of long bones, pelvic fractures, or multiple fractures.

EXPECTED PATIENT OUTCOMES

1. The patient's neurovascular status does not deteriorate.
2. The patient reports a decrease in pain.

3. Hemorrhage is controlled.
4. Open wounds are protected from further contamination.
5. No further tissue damage occurs.
6. The alert patient articulates an understanding of procedures to be performed in the ED.
7. Patients with open fractures that require operative intervention (open pelvic or femur fractures) undergo surgery within 6 hours.
8. Patients with fractures that benefit from operative intervention undergo surgery within 24 hours.

References

1. Reed LJ, Keegan MJ: Fat embolism syndrome: a complication
   of trauma, *Crit Care Nurs* 13(3):33-38, 1993.
2. American College of Surgeons: *Advanced trauma life support:
   student manual,* ed 6, Chicago, 1997, The College.
3. Holleran RS, editor: Orthopedic and vascular emergencies. In
   Flight nursing principle and practice, ed 2, St Louis, 1996, Mosby.
4. Good LP: Compartment syndrome: a closer look at etiology
   treatment, *AORN J* 56(5):904-911, 1992.
5. Syle DA: Orthopedic complications: compartment syndrome,
   fat embolism syndrome, and venous thromboembolism, *Nurs
   Clin North Am* 26(1):113-132, 1991.
6. Geiderman JM: Orthopedic injuries: management principles.
   In Rosen P et al, editors: *Emergency medicine concepts and clinical
   practice,* ed 4, St Louis, 1998, Mosby.
7. Schlenker JD, Koulis CP: Amputations and replantations,
   Emerg Med Clin North Am 11(3):739-753, 1993.
8. Schriger D, Baroff L: Defining normal capillary refill: variations with age, sex, and temperature, *Ann Emerg Med* 17:932-
   935, 1988.
9. Bachman D, Santora S: Orthopedic trauma. In Fleisher GR,
   Ludwig S, editors: *Textbook of pediatric emergency medicine,* ed 3,
   Baltimore, 1993, Williams & Wilkins.
10. Wolinsky PR: Assessment and management of pelvic fracture
    in the hemodynamically unstable patient, *Orthop Clin North
    Am* 28(3):321-329, 1997.
11. Ada JR, Miller ME: Scapular fractures: analysis of 113 cases,
    Clin Orthop 269:174-180, 1991.
12. Overton DT, Uehara DT: Evaluation of the injured hand,
    Emerg Med Clin North Am 11(3):585-600, 1993.
13. Graeme KA, Jackimczyk KC: The extremities and spine, *Emerg
    Med Clin North Am* 15(2):365-379, 1997.
14. Gulli B, Templeman D: Compartment syndrome of the lower
    extremity, *Orthop Clin North Am* 25(4):677-684, 1994.
15. Gluchacki BK: Recognizing compartment syndrome, *Nursing
    91* 21(10):33, 1991.

Eye Conditions

Mark Parshall

E

For the purposes of this chapter, eye conditions are organized according to the degree of risk for permanent visual impairment, rather than according to whether their etiology is traumatic.

OCULAR ANATOMY

A detailed description of the anatomy and physiology of the eye is beyond the scope of this chapter, but a brief summary is necessary for understanding the risk of visual impairment associated with various conditions.

The interior of the globe is divided into aqueous and vitreous compartments. The vitreous compartment is bounded anteriorly by the back of the lens[1] and contains a clear, colloidal gel called vitreous humor. This compartment is lined by the retina, a continuation of the optic nerve. The retina extends in all directions and lines the entire vitreous compartment, including the posterior aspects

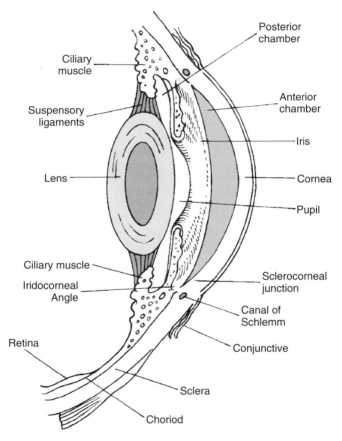

Figure 11-1 Ocular anatomy. (Modified from Thompson JM et al: Mosby's Clinical Nursing, ed 4, St Louis, 1997, Mosby.)

of the ciliary body and iris.[2] The choroid is a thin, pigmented, vascular layer sandwiched between the retina and sclera. The sclera is the fibrous outer shell of the globe. It is continuous with the outer sheath of the optic nerve posteriorly and with the cornea anteriorly.[1] The aqueous compartment contains aqueous humor and is separated from the vitreous compartment by the lens and its suspensory ligaments.[2] The aqueous compartment is divided into anterior and posterior chambers. The anterior chamber is bounded anteriorly by the cornea and posteriorly by the visible surface of the iris.[1,2] Aqueous humor is secreted by cells in the ciliary body[3] and drains via the canals of Schlemm, which are located in the anterior chamber angle, near the corneoscleral junction.[2] The posterior chamber is bounded anteriorly by the back of the iris and ciliary body and posteriorly by the front of the lens and its suspensory ligaments[1] (Figure 11-1). The uveal layer of the eye consists of the iris, the ciliary body and muscle, and the choroid.[1] The corneoscleral junction is called the limbus.

TRIAGE ASSESSMENT

NURSING ALERT

- True eye emergencies are those in which immediate triage to the treatment area and immediate intervention are necessary to preserve vision. In terms of triage priority, they are second only to immediate threats to life.
- True eye emergencies include (1) corrosive chemical burns from acids and alkali, (2) ruptured globe and penetrating ocular injuries, and (3) abrupt-onset visual loss (e.g., central retinal artery occlusion).

Chemical burns

In the case of corrosive acid or alkaline chemical burns, high-volume irrigation, preferably with an eye shower, should begin immediately. It is acceptable at this stage to assess gross visual acuity (e.g., finger-counting, hand motion perception, or light perception), but no time should be lost before commencing irrigation. If there is any doubt as to the corrosiveness or pH of a chemical injury, it is safest to initiate immediate high-volume irrigation, during which time consultation with a poison center may take place. Following adequate irrigation, a more detailed assessment of visual acuity may be undertaken if the patient is otherwise stable.

Open globe injuries and ocular impalement

Treatment for an open globe should not be delayed for formal visual acuity (VA) testing (e.g., Snellen chart or near card). However, it is important initially to determine and document whether the patient can count fingers, perceive hand motion, or perceive light with each eye[7] because initial gross acuity has prognostic value (in a majority of penetrating ocular injuries, initial VA is hand motion perception or worse).[7,8] It is also helpful to document the nature of the penetrating object (e.g., organic, metal, or glass) because this may influence diagnostic and treatment decisions.[7]

The patient should be brought to an acute treatment area immediately. If possible, the head should be elevated. No attempt should be made to assess ocular motility. Topical anesthetics should not be administered if an open globe is suspected. The injured eye should be shielded at the earliest opportunity (see Initial Interventions).

Sudden, atraumatic visual loss

A patient with sudden, atraumatic loss of vision should be brought to an examination area for immediate examination and treatment. The patient can be screened in the treatment area for light perception and consensual pupillary response.

NURSING ALERT

- Triage assessment should include the gross appearance of the eyes, particularly any obvious abnormalities of the globe, pupil, iris, lens, anterior chamber, lids, or periorbital tissues of either eye. Except in the case of a true eye emergency, visual acuity, ocular motility, the severity and quality of pain, and any pattern of redness should be assessed and documented during triage.

- The patient with unequal pupil size or reactivity should be asked about any history of eye injury or surgery as well as the use of any eye drops or motion-sickness patches. If there is no history that accounts for the inequality, the patient should be assigned a higher triage priority.

- Depending on the amount of pain and usual and current waiting times for urgent problems, it may be necessary to raise eye conditions to a higher triage category.

> • It is prudent to assign greater urgency to any eye problem in the "better" eye of a patient with useful vision in only one eye, or in an eye that previously has had surgery or significant injury.

Eye pain
• Pain from uveal structures (e.g., in iritis or acute glaucoma) is generally unilateral and deep and may be described as a boring or aching sensation or as a headache behind or in the affected eye.[9,10] Uveal pain is often associated with photophobia and is not relieved by topical anesthetics. In general, the patient with pain of this character should be accorded a higher priority than the patient whose eye pain is readily relieved by a topical anesthetic.
• Corneal pain is typically described as burning or searing.[9,11] Pain caused by a corneal abrasion is generally described as a scratching, foreign-body sensation. Pain resulting from a corneal injury is relieved promptly by topical anesthetics.
• Pain from conjunctivitis may be described as burning or itching, or it may mimic corneal pain.

Redness
• Redness associated with anterior uveitis—iritis or iridocyclitis—is often characterized by a "ciliary flush," a circular band of deeper redness at the corneoscleral limbus.[10-13]
• Redness (injection) from corneal injury or conjunctival inflammation or infection is diffuse with no ciliary flush.
• Ciliary flush generally suggests a more urgent condition than diffuse injection.
• Conjunctival edema (chemosis), as well as injection, may be present in conjunctivitis. Table 11-1 summarizes common presentations of the painful and red eye to facilitate triage.

FOCUSED NURSING ASSESSMENT
Visual Acuity Testing
Depending on the layout of the emergency department (ED), it may not always be feasible to conduct a full VA examination in the triage area. Emergency problems that carry an immediate threat to vision can usually be identified in triage without a complete VA examination. However, all patients with eye complaints must have a VA examination of

TABLE 11-1 Triage of the Painful, Red Eye

Problem	Pain onset	Quality	Redness	Discharge	Other	Category
Noncorrosive chemical	Immediate	Intense burning	Diffuse	Watery, unilateral or bilateral	Unilateral or bilateral Blepharospasm	Urgent
Corneal foreign body (FB)	Immediate, progressive, worsening	Scratching, FB sensation	Diffuse, but may have localized intensity	Tearing, watery Usually unilateral	Usually unilateral Blepharospasm	Urgent
Hyphema	Immediate, progressive, worsening	Dull, pressure (boring)	Blood in anterior chamber, +/− ciliary flush	+/− Symptom may be present or absent	Unilateral Often with periorbital hematoma Lethargy	Urgent
Acute (angle closure) glaucoma	Gradual	Dull, like headache or pressure	Diffuse, often with ciliary flush Steamy cornea	+/− Symptom may be present or absent	Headache, nausea/vomiting Scotoma Pupil dilated or midsize, possibly sluggish	Urgent
Anterior uveitis (iritis, iridocyclitis)	Gradual	Dull, intense, boring	Ciliary flush	Profuse tearing Usually unilateral	Pupil constricted, photophobia Usually unilateral	Urgent

E

Corneal abrasion	FB sensation that may have improved before worsening	Intense, burning	Diffuse, may have localized intensity	Tearing, watery Unilateral	Unilateral Blepharospasm Eye rubbing	Nonurgent as long as FB no longer present
Actinic keratitis (UV exposure)	Gradual onset, 8-12 hr after welding or sunlight exposure	Searing, burning, very intense, bilateral	Diffuse, bilateral	Tearing, watery Usually bilateral	Photophobia, eye rubbing	Nonurgent
Conjunctivitis	Gradual	Burning +/− photophobia Itching (allergic)	Diffuse, unilateral or bilateral	Allergic—watery Viral—mucoid Bacterial—purulent	Chemosis, blepharospasm, possible fever, URI Angioedema	Nonurgent
Subconjunctival hemorrhage	Usually painless	If pain present, consider other cause	Bloody, often localized	None	Usually asymptomatic, unless other problem present	Nonurgent

Data from Lawlor MC: *J Emerg Nurs* 15:32, 1989; Miller SJH, editor: *Parson's diseases of the eye*, ed 18, Edinburgh, 1990, Churchill Livingstone; O'Brien JM, Albert DM, Foster CS: Anterior uveitis. In Albert DM, Jakobiec FA, editors: *Principles and practice of ophthalmology: clinical practice*, Philadelphia, 1994, WB Saunders; and Wagoner MD, Sadun AA, Beinfang DC: Acute disorders of the eye. In May HL et al, editors: *Emergency medicine*, ed 2, Boston, 1992, Little, Brown.
FB, Foreign body.

each eye separately at the earliest feasible time.[14-16] Assessment may be via a standard (Snellen, Allen, or "E") far chart (at 20 feet) or a handheld (Rosenbaum) near card at 14 inches.[14] Patients with glasses or contact lenses should have their VA tested as corrected, if feasible. If their usual correction is unavailable or unusable, having the patients look through a pinhole (made with an 18-gauge needle) in a note card, or through the holes in a metal or plastic eye shield, can improve most refractive errors to approximately 20/30.[14,17] If a near card is used, adults over approximately 40 years of age may require reading correction.[17] Except in cases of suspected penetrating trauma to the globe, it is acceptable under physician order or written protocol to administer a topical anesthetic before VA testing.

Each eye should be tested separately before the testing of consensual (OU) vision. It is helpful to adopt a standard sequence for conducting a VA examination, usually OD, OS, OU.[5,16] In conditions that affect one eye predominantly, it is acceptable to test either the "good" eye or the "bad" eye first. Some authorities maintain that it is best to start with the bad eye in order to prevent the patient from memorizing the chart.[14,16] The author's preference is to start with the "good" eye first, since this is less stressful to the patient; memorization can be inhibited by having the patient start on a different line of the chart or by having the patient read left to right with one eye and right to left with the other. It is important to reassure the patient that the purpose of the VA examination is to establish a baseline for subsequent examination or follow-up; a change from the patient's usual VA does not necessarily imply permanent impairment.

Documentation should include the best line the patient can discern with each eye and with both together, whether corrective lenses were used, and the time at which the examination was performed. Conventional notation for VA testing records the distance from the far chart (or its equivalent if a near card is used) in the "numerator" and the distance at which a person with normal vision could read the line in the "denominator." Missed letters and symbols on a line the patient is otherwise able to read can be indicated by a minus sign after the VA (e.g., OD: 20/40-2). If VA is <20/200 in either eye (i.e., unable to read the top line), the distance to the chart can be reduced until the patient is able to read the top line. For example, if the patient could not read the top line at 20 feet (20/200) but

could at 10 feet, VA would be 10/200. If the patient is unable
to read the top line at any distance, acuity should be assessed
and documented according to the following sequence: finger
counting at 3 feet; hand motion perception; light perception
with or without projection (i.e., able or unable to determine
the direction of the light source); no light perception.[14]

Risk Factors

1. *Occupation:* A high proportion of serious eye injuries are
   related to occupational activities and could be prevented by the use of protective eyewear.[18-20] Between
   20% and 25% of penetrating eye injuries are work related.[21] The highest-risk occupations are construction,
   auto repair, and agriculture work.[19-21] Approximately
   15% of people with serious work-related eye injuries
   have a history of on-the-job eye injuries.[20,21] Activities
   such as grinding or hammering may generate enough
   force to cause shrapnel to penetrate the globe.
2. *Sports:* Recreational and sports activities are associated
   with hyphema, retinal detachment, and globe rupture.[19,20,22] The risk of injury is not reduced by the skill
   or experience of the individual but can be sharply reduced with proper protective eyewear and headgear.[20,23]
3. *Vehicular collisions and interpersonal violence:* Vehicular collisions are another common cause of eye injuries, both
   minor and serious. The use of restraint devices reduces
   the risk of an eye injury.[19,20] Eye injuries resulting from
   intentional battery are among the most common seen in
   the ED. A high proportion of serious eye injuries caused
   by vehicular collisions and fights are alcohol related.[8,18]
   The risk of a serious eye injury is increased if an orbital
   or midfacial fracture is present.[24]
4. *Gender:* Males are at two to six times greater risk for an
   eye injury across all ages.[18,20] The highest incidence of
   eye injuries is among young adult males, which reflects
   an aggregated risk from occupational and recreational
   causes, vehicular crashes, and battery.[21]

NURSING ALERT

Anyone with a history of eye surgery or a prior significant
eye injury has a higher risk for serious ocular injury for any
given energy level or mechanism of injury.[20,24,25]

5. *Medical history:* Iritis is commonly idiopathic but may be related to trauma or a wide variety of autoimmune, infectious, granulomatous, or neoplastic processes, including juvenile rheumatoid arthritis, ankylosing spondylitis, Crohn's disease, Reiter's syndrome, Sjögren's syndrome, sarcoidosis, herpes, cytomegalovirus, syphilis, tuberculosis, chlamydia, leukemia, lymphoma, and malignant melanoma.[10] Recreational nasal cocaine use has also been reported as a cause.[26]

Life Span Issues
Children

Young children, especially toddlers, are relatively uncoordinated, lack judgment about hazards, and have a developmental need to explore their world. These factors contribute to an increased risk of eye injury.[19,20,23,27] Inadequate adult supervision is commonly related to pediatric eye injuries. BB gun and fireworks injuries often cause devastating eye damage in children.[9] Eye injuries are also commonly seen in cases of child abuse and may be related to direct blows or shaking. Intraocular or retinal hemorrhage from accidental head trauma in children is rare and should heighten the suspicion of child abuse.[12,27,28] There are some reports of retinal hemorrhage following prolonged cardiopulmonary resuscitation (CPR) in children, but there is little evidence that this is caused by CPR alone; usually there is a concomitant head injury that is most commonly intentional.[28] On occasion, children with sickle-cell disease, some leukemias, cytomegalovirus retinitis, rickettsial diseases (e.g., Rocky Mountain spotted fever), and malaria may have a retinal hemorrhage.[28]

Conjunctivitis may occur in any age group, but the viral and bacterial forms are far more prevalent in small children, probably related to droplet transmission and hand-to-face contact with inadequate hand washing.[15,29]

Geriatric patients

Adults over the age of 65 have an increased risk of eye injuries because of diminished visual and auditory acuity, changes in coordination and reflexes,[30] and the greater likelihood of earlier eye surgery.[25] Falls are the most common cause of serious eye injuries for geriatric patients.

Although glaucoma is most commonly a disease affecting the geriatric population, it may occur in younger persons, particularly if hyphema or iritis is present or if there is a history of eye injury or eye surgery. Central retinal artery or vein occlusion is also more common in the geriatric population, especially in hypertensive patients, but may occasionally occur as a complication of certain types of eye surgery. Giant cell arteritis (which can cause blindness) is primarily a disease affecting persons who are more than 60 years of age.[31]

INITIAL INTERVENTIONS

1. *Removal of contact lenses:* Patients who are alert and oriented generally prefer to remove their own lenses. If the patient does not have a lens holder, the lenses should be covered in plain sterile saline in separate, labeled (left and right) sterile containers. If the patient is unable, or too distressed, to remove the lenses, the lenses can be removed manually or by means of a small suction cup. To remove hard lenses manually, open the lids beyond the margins of the contact lens and then close the lids with gentle, digital pressure that should pop the lens off the ocular surface. Soft lenses can be removed by gently pinching up the soft lens itself; the eye should be moist before removal.

NURSING ALERT

Topical anesthetics and fluorescein should not be administered until contact lenses have been removed.

2. *Eye irrigation:* Irrigation of one or both eyes is commonly performed. Except in corrosive chemical injuries, the eyes should be anesthetized topically before commencing and at intervals as needed (Table 11-2). An eye fountain (eye shower) is preferred for rapid decontamination of chemical injuries. Irrigation (a minimum of 1 to 2 L) may also be performed with IV normal saline or Ringer's lactate via irrigating lenses (Morgan lens) or manually via standard drip IV tubing (see Procedure 16). Small foreign bodies may be irrigated out with a small volume of ophthalmic irrigant such as Eye Stream.

3. *Eye shielding:* An open-globe injury or hyphema should be protected by the securing of a metal or plastic eye shield or a disposable cup over the injured eye as soon as possible. The purpose of the shield is the prevention of further injury as a result of rubbing or inadvertent contact and the reduction of stimulation from light or

TABLE 11-2 Topical Ophthalmic Agents Commonly Used In Eye Emergencies

Generic name	Proprietary name	Drug class/ mechanism	% Solution	Dosage	Special considerations
Proparacaine HCl	Ophthaine Ophthetic	Topical anesthetic	0.5%	1 gtt, repeat prn	Onset 20 sec, lasts 10-15 min
Tetracaine HCl	Pontocaine	Topical anesthetic	0.5%	1 gtt, repeat prn	Onset 1 min, lasts 15-20 min
Phenylephrine HCl	Neo-Synephrine	Mydriatic/ sympathomimetic	2.5% and 10%	1 gtt, repeat in 5-10 min	Onset <30 min, duration 2-3 hr 10% solution contraindicated for infants and for patients with hypertension, heart disease, or on TCAs
Homatropine HBr		Cycloplegic/ parasympatholytic	2% and 5%	1 gtt, repeat q10-15min × 2-3 doses	Onset 30 min, peak effect lasts for about 3 hr; some residual effect up to 48 hr

Drug	Brand	Classification	Concentration	Dosage	Comments
Cyclopentolate HCl	Cyclogyl	Cycloplegic/parasympatholytic	0.5%, 1%, and 2%	1 gtt, repeat × 1 in 10 min	Onset 30-60 min, duration <24 hr. Risk of neurotoxicity, especially in children
Tropicamide	Mydriacyl	Cycloplegic/parasympatholytic	0.5% and 1%	1 gtt q5min × 2-3 doses	Maximum effect in 20-25 min which lasts for only 15-20 min. Usually used only to facilitate examination
Pilocarpine HCl	Pilocar, numerous others	Miotic/cholinergic/parasympathomimetic	0.25% to 10%	1 gtt up to 6 times/day	Decreases IOP by promoting drainage of aqueous (secondary to miosis)
Timolol maleate	Timoptic	Beta-adrenergic blocking agent	0.25% and 0.5%	1 gtt daily or bid	Decreases IOP for up to 24 hr. Does not affect pupil or VA. Caution in CHF, asthma, COPD or for patients already on systemic beta-blockers

Data from Ellis PP: Commonly used eye medications. In Vaughan DV, Asbury T, Riordan-Eva P, editors: *General ophthalmology*, ed 13, Norwalk, Conn, 1992, Appleton & Lange; Lawlor MC: *J Emerg Nurs* 15:32, 1989; and Wagoner MD, Sadun AA, Bienfang DC: Acute disorders of the eye. In May HL et al, editors: *Emergency medicine*, ed 2, Boston, 1992, Little, Brown.

CHF, Congestive heart failure; *COPD*, chronic obstructive pulmonary disease; *IOP*, intraocular pressure; *TCA*, tricyclic antidepressants; *VA*, visual acuity.

movement. The shield should be taped lightly to the adjacent skin in a manner that does not exert pressure on the injured eye. The unaffected eye should be patched lightly to reduce consensual movement in the injured eye.

3. *Comfort measures:* Patients with suspected iritis, glaucoma, hyphema, or retinal detachment or whose complaints involve photophobia should be placed, if possible, in an examination room that is quiet and can be darkened.

Patients with corneal injuries or conjunctival inflammation may have anesthetic drops administered while awaiting examination if standing protocols exist or if the nurse obtains an order. Excessive use of topical anesthetics can aggravate corneal injuries and delay recognition of a worsening condition. Therefore patients are never discharged with topical anesthetics for self-administration; however, serial doses at appropriate intervals may be administered safely while the patient is in the ED.

PRIORITY NURSING DIAGNOSES*

♦ **Acute visual impairment†** related to injury or impaired ocular perfusion:
RISK FACTORS
- Penetrating, chemical, or high-energy blunt mechanism of injury
- Previous eye injury or eye surgery
- Age (<10 years old or >65 years old)[24,25,27]
- Nonuse of safety equipment (e.g., goggles, helmet, or vehicle restraints)
- Increased intraocular pressure (IOP)
- Inflammatory or infectious processes of the cornea or uveal structures
- Knowledge deficit‡

*Because of the variety of specific eye conditions, nursing diagnoses in this chapter are stated in terms of related factors or risk factors. Interventions are discussed under Clinical Conditions.
†The NANDA-approved nursing diagnosis "Sensory-perceptual alteration: visual" is extremely broad and subsumes problems as diverse as hemianopia, diabetic retinopathy, and visual hallucinations.[32] The primary concerns in emergency care are limitation or prevention of visual impairment.
‡Because of the variety and complexity of patients' individual circumstances, it may be more useful to consider "knowledge deficit" as a risk factor pertaining to either the current problem or the potential for recurrent injury, rather than as a separate nursing diagnosis.

◆ **Infection (or risk for infection):**
RISK FACTORS
- Corneal injuries
- Penetrating injuries
- Infectious lesions of the lids or periorbital tissues (e.g., shingles)
- Inadequate hand washing and infection control behaviors (e.g., conjunctivitis)
- Contact lenses (e.g., bacterial corneal ulcers)

◆ **Injury:**
RISK FACTORS
- Impaired visual acuity
- Impaired depth perception resulting from patching
- Risk-taking behavior or nonuse of protective eyewear
- Previous eye injury or eye surgery
- Knowledge deficit

◆ **Pain** related to injury, inflammation, or infection
◆ **Fear** related to visual impairment or loss, pain, or circumstances surrounding injury
◆ **Anxiety** related to potential interference with usual activities or loss of independence

PRIORITY DIAGNOSTIC TESTS

Slit lamp examination: A slit lamp (biomicroscope) is a binocular microscope that is used to diagnose an anterior chamber inflammation and injury or the depth of a corneal injury. The patient must be cooperative and able to sit up for a slit lamp examination.* Children and toddlers usually need to be held in a parent's lap for this examination to be accomplished.

Direct ophthalmoscopy: A direct ophthalmoscopic examination is used to diagnose conditions of the vitreous compartment and retina, as well as intraocular manifestations of other conditions (e.g., papilledema).

Tonometry (Schiøtz or applanation): Normal IOP is 12 to 21 mm Hg. IOP can be measured by any of several applanation tonometry devices or by a Schiøtz tonometer. Before tonometry, a topical anesthetic should be administered and the patient should be instructed not to rub the eye. Applanation tonometers, such as on a slit lamp, measure pressure directly and are most accurate.

---

*For bedside examination, a Wood's lamp and magnifying loupe may be used.

Fluorescein should be administered before the examination. Several handheld applanation tonometers are currently available that are more accurate than a Schiøtz tonometer for bedside use, although they are also more expensive.* A Schiøtz tonometer measures pressure indirectly by the displacement of a weighted plunger that moves an indicator needle along a calibrated scale. A conversion table, based on the plunger weight and scale reading, is necessary to determine the IOP in mm Hg. An applanation tonometry cone can be decontaminated by soaking for 10 minutes in a 1:10 bleach solution, after which it should be rinsed off, blotted dry, and replaced. A Schiøtz tonometer can be swabbed off and decontaminated in its own sterilization unit. Department policies should indicate whether tonometer decontamination is a physician or a nursing responsibility.

Fluorescein staining for cobalt blue, Wood's lamp, or slit lamp examination: Fluorescein dye has increased uptake in an area of corneal epithelial defect (e.g., abrasion and keratitis). Fluorescein strips are preferred to drops for infection control reasons. A drop of topical anesthetic is placed on the end of the strip, the lower lid is retracted, and the strip is touched to the palpebral conjunctiva.

Plain radiographs: Plain films are helpful in the diagnosis of some orbital and midfacial injuries, but a computed tomography (CT) scan is more definitive.

CT scan: A CT scan is preferred for complex facial injuries, orbital cellulitis, or suspected optic nerve trauma.

Cultures: Conjunctival cultures are helpful in cases of rapidly progressing conjunctivitis or chronic conjunctivitis that has been refractory to treatment.[29]

COLLABORATIVE INTERVENTIONS

Eye Patching

Patching traditionally has been a common method in the treatment of corneal epithelial defects (e.g., corneal abrasion or foreign-body removal). Patching keeps the lids shut over the cornea, which theoretically prevents lid move-

---

*A Perkins tonometer (Midwest Ophthalmics, 1237 Naperville Dr., Romeoville, IL 60441; 1-800-831-1194) uses the same kind of cone as a slit-lamp tonometer. A Tono-Pen (Mentor O & O, 3000 Longwater Dr., Norwell, MA 02061; 1-800-927-0250) has single-use disposable tips and does not require fluorescein instillation.

ments from interfering with corneal reepithelialization. Antibiotic ointment and mydriatic or cycloplegic drops are commonly ordered immediately before patching for prophylaxis against infection and ciliary spasm and iritis, respectively.[33,34] A double-patch technique is used. The first patch should be folded in half and placed on the closed eyelid. A second patch (or more if the eye is deep-set) is placed flat on top of the folded patch. The patch is taped obliquely from the forehead to the cheek or angle of the jaw with sufficient tension that the patient cannot open the eyelid beneath the patch. A prefabricated plastic and foam patch that is secured by elastic straps (Press-Patch) is an acceptable alternative. If ordered, a patch should be left in place for approximately 24 hours. A follow-up examination in the ED or with an ophthalmologist should be arranged to document evidence of healing and to determine the need for further consultation. For medicolegal and safety reasons, the patient should be instructed not to drive while the eye is patched because of diminished depth perception. Reading should be discouraged while the eye is patched because scanning movements of the unaffected eye elicit consensual movements of the affected eye. Patients with corneal injuries may also need oral antiinflammatory or narcotic pain medication and the appropriate precautions for these medications. An infected eye should not be patched because of the risk of a worsening infection or corneal ulceration. Also, some authorities maintain that corneal abrasions from contact lenses should not be patched because of the increased risk of a *Pseudomonas* infection.[34,35] Recently, several randomized clinical trials have compared patients who were assigned to conventional patch and antibiotic treatment with patients assigned to a "no-patch" group, who used antibiotic drops or ointment every 4 to 6 hours for the first 24 hours of treatment. The patients in the no-patch group have shown no difference in the amount of pain[36] or the rate or completeness of healing of uncomplicated corneal epithelial defects.[33,36-38]

Expediting Treatment, Consultation, and Transfer

Early nursing recognition (i.e., during triage or initial assessment) of presentations likely to require ophthalmologic or other specialty consultation expedites consultation and, when indicated, transfer. Any of the true eye emergencies will require immediate ophthalmologic consultation (or emergent transfer if no such capability exists locally). Presentations that generally require urgent specialty consultation or transfer include hyphema, retinal detachment, corneal or scleral lacerations, complex lid lacerations (e.g., disrupting a lid margin or canthal region), orbital cellulitis, ophthalmic shingles, and blowout fractures. Adherence to legal and institutional requirements for interfacility transfers is both an ethical and a medicolegal duty.

Clinical Conditions
Chemical burns
SIGNS AND SYMPTOMS
- The principal signs and symptoms of a corrosive chemical burn to the eye(s) are severe, burning pain, rapid onset of visual impairment, inflammation and swelling of the lids, and severe chemosis of the eye(s).
- Corneal haziness or opacification may be evident.[39]

DIAGNOSIS
- Initial diagnosis of a chemical burn is presumptive, based on symptoms and known or suspected exposure.
- Common acids include sulfuric acid (car batteries), hydrochloric acid (drain openers), and muriatic acid (swimming pool chemicals).
- Common alkalis include lye (drain openers and oven cleaners), lime (plaster and concrete), and ammonia.[39]
- Some detergents used for restaurant or institutional dishwashing contain bleach or alkaline corrosives; if constituents are not immediately known, they should be presumed corrosive.

TREATMENT
- If the chemical is in powder or crystalline form, it should be rapidly, but gently, brushed from the ocular region and face before irrigating.
- Initial decontamination should employ whatever method of irrigation that achieves the highest volume in light of concomitant injuries (e.g., an eye shower would not be feasible if the patient is unconscious or if a cervical spine fracture has not been ruled out).
- Strong acids cause the coagulation of proteins with which they come into contact, which limits the depth of injury.[39] An exception is hydrofluoric acid, which burns more deeply than other acids.[11,12,39]

- Strong alkaline chemicals cause liquefaction of proteins with which they come into contact and so have a tendency to penetrate through to the anterior chamber where they can damage the iris, ciliary body, and lens.[39] Therefore alkaline ocular exposures often need a longer period of irrigation than acids.
- The patient with a chemical burn should be attended to continuously during irrigation to provide emotional support and ensure the adequacy of irrigation.
- Irrigation should be continued for as long as it takes to get the conjunctival pH to normal range (7.4 to 7.6).[12]
- The pH is tested by retracting the lower lid gently and touching a test strip to the conjunctiva (much in the manner of a fluorescein strip).
- After initial decontamination, anesthetic drops may be instilled as needed until the irrigation and initial examination are complete.
- The pH should be retested several times after irrigation to make sure the pH is not changing.
- Some particulates (e.g., plaster and concrete powders) may embed in the lids or conjunctival fornices and cause ongoing release. Fine forceps debridement of such particles by the physician may be necessary.[39]
- Cycloplegic agents are generally ordered to reduce pain from a ciliary spasm. Topical steroids are helpful in this setting but should be administered only on the recommendation of the ophthalmologist.[11,39]
- Acetazolamide (PO or IV) or topical beta-blockers may be ordered after irrigation to decrease IOP.[39]
- Topical antibiotics and patching are commonly ordered.
- Systemic narcotic analgesics are often necessary.[12]
- Tetanus prophylaxis should be administered if indicated.

Open or ruptured globe and impalement injuries
SIGNS AND SYMPTOMS

- Signs of an open globe may include enophthalmos, proptosis (a globe protrusion caused by retrobulbar hemorrhage), obvious asymmetry of the globe, iridodialysis or pupil herniation (disruption of the iris at, respectively, the ciliary or pupillary margin), complete ("eight ball") hyphema, severe chemosis, and extrusion of aqueous or vitreous humor.
- Symptoms include severe pain and sudden, severe visual impairment or loss in the affected eye.[8,22] Small, intraoc-

ular foreign bodies may be attended by a more subtle visual impairment.

DIAGNOSIS

- The diagnosis of an open globe is based primarily on gross appearance, history, and the mechanism of injury.
- The IOP may be decreased below 10 mm Hg.
- Intraocular metal or glass foreign bodies can be diagnosed radiographically.
- CT scanning is helpful to determine whether the optic nerve has been severed or avulsed.

TREATMENT

- Open-globe injuries should be covered with a metal or plastic eye shield or a paper cup.[12]
- The unaffected eye should be patched or shielded to reduce consensual movement.[12,40]
- Tetanus and preoperative antibiotic prophylaxis are indicated.
- If the patient has an impalement of the globe or orbit, manual stabilization of the impaling object should be immediate.
- As soon as concomitant threats to ABCs have been ruled out, or as they are being treated, dressings may be applied to stabilize the object in a manner that does not put pressure on the object or the globe.
- Removal should be undertaken only by the appropriate surgical specialist in the operating room.

Central retinal artery occlusion

SIGNS AND SYMPTOMS

- Central retinal artery occlusion (CRAO) is a sudden, painless, unilateral visual loss caused by an embolus lodging in the central retinal artery. Patients are most commonly elderly and the prevalence is higher among men. Episodes are more common at night and in the early morning.[17]
- A sign of this condition is the absence of direct, but normal, consensual light reflex in the affected eye.[11]

DIAGNOSIS

- The diagnosis is based on the patient's description of the sudden onset of unilateral visual loss that did not resolve within a few minutes of onset, associated with characteristic funduscopic findings (e.g., an edematous, pale-milky retina with a "cherry red" fovea).[17]
- If the visual loss is associated with head pain, migraine or

temporal (giant cell) arteritis should be considered; an elevated erythrocyte sedimentation rate may suggest the latter.[17]

- Cerebrovascular disease, methanol ingestion, or hysterical blindness should be considered if the visual loss is bilateral.[15]

TREATMENT

- A small percentage of patients can have useful vision restored with prompt recognition and treatment, but salvage is rare after 2 hours from onset. Therefore CRAO is a true ophthalmic emergency.
- Firm ocular massage through closed lids may be performed by the physician for 3 to 4 seconds with abrupt release of pressure in an attempt to dislodge a thrombus.[11,17]
- If carbogen gas (95% O_2 + 5% CO_2) is available, it can be administered as a vasodilator for three 10-minute intervals with 5 minutes off between administrations. Otherwise, rebreathing into a paper bag for 10 to 15 minutes each hour may raise the patient's $Paco_2$.[17]
- Anterior chamber paracentesis, a pinhole puncture of the cornea at the limbal margin with a hypodermic needle or no. 11 scalpel blade, may also be attempted.[11,17] The purpose is to extrude a small amount of aqueous humor, thereby suddenly lowering IOP. This should only be performed by a physician experienced in the procedure.[17]

Noncorrosive chemical exposures

SIGNS AND SYMPTOMS

- Noncorrosive chemicals are painful and irritating to the eyes but are less likely to cause permanent visual impairment than corrosive chemicals (e.g., acids and alkalis).
- Symptoms generally include burning pain, blepharospasm, and tearing.
- Visual acuity may be unaffected or mildly diminished.
- Hyperemia (injection) is usually present, but chemosis is usually not.

DIAGNOSIS

- Common noncorrosive exposures involve petroleum distillates, alcohol-based products, and detergents. Even though the triage classification of noncorrosive chemical exposures is theoretically at a less emergent level, as a practical matter the pain and emotional distress they

E

cause may necessitate relatively rapid initiation of
treatment.

TREATMENT

- Again, if an eye shower is available, it is the best method
  of initial decontamination, followed by Morgan lens
  irrigation.
- The physician may order a topical antibiotic and patch,
  as in a corneal abrasion or actinic injury.
- A patient may have gotten "super glue" in the eye, which
  can cause the lids to adhere together. Usually, this can be
  manually debrided by the physician.

Amaurosis fugax (fleeting blindness)

SIGNS AND SYMPTOMS

- Amaurosis fugax is a transient, painless, unilateral loss of
  vision ("transient monocular blindness") most commonly
  related to ipsilateral carotid stenosis or microemboli.
- The patient describes the sensation of a curtain descending and then being raised,[31] or visual field constriction
  and expansion.
- Unlike CRAO, there is spontaneous improvement, generally within minutes of onset.
- Unlike migraine, amaurosis fugax is generally painless and
  not associated with fortification spectra (the scintillating,
  zigzag scotoma of classic migraine).[31] Episodes of amaurosis fugax are generally shorter than migraine episodes.

DIAGNOSIS

- The diagnosis is based on the rapid onset and resolution
  of the episode and on funduscopic examination.

TREATMENT

- Amaurosis fugax is a symptom, not a disease. In essence,
  it is a visual transient ischemic attack (TIA) that indicates
  a need for evaluation of the underlying cause, most commonly ipsilateral carotid disease (e.g., an ulcerated
  plaque).
- For patients with carotid stenosis, there is an increased
  risk of stroke, although this risk is not as great as with
  hemispheric TIA.
- Noninvasive carotid flow studies may be ordered or
  scheduled, and the patient may be started on one
  325-mg ASA per day.[31]
- Vascular and ophthalmologic consultations or referral is
  indicated.

- Other less common causes of transient, monocular blindness (e.g., giant cell arteritis) may call for different workups (e.g., an erythrocyte sedimentation rate for screening purposes) and referral.[15,31]

Retinal detachment

Signs and Symptoms

- Retinal detachment may be caused by trauma or degenerative changes associated with aging.
- The detachment is painless and gradual in onset unless it is associated with an acute injury.
- The classic symptom description is clouded vision or the sensation of a veil or curtain interfering with vision[40]; visual alterations can range from total loss of vision to relatively minor decreases in visual field and VA.[17] Patients also may indicate that they are perceiving "floaters" or flashing lights.[17]

Diagnosis

- Diagnosis is based primarily on history, progression, and a funduscopic examination.
- Specific funduscopic findings are beyond the scope of this chapter.

Treatment

- The treatment for retinal detachment is ultimately surgical, but it may be delayed.
- Guidelines for treatment will depend, to some degree, on the preferences of the consultant, but the guidelines may involve the patching or shielding of both eyes to reduce eye movements.[40]
- If the patient is to be discharged, a careful assessment must be made of what resources are available to the patient at home for assistance with self-care.

Hyphema

Signs and Symptoms

- Hyphema is a collection of blood in the anterior chamber, usually caused by a direct blow to the globe, such as by a ball or a fist, that causes bleeding from the vessels of the ciliary body. Since the blood is denser than the aqueous humor, it tends to settle in the lower half of the anterior chamber and is generally visible as a distinct blood fluid level.
- Hyphema is graded according to how much of the anterior chamber is filled with blood (Table 11-3).

TABLE 11-3 Grades of Hyphema

Grade	Blood level in anterior chamber
Microscopic	Blood-tinged aqueous humor—no layering
Grade I	$\leq \frac{1}{3}$ anterior chamber height
Grade II	$> \frac{1}{3}$, but $< \frac{1}{2}$ of anterior chamber height
Grade III	$\geq \frac{1}{2}$ of anterior chamber but not complete
Grade IV	Complete ("eight ball") hyphema

Data from Kitt S, Kaiser J: *Emergency nursing: a physiologic and clinical perspective,* Philadelphia, 1990, WB Saunders; Shingleton BJ, Hersh PS: Traumatic hyphema. In Shingleton BJ, Hersh PS, Kenyon KR, editors: *Eye trauma,* St Louis, 1991, Mosby.

- Pain resulting from hyphema is a deep aching, but concomitant injury to the cornea or orbit may cause mixed pain presentations.[9,41] The degree of visual impairment is proportional to the grade of hyphema.
- Hyphema is frequently accompanied by somnolence, especially with children. The etiology of this association is not certain.[41]

DIAGNOSIS
- Although hyphema is usually easy to identify, a few confounding circumstances may occur. Hyphema is, at times, difficult to discern if a patient has dark brown eyes because there is less contrast. Since it is a unilateral injury, comparison with the uninjured eye is always helpful.
- A second difficulty occurs if a patient is under spinal precautions or has been lying supine. In this instance the blood may settle more diffusely in the anterior chamber, with a less distinct layering.

TREATMENT
- Clinical management of hyphema is directed toward preventing complications and reducing the risk of rebleeding.
- The injured eye should be shielded (not patched) to prevent further injury (e.g., from rubbing).
- If possible, the patient should be positioned sitting upright or with the head of the bed elevated.
- There is a risk of renewed bleeding. This risk is greatest 2 to 5 days after the injury.
- Although the blood is usually reabsorbed spontaneously, it can cause staining of the cornea.

- Cycloplegic or mydriatic drops may be ordered to reduce or prevent a ciliary spasm.[41]
- A patient with hyphema requires urgent ophthalmologic consultation.
- A patient with higher-grade hyphema is hospitalized on bed rest.
- Some ophthalmologists will treat lesser grades of hyphema at home if the patient will comply with activity restriction and daily follow-up visits and is not taking anticoagulants.[12,41]
- A patient being discharged home should be advised not to take aspirin or nonsteroidal antiinflammatory medications.[12]
- Anyone who has suffered hyphema has an increased lifetime risk of glaucoma in the injured eye.[41]

Orbital blowout fracture
Signs and Symptoms
- The classic symptoms of a blowout fracture are binocular diplopia and infraorbital anesthesia.
- Signs may include a gaze limitation as a result of the entrapment of ocular muscles or enophthalmos resulting from herniation of periorbital fat.
- Gaze limitation and enophthalmos may occur as late signs that may not be evident acutely, and they may occur independently or in combination.
- The mechanism of injury is a blunt retrograde displacement of the globe that is relatively noncompressible because it is fluid filled. This can cause the orbital floor (ethmoid bone) or the lateral or medial orbital walls to fracture.

Diagnosis
- A blowout fracture is suspected on the basis of the mechanism of injury and on signs and symptoms and is confirmed radiographically by plain films or a CT scan.

Treatment
- An ice pack applied to the orbital area is helpful.
- After the cervical spine has been cleared, the head should be elevated to reduce swelling.
- The patient should be instructed not to blow his or her nose.
- Specialty consultation by a plastic or maxillofacial surgeon is indicated, but surgical repair is not always neces-

sary. Surgical repair is often performed on an elective basis after swelling has gone down.

Eyelid lacerations

The priority given to eyelid lacerations depends on their complexity and on whether a facility has appropriate consultants (e.g., ophthalmology or plastic surgery). Lid lacerations that disrupt the tarsal plate or lid margin, as well as those that involve the lacrimal drainage system or lateral or medial canthus of the eye, usually require specialty consultation.[12]

Iritis and iridocyclitis (anterior uveitis)

SIGNS AND SYMPTOMS

- Anterior uveitis is generally unilateral and associated with an acute decrease in pupillary responsiveness.
- The pupil of the affected eye is constricted and may be irregular.
- The affected iris may have a muddy, grayish cast relative to the unaffected eye.[13]
- The pain is of gradual onset, aching in nature, and associated with intense photophobia and watery discharge. The pain may also be increased in the affected eye when it responds consensually to elicitation of the light reflex in the unaffected eye.[10,13,42]
- In severe cases, aqueous humor may be cloudy and associated with a complaint of blurred vision.[42]

DIAGNOSIS

- Patients with anterior uveitis will have inflammatory vasodilation and increased vascular permeability of the iris and ciliary body, causing protein and fibrin exudation into the anterior chamber. This causes a characteristic flare on slit lamp examination that is diagnostic for the condition.[10,11,13,42]
- A diagnosis of iridocyclitis implies that the ciliary body and iris are both involved. Although this is more serious, there is little difference in terms of initial evaluation and treatment.[10,13]
- Most cases of anterior uveitis in young adults are idiopathic, but the uveitis can also be associated with ocular trauma or inflammation or a manifestation of infectious, autoimmune, or neoplastic disease.[42]

TREATMENT

- Fibrin deposits may cause the formation of synechiae (adhesions) of the iris and ciliary body that can interfere

with the drainage of aqueous humor and lead to acute
angle closure glaucoma[10,11,13,42] or chronic glaucoma.[42]

- Treatment involves the administration of a long-acting
cycloplegic agent such as homatropine hydrobromate
5% (Isopto-homatropine) or cyclopentolate HCl 1%
(Cyclogyl) and referral for prompt ophthalmologic
consultation.
- The eye should not be patched but may be shielded; the
patient may instead use dark glasses to decrease discomfort from light.[11]
- Warm compresses may afford some symptomatic
relief.[11]
- Topical steroids may be ordered.[42]
- The patient may need oral narcotics and should be counseled not to drive while the eye is shielded or while the
pupil is dilated by cycloplegic medication.

Acute (angle closure) glaucoma
SIGNS AND SYMPTOMS

- Acute glaucoma is often attended by conjunctival injection and a ciliary flush. In contrast to iritis, however, the
pupil of the affected eye tends to be moderately dilated,
or midposition, and poorly reactive.
- The cornea may be edematous, giving rise to a clouded,
hazy, or "steamy" appearance.[42]
- The patient may report visual alterations such as diminished acuity, blurred vision, or halos around light
sources.
- Often the pain is described as an intense, periorbital
headache and may be associated with nausea and vomiting. As such, it will also need to be discriminated from
migraine headache, which may also have symptoms of
nausea, vomiting, and visual disturbance, but is not associated with altered appearance of the eye or increased
IOP.[15,42]
- An acute episode may be precipitated by anticholinergic
or sympathomimetic (beta-agonist) medications (e.g., in
patients with asthma or chronic obstructive pulmonary
disease) or by the administration of topical mydriatic
agents.[42]

DIAGNOSIS

- An acute elevation of IOP above 20 mm Hg is diagnostic
for acute glaucoma.
- Determination of the acuity of the elevation is based on

the history and progression of symptoms. The outcome of an episode is less dependent on the degree of pressure elevation than on its duration.[42]

TREATMENT

- Therapy is directed toward reducing IOP by decreasing the production and improving the outflow of aqueous humor, as well as by osmotically decreasing the volume of vitreous humor.[42]
- A topical beta-blocker such as timolol or betaxolol may be ordered to decrease the production of aqueous humor, thus decreasing IOP. The pressure decrease onset takes approximately 30 minutes, with maximal decrease in 1 to 2 hours. Caution is advised for patients with chronic obstructive pulmonary disease or reactive airway disease and for patients with a heart block.[42]
- The carbonic anhydrase inhibitor acetazolamide (Diamox), up to 500 mg PO, IM, or IV, may also be ordered to reduce the rate of production of aqueous humor,[42,43] often in conjunction with a topical beta-blocker.[42]
- If IOP has been found to be elevated and the patient is not vomiting, oral glycerol (1 to 1.5 g/kg) may be ordered for its osmotic effect.[4] Because glycerol is metabolized to glucose, it should be used cautiously in diabetics.[42]
- If the patient is vomiting, IV mannitol (20%; 1.5 to 2 g/kg) may be administered.[42,43] Both glycerol and mannitol draw water from vitreous humor, thus decreasing its volume. Because both are nonspecific in their osmotic effects, they increase the circulating blood volume. Therefore they should be used cautiously in patients with congestive heart failure (CHF) or chronic renal failure.[42]
- Pilocarpine drops (1% to 4%) may be ordered (acutely, 1 gtt every 15 minutes for 1 to 2 hours[42]) to constrict the pupil, thus improving the outflow of aqueous humor.[11,43] IOP may begin to decrease before miosis is evident.[42]
- Cycloplegic or mydriatic medications are contraindicated.
- Ophthalmologic consultation is necessary and may require the transfer of the patient, but ultimately the patient may be discharged.
- Specific guidelines regarding medications, activity restrictions, and follow-up should be clarified with the consultant before discharge.
- Following the acute episode of angle closure, definitive treatment is surgical.[42]

Periorbital and orbital cellulitis
SIGNS AND SYMPTOMS
- Periorbital (preseptal) cellulitis is an infection of the eyelids and surrounding tissues anterior to the orbital septum. Preseptal cellulitis is most commonly caused by trauma to the lids and surrounding tissues or as a sequel to an upper respiratory infection. It is common in children. In general, VA, pupil reflexes, and extraocular movements (EOM) are unaffected. Proptosis and chemosis are absent.[44]
- If the infection affects structures posterior to the orbital septum, it is referred to as orbital cellulitis. This is a potentially life-threatening infection that can lead to blindness, cavernous sinus thrombosis, or an intracranial abscess. Orbital cellulitis may result from dental infection, sinusitis, periorbital trauma, or an infection of the eyelids or lacrimal system. Because structures anterior to the orbital septum may also be involved, look for signs that may distinguish orbital cellulitis from preseptal infection. These include fever, pain on eye movement, limitation of EOM, abnormal pupil reflexes, diminished VA, chemosis, and proptosis.[44]

DIAGNOSIS
- A CT scan of the orbit is often necessary to evaluate the depth of the infection.

TREATMENT
- Infants and young children with periorbital cellulitis should be hospitalized, because the condition may be associated with sepsis or meningitis.
- For adult patients with periorbital cellulitis, the condition can be managed on an outpatient basis if the patients are capable of complying with antibiotic therapy and follow-up. If it is managed on an outpatient basis, the patients should be reevaluated within 24 hours. If there is no evidence of improvement, they may require a CT scan to ascertain the depth of the infection. They also may require admission.[44]
- Patients of any age with orbital cellulitis require admission for administration of IV antibiotics.[11,15,44]

Superficial injuries (corneal foreign bodies, abrasions, and actinic keratitis)
SIGNS AND SYMPTOMS
- See Table 11-1.

DIAGNOSIS
- Diagnosis is based on fluorescein staining and Wood's lamp, cobalt blue light, or slit lamp examination.

TREATMENT
- Superficial corneal foreign bodies may be removed by irrigation or with a cotton swab.
- The physician can remove embedded foreign bodies with a spud or the bevel of a 25-gauge hypodermic needle. Often this is done under slit lamp visualization. This can be disquieting to the patient even though the cornea is anesthetized. It is often helpful for the nurse to remain with the patient during the removal to assist the patient to sit still.
- If the foreign body was metallic, it can leave a rust ring behind; rust rings are often removed in the ED with a rotary burr.
- If the patient is deemed reliable and understands the necessity of follow-up, the eye can be patched with antibiotic ointment for 24 to 36 hours and the ring can be removed by an ophthalmologist the following day.[12]
- Treatment for a corneal abrasion or actinic injury involves antibiotic ointment, oral analgesics, and patching.
- Patients with contact lenses should be advised not to reinsert them until cleared by an ophthalmologist or optometrist.

Ophthalmic shingles (herpes zoster)

SIGNS AND SYMPTOMS
- Ophthalmic shingles is characterized by unilateral, intense pain with herpetic lesions disposed linearly along the distribution of one of the facial nerves.

DIAGNOSIS
- The distribution of the pain and lesions and the characteristic appearance of the lesions are diagnostic.
- A history of chickenpox supports, but does not make, the diagnosis.

TREATMENT
- Although it may be confined to extraocular tissues, there is a risk of corneal involvement that can lead to blindness.
- Ophthalmologic consultation is essential; hospitalization may be necessary.
- Treatment with oral acyclovir is common.[43]
- While awaiting consultation, the patient will be more comfortable in a darkened room.

Conjunctivitis

SIGNS AND SYMPTOMS

- Bacterial conjunctivitis is usually bilateral, with a purulent, matting discharge that is usually worse upon awakening.
- Viral conjunctivitis usually begins in one eye but often spreads to the other. It has a more mucoid discharge and is often associated with fever and sore throat.[11,15,29]
- Pain from infectious conjunctivitis is burning or itching but is generally less intense than corneal pain.
- The patient may complain of blurry vision resulting from a blepharospasm or discharge, but visual acuity is generally unaffected.[15]
- Allergic conjunctivitis may be unilateral or bilateral and is generally associated with itching, puffy eyelids and a watery to mucoid discharge.[15,29]

DIAGNOSIS

- Diagnosis is made by clinical presentation and progression.
- Cultures are indicated for infants, for conjunctivitis of rapid onset or progression, and for chronic cases.[22]

TREATMENT

- Viral conjunctivitis is self-limiting but highly contagious. Treatment is focused on alleviation of discomfort with warm compresses and topical decongestants. Some practitioners prescribe topical antibiotic prophylaxis. Steroids and patching are contraindicated. Patients or parents should be advised of the importance of careful hand washing and of not sharing towels.[29] Medical and nursing staff also need to be scrupulous about hand washing and disinfection.
- Bacterial conjunctivitis is treated with antibiotic drops or ointments and warm compresses. Steroids and patching are contraindicated.[29]
- Allergic conjunctivitis is treated with antihistamines and topical decongestants. Steroids are controversial, and their use is discouraged in episodic care.[29]

Hordeolum (stye)

SIGNS AND SYMPTOMS

- A stye is a localized infection, usually staphylococcal, of any of several glands of the eyelid.
- It may involve the glands of Zeis or Moll's glands (external) or the meibomian glands (internal).
- The patient has a localized, tender erythematous swelling of the underside of the lid or lid margin.

Diagnosis
- Diagnosis is based on clinical presentation.

Treatment
- Treatment involves an antibiotic ointment and warm compresses.

NURSING SURVEILLANCE

1. Monitor pain relief and administer an analgesic or topical aesthetic as ordered.
2. Expedite examination and treatment.
3. Coaching, guiding, and teaching the patient and family throughout the emergency visit are essential. Concrete information about the eye examination and what sensations the patient is likely to experience facilitates coping by providing the patient with objective expectations against which the experience and any uncomfortable sensations can be gauged. Offering clear information about the nature of the eye problem and usual functional outcomes helps to reduce uncertainty about what is in store in the short and long term.

EXPECTED PATIENT OUTCOMES

1. Pain and emotional distress (e.g., fear and anxiety) are reduced.
2. Ocular pH is normal (7.4 to 7.6) in chemical injury.
3. There is no evidence of rebleeding in hyphema.
4. IOP is stabilized.
5. The patient should feel secure in the ability to cope with the problem and in treatment expectations.
6. The patient understands functional limitations imposed by treatment (e.g., cycloplegia or patching), as well as the plan of treatment and follow-up.

DISCHARGE IMPLICATIONS

1. The patient and family should understand expected time frames for improvement and the significance of any signs or symptoms that may represent a developing complication or other departure from the predicted course. It is important to establish with whom the patient should follow up (e.g., ED, family physician, and ophthalmologist) and whether follow-up is essential (e.g., hyphema) or merely "prn" (e.g., conjunctivitis).

2. The relation of the problem to risk-taking behaviors (such as the failure to use protective eyewear) and measures the patient can take to prevent recurrent injury should be explored in a nonjudgmental fashion.
3. Patients with corneal injuries who wear contact lenses should be instructed not to reinsert their contacts until they are cleared to do so in a follow-up examination.

References

1. *Dorland's illustrated medical dictionary,* ed 27, Philadelphia, 1988, WB Saunders.
2. Netter FH: *Atlas of human anatomy,* Summit, NJ, 1989, Ciba-Geigy.
3. Ganong WF: *Review of medical physiology,* ed 16, Norwalk, Conn, 1993, Appleton & Lange.
4. Emergency Nurses Association (Newberry L, editor): *Sheehy's emergency nursing: principles and practice,* ed 4, St Louis, 1998, Mosby.
5. Kitt S, Kaiser J: *Emergency nursing: a physiologic and clinical perspective,* Philadelphia, 1990, WB Saunders.
6. Robinson KS: Eye, ear, nose, throat, and dental emergencies. In Sheehy SB, Pisarcik-Lenehan G, editors: *Manual of emergency care,* ed 5, St Louis, 1999, Mosby.
7. Linden JA, Renner GS: Trauma to the globe, *Emerg Med Clin North Am* 13:581, 1995.
8. Parver LM et al: Characteristics and causes of penetrating eye injuries reported to the national eye trauma system registry, 1985-1991, *Public Health Rep* 108:625, 1993.
9. Hitchings R: Eye pain. In Wall PD, Melzack R, editors: *Textbook of pain,* ed 2, Edinburgh, Scotland, 1989, Churchill Livingstone.
10. O'Brien JM, Albert DM, Foster CS: Anterior uveitis. In Albert DM, Jakobiec FA, editors: *Principles and practice of ophthalmology: clinical practice,* Philadelphia, 1994, WB Saunders.
11. Goodenberger D, Greer D: Ophthalmic emergencies, *Top Emerg Med* 6(3):1, 1984.
12. Janda AM: Ocular trauma: triage and treatment, *Postgrad Med* 90(7):51, 1991.
13. Miller SJH, editor: *Parson's diseases of the eye,* ed 18, Edinburgh, Scotland, 1990, Churchill Livingstone.
14. Handler JA, Gheezi KT: General ophthalmologic examination, *Emerg Med Clin North Am* 13:521, 1995.
15. Lawlor MC: Common ocular injuries and disorders, *J Emerg Nurs* 15:32, 1989.
16. Neff JA: Visual acuity testing, *J Emerg Nurs* 17:431, 1991.

17. LaVene D, Halpern J, Jagoda A: Loss of vision, *Emerg Med Clin North Am* 13:539, 1995.

18. Feist RM, Farber MD: Ocular trauma epidemiology, *Arch Ophthalmol* 107:503, 1989.

19. Schein OD et al: The spectrum and burden of ocular injury, *Ophthalmology* 95:300, 1989.

20. Schein OD, Vinger PF: Epidemiology and prevention. In Shingleton BJ, Hersh PS, Kenyon KR, editors: *Eye trauma,* St Louis, 1991, Mosby.

21. Dannenberg AL et al: Penetrating eye injuries in the workplace: the national eye trauma system registry, *Arch Ophthalmol* 110:843, 1992.

22. Sternberg P: Prognosis and outcomes for penetrating ocular trauma. In Shingleton BJ, Hersh PS, Kenyon KR, editors: *Eye trauma,* St Louis, 1991, Mosby.

23. Semonin-Holleran R: Trauma in childhood. In Neff JA, Kidd PS, editors: *Trauma nursing: the art and science,* St Louis, 1993, Mosby.

24. Joseph E et al: Predictors of blinding or serious eye injury in blunt trauma, *J Trauma* 33:19, 1992.

25. Klopfer J et al: Ocular trauma in the United States: eye injuries resulting in hospitalization: 1984 through 1987, *Arch Ophthalmol* 110:838, 1992.

26. Wang ESJ: Cocaine induced iritis, *Ann Emerg Med* 20:192, 1991.

27. Hoover DL, Smith LEH: Evaluation and management strategies for the pediatric eye trauma patient. In Shingleton BJ, Hersh PS, Kenyon KR, editors: *Eye trauma,* St Louis, 1991, Mosby.

28. Gayle MO et al: Retinal hemorrhage in the young child: a review of etiology, predisposed conditions, and clinical implications, *J Emerg Med* 13:233, 1995.

29. Wagoner MD, Sadun AA, Bienfang DC: Acute disorders of the eye. In May HL et al, editors: *Emergency medicine,* ed 2, Boston, 1992, Little, Brown.

30. Newman R: Trauma in the elderly. In Neff JA, Kidd PS, editors: *Trauma nursing: the art and science,* St Louis, 1993, Mosby.

31. Amaurosis Fugax Study Group: Current management of amaurosis fugax, *Stroke* 21:201, 1990.

32. McFarland GK, McFarlane EA, editors: *Nursing diagnosis and intervention,* ed 2, St Louis, 1992, Mosby.

33. Campanile TM, St Clair DA, Benaim M: The evaluation of eye patching in the treatment of traumatic corneal epithelial defects, *J Emerg Med* 15:769, 1997.

34. Bertolini J, Pelucio M: The red eye, *Emerg Med Clin North Am* 13:561, 1995.

35. Schein OD: Contact lens abrasions and the nonophthalmologist, *Am J Emerg Med* 11:606, 1993.

36. Patterson J et al: Eye patch treatment for the control of corneal abrasion, *South Med J* 89:227, 1996.

37. Kirkpatrick JN, Hoh HB, Cook SD: No eye pad for corneal abrasions, *Eye* 7:468, 1993.

38. Hulbert MF: Efficacy of eye pad in corneal healing after corneal foreign body removal, *Lancet* 337:643, 1991.

39. Wagoner MD, Kenyon KR: Chemical injuries. In Shingleton BJ, Hersh PS, Kenyon KR, editors: *Eye trauma,* St Louis, 1991, Mosby.

40. Emergency Nurses Association: *Emergency nursing core curriculum,* ed 4, Philadelphia, 1994, WB Saunders.

41. Shingleton BJ, Hersh PS: Traumatic hyphema. In Singleton BJ, Hersh PS, Kenyon KR, editors: *Eye trauma,* St Louis, 1991, Mosby.

42. Bertolini J, Pelucio M: The red eye, *Emerg Med Clin North Am* 13:561, 1995.

43. Ellis PP: Commonly used eye medications. In Vaughan DV, Asbury T, Riordan-Eva P, editors: *General ophthalmology,* ed 13, Norwalk, Conn, 1992, Appleton & Lange.

44. Rubin S, Hallagan L: Lids, lacrimals, and lashes, *Emerg Med Clin North Am* 13:631, 1995.

E

Chapter 12

Genitourinary and Renal Conditions

Pamela S. Kidd

TRIAGE ASSESSMENT

The most common genitourinary (GU) conditions encountered in the emergency department (ED) are genitourinary trauma, urinary tract infections (UTIs), renal calculi, renal failure, and epididymitis. To differentiate among these conditions, you should elicit the following information from the patient at triage:

- History of fever (suspect infection)
- History of injury (suspect trauma)
- History of rapid weight gain, edema, or increasing dyspnea (suspect renal failure)
- History of penile discharge (suspect genital problem)
- History of acute onset of pain or nausea and vomiting (N/V) (suspect renal calculi or trauma)
- History of renal transplant
- History of recent infection or sore throat (suspect strep-induced acute renal failure [ARF])
- Pain changes with position (suspect genital problem)
- Bloody urine (suspect infection, trauma, or calculi)

Vital Signs

- *Tachycardia:* Related to pain and increased fluid volume
- *Hypertension:* Related to increased fluid volume
- *Fever:* Related to infection
- *Tachypnea:* Related to increased fluid volume

General Observations

- Presence of jugular venous distention (suspect renal failure)
- Audible crackles or rales with or without foamy sputum (suspect renal failure)
- Deep and rapid respirations (may indicate metabolic acidosis secondary to renal failure)
- Presence of diaphoresis, pale, clammy skin secondary to sympathetic nervous system action (suspect renal calculi, testicular torsion, epididymitis, and GU trauma)

G

NURSING ALERT

Few GU conditions are medical emergencies. Patients with severe pain, tachypnea, or hypertension should be triaged immediately to the treatment area.

FOCUSED NURSING ASSESSMENT

Nursing assessment centers on perfusion, elimination, and sexuality.

Perfusion
Heart sounds
The presence of S_3 or S_4 may indicate acute heart failure related to fluid overload.
Breath sounds
The presence of rales or crackles that do not clear with coughing may indicate pulmonary edema related to heart failure secondary to fluid overload.
Mental status
Disorientation may occur related to decreased cerebral circulation secondary to heart failure and fluid overload or as a result of accumulated toxins.
Peripheral pulses
Weak peripheral pulses and moderate (3 to 4+) peripheral edema may be present as a result of fluid overload.

Vascular access devices

The presence of current or past vascular access devices may indicate previous renal deficiency. Assess patency if appropriate. Palpate the length of a graft for a strong thrill (constant vibration) indicating adequate blood flow. Auscultate for a bruit produced by blood flow through the graft. Maintain the integrity of peripheral devices by not using the extremity for obtaining blood pressure (BP) measurement, a blood specimen, or venous access.

Elimination
Pattern of elimination

A stopped urination stream may indicate obstruction. Increased frequency may indicate infection. Decreased urination (<400 ml in 24 hr) or diuresis (>4 to 5 L/24 hr) may indicate ARF.

Pain on urination

If the pain is suprapubic in location, it may indicate bladder or urethral trauma or a lower UTI. If the pain is located in the flank, it may indicate renal or ureter trauma, an upper UTI, or renal calculi.

Pain

Pain radiating to the shoulder may indicate intraperitoneal extravasation of urine. Pain from urine colic occurs most frequently at night or in the early morning.

Hematuria

Hematuria may be present in cases of infection, calculi, or trauma.

Retroperitoneal bleeding

Inspect the flanks for ecchymotic areas and abrasions suggestive of renal trauma. If these are present, auscultate the flank for the presence of a bruit suggestive of renal vascular trauma. Mark the size of any hematoma.

Urinary meatus

Inspect the urinary meatus for sign of bleeding associated with urethral injury.

Bruising

Inspect for bruising around the umbilicus and bruising over the flank resulting from a retroperitoneal hemorrhage (Grey Turner's sign). Positive bruising suggests renal trauma.

Bladder

Palpate the bladder to determine if distention is present. Urgency, pain on voiding, and bladder distention suggest a bladder or urethral injury.

Sexuality
Pain during or after intercourse
Pain during or after intercourse may be present with sexually transmitted diseases (STDs) (see Chapter 17) and in epididymitis.
Testicles
Unilateral testicular pain is associated with testicular torsion.
Scrotum
Scrotal pain occurs in epididymitis.
Penile discharge
Penile discharge may be present in STDs and epididymitis.
Testicular swelling
Swelling may be present in testicular torsion. Table 12-1 contrasts symptoms of torsion and epididymitis.

G

TABLE 12-1 Differentiating Testicular Torsion and Epididymitis

	Torsion	Epididymitis
History	Previous episode common	Recent sexual activity
Age	Most common from 12-18 years	Age at onset of sexual activity and older
Pain	Sharp, sudden onset	Gradual onset
Fever	Absent (usually)	Present
Edema	Elevated testis (in order to assess this, stand at foot of patient's bed and have patient fold his arms over his chest)	Swollen scrotum
Urethral discharge	Absent	Possible
CBC	Normal	Elevated WBC count
Urinalysis	Normal	Bacteriuria
Testicular scan	Hypoperfused	Hyperperfused
Prehn's sign (amount of pain elicited on testis elevation)	Negative (pain increases)	Positive (pain decreases)

Genitalia

Inspect the genitalia for the presence of vaginal bleeding, penile discharge, or evidence of incontinence.

Trauma

A patient with multiple injuries will have myoglobulinuria. Aggressive volume replacement, alkalinization of the urine, and mannitol should decrease the incidence of ARF.[1]

Risk Factors

1. **Exposure risk:** Multiple partners, bisexuality, and homosexuality may expose the patient to HIV and STDs (see Chapters 6 and 17, respectively).
2. **Gender:** Genital trauma is more common among males.
3. **Contact sports, heavy lifting:** Contact sports and heavy lifting are associated with renal trauma, bladder trauma, and testicular torsion.
4. **Acceleration and deceleration forces:** These types of forces (e.g., falls or a one-car motor vehicle crash where the car hits a stationary object such as a tree) are associated with renal trauma.
5. **Medical history:** Diabetes, repeated UTIs, autoimmune disease, congenital renal abnormalities, and previous trauma are associated with chronic renal failure.
6. **Medication history:** Antibiotics (especially aminoglycosides), pesticide exposure (agricultural workers), and contrast media (recent diagnostic test) are associated with ARF.

Life Span Issues

1. **Youth:** Testicular torsion is most common in adolescence. Ureter rupture is most common in pediatric patients with blunt injuries (e.g., pedestrian rolled over by motor vehicle).
2. **Postmenopausal:** UTIs are more common among young females and postmenopausal women.
3. **Children:** Children with symptoms of UTI may also be victims of sexual abuse.

INITIAL INTERVENTIONS

Regardless of the source of the GU condition, the following interventions will not harm the patient and may be beneficial:

1. Raise the head of the patient's bed 30 degrees if cervical spine injuries have been ruled out.
2. If the patient can void, obtain a midstream clean-catch specimen. Split the specimen with sterile technique to provide for a urinalysis (UA) and a specimen for culture and sensitivity if the UA result is positive for infection. Examine the specimen for hematuria, protein, glucose, and pH using a clinical reagent strip. If possible, examine it for the presence of leukocytes using a clinical reagent strip. Females during their menses should have a catheterized specimen obtained if no sign of urethral injury is present. If the urine test result is negative for hematuria, a UA may not be obtained.
3. Initiate I/O recording.
4. In cases of testicular swelling, elevate the scrotum on a pillow or towel and apply ice. Place a protective barrier between the ice and the skin.
5. If renal failure is suspected, record the patient's weight. Measure the circumference of edematous extremities. Initiate neurovascular checks of edematous extremities. Keep the patient NPO until a physician examines him or her.
6. Monitor vital signs every 30 minutes (or by policy) if renal failure is suspected.

PRIORITY NURSING DIAGNOSES

Risk for fluid volume excess
Risk for pain
Risk for altered patterns of urinary elimination: urge incontinence
Risk for urinary retention
Risk for infection

♦ **Fluid volume excess** related to primary renal damage or decreased cardiac output as demonstrated by pulmonary, peripheral or generalized edema, hypertension, tachypnea, hyperphosphatemia, hyperkalemia, metabolic acidosis, jugular venous distention, or oliguria:

INTERVENTIONS

• Monitor breath sounds and oxygen saturation levels.
• Initiate intake and output measurement.
• Either insert an intermittent IV infusion device or limit IV fluids to a keep-vein-open rate (30 ml/hr) per physician order.

- Anticipate the administration of diuretics and urinary catheter insertion.
◆ **Pain** related to inflammation, tissue trauma, and spasms, as demonstrated by tachycardia, facial expressions, frequent changes in position, or refusal to change position:
  INTERVENTIONS
  - Place the patient in a position of comfort.
  - Initiate imagery, relaxation exercises, or other coping mechanisms previously identified by the patient.
  - Administer nonsteroidal antiinflammatory agents and narcotics per physician order.
◆ **Altered patterns of urinary elimination: urge incontinence** related to infection and trauma, as demonstrated by involuntary urine loss associated with urge to void:
  INTERVENTIONS
  - Monitor voiding patterns (precipitating factors, amount, and time).
  - Document any voiding mishaps (e.g., wet sheets).
  - Assess symptoms associated with voiding.
◆ **Urinary retention** related to chronic obstruction, as demonstrated by bladder distention and decreased urine output:
  INTERVENTIONS
  - Assess breath sounds for crackles.
  - Assess edema.
  - Percuss or palpate the bladder to determine the degree of distention.
  - Initiate intake and output measurement.
  - Insert a urinary catheter per physician order.
◆ **Risk for infection** related to anticipated invasive procedures, retention of urine, insertion of urinary catheter, and decreased immunocompetence:
  INTERVENTIONS
  - Maintain sterile technique for all invasive procedures.
  - Document a baseline temperature and the route by which it was obtained.
  - Assess for evidence of infection (urine integrity, quality of breath sounds, wound healing) as appropriate.

PRIORITY DIAGNOSTIC TESTS
Laboratory Tests
If renal failure or fluid volume excess is suspected, obtain enough blood for a complete blood count (purple-top tube) and electrolytes (red-top tube). If possible, fill an ad-

ditional red-top tube for potential type and crossmatch (transfusion may be necessary if anemia is severe). Clotting profiles may be needed: if so, fill a blue-top tube. If an infection or obstruction is suspected, a complete blood count (purple-top tube) should be adequate.

Complete blood count: Expect a decreased hematocrit in chronic renal failure and an increased white blood cell count in infection. If the infection is acute and bacterial in origin, an increased level of neutrophils and a decreased level of lymphocytes will be present.

Urinalysis and urine culture and sensitivity: The presence of casts indicates pyelonephritis (upper UTI). The presence of white blood cells and RBCs is nonspecific for infection and calculi. A UTI may be the first manifestation of sepsis. Sepsis can be produced by gram-negative or gram-positive organisms. Urine-specific gravity and osmolality differ depending on the origin of renal failure. Table 12-2 contrasts these differences. Urine cultures are usually reserved for patients with chronic disease, patients who are pregnant, geriatric patients, pediatric patients, and immunosuppressed patients.

Blood urea nitrogen and creatinine: This differs according to the origin of the renal failure (see Table 12-2). A creatinine test is specific for renal function, since the amount of creatinine entering the blood remains constant. Changes in the glomerular filtration rate produce an increase in creatinine.

Electrolytes and basic metabolic profile: Hyperkalemia may be present in renal failure. If so, assess for hyperactive reflexes and electrocardiogram changes (peaked T-waves, a prolonged PR interval, and QRS duration).

Arterial blood gases: Metabolic acidosis (pH <7.35, HCO_3 <22, and $PaCO_2 \leq 35$) may be present in renal failure.

NURSING ALERT

If the hematocrit is low, anticipate obtaining a specimen for type and crossmatch and initiating IV access (heparin lock is useful, since fluid restriction may be necessary). Use an 18-gauge or larger IV catheter.

If hyperkalemia or metabolic acidosis is present, anticipate dialysis. Initiate cardiac monitoring. Anticipate the administration of sodium polystyrene sulfonate (Kayexalate),

Continued

NURSING ALERT—cont'd

glucose with insulin, and sodium bicarbonate. IV access is necessary. Hyperphosphatemia requires the administration of phosphate binders (aluminum hydroxide antacids [Amphojel]) or calcium antacids (ALTernaGEL).

If an increased number of white blood cells is noted, no action may be necessary. However, if an upper UTI or sepsis is suspected, IV antibiotics may be needed. Anticipate IV administration. Blood cultures may be ordered and can be initiated with IV insertion before antibiotic administration.

TABLE 12-2 Categories of Acute Renal Failure and Related Laboratory Values

	Prerenal (decreased renal perfusion)	Intrarenal (ATN) (renal vessel, nephron, tubule, glomerular damage)	Postrenal (obstruction)
Urine			
Volume	Low	Low or high	Low or high
Sodium	<20 mEq/L	>20 mEq/L	>40 mEq/L
Osmolality	>350 mOsm	<300 mOsm (fixed)	<350 mOsm (varies)
Specific gravity	>1.020	<1.010	
Creatinine	~Normal	Low	Low
FE na^{+1}	≤1%	1%	
Plasma			
Urea (BUN)	High	High	High
Creatinine	~Normal	High	High
BUN: creatinine	20:1 or more	10:1 to 15:1	10:1

From Stillwell SB: *Mosby's critical care nursing reference,* St Louis, 1996, ed, 2 Mosby.
ATN, Acute tubular necrosis: *BUN,* blood urea nitrogen; FE *na^{+1},* Fractional excretion of sodium.

Radiographic Tests

Intravenous pyelogram: This test is used to assess upper urinary tract function. A contrast medium is injected intravenously, and serial x-ray films are obtained. Expect a 30- to 45-minute procedure. If the patient's BP is unstable, the nurse or physician should accompany the patient if he or she is to be taken out of the department for test completion. A "one-shot" intravenous pyelogram (IVP) just before laparotomy is useful for patients too unstable to await CT scanning. This film checks for two functioning kidneys and gross renal trauma.[2]

NURSING ALERT

Assess any allergies. Iodine and seafood allergies may require cancellation of IVP or premedication (steroids, antihistamines, and acetaminophen) to minimize reaction.

Retrograde pyelogram: This test is used to assess ureter function. Dye is injected through catheters placed in ureters. Note the same concerns as with IVP.

Cystography: A cystography is used to assess bladder function. Radiopaque dye is injected through a urinary catheter. X-ray films are obtained to determine if the bladder is distended with dye or extravasated. Extravasation may be performed intraperitoneally or extraperitoneally. A cystogram is typically a 15- to 20-minute procedure.

NURSING ALERT

The patient may complain of severe burning and discomfort if a bladder laceration or rupture is present. Prepare the patient for this pain, and use distraction, imagery, and medication as appropriate to facilitate patient coping.

Retrograde urethrography: This test is usually performed in conjunction with cystography. Radiopaque dye is injected through a urinary catheter as the catheter is inserted to detect urethral lacerations. Note the same concerns as for an IVP.

CT/renal scan: This test is rapidly replacing the IVP and arteriography because it is noninvasive. Depending on the type of scanner, this procedure may take 15 to 30 minutes. It is difficult to use with an agitated patient because clear films cannot be obtained with patient movement. The test is used when gross hematuria is present on UA.

Renal angiography: This test is used when a renal vascular injury is suspected and when the patient has a mechanism of injury severe enough to cause renal damage (e.g., fracture of lower ribs) and unstable vital signs. If the IVP shows absent or poor visualization of contrast medium, an angiogram may be performed.

Renal ultrasonography: This test may be used to assess for obstruction and abscesses. The test is a noninvasive procedure performed at the bedside, using reflection of high-frequency sound waves to produce an organ image.

Radionuclide imaging: Radionuclide is IV administered, and a radioactivity-detecting device records the radionuclide uptake to evaluate alterations in blood flow. This test is used for both renal and testicular problems.

NURSING ALERT

Use gloves when handling the patient's urine after this procedure, since the excretion of the radionuclide may take 24 hours.

COLLABORATIVE INTERVENTIONS

1. The patient should assume the semi-Fowler's position to facilitate urine drainage in urinary tract trauma if cervical spine injury has been ruled out.
2. A urinary catheter may be ordered to monitor urine output. If blood is present at the urinary meatus, the patient may have a pelvic fracture. If the patient complains of suprapubic pain with or without perineal discoloration, do not pass the catheter until a retrograde urethrogram is performed.
3. In selecting a urinary catheter, examine the urethral opening and select an appropriate size for the opening (usually a size 12 to 16 Fr in adults). Age, weight, and gender are not useful criteria for choosing catheter size.

4. The patient may require rapid fluid removal using continuous arteriovenous hemofiltration, continuous venous-venous hemofiltration, hemodialysis, or peritoneal dialysis. Pulmonary edema, hyperkalemia, uncontrolled hypertension, and pericarditis are indicators for rapid fluid removal.
5. An ECG is usually obtained in acute or chronic renal failure to check for life-threatening arrhythmias secondary to hyperkalemia.

Clinical Conditions
Genitourinary conditions
Acute cystitis (lower urinary tract infection)
SYMPTOMS
- Symptoms include irritability in children, dysuria, urinary frequency, suprapubic tenderness, and a foul odor to urine.

DIAGNOSIS
- The UA shows an increased level of neutrophils. (A positive UA result has >2-5 leukocytes, >2-5 RBCs, and >1+ bacteria.[4])

TREATMENT
- Administer trimethoprim or trimethoprim-sulfamethoxazole PO (assess patient sensitivity to sulfa).
- Increased fluid intake and frequent resting periods may be ordered.

Acute pyelonephritis (upper urinary tract infection)
SYMPTOMS
- The symptoms are the same as those for cystitis, plus fever, nausea and vomiting, and flank pain.

DIAGNOSIS
- The patient will have casts in his or her urine. A complete blood count with differential will show an increased number of white blood cells. Electrolytes, blood urea nitrogen, and creatinine should also be measured.

TREATMENT
- Administer oral antibiotics if the case is mild.
- IV antibiotics are administered if the case is severe or if the patient cannot tolerate PO medications secondary to nausea and vomiting.
- Cephalosporins, ampicillin, quinoline drugs

(ciprofloxacin, ofloxacin, enoxacin, and norfloxacin), aminoglycosides, and IV trimethoprim may be ordered.
- Increased fluid intake and analgesics may be ordered.
- Children and pregnant females (because of an increased chance of premature labor) are usually hospitalized.

Sepsis

SYMPTOMS
- Symptoms include suprapubic pain, a fever, a change in vital signs without an obvious cause, and a change in mental status.

DIAGNOSIS
- Diagnosis is based on blood cultures. However, blood cultures may have a negative result and systemic infection may still be present.

TREATMENT
- Aminoglycosides may be ordered to treat urologic infections to reduce the frequency of gram-negative bacteremia.

Urinary calculi

SYMPTOMS
- The patient experiences sudden, severe pain and extreme restlessness with costovertebral angle tenderness.
- The patient experiences nausea and vomiting.
- Hematuria may be present.
- Fever is not present unless an infection accompanies the calculi.

DIAGNOSIS
- Diagnosis is based on a history of calculi.
- Perform an IVP to identify site and renal function.
- A renal ultrasound may be used.
- Perform a stone analysis if calculi pass.

TREATMENT
- Increase fluids to 2 qt/day.
- Administer IV pain medication.
- Administer a prostaglandin inhibitor (Ketorolac) to decrease ureteral peristalsis.[2]
- Administer penicillamine to dissolve stones. Stones up to 5 mm may pass spontaneously.
- Extracorporeal shock-wave lithotripsy may be used if calculi are in the renal collecting system or upper ureter and are <2 cm.
- Stones >2 cm in the upper renal poles or those >1 cm in the lower renal poles may be removed by percutaneous nephrolithotomy.

Testicular torsion
SYMPTOMS
See Table 12-1.
- The patient exhibits a positive Prehn's sign.
- The patient experiences an acute onset of pain and increased pain when the testis is elevated.
- The pain usually occurs after physical activity or during sleep.
- The patient experiences nausea and vomiting.
- The patient exhibits scrotal swelling.

DIAGNOSIS
- This condition is the result of a congenital defect.
- This is a surgical emergency and must be repaired within 6 hours to maintain testis viability.
- Diagnosis is based on a decreased image on testicular ultrasonography. A Doppler blood flow study shows diminished blood flow. A radionuclide testicular scan shows hypoperfused testis.

TREATMENT
- Administer IV pain medication.
- Prepare the patient for transfer to the operating suite.

Epididymitis
SYMPTOMS
See Table 12-1.
- The patient has a swollen scrotum.
- The patient has a fever.
- Urethral discharge is noted.
- Dysuria is present.
- The symptoms have a gradual onset.
- The patient has a recent history of sexual activity.

DIAGNOSIS
- Diagnosis is made with an enhanced image on a testicular ultrasound.
- An increased blood flow to the testicular area is seen, using a Doppler stethoscope.
- A hyperperfused testis is shown on a radionuclide testicular scan.

TREATMENT
- Administer oral antibiotics.
- Provide scrotal support.
- Apply ice packs to the testes.
- Elevate the testes.
- Pain medication may be ordered.

Genitourinary trauma
SYMPTOMS
- The patient experiences pain, swelling, or ecchymoses in the scrotum, perineum, or flank.
- The patient experiences bladder distention.
- The patient feels pain on voiding.
- Hematuria and blood at the urinary meatus are noted.
- Genitourinary trauma is associated with a pelvic fracture.
- The patient has renal vascular injuries that may present without hematuria (e.g., renal thrombosis).

Gross hematuria does not indicate the severity of the injury.

Table 12-3 compares symptoms for upper and lower urinary tract trauma.

DIAGNOSIS
- Diagnosis is based on an IVP, retrograde pyelogram, cystography, retrograde urethrogram, and CT scan.

TREATMENT
- Treatment is usually conservative, with drainage by urinary catheter or suprapubic catheter until the hematuria clears.
- Surgery is indicated when vital signs cannot be maintained with fluid or blood replacement, and when expanding flank mass, decreased urine output, decreased central venous pressure, and continuing gross hematuria are noted. Renal vascular emergencies require surgical intervention. Prepare these patients for transfer to the operating suite.
- When urinary tract trauma patients are conservatively managed with urinary catheter placement and no surgical exploration, expect these patients to be admitted.[3]
- Penetrating urinary tract trauma is usually surgically explored. Blunt bladder trauma with intraperitoneal extravasation is usually surgically explored.

Genitalia injuries
SYMPTOMS
- The patient experiences severe pain and nausea and vomiting.
DIAGNOSIS
- Most genitalia injuries are diagnosed by observation.
- A urethral injury may be present and is evaluated by retrograde urethrogram.
- Transillumination of the scrotum is performed to determine if the testis is ruptured.

TABLE 12-3 Comparison of Urologic Injuries

Nursing diagnosis	Renal injuries	Ureteral injuries	Bladder injuries	Urethral injuries
Pain	Mild, localized tenderness to severe discomfort in groin, flank, upper abdomen; may radiate to groin or thigh of affected side	Flank, lower abdomen on affected side	Pelvic area, lower abdomen, suprapubic region; may radiate to shoulder	Suprapubic region
	Abdominal guarding			
Altered patterns of urinary elimination	Hematuria may be present (gross or microscopic)	Hematuria may be present	Small amount of bloody urine on catheterization	May be slight hematuria initially
		Possible anuria	Associated with pelvic fracture or direct trauma	Difficulty voiding; high incidence of functional incontinence with urethral injuries in females and with posterior urethral injuries in males after trauma
		Rarely injured with blunt trauma	Strong urge to void but inability to do so	Associated with pelvic fracture or direct trauma

From Kidd P: Elimination, metabolism and sexuality: genitourinary. In Neff J, Kidd P, editors: *Trauma nursing: the art and science,* St Louis, 1993, Mosby.

G

Continued

TABLE 12-3 Comparison of Urologic Injuries—cont'd

Nursing diagnosis	Renal injuries	Ureteral injuries	Bladder injuries	Urethral injuries
Fluid volume deficit	Possible	Possible	Possible	Unlikely
Altered genitourinary tissue perfusion related to infection	Possible	Possible	Unlikely	Unlikely
Infection as demonstrated by nausea and vomiting, abdominal distention and rigidity, absent bowel sounds, soft mass in flank	Possible	Possible	Possible with laceration of bladder fundus and penetrating trauma	Possible
High risk for altered renal tissue perfusion	Arteriovenous fistula; hydronephrosis, hypertension	Ureteral compression leading to hydronephrosis	Unlikely	Unlikely
Sexual dysfunction	Unlikely	Unlikely	Unlikely	Higher incidence of impotence and infertility with posterior urethral injuries in males

From Kidd P: Elimination, metabolism and sexuality: genitourinary. In Neff J, Kidd P, editors: *Trauma nursing: the art and science*, St Louis, 1993, Mosby.

TREATMENT
- Lacerations are treated by direct pressure.
- Crush injuries are treated with elevation and ice.
- Foreign bodies surrounding the penis may be removed with a ring cutter after relieving penile edema by irrigating the distal penis with heparinized saline or by making small incisions to allow fluid drainage.
- Most scrotum and vaginal lacerations are cleansed and repaired under anesthetic in the operating suite.

Renal conditions
Renal failure
SYMPTOMS
- ARF may have a prerenal, intrarenal, or postrenal cause.
- In the ED, the patient may be in a shock state, and the ARF is secondary to hypoperfusion.
- Acute tubular necrosis is a form of intrarenal ARF. It may occur secondary to trauma or acute infection.
- Postrenal failure results from an obstruction to urine flow, and in a patient in the ED is usually related to a tumor or stone.
- Symptoms are diverse in nature with multisystem involvement. Table 12-4 lists systems, symptoms, and related pathophysiologies.
- Patients initially exhibit oliguria. However, this is followed by a diuretic phase in which urine output may increase to 3 to 5 L/24 hr.
- Patients in the diuretic phase have fluid volume deficit and hypotension.
- Prerenal origin is related to decreased renal perfusion.

DIAGNOSIS
- Diagnosis is confirmed by BUN and creatinine levels.
- Table 12-2 compares the laboratory values in the three categories of ARF.

TREATMENT
- Treatment depends on the type of ARF.
- In prerenal origin, enhancing cardiac output and renal perfusion is a goal.
- Fluid challenge, inotropes, and low-dose dopamine may be used to increase cardiac output enough to allow for continuous venous-venous hemofiltration or dialysis.
- Fluid restriction, diuretics, IV nitroglycerin, and dialysis may be used in intrarenal and postrenal etiologies.

TABLE 12-4 Clinical Manifestations of Acute Renal Failure

Symptom	Pathophysiology
Cardiovascular system	
Dysrhythmia	Hyperkalemia, hypocalcemia
Heart failure	Hypertension, fluid retention
	Decreased H^+ secretion
Metabolic acidosis	Decreased Na^+ reabsorption
	Decreased HCO_3 reabsorption/ generation
Hypertension	Increased Na^+ retention
	Activation of renin
Pulmonary system	
Pulmonary edema	Left ventricle dysfunction
	Increased capillary permeability
	Fluid retention
Kussmaul's respirations	Metabolic acidosis
Hematopoietic system	
Anemia	Decreased erythropoietin
Altered coagulation	Platelet dysfunction related to toxins
Immunosuppression	Decreased neutrophils
Gastrointestinal system	
Anorexia	Breakdown of urea, release of ammonia

- Electrolyte abnormalities and metabolic acidosis must be treated. Bicarbonate is given when the bicarbonate level is <10 mEq/L.
- The most serious electrolyte abnormality encountered in the ED is usually hyperkalemia (≥6.5 mEq/L). IV administration of calcium, insulin, and glucose will shift the potassium to the intracellular space. Potassium-binding ion exchange resins (Kayexalate) will be given. Albuterol by aerosol also shifts potassium intracellularly.[1]
- Hyperphosphatemia and hypocalcemia may also be present. Oral calcium-based antacids will bind phosphorus in the gut. IV calcium will be administered for hypocalcemia.

TABLE 12-4 Clinical Manifestations of Acute
Renal Failure—cont'd

Symptom	Pathophysiology
Gastrointestinal system—cont'd	
Nausea and vomiting	
Gastritis/gastrointestinal bleed	Ammonia produces ulcerations
Neuromuscular system	
Decreased level of consciousness	Metabolic acidosis
	Uremic toxin accumulation
Tremors, hyperreflexia	Hyperkalemia
Integumentary system	
Pallor	Anemia
Yellow skin	Urochrome excretion
Pruritus	Calcium and phosphate skin deposits
	Platelet dysfunction
Purpura	Terminal sign
Uremic frost	Urea skin crystals
Skeletal system	
Hypocalcemia	Hyperphosphatemia resulting from decreased excretion
	Decreased Ca^+ absorption resulting from decreased conservation of vitamin D

- If the patient is in the diuretic phase of ARF, hypokalemia may occur. Patients in this condition require volume and potassium replacement.

Renal transplant rejection

SYMPTOMS

- In addition to the symptoms seen in ARF, the patient will have a fever.
- Urine output may drop suddenly.
- A 2- to 3-lb weight gain may be noted in a 24-hour period.

DIAGNOSIS

- Diagnosis is confirmed by a renal biopsy, but a renal scan may be performed to assess blood flow while the patient is in the ED.

TREATMENT

- IV steroids may be administered.
- Immunosuppressant drug therapy is initiated.
- Drug therapy may include azathioprine (Imuran), cy-closporine (Sandimmune), and monoclonal antibodies. These drugs require careful patient monitoring. See the company's drug insert for information.

NURSING SURVEILLANCE

1. Monitor hematuria.
2. Monitor vital signs.
3. Monitor I/O to assess fluid balance.
4. Observe and mark ecchymotic areas and expanding masses.

EXPECTED PATIENT OUTCOMES

1. A urinary output of 30 ml/hr or 1 ml/kg/hr in children is maintained.
2. Mean arterial pressure is maintained between 70 and 105 mm Hg.
3. Fever decreases.
4. Pain decreases in severity as documented by a pain scale.
5. Nausea and vomiting are absent.
6. The patient has diminished crackles and rales upon auscultation.
7. Electrolyte values are within normal limits.

DISCHARGE IMPLICATIONS
Urinary Tract Infections

1. Teach good hygiene. Instruct the patient to void after intercourse.
2. Stress follow-up after treatment in 7 to 14 days to exam-ine for reinfection.
3. Vitamin C tablets (1 g/day) or three 8-oz glasses of cran-berry juice daily decrease bacterial adherence to the bladder wall and increase urine acidity.[4]
4. Increase fluids to 2 qt/day.
5. Instruct the patient to return if fever or chills persist or N/V precludes the taking of antibiotics.

Discharged with Indwelling Catheter

Patients with indwelling urinary catheters do not benefit from routine catheter changes.[5] Irrigate a catheter only if a decreased flow is noted. Catheters should be changed only if a blockage is present. To decrease the incidence of blockage, patients should consume 2 qt of fluids daily to dilute urine. Vitamin C tablets (1 g/day) or three 8-oz glasses of cranberry juice daily decrease encrustation on catheter surfaces, thus decreasing the incidence of blockage.

Renal Calculi

1. Stress increasing hydration to 2 qt/day.
2. Teach the patient how to strain urine, and provide a strainer.
3. Inform patients that after analysis of the stone is performed, dietary changes need to be made (e.g., decreased calcium intake, decreased oxalate intake, and a low purine diet).

Genitourinary Trauma

1. Instruct the patient to increase fluid intake.
2. The patient should return to the ED if decreased urine output occurs. The patient can measure urine at home.
3. Bed rest is suggested until the hematuria clears (if present).
4. Stress the need for follow-up to assess renal function and potential complications such as hypertension.

References

1. Wolfson A, Maenza R: Renal failure and dialysis. In Rund D et al, editors: *Essentials of emergency medicine,* St Louis, 1996, Mosby.
2. Bresler M, Sternbach GL: *Manual of emergency medicine,* St Louis, 1998, Mosby.
3. Hanno P, Cass A: The injured bladder, *Emerg Med* 22:347-351,1992.
4. Moyle R, White R: Is choice of catheter size an important factor in patient discomfort? *Inforum* 12:9-10, 1991.
5. Brechtelsbauer D: Care with an indwelling urinary catheter, *Postgrad Med* 92:127-132, 1992.

Bibliography

Mulholland S: UTI in women, *Consultant* April, 1995.

Chapter 13

Hematologic and Oncologic Conditions

Pamela S. Kidd
Patty Sturt

CLINICAL CONDITIONS
Hematologic Conditions
Disseminated Intravascular Coagulation
Hemophilia
Sickle-Cell Disease
   Acute Sickle-Cell Pain Crises
      Bone Crisis
      Joint Crisis
      Abdominal Crisis
      Splenic Sequestration Crisis
      Central Nervous System Crisis
      Aplastic Crisis
Oncologic Conditions
   Hypercalcemia
   Neoplastic Cardiac Tamponade
   Spinal Cord Compression
   Superior Vena Cava Syndrome
   Tumor Lysis Syndrome

TRIAGE ASSESSMENT

Most patients who come to the triage area with a hematologic or oncologic emergency need urgent or emergency treatment. Patients with blood dyscrasias are usually knowledgeable about their disease process and seek emergency services only after trying multiple treatment strategies at home. Rarely are these patients initially diagnosed in the emergency department (ED) (see Life Span Issues). Oncology patients may not be as familiar with complications associated with their disease or the treatment of their disease.

Hematologic and Oncologic Conditions
Level of consciousness

If the patient is disoriented, suspect an intracranial bleed, metastatic tumor, or electrolyte abnormality and triage immediately to the treatment area. Patients with sickle-cell anemia (SCA) are at risk for cerebrovascular attacks. Altered mental status or coma may occur as a result of cerebral hypoxia.

Pain

Back pain is a critical symptom for a patient with cancer. Back pain is the first symptom in neoplastic spinal cord compression (SCC). Rest does not relieve the pain (Table 13-1). In hemophilia, pain is present on rest and movement of the affected extremity or muscle group. Immobilization and the application of ice and a pressure dressing (elastic bandage) may relieve the pain. In SCA, pain may be precipitated by alcohol use, physical activity, changes in temperature or altitude, and emotional stress.

Vascular access device

Does the patient have an indwelling central venous catheter or vascular access device? Infection and thrombosis may occur when these devices are present.

Hematologic Conditions
Injury history

Patients with hemophilia and SCA have symptoms inconsistent with a minor trauma history. With hemophilic patients, any injury to the head and spinal column, no matter how trivial should be viewed as significant and triaged immediately to the treatment area.[1]

Treatment before arrival

Ask what type of care was given at home. Hemophilic patients may have administered several units of factor replacement at home, thus alerting ED personnel that additional medication or blood products may be necessary.

NURSING ALERT

Trust the patient. Many hemophiliacs will be able to detect bleeding before physical or radiographic signs are present. Because of the possibility of life-threatening or limb-threatening complications, triage the patient immediately to the treatment area.

TABLE 13-1 Oncologic Emergencies

Emergency	Symptoms	Triage clue
Acute tumor lysis syndrome		
Hyperuricemia	Dysuria, anuria, anorexia, vomiting, lethargy, pain and swelling of joints	Recent initiation of chemotherapy for treatment of leukemia or lymphoma
Hyperkalemia	Bradycardia, hypotension ECG changes: • Tall peaked T-waves • Depressed ST segment • Widening of QRS, diarrhea, muscle weakness	
Hyperphosphatemia/ hypocalcemia	Carpopedal spasms, hyperactive deep tendon reflexes, seizures, irritability, photophobia, diarrhea	
Hypercalcemia	N/V, constipation, abdominal pain, polyuria, bradycardia, mental changes ECG changes: • Prolonged PR interval	History of breast cancer with bony metastatic disease
Spinal cord compression		
Cervical region: symptoms listed in order of appearance	Motor impairment of arm Motor impairment of ipsilateral leg Motor impairment of contralateral leg Motor impairment of opposite arm	Pain is worse on lying down

H

Thoracic region	Stiff and weak legs	
	Altered pain and temperature sensation on opposite side from maximum motor weakness	
Radicular or nerve root	Pain over affected spinal process that is aggravated with coughing, sneezing, or straight-leg raising, spasms, loss of deep tendon reflexes	Symptoms are worse on awakening
Superior vena cava syndrome	Edema, erythema of face and neck, visual changes, headache, conjunctival hemorrhage, engorged neck veins, dyspnea	May have indwelling central venous catheter, since obstruction may be external from mass or internal from clot
Pericardial tamponade	Dyspnea, chest pain, cough, tachycardia, distant heart sounds (possible), jugular venous distension	Other typical symptoms of tamponade seen in traumatic injury (e.g., pulsus paradoxus or pericardial rub) may be absent
Anemia	Dyspnea, fatigue, dizziness, pallor, tachycardia	History of radiation to pelvis area or chemotherapy
Thrombocytopenia	Petechiae, GI/GU bleeding, epistaxis	History of radiation or chemotherapy
Disseminated intravascular coagulation	Fever, petechiae, conjunctival hemorrhage, melena, hematemesis, headache, change in mentation, hematuria	Bleeding from three unrelated sites

ECG, Electrocardiogram; *GI/GU,* gastrointestinal/genitourinary.

Factor type

If the patient is a hemophiliac, ask what type of factor preparation he or she uses. If possible, obtain the batch number from the patient. This reduces the number of plasma donors to whom the patient is exposed.

Medications

Ask the patient what medications he or she takes at home and whether he or she has run out of medication. SCA patients may visit the ED for a renewal of analgesics.

Oncologic Conditions
Radiation and chemotherapy

Determine whether the patient has had radiation therapy or outpatient, as well as home, chemotherapy agents. Disseminated intravascular coagulation (DIC) and tumor lysis syndrome (TLS) may occur quickly after initiation of chemotherapy or radiation, especially after first-time chemotherapy for leukemia. Symptoms may be related to chemotherapeutic agents that the patient is receiving (Table 13-2).

Medical history

Certain cancerous cell types and tumor sites are associated with particular complications (Table 13-3).

Vital Sign Changes for Both Hematologic and Oncologic Conditions

- *Respirations:* The patient's respiratory rate and pattern may be altered if airway compromise is occurring secondary to retropharyngeal bleeding. Tachypnea may indicate an acute chest crisis in SCA.
- *Blood pressure:* Hypotension may be present in acute sequestration syndrome in SCA. In this syndrome, blood pools in an organ, depleting circulating blood volume. DIC may produce hypotension as a result of excessive bleeding. Hypotension may also occur in cases of hypercalcemia because of the polyuria it produces.
- *Fever:* A low-grade fever may be present in sickle-cell crisis and indicate infection as an etiology. For the cancer patient, infection is defined as one temperature measurement $\geq 101°$ F ($38.5°$ C) or three readings $>100.4°$ F ($38°$ C) in a 24-hour period.[2]

Vital Signs (Oncologic Conditions)

- *Pulsus paradoxus:* An exaggerated decrease (>10 mm Hg) of the systolic blood pressure (BP) during inspira-

TABLE 13-2 Complications of Chemotherapeutic Agents

Agent	Side effects	Use
Doxorubicin	Chemical pericarditis and dysrhythmia	Leukemia, breast cancer
Daunomycin	Chemical pericarditis and dysrhythmia	Leukemia, breast cancer
Cisplatin	Nephrotoxicity, neurotoxicity, and ototoxicity	Oat cell lung cancer, ovarian and testicular cancer
Cyclophosphamide	Hemorrhagic cystitis	Breast cancer; lymphoma
Methotrexate	Nephrotoxicity and hepatic toxicity, pulmonary fibrosis	Breast cancer, osteogenic sarcoma, lymphoma, leukemia
Bleomycin	Pulmonary fibrosis, Raynaud's phenomenon	
Interferon	Neurotoxicity, congestive heart failure	
Interleukin-2	Hyperthermia, myocardial infarction, respiratory distress	Hairy-cell leukemia

H

TABLE 13-3 Complications of Cancer

Primary cancer site and type	Associated oncologic emergency
Breast cancer	Hypercalcemia, neoplastic cardiac tamponade, SCC, SVCS, pleural effusion, brain tumor
Lung cancer	
Squamous cell	Pleural effusion, SCC, brain tumor, SVCS
Adenocarcinoma	Pleural effusion, SCC, brain tumor
Oat cell	SVCS, pleural effusion
Multiple myeloma	Hypercalcemia
Lymphoma	Hyperkalemia, hypercalcemia, neoplastic cardiac tamponade, TLS, SCC, SVCS, pleural effusion
Leukemia	Hypercalcemia, TLS, hyperkalemia, thrombocytopenia, hemorrhage
Prostate	SCC, brain tumor, DIC
Pancreatic	DIC, thrombocytosis
Bone	Hypercalcemia

DIC, Disseminated intravascular coagulation; *SCC,* spinal cord compression; *SVCS,* superior vena cava syndrome; *TLS,* tumor lysis syndrome.

tion (pulsus paradoxus) may be present in neoplastic cardiac tamponade.

Vital Signs (Hematologic Conditions)
- *Heart rate:* Tachycardia will be present in acute sequestration syndrome to compensate for decreased circulating blood volume.

General Observations (Hematologic Conditions)
Hemorrhage
- Assess for signs of hemorrhage (petechiae, ecchymoses, hematomas, or swelling). If any of these are detected, pressure and cold should be applied to the site if possible. Elevation of the area is indicated, and extremities should be immobilized at the triage area. The degree of swelling present is not a good indicator of the degree of bleeding.
Hyphema
- Assess for blood in the anterior chamber of the eyes (hyphema). For patients with SCA, hyphema can have devastating complications because of the increased intraocular pressure (IOP) caused by the blockage of outflow tracts

by sickled cells. Triage these patients immediately to the treatment area.

General Observations (Oncologic Conditions)
Edema
- Assess for facial, neck, and periorbital edema. In superior vena cava syndrome (SVCS), edema in these areas may be present and may worsen with bending over or lying down.

FOCUSED NURSING ASSESSMENT (HEMATOLOGIC AND ONCOLOGIC CONDITIONS)
Perfusion
Heart sounds
Muffled heart sounds may be present in neoplastic cardiac tamponade. Tamponade may result from primary or secondary tumors and mediastinal radiation treatment. A systolic murmur may be present in SCA as a result of chronic anemia. The apical pulse may be shifted in SCA because of congestive heart failure (CHF) that develops from pulmonary hypertension secondary to repeated pulmonary infarcts.
Neck veins
With SCA patients, neck veins may be distended because of cor pulmonale. With cancer patients, distended neck veins may suggest neoplastic cardiac tamponade or SVCS.

Cognition
Perform a neurologic assessment and assign the patient a Glasgow Coma Scale score (see Reference Guide 10 and 18). A patient with a score of <15 may need CT brain scanning. Assess neck rigidity, since meningitis is common in pediatric patients with SCA. If the condition is present, anticipate a lumbar puncture (see Procedure 23) and cerebrospinal fluid cultures.

Mobility
Stiffness of the joints, a limited range of motion, and joint edema are common in hemarthroses (joint bleeding). Weakness on ambulation may be a sign of SCC and may be present for several weeks before the patient seeks treatment. Patients with SCC who are ambulatory at the time they seek treatment have a better chance of remaining mo-

bile. Numbness and tingling in the extremities may be another sign of SCC. Extension of the extremities may elicit an electrical sensation down the back.

FOCUSED NURSING ASSESSMENT (ONCOLOGIC CONDITIONS)

Ventilation
Breath sounds
Pleural effusions may develop in neoplastic cardiac tamponade and SVCS, diminishing breath sounds in the affected area.

Extremities
Examine the patient's extremities for deformity and angulation. Pathologic fractures may be present in malignancy. Pain is present on weight bearing.

FOCUSED NURSING ASSESSMENT (HEMATOLOGIC CONDITIONS)

Sexuality
Priapism
Priapism (a painful sustained erection) may be present in SCA. Because erectile dysfunction and impotence may occur if the condition is left untreated, hydration and analgesia are initiated quickly.

Risk Factors for Both Hematologic and Oncologic Conditions
Infection
Many hemophiliacs have human immunodeficiency virus (HIV) because they have received blood products from multiple donors (HIV-contaminated blood products were used between 1978 and 1985).[2] They may be immunosuppressed and have an active infection in addition to their presenting complaint.

Obstruction
SVCS is more likely to develop in a patient with right-sided vs. left-sided lung or bronchogenic cancer.

Life Span Issues (Hematologic Conditions)
Children
1. Hemophilia, when not diagnosed at birth, is usually detected when the child begins to walk and joint swelling occurs.

2. Cutting teeth and losing deciduous teeth may precipitate bleeding in hemophilia.
3. The death of patients with SCA between the ages of 1 and 3 years old is frequently related to pneumococcal sepsis and can be prevented with prophylactic penicillin. If the patient is receiving penicillin, this should be noted, since clinical presentation and bacterial studies may be altered in the presence of an infection.
4. Acute chest crisis is more common among pediatric patients with SCA.

Women

Postpartum bleeding may occur on a delayed basis after hospital discharge with women who have von Willebrand's disease.

Adults

1. With adult hemophiliac patients, intracranial bleeding may occur spontaneously (without an injury history).
2. Adult patients with SCA frequently die from bone marrow and fat embolization or the effects of excessive narcotic use.

Life Span Issues (Oncologic Conditions)
Children

Bladder control regression may be the first symptom for children who have SCC because of cancer.

INITIAL INTERVENTIONS (HEMATOLOGIC AND ONCOLOGIC CONDITIONS)

1. Initiate oxygen administration as needed to relieve dyspnea and impaired gas exchange. If dyspnea is present (as in suspected SVCS), elevate the head of the bed and administer low-flow oxygen. Initiate pulse oximetry.
2. Initiate IV access. Oncologic and hematologic emergencies require fluid resuscitation, factor replacement, pain control, electrolyte replacement or removal, or diuretics. Patients with SCA and hemophilia have had multiple IV catheters, and their veins may be sclerosed. Ask the patient for the "best vein site." Place the largest IV catheter that vein integrity will allow. Hydration in the SCA patient is initiated with D_5W or D_5 ½NS because these allow free water to enter the cells and thus decrease the hemoglobin concentration, improving tissue oxygenation.

> **NURSING ALERT**
>
> For unsuccessful IV attempts, apply pressure to the puncture or injection site for at least 10 minutes in hemophilic patients.

3. While starting the IV in hemophilic patients, obtain blood for a complete blood count (CBC) and coagulation studies. This allows for the prediction of the amount of factor replacement necessary based on the severity and location of the bleed and the degree of factor activity present.

4. Initiate pain control. Pain occurs in SCA from obstruction of the blood flow and its resulting hypoxia and ischemia. SCA pain may be relieved by IV hydration. Ask the patient what usually relieves the pain based on the severity of the episode. Distraction, imagery, and relaxation techniques can be initiated immediately. Seek an order for administration of acetaminophen, antiinflammatory agents, and narcotics.

> **NURSING ALERT**
>
> Aspirin products should not be administered to hemophilic patients because of their interference with platelet function. Meperidine (Demerol) is not used in SCA patients because repeated doses are usually necessary, resulting in accumulation of narcotic metabolites and subsequent respiratory depression. Ketorolac (Toradol) has had mixed success in treating SCA pain.

5. Use universal precautions. Hemophiliac patients have a high rate of HIV and hepatitis B infection. Cancer patients' white blood cell (WBC) count may be below 2000 cells/mm^3, increasing their susceptibility to opportunistic and nosocomial infections. Patients with a low WBC count should be placed in a private room. Wash your hands well before each patient contact.

6. If the patient is complaining of chest pain, obtain an electrocardiogram (ECG). Several oncologic emergencies produce the symptom of chest pain (e.g., neoplastic cardiac tamponade and hypercalcemia).

PRIORITY NURSING DIAGNOSES

Risk for impaired gas exchange
Risk for pain
Risk for injury
Risk for impaired physical mobility

✦ **Impaired gas exchange** related to pulmonary infiltrates from microinfarctions in SCA, pleural effusion in malignancy, and cor pulmonale in SVCS:

INTERVENTIONS

• Administer antibiotics as ordered.
• Administer diuretics, oxygen, and vasoactive drugs as ordered.

✦ **Pain** related to nerve compression, inadequate cardiac output, or ischemia:

INTERVENTIONS

• Administer IV fluids and oxygen in cases of suspected ischemia.
• Use imagery, distraction, or relaxation techniques.
• Administer narcotics, acetaminophen, or antiinflammatory drugs.

✦ **Injury** related to bleeding:

INTERVENTIONS

• Observe for hemorrhage.
• Monitor the mucous membranes, urine, sputum, and stool for blood.
• Perform frequent neurologic and abdominal assessments.

✦ **Impaired physical mobility** related to joint bleeding and stiffness or SCC:

INTERVENTIONS

• Immobilize and elevate joints.
• Apply cold compresses to affected areas.
• Initiate and maintain spinal immobilization until radiographic tests are completed and the results are returned.

PRIORITY DIAGNOSTIC TESTS

Laboratory Tests

Laboratory data that is diagnostic for hemophilia is located in Table 13-4.

Complete blood count: A CBC may be ordered to detect dehydration (high hematocrit) and infection in SCA. A

TABLE 13-4 Laboratory Values in Bleeding Disorders

Condition	aPTT	Bleeding time	Factor VIII	Factor IX	vWF
Hemophilia A	Increased	Normal	Decreased	Normal	Normal
Hemophilia B	Increased	Normal	Normal	Decreased	Normal
von Willebrand's disease	Normal or increased	Increased	Decreased	Normal	Decreased

aPTT, Activated partial thromboplastin time; *vWF*, von Willebrand's factor.

WBC count >20,000 has been associated with a higher infection and death rate in SCA. Hemoglobin levels will be extremely low in acute sequestration syndrome in SCA.

Electrolytes: The potassium and phosphorus levels may be elevated in TLS. The calcium level may be increased in malignancy and decreased in TLS.

Fibrin split products: This level will be increased in DIC.

Hemoglobin S level: This level will be elevated in cases of acute crisis in SCA.

Platelets: The level of platelets will be decreased in DIC.

Prothrombin time: This time will be increased in DIC.

Partial thromboplastin time: This time will be increased in DIC.

Reticulocyte count: A reticulocyte count may be ordered in SCA to detect an aplastic crisis.

Uric acid: This level will be increased in TLS.

Urinalysis: A urinalysis may be ordered to detect dehydration or infection in the patient with SCA.

Radiographic Tests

Lateral soft tissue neck films: These films may be ordered to rule out retropharyngeal bleeding in hemophilia.

Chest film: A chest film may be ordered to rule out infection and infiltrates in SCA. A widened mediastinum may be present with SVCS.

CT scan: A scan of the head may be used to detect intracranial bleeding in hemophilia and SCA. A scan of the chest may show collateral circulation in SVCS.

Long bone films: These films may be obtained in hemophilia and SCA to detect acute joint effusions.

Spinal films: Most cases of vertebral body involvement by tumor (and SCC) can be identified using spinal films.

Other Tests

Abdominal ultrasound: An ultrasound may be ordered to evaluate abdominal pain in SCA.

ECG: The direction of the QRS complex and T-wave may change with every other beat in cardiac tamponade. In hypercalcemia, first- or second-degree heart block may be present. In hyperkalemia associated with TLS, tall, peaked T-waves may be present.

Echocardiogram: This test may be useful in diagnosing the degree of pericardial effusions.

Venography: Venography may be used to identify the degree of obstruction in SVCS.

COLLABORATIVE INTERVENTIONS

1. Initiate blood product replacement. Hemophilic patients may need factor replacement in cases in which they come to the ED with a primary problem (e.g., laceration) and will require an invasive procedure (e.g., suturing). When in doubt, initiate factor replacement while awaiting laboratory results.
2. Simple or partial exchange transfusions may be administered in SCA to improve local blood flow to infarcted areas. A hemoglobin S level of <30% is desired.
3. In DIC, clotting factors may be replenished using platelets, fresh frozen plasma, or packed cells.

Clinical Conditions
Hematologic conditions
Disseminated intravascular coagulation

DIC may be associated with infection or may be a complication of malignancy in which tumors secrete substances that activate the clotting cascade or in which antineoplastic therapy is lysing necrotic tumor cells. In DIC the pace of the clotting cascade is accelerated and fibrinolysis is unable to keep pace with thrombus formation. Injury occurs from thrombi in the microcirculation and from bleeding as a result of the consumption of clotting factors in the microcirculation.

SYMPTOMS
- Bleeding generally occurs from three or more sites.
- Petechiae, epistaxis, abdominal pain and distention, melena, hematuria, hemoptysis, and level-of-consciousness (LOC) changes may be present.
- The bleeding site(s) determine the symptoms.

DIAGNOSIS
- Laboratory data show increased prothrombin and partial thromboplastin times.
- Levels of fibrin split products are elevated.
- The level of platelets and fibrinogen is decreased.

TREATMENT
- Heparin therapy is used to block microthrombus formation.
- In malignancy, patients may be resistant to heparin therapy. Oncology patients with solid tumors usually suffer

greater problems from hypercoagulability.[3] Aspirin and dipyridamole may be used.

- Platelets (when the platelet count is <5000/mm³), packed red blood cells, fresh frozen plasma, or factor VIII may be given. (See the "How to Calculate Factor Replacement" box.)

Hemophilia

Hemophilia is a genetic disorder characterized by a clotting factor deficiency. Hemophilia primarily affects males, but females carry the trait. It results in prolonged or excessive bleeding in response to varying degrees of physical injury. Hemophilia A is the most common type and results from a factor VIII deficiency. Hemophilia B results from a factor IX deficiency. In von Willebrand's disease, factor VIII is synthesized but in inadequate amounts.

SYMPTOMS

- The bleeding site and respective symptoms are listed in Table 13-5.

DIAGNOSIS

- Table 13-4 clarifies the laboratory values in most types of hemophilia.
- Factor levels should be determined to calculate the factor replacement that is adequate for the type and severity of factor deficiency and the type, severity, and location of the bleeding.

TREATMENT

- Table 13-6 describes treatment alternatives based on the location of the bleeding.
- Bleeding of the mucous membranes of the mouth and nose is treated with both factor replacement and

---

HOW TO CALCULATE FACTOR REPLACEMENT

Amount of factor VIII required = (wt in kg) × (0.5) × (% change desired in factor activity).*

Amount of factor IX required = (wt in kg) × (1.0) × (% change desired in factor activity).*

---

*Table 13-5 includes factor activity treatment goals. Percent (%) change is based on the difference between the degree of factor activity present (by laboratory testing) and the treatment goal.

Text continued on p. 471

TABLE 13-5 Common Manifestations of Bleeding in Hemophilia Disorders

Bleeding site	Symptoms	Special considerations
Muscle	Pain at site on movement or rest Numbness, tingling if nerve compression occurs Decreased or absent DTRs	Potential for compartment syndrome
Hemarthrosis	Edema at site Pain is usually in knee, elbow, shoulder, ankle, or wrist Limited range of motion	More factor replacement is required for weight-bearing joints Hypovolemia may occur if bleeding into shoulder or hips
Central nervous system	Altered LOC, headache, vomiting, seizures	May have 24-hr symptom-free interval after injury
Gastrointestinal	Melena, hematemesis	
Retropharyngeal	Sore throat, dysphagia, dyspnea, change in voice quality	Usually occurs after dental procedures
Retroperitoneal	Tender RLQ Absent bowel sounds Rigid abdomen Flank pain with hematoma Hypovolemic signs	

DTRs, Deep tendon reflexes; *LOC,* level of consciousness.

TABLE 13-6 Comparison of Hemophilia Disorders

Condition	Treatment goal	von Willebrand's disease	Hemophilia A with inhibitors	Hemophilia A	Hemophilia B	Special considerations
Hematoma	Increase factor VIII to 30%	FFP: 10 ml/kg Cryo: 2 bags/10 kg Factor VIII conc: 10 IU/kg DDAVP × 4 days	Factor IX conc: 50 IU/kg	Cryo: 2 bags/10 kg Factor VIII conc: 10 IU/kg*	FFP: 10 ml/kg Factor IX conc: 10 IU/kg	Cryo contains 60-125 U factor VIII/bag Use microaggregate filter
Hematuria	Increase factor VIII to 30%	Steroids: 2 mg/kg FFP: 10 ml/kg DDAVP × 3 days Factor VIII conc: 10 IU/kg	Factor IX conc: 100 IU/kg Autoplex: 80-100 IU/kg Factor VIII: inhibitor bypass activity (FEIBA) 80-100 IU/kg Steroids: 2 mg/kg	Steroids: 2 mg/kg Cryo: 4 bags/10 kg Factor VIII conc: 40 IU/kg	Steroids: 2 mg/kg Factor VIII conc: 40 IU/kg	Factor VIII conc must be drawn up through a special filter needle

Amicar is a trade name for E-aminocaproic acid. Cyklokapron is a trade name for tranexamic acid.

*This dose can be increased to a loading dose of 50 IU/kg

Cryo, Cryoprecipitate; *DDAVP*, desmopressin, can be administered IV, subcutaneously, intranasally; if given IV, dilute in 50 ml saline and give over 15 to 30 minutes; *factor VIII conc*, factor VIII concentrate (Humate P, Hemofil, Koate); *FFP*, fresh frozen plasma. *Continued*

Continued

TABLE 13-6 Comparison of Hemophilia Disorders—cont'd

Condition	Treatment goal	von Willebrand's disease	Hemophilia A with inhibitors	Hemophilia A	Hemophilia B	Special considerations
Hemarthrosis	Increase factor VIII to 30%	FFP: 5-10 ml/kg Cryo: 2 bags/ 10 kg DDAVP × 3 days Factor VIII conc: 10 IU/kg	Factor XI conc: 100-150 IU/kg Autoplex: 80-100 IU/kg Factor VIII: (FEIBA) 80-100 IU/kg Steroids: 2 mg/kg	Cryo: 3-4 bags/ 10 kg Factor VIII conc: 15-20 IU/kg	Factor IX conc: 15 IU/kg Prednisone: 2 mg/kg/day	—
Mouth	Increase factor VIII to 30%	DDAVP × 3 days Factor VIII conc: 20 IU/kg FFP: 20 ml/kg Amicar: 100 mg/ kg q6hr	Amicar: 100 mg/kg q6hr Factor IX: 100 IU/kg Cyklokapron: 25 mg/kg q6hr	Cryo: 6 bags/ 10 kg Factor VIII conc: 40 IU/kg Amicar: 100 mg/kg q6hr Cyklokapron: 25 mg/kg q6hr	Factor IX conc: 20 IU/kg Amicar: 100 mg/ kg q6hr Cyklokapron: 25 mg/kg q6hr	Amicar must be given slowly when given IV; do not push

Epistaxis	Increase factor VIII to 30%	FDDAVP × 5 days Factor VIII conc: 20 IU/kg FFP: 20 ml/kg Amicar: 100 mg/kg q6hr Cyklokapron: 25 mg/kg q6hr	Amicar: 100 mg/kg q6hr Factor IX: 100 IU/kg Cyklokapron: 25 mg/kg q6hr	Cryo: 6 bags/10 kg Factor VIII conc: 40 IU/kg Amicar: 100 mg/kg q6hr Cyklokapron: 25 mg/kg q6hr	Factor IX conc: 20 IU/kg Amicar: 100 mg/kg q6hr Cyklokapron: 25 mg/kg q6hr
Gastro-intestinal	Increase factor VIII to 80%	FFP: 10 ml/kg Cryo: 2 bags/10 kg Factor VIII conc: 10 IU/bag	Factor IX conc: 100-150 IU/kg FEIBA or Autoplex: 50 IU/kg q8hr	Cryo: 6 bags/10 kg Factor VIII conc: 50 IU/kg	Factor IX conc: 40 IU/kg
Central nervous system	Increase factor VIII to 100%	FFP: 15 ml/kg Cryo: 3 bags/10 kg Factor VIII conc: 15 IU/kg	Factor IX conc: 100-150 IU/kg FEIBA or Autoplex: 50 IU/kg q8hr	Cryo: 6 bags/10 kg Factor VIII conc: 50 IU/kg	Factor IX conc: 40 IU/kg

Amicar is a trade name for E-aminocaproic acid. Cyklokapron is a trade name for tranexamic acid.

Continued

TABLE 13-6 Comparison of Hemophilia Disorders—cont'd

Condition	Treatment goal	von Willebrand's disease	Hemophilia A with inhibitors	Hemophilia A	Hemophilia B	Special considerations
Retro-pharyngeal	Increase factor VIII to 100 %	FFP: 15 ml/kg Cryo: 3 bags/ 10 kg Factor VIII conc: 15 IU/kg	Factor IX conc: 100-150 IU/kg FEIBA or Autoplex: 50 IU/kg q8hr	Cryo: 6 bags/ 10 kg Factor VIII conc: 50 IU/kg	Factor IX conc: 40 IU/kg	Factor IX conc: 40 IU/kg
Retro-peritoneal	Increase factor VIII to 100%	FFP: 15 ml/kg Cryo: 3 bags/ 10 kg Factor VIII conc: 15 IU/kg	Factor IX conc: 100-150 IU/kg FEIBA or Autoplex: 50 IU/kg q8hr	Cryo: 6 bags / 10 kg Factor VIII conc: 50 IU/kg	Factor IX conc: 40 IU/kg	

Amicar is a trade name for E-aminocaproic acid. Cyklokapron is a trade name for tranexamic acid.

antifibrinolytic agents (e.g., Amicar) because saliva contains high levels of fibrinolytic enzymes, making clots unstable.
- Ice, elastic bandages (pressure dressings), packing, and immobilization and elevation may be used in addition to medication and factor administration to control bleeding in joints, muscles, and the nose.

Sickle-cell disease

SCA occurs predominantly among the black population. It is characterized by the presence of an abnormal type of hemoglobin in the red blood cell, termed hemoglobin S.[4] When the cell becomes hypoxic, these red blood cells assume an irregular, crescent shape, causing an increase in blood viscosity that results in stasis of blood flow and in sludging. This leads to microvascular obstruction and to tissue ischemia. The sickling process occurs with local tissue hypoxia, dehydration, and acidosis and with exposure to cold, infection, or emotional stress.

Sickle-cell crisis refers to a variety of acute symptomatic events that occur because of the sickling process associated with SCA. The most common emergency is the pain associated with vascular occlusion. Aplastic crises normally follow a viral infection, causing bone marrow suppression with worsening anemia. Splenic sequestration crises occur from sudden trapping of blood in the spleen. Splenic function may be altered, which increases the patient's susceptibility to infection.

SYMPTOMS

Bone crises caused by sludging of blood
- Acute long bone pain
- Back pain (common in pediatric patients)
- Nonpitting edema

Joint crises caused by pulmonary microinfarction
- Chest pain
- Dyspnea and tachypnea
- Pleural effusions
- Nonproductive cough
- Hemoptysis (suggests a pulmonary infarction)

Abdominal crises caused by ischemia or infarcts of the mesenteric and abdominal viscera
- Abdominal pain
- Nausea, vomiting, and diarrhea

Splenic sequestration crises
- Left upper quadrant tenderness and enlarged spleen
- Infections

Central nervous system crises related to thrombotic stroke
- Headache
- Visual changes
- Change in LOC

Aplastic crisis
- Fatigue and dyspnea
- Decreased number of RBCs and hemoglobin
- Decreased number of or absence of reticulocytes

Other symptoms
- Priapism

DIAGNOSIS
- Diagnosis is based on the patient's history of SCA, clinical presentation, and laboratory values (CBC and reticulocyte count).

TREATMENT
- Begin hydration with oral or IV fluids or both. D_5W or $D_5\frac{1}{2}NS$ is recommended. Begin at a rate of 150 to 200 ml/hr for adults.[2]
- Provide oxygen therapy at 2 to 4 L/min per nasal cannula.
- Administer pain medications as ordered. Narcotic analgesics are frequently used for pain management.
- Administer antiemetics as ordered for nausea.
- Administer antibiotics as ordered by the physician if an underlying infection is present.
- Patients with aplastic or splenic sequestration crises may need blood transfusions.
- Administer folate per physician order for anemia.

Oncologic conditions

Hypercalcemia
Hypercalcemia in cancer may occur for the following reasons: the tumor produces a parathyroid hormone–like substance; hormonal treatment of primary cancer (e.g., tamoxifen) may cause progression of hypercalcemia; or the tumor produces direct bone destruction. The incidence of hypercalcemia is higher among patients with breast or lung tumors.[4]

SYMPTOMS
- Nausea, vomiting, and polyuria are the initial signs and contribute to the hypovolemia associated with hypercalcemia.

- The patient experiences abdominal pain and distention.
- The patient experiences muscle weakness.
- Deep tendon reflexes (DTRs) are diminished or absent.
- The patient experiences confusion or a decreased LOC.

DIAGNOSIS

- Serum calcium levels are elevated (greater than 12 mg/dl).
- ECG changes of short ST segments, first- or second-degree heart block, and wide T-waves may be present.

TREATMENT

- Medications used to treat hypercalcemia are discussed in Table 13-7.
- IV saline (0.9% alternating with 0.5%) is administered (2 to 5 L/day or 250 to 500 ml/hr).
- After volume is restored, diuretics are given to assist in eliminating calcium.
- Medications aimed at preventing bone breakdown (e.g., calcitonin, plicamycin, and gallium nitrate) are administered.
- Radiation and chemotherapy aimed at the primary tumor may be instituted.
- Dialysis may be used for patients with hypercalcemia and renal failure.

H

NURSING ALERT

Hypokalemia may occur with saline hydration and diuretic use in treating hypercalcemia. Monitor the patient for muscle weakness, paralytic ileus, and flattening of the T-wave (T-wave inversion) on an ECG.

Neoplastic cardiac tamponade

Neoplastic cardiac tamponade occurs when a malignancy causes fluid to accumulate within the pericardial sac. This fluid accumulation then causes a marked rise in intrapericardial pressure. The heart is unable to pump against this increased pressure (tamponade).

SYMPTOMS

- Pallor
- Decreased LOC
- Hypotension
- Elevated central venous pressure
- Muffled heart tones
- Oliguria

TABLE 13-7 Drug Summary

Drug	Dose/route	Special considerations	Use
Plicamycin	10-25 μg/kg IV		Hypercalcemia
Mithramycin	15-25 μg/kg IV q day × 2 days	Produces thrombocytopenia and rapid rebound of Ca^+	Hypercalcemia
Etidronate disodium (Didronel)	7.5 mg/kg IV q day × 3 days 400 mg PO bid		Hypercalcemia
Calcitonin	4-8 IV/kg IM q6-12h		Hypercalcemia
Allopurinol	300-800 mg PO q day		Hyperuricemia
Sodium polystyrene sulfonate (Kayexalate)	20-50 g PO	Potassium-binding resin	Hyperkalemia
Calcium gluconate	5-10 ml of a 10% solution IV		Hyperkalemia

Sodium bicarbonate	44 mEq IVP over 5 min or 50-100 mEq in 1 L of 0.25% NS at 100-200 ml/hr IV	Encourages cellular export of hydrogen and import of potassium	Hyperkalemia
Insulin and glucose	5-20 U regular insulin plus 25 g glucose IV (250 ml of 10%-20% glucose solution)	Glucose will import potassium into the cell	Hyperkalemia
Aluminum hydroxide	500 mg–2 g bid-qid PO		Hyperphosphatemia
Furosemide	40-80 mg PO or IV q4-6hr	Must be titrated with normal saline IV administration	Hypercalcemia
Metoclopramide hydrochloride	2 mg/kg IV q4-6hr		Antiemetic for vomiting associated with chemotherapy
Gallium nitrate	100-200 mg/m² q day, infuse over 24 hr continuous IV infusion for 5 days	Do not use with other nephrotoxic drugs or in renal failure	Hypercalcemia

DIAGNOSIS
- Diagnosis is made based on clinical presentation, an ECG, and an echocardiogram.

TREATMENT
- Pericardiocentesis is the treatment of choice (see Procedure 25).
- Continuous drainage by an indwelling catheter may be initiated until surgery can be performed.
- IV fluid administration and vasoactive medications (e.g., dopamine) may be used.
- Pericardial sclerosis may be instituted using chemotherapeutic agents.

Spinal cord compression
SCC usually occurs from metastatic tumors. Cancers of the lung, breast, prostate, and kidney carry the highest risk.

SYMPTOMS
- Back pain is localized, unrelieved by rest, and exacerbated by lying flat.
- Straining and coughing also worsens the pain.
- The patient experiences decreased motor function.
- The patient experiences decreased sensation to pain and touch.
- The patient experiences bowel and bladder dysfunction.
- The patient's DTRs initially may be hyperreflexic, but eventually DTRs diminish.

DIAGNOSIS
- Diagnosis is made based on clinical history, spine films, myelography, and an MRI in some cases.

TREATMENT
- High-dose steroids may be given (dexamethasone 100 mg/day IV).
- Radiation and surgery may be used.

Superior vena cava syndrome
The superior vena cava may be compressed externally by a mass or internally by a thrombus (as in cases of indwelling central venous catheters) or by direct invasion by the disease process.

SYMPTOMS
- The patient experiences dyspnea, cough, dysphagia, hoarseness, and chest pain.
- Edema of the face and neck occurs.
- In severe obstruction, syncope and a decreased LOC occur.

- Symptoms are worse upon rising in the morning or when bending over.

DIAGNOSIS
- Diagnosis is confirmed by chest film and venography.

TREATMENT
- If SVCS is caused by external compression, chemotherapy and radiation are used.
- If thrombosis is present, urokinase (4400 U/kg IV bolus followed by 4400 U/kg/hr), streptokinase (250,000 U IV bolus followed by 100,000 U/hr), or a tissue plasminogen activator (check drug insert for proper dosage, since dosage varies) may be given.
- Surgery may be indicated.
- Diuretics may be given as a temporary measure.

Tumor lysis syndrome

TLS is a positive indicator that therapy is effective. As tumor cells are killed, potassium, phosphate, and uric acid levels rise. Calcium levels will fall in response to the elevated phosphate levels.

SYMPTOMS
- Symptoms are listed in Table 13-1.
- Joint pain may occur secondary to accumulation of uric acid.
- Renal function may decrease because of uric acid crystal formation.
- Cardiac symptoms of tachycardia, hypotension, tall T-waves, prolonged ST segment, and delayed conduction occur because of hypocalcemia and hyperkalemia.
- Hyperactive DTRs and muscle cramps may be present.

DIAGNOSIS
- Diagnosis is based on serum electrolyte levels and the uric acid level.

TREATMENT
- IV hydration is started using 250 ml of 10% to 20% glucose with 10 to 20 U of regular insulin.
- Potassium is restricted in both IV fluids and diet.
- Calcium gluconate may be given.
- Cation exchange resins (Kayexalate and aluminum hydroxide) may be used to remove potassium and phosphate, respectively, and allopurinol is used to remove the uric acid.
- Sodium bicarbonate may be given to decrease the likelihood of uric acid precipitation.

NURSING SURVEILLANCE

1. Monitor the patient for complications of factor or blood replacement. Allergic reactions may range from wheezing, fever, chills, and hives to dyspnea. Flushing, tachycardia, nausea, and headaches may occur if the drugs are infused too rapidly.
2. Monitor the patient for response to fluid administration. Fluid overload can quickly occur, especially in malignancy where radiation treatment has been administered to the mediastinum and chest. Hydration is a common treatment for oncologic emergencies (e.g., hypercalcemia, TLS, and cardiac tamponade). Fluid overload can also occur in SCA in cases of multiple pulmonary infarcts and pulmonary hypertension.
3. Monitor the patient for changes in the LOC.

EXPECTED PATIENT OUTCOMES

1. Factor activity levels are at least 50% (in cases of hemophilia).
2. The hemoglobin S level is 30% or less.
3. The LOC remains unchanged or improves.
4. Seizure activity is diminished.
5. Serum electrolyte levels normalize.
6. Pain diminishes.

DISCHARGE IMPLICATIONS

Hematologic Conditions

1. Teach prevention of acute episodes.
2. In SCA, avoid changes in temperature, hydration, and stressful situations.
3. In hemophilia, avoid injury (e.g., wear protective devices such as helmets and kneepads, as appropriate for activity) and use of products that contain aspirin. Home environments (e.g., playground areas) may need alteration to promote safety. Only electric razors should be used. Good dental hygiene may prevent the need for tooth extractions and subsequent bleeding.
4. Teach recognition of acute episodes. Hemophiliacs should be taught how to examine their urine for microscopic hematuria (using urine reagent strips). A tingling sensation may precede any objective signs of bleeding. A change in the LOC, vomiting, severe headache, mood

changes, and gait changes may signal intracranial bleeding. Pallor, weakness, and restlessness may indicate internal bleeding.

5. Encourage health care evaluation after what is perceived to be a "minor" injury. Major bleeding may occur hours after minor trauma.
6. Help the patient obtain a "Medic Alert" tag.

Oncologic Conditions

1. Teach prevention of acute episodes.
2. Encourage patient mobility and fluid intake of 3 to 4 L of fluid/day to prevent hypercalcemia.

References

1. Medical Advisory Council of the Florida State Chapter of the National Hemophilia Foundation (1993): Emergency room care for hemophiliac patients, *J Fla Med Assoc* 80:250-254, 1993.
2. Hamilton G: Anemia, polycythemia, and white blood cell disorders. In Rosen P, Barkin R, editors: *Emergency medicine*, ed 4, 1998, St Louis, Mosby.
3. Bick R: Coagulation abnormalities in malignancy: a review, *Semin Thromb Hemost* 18:353-372, 1992.
4. Gross J, Johnson B: *Handbook of oncology nursing*, ed 2, 1994, Jones & Bartlett.

Chapter 14

Neurologic Conditions

Patty Sturt
Steve Talbert

TRIAGE ASSESSMENT

Neurologic emergencies can occur because of trauma or disease processes that impair functioning of the brain and spinal cord. If the patient is not alert or oriented, it may be necessary to obtain the history from EMS personnel, family, friends, or witnesses. If the primary functions of airway, breathing, and circulation (ABCs) are intact, obtain the following data:

Recent trauma

A history of any recent trauma involving the head, face, or spine should be elicited. Determine if there was a loss of consciousness. Suspect increased intracranial pressure (ICP) from bleeding and edema with brain trauma. Suspect spinal cord edema or partial or complete cord transection with spine trauma.

Neurologic history

Determine if there is a history of hemorrhagic or ischemic strokes, transient ischemic attacks (TIAs), seizures, syncope, or tumors or masses involving the brain or spinal cord. Patients with these conditions have a higher risk of cerebral edema, ischemia, or infarction.

Behavior

Behavior changes, sleepiness, memory loss, or confusion may indicate an increase in the ICP.

Headache

Headache is a symptom often associated with increased ICP caused by a subarachnoid hemorrhage, brain trauma, or an intracranial mass.

Sensation and movement

Numbness, decreased sensation, weakness, or paralysis in one or more extremities frequently occurs in patients experiencing a stroke or a TIA.

Vomiting

Vomiting can occur because of increased ICP resulting from a mass, intracranial hemorrhage, or brain trauma.

Speech

Suspect a stroke, a TIA, or an intracranial mass if the patient has slurred speech or difficulty speaking.

Gait

A staggered gait and uncoordinated movements may be seen with patients who have cerebellar dysfunction.

Ventricular peritoneal shunt

Increased ICP caused by excess cerebrospinal fluid (CSF) in the ventricles can occur if the shunt becomes dislodged, infected, or blocked.

Infections

Suspect meningitis or a brain abscess with patients who have a recent history of infection involving the ears, sinuses, or respiratory tract.

Medications

Determine the current medications the patient is using. Ask about the patient's compliance with antihypertensives or anticonvulsants. Suspect ischemic stroke if the patient is noncompliant with antihypertensives. Suspect status epilepticus if the patient is noncompliant with anticonvulsant medications.

Vital Signs

- *Bradycardia* is a late finding of increased ICP. Bradycardia related to unopposed parasympathetic nervous system stimulation occurs in cases of spinal shock.
- *Hypertension* is a late finding of increased ICP. As ICP rises, the blood pressure rises reflexively to maintain cerebral blood flow.
- *Hypotension* is a symptom of spinal shock. A loss of vasomotor tone below the level of the injury causes vasodilation.
- *Respirations:* Respiratory irregularities are a late sign of increased ICP. An abnormal respiratory rate and pattern indicates impending herniation of the respiratory centers located in the brainstem.
- *Fever* is a symptom associated with lesions of the hypothalamus, increased ICP affecting the hypothalamus, central nervous system infections (meningitis or encephalitis), or status epilepticus.
- *Hypothermia* may occur in cases of spinal shock because of vasodilation and a loss of the ability to shiver below the level of the injury.

General Observations

- **Pupil size and reaction:** See Focused Nursing Assessment.
- **Gait:** A staggered gait, uncoordinated movements, and ataxia are often indicative of cerebellar lesions.
- **Speech:** Slurred speech or difficulty expressing thoughts may indicate an impairment of the Broca's area in the frontal lobe.
- **Eye movements:** Abnormal movements often occur with seizure activity.
- **Ecchymosis:** Ecchymosis around the eyes or behind the ear may be seen in some patients with a basilar skull fracture.
- **Drainage:** Basal skull fractures can transverse the paranasal air sinuses of the frontal bone or the middle ear within the temporal bone, resulting in a dural tear.

CSF can leak through the dural tear and drain from an ear or the nose.

FOCUSED NURSING ASSESSMENT

Nursing assessment should focus on perfusion, ventilation, mobility, and sensation.

Perfusion
Level of consciousness

The level of consciousness (LOC) is the most important factor in the neurologic assessment. The Glasgow Coma Scale is a tool that allows objective measurement of the LOC. There are three categories to be assessed—best eye opening, best motor response, and best verbal response. The range of possible scores is from 3 to 15. A score of 15 indicates a fully alert and oriented person. A score of three indicates a deep coma. Table 14-1 describes the three categories, possible findings in each category, and the scores.

NURSING ALERT

Inform the physician immediately if there is a decrease in the score on the Glasgow Coma Scale. This may indicate an increase in ICP.

Pupils

Assess pupil size and reactivity to light. The millimeter scale is frequently used to record pupil size (Figure 14-1).

When light is shone into the eye, the pupil should immediately constrict. The terms used to describe the pupillary reaction include brisk, sluggish, nonreactive, or fixed.

Pupils are normally equal. The "Common Abnormal Pupillary Responses" box describes various pupil findings and their significance.

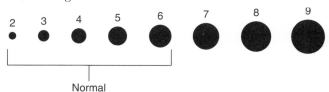

Figure 14-1   Pupil gauge in millimeters. (From Stillwell SB: *Mosby's critical care nursing reference,* ed 2, St Louis, 1996, Mosby.)

Text continued on p. 490

TABLE 14-1 Glasgow Coma Scale

Category	Response	Description and technique	Score
Best eye response	Opens eyes spontaneously	Opens eyes without verbal or tactile stimuli	4
	Opens eyes to verbal stimuli	Opens eyes on command or when called by name	3
	Opens eyes to painful stimuli	Start with a normal tone of voice and increase the loudness as necessary	2
		Squeeze the trapezius muscle, or squeeze the inner aspect of the arm or thigh; do not rub the sternum with your knuckle, since the skin in this area is thin and fragile and bruises easily (especially in a geriatric patient); avoid twisting or pinching the nipples; do not apply pressure to the supraorbital area in head-injured patients. NOTE: These techniques to elicit pain also apply to the motor and verbal categories.	
	No eye opening	Does not open eyes to painful stimuli	1
Best motor response	Obeys simple commands	Raises arms or holds up specific number of fingers on request	6
		Do not ask patients to grasp hand; hand grasp may be a reflexive response	
	Localizes pain	Cannot follow commands but locates the painful stimulus and attempts to remove it with hand	5

	Withdraws from pain	Does not actually locate the source of pain with a hand but does withdraw from the pain; for example, may flex arm to withdraw from the painful stimulus of a pinch	4
	Abnormal flexion (to noxious or painful stimuli)	Adducts shoulders, flexes and pronates arms, flexes wrist, and makes a fist (decorticate posturing)	3
	Abnormal extension (to noxious or painful stimuli)	Adducts and internally rotates shoulders, extends forearm, and flexes wrist (decerebrate posturing)	2
	No motor response	Flaccid	1
Best verbal response	Oriented	No response to maximally applied painful stimuli Able to converse and oriented to person, place, and time	5
	Confused	Able to converse but is not fully oriented or demonstrates confusion	4
	Inappropriate words	Words are recognizable but make little or no sense; words verbalized in a disorganized manner	3
	Incomprehensible words	Words are not recognizable—moans, groans	2
	None	Does not make any sound in response to pain	1

N

COMMON ABNORMAL PUPILLARY RESPONSES

Oculomotor nerve compression

Observation

One pupil (R) is larger than the other (L), which is of normal size. The dilated pupil (R) does not react to light, although the other (L) pupil reacts normally.

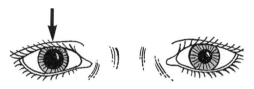

Meaning

A dilated, nonreactive (fixed) pupil indicates that the controls for pupillary constriction are not functioning. The parasympathetic fibers of the oculomotor nerve control pupillary constriction. The most common cause of interruption of this function is compression of the oculomotor nerve, usually against the tentorium or posterior cerebral artery. The compression of the oculomotor nerve against these structures is caused by a lesion, such as a hematoma, tumor, or cerebral edema, on the same side of the brain as the dilated pupil. This causes downward pressure so that the uncus of the temporal lobe herniates, trapping the oculomotor nerve between it and the tentorium.

Action

The nurse will need to check previous assessments to determine what the pupil size and reaction to light have been in the past. If the dilated pupil is a new finding, it should immediately be reported to the physician because the process of rostral-caudal downward pressure must be treated without delay. Changes can also be expected in the level of consciousness, motor function, and other parameters of the neurologic assessment.

From Hickey JV: *The clinical practice of neurological and neurosurgical nursing,* Philadelphia, 1992, JB Lippincott.

COMMON ABNORMAL
PUPILLARY RESPONSES—cont'd

Bilateral diencephalic damage

Observation

Upon examination the pupils appear small but equal in size, and both react briskly to direct light, contracting when light is introduced and dilating when light is withdrawn.

Meaning

The sympathetic pathway that begins in the hypothalamus is affected. Because both pupils are equal in size and respond equally to light, the damage is bilateral. Therefore it can be assumed that there is bilateral injury in the diencephalon (thalamus and hypothalamus).

Because metabolic coma can also cause bilaterally small pupils that react to light, this diagnostic possibility must be ruled out.

Action

The findings should be compared to previous assessments to determine whether this is a new development. The possibility of metabolic coma should be considered by reviewing blood electrolyte and blood glucose levels. For example, diabetic acidosis may cause a metabolic coma because of an excessive amount of glucose in the blood. The abnormal glucose level would be evident upon checking.

A review of blood chemistry values is particularly important if the patient was a recent emergency admission, for whom an adequate history may not have been collected. If the small, reactive pupils are a new finding, this information should be reported.

N

Continued

COMMON ABNORMAL
PUPILLARY RESPONSES—cont'd

Horner's syndrome

Observation

One pupil (L) is smaller than the other (R), although both pupils react to light. The eyelid on the same side as the small pupil droops (ptosis). There may be a sweating deficiency (anhidrosis) on the same side of the face as the ptosis. The collective symptoms of a small reactive pupil, ptosis, and anhidrosis are called Horner's syndrome.

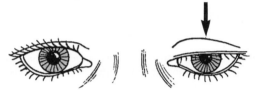

Meaning

An interruption of the ipsilateral sympathetic innervation to the pupil can be caused by hypothalamic damage (posterior or ventrolateral portion), a lesion involving the lateral medulla or the ventrolateral cervical spinal cord, and sometimes occlusion of the internal carotid artery. Downward displacement of the hypothalamus along with a unilateral Horner's syndrome may be an early sign of transtentorial herniation.

Action

If this is a new finding, it should be reported.

Midbrain damage

Observation

Both pupils are at midposition and are nonreactive to light.

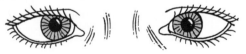

From Hickey JV: *The clinical practice of neurological and neurosurgical nursing,* Philadelphia, 1992, JB Lippincott.

COMMON ABNORMAL
PUPILLARY RESPONSES—cont'd

Meaning

When the pupils are midposition in size and nonreactive, neither the sympathetic nor parasympathetic innervation is operational. This finding is often associated with midbrain infarction or transtentorial herniation.

Action

The pupils should be evaluated in conjunction with other neurologic assessments. The change in pupil size and reaction should be reported if this represents a new finding.

Pontine damage
Observation

Very small (pinpoint), nonreactive pupils are seen.

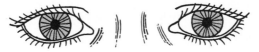

Meaning

Most often, this finding indicates hemorrhage into the pons, a grave occurrence because the pons controls many motor pathways and vital functions. Bilateral pinpoint pupils may also occur with opiate drug overdose, so this possibility should be ruled out.

Action

Report this finding if it is new. The prognosis for patients with pontine damage is grave. Other changes in neurologic status, such as a decreased LOC and respiratory abnormalities, would also be expected.

N

Continued

COMMON ABNORMAL PUPILLARY RESPONSES—cont'd

Dilated unreactive pupils

Observation

Both pupils are dilated and nonreactive (fixed).

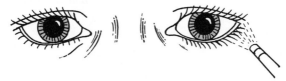

Meaning

This finding is characteristic of the terminal stages of severe anoxia, ischemia, and death. Since atropine-like drugs cause dilated pupils, this possibility must be ruled out. An intact ciliospinal reflex can produce momentary bilateral dilation.

Action

Emergency action is necessary to reverse the anoxic state and prevent death. Oxygen therapy at high concentrations and a patent airway must be ensured to provide oxygen for the ischemic cerebral cells.

From Hickey JV: *The clinical practice of neurological and neurosurgical nursing*, Philadelphia, 1992, JB Lippincott.

Respirations

Assess respiratory rate, depth, and rhythm. Abnormal respiratory patterns are frequently seen with lesions involving the pons and midbrain (respiratory centers of the brain).

Cheyne-Stokes: Rhythmic waxing and waning in the depth and rate of the respirations are followed by apnea. Lesions are often bilateral and involve the basal ganglia, thalamus, or hypothalamus.

Central neurogenic hyperventilation: Respirations are increased in depth and rate. Lesions are usually in the midbrain or upper pons.

Apneustic breathing: The patient pauses 2 to 3 seconds after a full or prolonged inspiration. The lesion is located in the lower pons.

Cluster breathing: There are clusters of irregular breaths with periods of apnea at irregular intervals. The lesion is located in the lower pons or upper medulla.

Biot's (ataxic) breathing: There is a completely irregular, unpredictable pattern with deep and shallow random breaths and pauses. The lesion is located in the medulla.

Circulation

Note the rate and quality of the pulses. Bradycardia can be seen in cases of spinal shock. Atrial and ventricular arrhythmias can occur with patients who have a subarachnoid hemorrhage.[1] Obtain a blood pressure (BP). Hypotension is seen in cases of spinal shock.

Ventilation

Assess breath sounds for crackles and wheezes. Decreased breath sounds may indicate hypoventilation.

Assess chest and abdominal movement. Respiratory assessment is extremely important for patients with cervical spine injuries. An injury at C4 or above will impair phrenic nerve innervation and will result in paralysis of the diaphragm. In these cases, air movement will be inadequate and mechanical ventilation will be necessary. Injuries involving T1 to T6 spare the diaphragm but impair the intercostal muscles, placing the patient at increased risk for respiratory problems. Injuries involving T6 to T12 may impair the abdominal muscles and decrease the ability to generate a cough.

N

Mobility

Assess motor ability and strength. The motor assessment usually focuses on the arms and legs. The identification of changes is important for noting deterioration, improvement, or stabilization in the patient's condition. Always compare motor strength on one side with strength on the other. To assess the upper extremities, extend the middle and index finger of your hands and ask the patient to squeeze with his or her hands. The grasps should be strong and equal. Next, have the patient attempt to move his or her shoulders, forearms, and wrists against resistance. To assess strength in the patient's lower extremities, have the patient flex and extend the upper leg, knee, and ankle on each side against gravity and against resistance. Instruct the patient to press his or her feet against your hands. The fol-

TABLE 14-2 Motor Assessment of the
Corticospinal Tract

Spinal level	Motor assessment
C5	Shoulder abduction
C5-6	Elbow flexion
C7	Finger and elbow extension
C6-7	Wrist dorsiflexion
C8	Thumb-finger pinch
L2-4	Hip flexion
L5-S1	Knee flexion
L2-4	Knee extension
L5	Foot dorsiflexion
S1	Foot plantar flexion

lowing scale can be used to measure motor strength and
movement:

0 = None	3 = Against gravity
1 = Trace	4 = Against some resistance
2 = Not against gravity	5 = Against strong resistance

For spinal cord injury (SCI) patients, the motor assessment
helps identify the level of injury and assess the function of
the corticospinal tract within the cord. Table 14-2 indicates
the level of the spinal cord and associated muscle function.

Sensation

Assessing the sensory function is helpful in identifying the
level of involvement for SCI patients. Starting at the feet
and systematically working upward and comparing both
sides, determine the patient's ability to detect light touch
and pain (pinprick). Ask the patient to tell you when the
sensation is felt. Record the highest level of function on
each side of the body. Figure 14-2 indicates the area of sensation with the level of the cord.

Risk Factors

1. TIAs, hypertension, hypercholesteremia, hypertriglyc-
   eridemia, diabetes mellitus, cigarette smoking, and alcoholism are all considered risk factors for strokes.

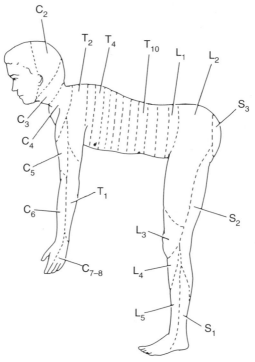

Figure 14-2 Arrangement of dermatomes is more easily understood when an individual is considered in quadruped (crouched) position. It is important to correlate the level of injury with the area of the body surface that is affected (dermatome). (Adapted from Zejdlik CP: *Management of spinal cord injury,* Boston, 1992, Jones & Bartlett.)

2. A history of atrial fibrillation increases the risk of cerebral emboli.
3. Medications such as anticoagulants and oral contraceptives place the patient at increased risk for strokes and epidural and subdural hematomas.
4. Driving while under the influence of alcohol or drugs increases the risk of motor vehicle crashes. Motor vehicle crashes are the most frequent cause of head injuries and SCIs.

Life Span Issues

1. Brain injury occurs most often among the 15- to 30-year-old age group. Males are affected more often than females.[2]
2. Home falls contribute significantly to the incidence of head trauma, particularly among the geriatric population.
3. Sixty percent of SCIs occur with persons 16 to 30 years of age. The majority of those affected are males.

INITIAL INTERVENTIONS

1. Maintenance of a patent airway is the highest priority. Assume that the head-injured patient has a cervical spine injury. Open the airway with techniques that require no movement of the head. Such techniques include the jaw thrust maneuver, nasotracheal intubation, or placement of an oral or nasopharyngeal airway. A cricothyrotomy may be necessary if attempts at nasotracheal intubation fail.

NURSING ALERT

Any patient with an altered level of consciousness needs to be monitored carefully for airway compromise.

2. Support breathing with 100% oxygen per bag-valve mask device if the patient is hypoventilating or apneic. For patients not requiring intubation, 100% oxygen per nonrebreather mask should be used.
3. Maintain the patient in spinal immobilization until a spinal cord injury has been ruled out by a physician. Patients should not be left on backboards for long periods of time. This promotes decubitus formation.
4. Have suction available at all times.
5. Insert two large-bore IVs.
6. Anticipate the need for the insertion of a ventricular drainage catheter for patients with signs and symptoms of increased ICP. The signs and symptoms of increased ICP include a decreased LOC, pupil changes, weakness, nausea, vomiting, headache, seizures, and an abnormal respiratory pattern.
7. Anticipate the need for cervical traction for patients with a cervical fracture.

8. Anticipate the need for a computed tomography (CT) scan. Notify the CT scan technician.

NURSING ALERT

Complete spinal immobilization requires a rigid cervical collar of appropriate size, head immobilization devices, tape or straps across the forehead, straps across the shoulders, hips, and above the knees if the patient is on a backboard, and in-line spinal alignment.

PRIORITY NURSING DIAGNOSES

Risk for ineffective airway clearance
Risk for ineffective breathing pattern
Risk for altered cerebral tissue perfusion
Risk for injury
Risk for altered tissue perfusion: peripheral, renal

◆ **Ineffective airway clearance** related to a decreased LOC and seizure activity:
   INTERVENTIONS
   • Maintain a patent airway (jaw thrust, oral airway, nasopharyngeal airway, or intubation).
   • Provide suction for the patient as needed.

◆ **Ineffective breathing pattern** related to increased ICP affecting the respiratory centers of the brain and to SCI with impairment of the diaphragm or intercostal muscles:
   INTERVENTIONS
   • Administer 100% oxygen.
   • Assist breathing with a bag-valve mask device as needed.
   • Prepare to assist with intubation if the patient is hypoventilating or is in respiratory distress.

◆ **Altered cerebral tissue perfusion** related to increased ICP:
   INTERVENTIONS
   • Maintain P_{CO_2} at 30 to 35 mm Hg.[1,3]
   • Anticipate the need to insert a ventricular drainage catheter.
   • Closely monitor the patient's score on the Glasgow Coma Scale.

◆ **Risk for injury** related to cerebral edema, seizure activity, and noncompliance with anticonvulsants:

N

INTERVENTIONS
- Pad the side rails of the bed.
- Have suction and oxygen available at all times.
- Administer anticonvulsants as ordered by the physician.

◆ **Altered tissue perfusion: peripheral, renal** related to hypotension associated with spinal shock:

INTERVENTIONS
- Insert two large-bore IVs.
- Administer fluid boluses and vasopressors as ordered by the physician.

PRIORITY DIAGNOSTIC TESTS

Laboratory Tests

ABG: A P_{CO_2} of 30 to 35 mm Hg should be maintained. Reducing the P_{CO_2} results in vasoconstriction of the cerebral vessels, which reduces cerebral blood volume and ICP.

Complete blood count: Expect an increase in the white blood cell count with central nervous system (CNS) infections such as meningitis.

Electrolyte levels: Mannitol (Table 14-3) can cause electrolyte imbalances (especially hypokalemia). Vomiting can cause hypokalemia and other electrolyte imbalances.

Type and crossmatch: This is necessary if the patient has other system involvement such as chest or pelvic injuries. Patients do not become hypovolemic from a closed-head injury.

Blood alcohol level: A high serum alcohol level may alter the LOC and decrease the patient's ability to cooperate with the examination and treatment.

Urine and serum drug screen: Many drugs can alter the LOC and pupil size.

Cerebrospinal fluid (CSF): CSF may be obtained via a lumbar puncture or intraventricular catheter (IVC) to assess color, white blood cell count, protein content, glucose content, and culture and sensitivity.
- The presence of more than 5 to 10 white blood cells/mm³ indicates an inflammatory process such as meningitis. Cloudy fluid indicates infection.
- Normally, CSF glucose is approximately 80% of the blood glucose. A decreased CSF glucose level is suggestive of bacterial meningitis.
- The normal protein count is 15 to 45 mg/100 ml. The

TABLE 14-3 Drug Summary

Drug	Dose and route	Special considerations
Cefotaxime (third-generation cephalosporin)	150-200 mg/kg in 4 divided doses or 1-2 g every 6 hr, not to exceed 12 g daily *Pediatric:* 50-180 mg/kg/day in 4-6 divided doses; dilute 50-100 mg/ml and administer IVPB over 15-30 min	Lower dose may be needed for renal impaired patients
Ceftriaxone (cephalosporin)	4 g in 2 divided doses; total daily dose should not exceed 4 g *Pediatric:* 50-100 mg/kg in 2 divided doses; administer IVPB	—
Diazepam (benzodiazepine)	5-10 mg, may be repeated every 5-10 min *Pediatric:* 0.1-0.3 mg/kg slow IV push 5 mg/min	Antagonist is Romazicon Monitor for respiratory depression
Furosemide (diuretic)	20-40 mg IV push over 1-2 min	Frequent administration may cause dehydration
Hydralazine (antihypertensive)	10-20 mg slow IV push at a rate of 10 mg/min	Continuously monitor BP

IVP, IV push; *IVPB,* IV piggyback.

Continued

TABLE 14-3 Drug Summary—cont'd

Drug	Dose and route	Special considerations
Lorazepam (benzodiazepine)	2-4 mg IV push; rate should not exceed 2 mg/min	Romazicon is antagonist
Mannitol 20% (osmotic diuretic)	0.25 to 1 g/kg over 15-30 min IVPB	Must be given in a line with a filter Monitor for potential dehydration and increased serum osmolarity
Methylprednisolone (steroid)	For SCI patients: 30 mg/kg loading dose followed by 5.4 mg/kg every hr for the next 23 hr Loading dose is IVP Hourly infusion on pump	Must be given within 8 hr of the injury
Nitroprusside (vasodilator)	50 mg in 250 ml of 5% dextrose in water for concentration of 200 µg/ml Start infusion of 0.5 µg/kg/min; titrate to desired BP; maximum infusion rate is 10 µg/kg/min; must be given with a continuous infusion pump	IV bag must be wrapped with an opaque material or aluminum foil to protect it from light
Penicillin G	20-24 million U in 6 divided doses Administer IVPB over 30 min	—
Phenobarbital (anticonvulsant)	Pediatric: 20 mg/kg IV Do not exceed 50 mg/min	Monitor for respiratory depression and hypotension
Phenytoin (anticonvulsant)	15-18 mg/kg 50 mg/min or slower by IV infusion*	Rapid infusion can precipitate cardiac arrhythmias and hypotension Must be given in IV solution of normal saline

*From Gahart BL: *Intravenous medications*, St Louis, 1994, Mosby.

protein count may be elevated with tumors, viral meningitis, and hemorrhage.
- A culture can be obtained to identify the invading organism. Sensitivity can also be determined to identify the most effective drug therapy.

Radiographic Tests

Spine films: Cervical, thoracic, lumbar, and sacral views may be ordered to determine the presence of fractures and dislocations. C7 to T1 is often difficult to visualize in obese or heavily muscled patients. It may be necessary to pull the shoulders downward toward the feet while the x-ray examination is being conducted. The swimmer's view (one arm above the head) can also be helpful in visualizing the cervical spine. An open-mouth view can be used to visualize the odontoid process. The odontoid process is an upward extension of the body of C2.

Skull films: Skull films are used to rule out skull fractures. The films include anteroposterior and lateral views.

CT scan: The CT scan is extremely useful in locating and diagnosing various cranial lesions such as abscesses, cysts, infarctions, hematomas, and tumors. IV radiopaque material (contrast) may be given to improve the clarity of images.

MRI: The MRI is efficient in identifying cerebral and spinal cord edema, CNS ischemia or infarcted areas, hemorrhage, and tumors in the brainstem, basal skull, and spinal cord.

COLLABORATIVE INTERVENTIONS

Overview

Increased intracranial pressure

There are three main components (volumes) creating ICP—brain tissue, blood volume, and CSF. Brain tissue constitutes 80% of the volume, whereas blood and CSF account for 10% each. An increase in one volume (e.g., edema or hyperemia) may increase ICP unless it is accompanied by an equal decrease in one or more of the other components. The body is able to compensate for mild to moderate ICP elevations (increased intracranial volume) by increased absorption of CSF and shunting cerebral blood volume. Rapid or significant elevations in ICP are not tolerated well and may result in herniation—a terminal event.

Brain tissue volume can be increased by cerebral edema, intracranial blood, tumors, and abscesses. Blood volume can be increased by hypercapnia and hyperthermia. Overproduction or decreased absorption of CSF can result in hydrocephalus. Conditions associated with hydrocephalus are tumors, subarachnoid hemorrhage, meningitis, and Guillain-Barré syndrome.

Normal ICP is 0 to 14 mm Hg.

NURSING ALERT

Early recognition of elevated ICP accompanied by measures to maintain cerebral perfusion is important to maintaining brain function.

SYMPTOMS

Symptoms vary with the magnitude of the insult, the time over which the insult occurs, and the effectiveness of compensatory mechanisms.

Early symptoms of increased ICP may include the following:
- Headache
- Nausea and vomiting
- Muscle weakness
- Hemiplegia
- Hemiparesis

As cerebral perfusion is further compromised, symptoms will include the following:
- A decrease in the LOC (Table 14-1)
- Seizures
- Pupillary changes (see "Common Abnormal Pupillary Responses" box)

Severe increases in ICP cause the following results:
- Profoundly abnormal motor response (flexing, extending, or absent)
- Changes in respiratory rate and depth
- Hypertension
- Hyperthermia
- Bradycardia

Loss of brainstem reflexes occurs, including the corneal, oculocephalic, and oculovestibular reflexes. The physician assesses the oculocephalic reflex (doll's eyes phenomenon) by rotating the head while holding the eyelids open. The reflex is intact if the eyes move in the opposite direction of the head. The oculovestibular reflex is assessed by injecting cold water into the external auditory canal. If the reflex is intact, the eyes will move toward the side being irrigated. This examination should be performed by the physician and not by the nurse.

DIAGNOSIS

- The preferred method for monitoring ICP is through an IVC (see Procedure 21). The catheter affords the opportunity to drain CSF if necessary to maintain an appropriate ICP and facilitate cerebral perfusion pressure (CPP) management.
- The CPP may also be calculated and monitored if an IVC has been inserted. The CPP is an indirect measurement of cerebral blood flow and is determined by subtracting the ICP from the mean arterial pressure (MAP) (CPP = MAP − ICP). Normal CPP is 60 to 100 mm Hg. A CPP of 70 mm Hg is generally the therapeutic goal.

TREATMENT

General treatment principles include the following:

- Maintain the head in a neutral position to facilitate venous outflow.
- Avoid extreme hip and knee flexion. This can increase intraabdominal and intrathoracic pressures.
- Use the logroll technique to position the patient.
- Suction the endotracheal tube for no longer than 10 to 15 seconds at a time. The number of suction passes should be limited to a maximum of two during any one suction episode.[4]
- The position of the head of the bed is controversial. The head of the bed should be positioned based on the individual's ICP and CPP.[5] If a spinal injury has been ruled out, elevating the head of the bed 30 to 45 degrees may facilitate venous outflow.
- Decrease loud stimuli and bright lights.

TREATMENT OF MILD HEAD INJURY (GCS SCORE 14-15)

- Perform an ongoing neurologic evaluation.
- The patient may be discharged or admitted.

TREATMENT OF MODERATE HEAD INJURY (GCS SCORE 9-13)

- Perform a neurosurgical evaluation.
- Perform an ongoing neurologic evaluation.
- Obtain a CT examination of the head.

- Be prepared to intubate should neurologic status deteriorate.
- Prepare the patient for admission or transfer.

TREATMENT OF SEVERE HEAD INJURY (GCS SCORE ≤8)[3,6]

- Perform an endotracheal intubation (consider rapid sequence induction protocol—see Procedure 15).
- Obtain a neurosurgical consult.
- Obtain a CT examination of the head.
- Maintain adequate oxygen saturation (≥95%).
- Maintain an adequate MAP (≥90 mm Hg).
- Maintain adequate CPP as prescribed (usually 70 mm Hg in adults and 50 mm Hg in children).
- Control ventilations to maintain adequate oxygenation and a $PaCO_2$ of 30 to 35 mm Hg.
- Prophylactic use of hyperventilation should be avoided. Hyperventilation may be used acutely if signs of impending herniation are present. Other measures to improve cerebral perfusion (adequate oxygenation and adequate MAP) should accompany hyperventilation efforts. If hyperventilation is used, it should be short term only.
- Administer osmotic diuretic (mannitol) as an IV bolus (0.25 to 1.0 g/kg).
- Perform gastric decompression (oral or nasal gastric tube).
- Place an indwelling urinary catheter.
- Perform a ongoing neurologic evaluation.
- Prepare the patient for admission or transfer.
- Prepare for placement of an IVC to monitor ICP and CPP and to drain CSF.
- Sedate the patient as prescribed by the physician. Monitor BP closely because many sedatives may cause hypotension.
- The use of steroids has not proved beneficial in clinical studies, and their administration is not recommended.

Clinical Conditions
Herniation syndrome
Herniation is the protrusion of brain tissue outside of its normal compartment.[7]

SYMPTOMS

- See Table 14-4.

TABLE 14-4 Herniation Syndrome

Type of herniation	Description	Symptoms
Supratentorial cingulate herniation	An expanding lesion in one cerebral hemisphere causes pressure medially, forcing the cingulate gyrus under the falx cerebri; displacement of the falx compresses the internal cerebral vein; if untreated, can lead to central or uncal herniation	Changes in mental status and level of consciousness A midline shift may be present on the CT scan
Central (transtentorial) herniation	Downward displacement of the cerebral hemispheres, basal ganglia, diencephalon, and midbrain through the tentorial notch	Early signs: decreased level of consciousness, small but reactive pupils, Cheyne-Stokes respirations, increased motor spasticity; hemiparesis Late signs: decorticate or decerebrate posturing, pupils progress from unequal and nonreactive to dilated and fixed

Continued

TABLE 14-4 Herniation Syndrome—cont'd

Type of herniation	Description	Symptoms
Uncal (lateral transtentorial) herniation	A large lateral lesion at the middle fossa causes lateral displacement of the medial portion of the temporal lobe through the tentorial notch	Early signs: Ipsilateral dilated pupil from pressure on the oculomotor nerve, contralateral hemiplegia, or hemiparesis, decreased level of consciousness, respiratory changes Late signs: Unconsciousness, bilateral fixed dilated pupils, decorticate or decerebrate posturing, absence of oculocephalic and oculovestibular reflexes
Subtentorial herniation	Can occur by either upward displacement of the cerebellum through the tentorial notch or downward movement of brain tissue (brainstem or cerebellar tonsils) through the foramen magnum	Abnormal respiratory patterns and pupillary changes depending on area involved, coma, hemiparesis, hemiplegia, and decorticate or decerebrate posturing

DIAGNOSIS
- Diagnosis is based on symptoms and the results of a CT scan.

TREATMENT
- Treatment is the same as for increased ICP. Specific treatment is based on the location and cause of the increased ICP.

Seizures

Seizures are produced by intermittent, sudden, massive neuronal discharge (electrical activity) in various parts of the brain. The clinical manifestations depend on the type.

Generalized tonic-clonic (grand mal):

SYMPTOMS
- A generalized tonic-clonic (grand mal) seizure is manifested by a sudden loss of consciousness with rigidity of the trunk and extremities, followed by a clonic phase with violent rhythmic muscular contractions. Apnea and cyanosis frequently occur. The seizure lasts approximately 2 to 5 minutes. Afterward, the patient may experience a headache, confusion, weakness, and motor or sensory deficits. These symptoms persist for minutes to hours.

DIAGNOSIS
- Diagnosis is based on history (tonic-clonic seizures may occur with tumors, head injuries, overdoses, infections, electrolyte imbalances, ventriculoperitoneal shunt malfunction, febrile illness with children, subtherapeutic anticonvulsant levels, or hypoxic events) and symptoms.
- Carefully observe and record the activity associated with the seizure.

TREATMENT
- Turn the patient to the side to facilitate drainage of secretions.
- If the cause of the seizure is unknown, administer Narcan as ordered. Dextrose 50% (dextrose 25% for children) may be administered if a finger-stick blood glucose test reveals hypoglycemia.
- Pad side rails to prevent injury. Keep the bed in a low position.
- Establish IV access for medication administration.
- Administer anticonvulsants such as diazepam, lorazepam, and phenytoin as ordered. Phenobarbital is frequently used for children (Table 14-3).

- Administer acetaminophen 10 to 15 mg/kg for the febrile child.

Status epilepticus

Status epilepticus is defined as continuous seizures or seizures that occur at a frequency that prevents the patient from fully recovering from one seizure before having another.

DIAGNOSIS

- Diagnosis is based on history and examination.
- Common causes include the sudden withdrawal of anticonvulsants, subtherapeutic levels of anticonvulsants, meningitis, encephalitis, hypoxia, or withdrawal from alcohol.

TREATMENT

- The treatment is the same as for generalized tonic-clonic seizures.

Petit mal seizures

Petit mal seizures generally occur with children who are between 4 and 12 years of age. There is an abrupt cessation of activity and a glassy stare (the child may stare straight ahead for 5 to 30 seconds). The child resumes activity after the seizure.

DIAGNOSIS

- Diagnosis is based on history and symptoms.

TREATMENT

- Administer anticonvulsant medication as prescribed by a physician.

Focal (jacksonian) seizures

Focal (jacksonian) seizures begin with slow, repetitive jerking of a body part that increases in strength and rate over a period of 5 to 15 seconds.[8]

DIAGNOSIS

- Diagnosis is based on history and symptoms.

TREATMENT

- Protect the patient from injury.
- Anticipate the need for anticonvulsants.

Central nervous system infections

Meningitis

Meningitis is an inflammation of the meninges (coverings of the brain and spinal cord) as a result of viral or bacterial invasion.

SYMPTOMS

- Symptoms may include fever, a severe headache, changes in the LOC, stiff neck, photophobia, seizure activity, in-

creased ICP (because of cerebral exudate, cerebral edema, and hydrocephalus), and petechiae (seen in meningococcal meningitis).
- Infants may have bulging fontanels, irritability, temperature instability, and poor feeding.
- Geriatric patients may experience only low-grade fever and confusion.[9]

DIAGNOSIS
- Diagnosis is based on history (a recent history of head trauma, ear infections, sinus infection, or respiratory illness), symptoms, and CSF analysis.

TREATMENT
- Maintain the ABCs.
- Initiate IV antibiotic therapy as soon as possible. Antibiotics used for bacterial meningitis may include penicillin, cefotaxime, or ceftriaxone. Ampicillin may be used for infants and children.
- Decrease stimuli such as noise and lights.
- Initiate seizure precautions.
- Administer antipyretics and analgesics.

Encephalitis

Encephalitis is an inflammation of the brain caused by viruses, bacteria, or parasites. Viruses are the most common cause.

SYMPTOMS
- Symptoms may include a fever, a headache, a stiff neck, changes in the LOC, hemiparesis, facial weakness, ataxia, nystagmus, and generalized seizures.

DIAGNOSIS
- Diagnosis is based on symptoms and CSF analysis.

TREATMENT
- Decrease stimuli such as noise and lights.
- Administer analgesics and antipyretics.
- Initiate seizure precautions.
- Treat any increased ICP.
- There is no definitive drug treatment for viral encephalitis. Steroids may decrease cerebral edema. Prophylactic anticonvulsants are frequently used to prevent seizures.

Head injuries
Concussion

Concussion is a transient, temporary loss of consciousness caused by mechanical force to the brain. Consciousness returns within minutes after the impact.[10]

SYMPTOMS
- The patient experiences a temporary loss of consciousness.
- Other symptoms may include amnesia, a headache, dizziness, drowsiness, irritability, and visual disturbances. These symptoms may last several minutes to days.

DIAGNOSIS
- Diagnosis is based on history and symptoms.
- The result of a CT scan will be normal.

TREATMENT
- Monitor the patient for changes in neurologic status.
- Administer nonnarcotic analgesics for any headache.
- Give head injury instructions if the patient is discharged from the ED (see Procedure 20).

Contusion

A contusion is a bruising of the brain. Edema of brain tissue is a concern.

SYMPTOMS
- Symptoms are related to the amount of bruising and swelling and to the area involved.
- Symptoms may include an altered LOC, a headache, nausea, vomiting, visual disturbances, seizures, and hemiparesis.

DIAGNOSIS
- Diagnosis is based on a history of head trauma and on symptoms and CT scan findings.

TREATMENT
- Treat any increased ICP. Maintain CPP of at least 70 mm Hg.
- Anticipate the need for anticonvulsants.
- Initiate seizure precautions.

Epidural hematoma

An epidural hematoma is caused by bleeding between the skull and dura mater (outer meningeal layer). Many patients have a skull fracture. Often there is a fracture in the temporal bone with a tear in the meningeal artery or vein under the bone.

SYMPTOMS
- Symptoms may include an initial loss of consciousness followed by a lucid interval that lasts a few hours.
- The lucid interval is followed by a rapid deterioration in the LOC. At least 15% of patients do not have a lucid interval.

- A headache, dilated pupil, hemiparesis, and other symptoms of increased ICP may be present.

DIAGNOSIS
- Diagnosis is based on history, symptoms, and CT scan findings.

TREATMENT
- Treat any increased ICP. Maintain CPP of at least 70 mm Hg.
- Prepare the patient for surgical evacuation of the clot.

NURSING ALERT

The ICP can increase quickly to a dangerous level with arterial epidural bleeds. Herniation is a concern. Death may result if surgery is delayed.

Subdural hematoma

A subdural hematoma occurs when blood collects between the dura and arachnoid meningeal layers. The hematoma can develop from the rupture of vessels or from bleeding from contused or lacerated areas. Subdural hematomas are common in the geriatric population. There are three categories—acute, subacute, and chronic.

1. Acute: Associated with major cerebral trauma. Symptoms occur within 48 hours.
2. Subacute: Associated with less severe contusions. Symptoms appear within 2 days to 2 weeks.
3. Chronic: Symptoms occur from 2 weeks to several months. Chronic hematomas are seen in patients who fall frequently because of alcohol abuse.

SYMPTOMS
- Symptoms include a headache (which gradually worsens), drowsiness, confusion, slow thought processes, hemiparesis (late sign), and seizures.

DIAGNOSIS
- Diagnosis is based on history, symptoms, and CT scan findings.

TREATMENT
- Treat any increased ICP.
- Administer nonnarcotic and nonaspirin analgesics.
- Small hematomas rarely require surgery, since they are frequently absorbed.
- Larger hematomas require surgical evacuation.

Diffuse axonal injury

A diffuse axonal injury is a severe injury that involves widespread brain damage. Shearing forces disrupt axons in the cerebral white matter.

SYMPTOMS
- A GCS score of 3 to 5
- Hypertension
- Hyperthermia
- Decerebrate or decorticate posturing

DIAGNOSIS
- Diagnosis is based on CT scan findings and symptoms.

TREATMENT
- Intubate the patient. Maintain adequate oxygenation and ventilation.
- Measures to control ICP and maintain CPP >70 mm Hg.

Basal skull fractures

Basal skull fractures involve the base of the skull. The frontal and temporal bones are frequently affected. The fracture can be linear, comminuted, or depressed. Fractures involving the sinus areas frequently result in CSF leaks.

SYMPTOMS
- Symptoms include drainage from the ears or nose, periorbital ecchymosis (raccoon's eyes), ecchymosis over the mastoid bone (Battle's sign, does not usually develop for 24 hours), subconjunctival hemorrhage, hearing loss, agitation, headache, nausea, and vomiting.

DIAGNOSIS
- Diagnosis is based on history, symptoms, results of a skull x-ray examination, and CT scan findings.
- The halo sign (blood encircled by a yellow stain on bed linens) is highly suggestive of a CSF leak. Most leaks resolve in 2 to 10 days.

TREATMENT
- Anticipate the need for prophylactic antibiotics if there is a CSF leak (prevent meningitis).
- Do not pack the ears or nose.
- Instruct the patient not to blow his or her nose.
- Ensure tetanus and diphtheria prophylaxis.
- Admit the patient for observation.
- Monitor the patient for symptoms of an epidural hematoma if the fracture involves the temporal bone.
- Monitor the patient for increased ICP from a possible underlying tissue injury.

NURSING ALERT

Never insert a nasogastric tube in a patient with head or facial injuries with nasal drainage. The tube may transverse the sinuses and cribriform plate and enter the brain.

Vascular injuries
Hemorrhagic stroke and injury

Subarachnoid hemorrhage is the most common hemorrhagic stroke. This condition, a sudden bleeding into the subarachnoid space, most often results from the rupture of an aneurysm.[6] An aneurysm is an outpouching of the wall of a blood vessel. Other causes include severe brain injury and the rupture of an arteriovenous malformation.

SYMPTOMS
- Symptoms include a sudden and severe headache, a sudden transient loss of consciousness (occurs in 45% of all subarachnoid hemorrhage patients), nausea, vomiting, a stiff neck, photophobia, signs of increased ICP, elevated temperature, and an elevated blood pressure (BP).

DIAGNOSIS
- Diagnosis is based on symptoms and CT scan findings.

TREATMENT
- Treatment is geared toward controlling the BP and ICP to prevent an aneurysmal rebleed until the patient goes to surgery (1 to 3 days after hemorrhage).
- The patient must have bed rest.
- The patient should remain in a quiet environment.
- Maintain systolic BP at no more than 150 mm Hg. Systolic pressures above this level can be treated with hydralazine or nitroprusside (Table 14-4).
- Use anticonvulsants as prophylaxis against seizures.
- Use analgesics to control any headaches.
- Monitor the patient for complications such as diabetes insipidus.
- Treat increased ICP.

Ischemic stroke

Ischemic strokes occur when a blood vessel supplying the brain is occluded. The majority of ischemic strokes are caused by blood clots that develop within the brain artery itself (cerebral thrombosis). Ischemic strokes also occur when clots arise elsewhere in the body and migrate to the brain (embolic stroke). The result is ischemia to the cerebral tissue.

N

CORRELATION OF CEREBRAL ARTERY INVOLVEMENT AND COMMON MANIFESTATIONS

Internal carotid artery

Contralateral paresthesia (abnormal sensations) and hemiparesis (weakness) of arm, face, and leg

Eventually complete contralateral hemiplegia (paralysis) and hemianesthesia (loss of sensation)

Visual blurring or changes, hemianopsia (loss of half of visual field), repeated attacks of blindness in the ipsilateral eye

Dysphasia with dominant hemisphere involvement

Anterior cerebral artery

Mental impairment such as perseveration, confusion, amnesia, and personality changes

Contralateral hemiparesis or hemiplegia with leg loss greater than arm loss

Sensory loss over toes, foot, and leg

Ataxia (motor incoordination), impaired gait, incontinence, and akinetic mutism

Middle cerebral artery

Level of consciousness varies from confusion to coma

Contralateral hemiparesis or hemiplegia with face and arm loss greater than leg loss

---

From Stillwell SB: *Mosby's Critical Care Nursing Reference,* St Louis, 1992, Mosby.

SYMPTOMS
- The box "Correlation of Cerebral Artery Involvement and Common Manifestations" describes the symptoms based on the cerebral artery occluded.

DIAGNOSIS
- Diagnosis is based on history or risk factors for stroke, on symptoms, and on the results of diagnostic procedures, including a CT scan, angiography, and carotid studies.
- The CT scan may be normal initially.

TREATMENT
- Anticoagulant therapy with heparin may be needed to decrease further development of thrombi.
- Treat increased ICP as necessary.

CORRELATION OF CEREBRAL ARTERY INVOLVEMENT AND COMMON MANIFESTATIONS—cont'd

Middle cerebral artery—cont'd

Sensory impairment over same areas of hemiplegia

Aphasia (inability to express or interpret speech) or dysphasia (impaired speech) with dominant hemisphere involvement

Homonymous hemianopsia (loss of vision on the same side of both visual fields) and inability to turn eyes toward the paralyzed side

Posterior cerebral artery

Contralateral hemiplegia with sensory loss

Confusion, memory involvement, and receptive speech deficits with dominant hemisphere involvement

Homonymous hemianopsia

Vertebrobasilar artery

Dizziness, vertigo, nausea, ataxia, and syncope

Visual disturbances, nystagmus, diplopia, field deficits, and blindness

Numbness and paresis (face, tongue, mouth, one or more limbs), dysphagia (inability to swallow), and dysarthria (difficulty in articulation)

N

- Supportive therapy such as supporting flaccid limbs and proper body alignment should be implemented.
- Elevate the head of the bed to facilitate the drainage of oropharyngeal secretions.
- Thrombolytics should be considered for patients who have had symptoms <3 hours. A CT scan of the head should be obtained within 25 minutes of arrival at the ED to rule out hemorrhagic stroke. Hypertension (systolic BP >185 or diastolic BP >110) should be controlled before administration of thrombolytics. One to two inches of nitropaste or one to two doses of 10 to 20 mg of labetalol may reduce the BP. Heparin should not be given before or 24 hours after thrombolytic administration.

Spinal injuries
Cord transection

Complete transection of the spinal cord results in spinal shock with a complete loss of motor, sensory, reflex, and autonomic function below the level of the injury. The severity of spinal shock is influenced by the level of the injury. Injuries above T6 disrupt sympathetic nervous system activity below the level of the injury. Thus there is unopposed parasympathetic nervous system activity. The extent of the loss of function is less with partial cord transections. Varying degrees of spinal shock may be seen with cord injuries from contusions, compression, lacerations, and hemorrhage.

SYMPTOMS

- Loss of sensation below the level of the injury
- Flaccid paralysis below the level of the injury
- Hypotension
- Vasodilation below level of injury
- Bradycardia
- Lack of sweating below the level of injury
- Loss of all spinal reflexes below the level of injury
- Atonic bladder and bowel

TREATMENT

- Maintain spinal immobilization.
- Maintain a patent airway.
- Prepare to intubate patients who have cervical cord injuries above C4.
- Administer 100% oxygen.
- Apply two large-bore IVs with Ringer's lactate or normal saline.
- Maintain systolic BP of at least 80 to 90 mm Hg. Mental status and urine output are useful parameters in evaluating perfusion.
- Administer an IV fluid bolus if BP is <90 mm Hg or inadequate to maintain perfusion.
- Titrate vasopressor agents such as dopamine or dobutamine if IV fluids are not successful in maintaining BP.
- Initiate cardiac monitoring.
- Treat bradycardia with atropine.
- Insert a nasogastric tube to decrease the risk of vomiting and aspiration.
- Insert a urinary catheter to monitor urine output.
- Implement measures to keep the patient warm (vasodila-

tion and a lack of the ability to shiver can decrease body temperature).

- Assist with the application of cervical skeletal traction. A general rule is to use 5 lb of weight for each level of injury beginning with C1 (e.g., a fracture of C3 would require 15 lb of weight). Weights should be free hanging.

Cord syndromes

See Figures 14-3 to 14-5.

DIAGNOSIS

- Diagnosis is based on a history of spinal trauma and on symptoms.

TREATMENT

- Maintain spinal immobilization.
- Administer 100% oxygen.
- Initiate two large-bore IVs.
- Insert a nasogastric tube and urinary catheter.
- Administer IV methylprednisolone (Table 14-4).
- Assist with the application of cervical skeletal traction or the halo immobilization device.

Autonomic hyperreflexia

Autonomic hyperreflexia (also known as autonomic dysreflexia) is a serious hypertensive emergency that arises in the postacute phase of SCI. This occurs once reflex activity has returned in patients who have injuries at or above T6. Autonomic hyperreflexia is caused by noxious stimuli that result in mass reflex stimulation of the sympathetic nerves below the level of the injury. Noxious stimuli are often caused by a distended bladder, constipation, fecal impaction, cystitis, urinary calculi, pressure ulcers, and stimulation from skin lesions. If left untreated, this condition can lead to a CVA, seizure activity, or myocardial infarction.

SYMPTOMS

- Sudden hypertension is a primary symptom; systolic BP as high as 240 to 300 mm Hg; may be significant rise in the patient's BP when compared with usual baseline
- Anxious appearance
- Pounding headache
- Blurred vision
- Flushed face and neck
- Profuse sweating above level of injury
- Nasal congestion
- Nausea

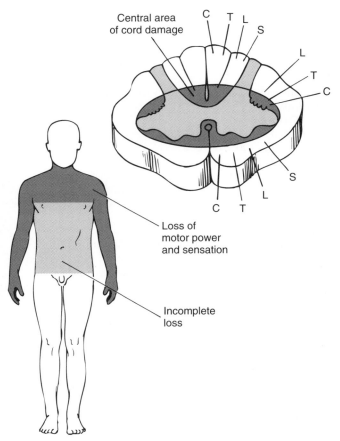

Figure 14-3   Central cord syndrome. A cross section of the cord shows central damage and the associated motor and sensory loss. *C,* Cervical; *T,* thoracic; *L,* lumbar; *S,* sacral. (Modified from Hickey JV: *The clinical practice of neurological and neurosurgical nursing,* Philadelphia, 1992, JB Lippincott.)

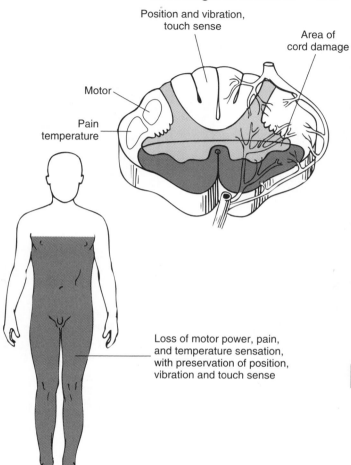

Position and vibration, touch sense

Area of cord damage

Motor

Pain temperature

Loss of motor power, pain, and temperature sensation, with preservation of position, vibration and touch sense

Figure 14-4 Anterior cord syndrome. Cord damage and associated motor and sensory loss. (Modified from Hickey JV: *The clinical practice of neurological and neurosurgical nursing,* Philadelphia, 1992, JB Lippincott.)

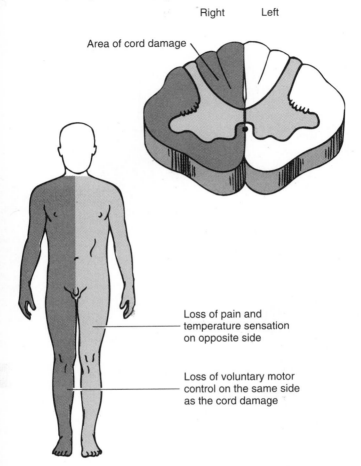

Right   Left

Area of cord damage

Loss of pain and
temperature sensation
on opposite side

Loss of voluntary motor
control on the same side
as the cord damage

Figure 14-5   Brown-Séquard syndrome. Cord damage and associated
motor and sensory loss. (Modified from Hickey JV: *The clinical practice
of neurological and neurosurgical nursing,* Philadelphia, 1992, JB
Lippincott.)

DIAGNOSIS
- Diagnosis is based on a history of previous SCI and on symptoms.

TREATMENT
- Treatment is directed toward removing the noxious stimuli and lowering the BP.
- If a urinary catheter is in place, attempt to irrigate if a plug or obstruction is suspected.
- Replace the catheter if irrigation does not remove the obstruction.
- Other treatment measures that should be considered include digital removal of any fecal impaction and removal of pressure from areas of irritated or broken skin.
- Elevate the head of the bed and administer an antihypertensive as ordered by the physician.

NURSING SURVEILLANCE

1. Monitor the trend of the patient's vital signs.
2. Monitor the trend of the patient's GCS score.
3. Monitor the trend of the patient's pupil size and reactivity to light.
4. Monitor the trend of the patient's ICP and CPP.
5. Monitor the trend of the patient's motor and sensory function.
6. Monitor the trend of the patient's urine output.

EXPECTED PATIENT OUTCOMES

1. Patent airway
2. Bilateral equal breath sounds
3. Systolic BP between 80 and 150 mm Hg or as needed to maintain perfusion
4. Heart rate between 60 and 100 beats/min
5. Equal and reactive pupils
6. No deterioration in the LOC
7. ICP of 0 to 15 mm Hg
8. CPP of 70 to 100 mm Hg
9. Urine output of at least 30 ml/hr
10. Normothermic
11. No seizure activity

DISCHARGE IMPLICATIONS

1. Instruct the patient on the importance of medication (anticonvulsant) compliance.

520   Chapter Fourteen

2. Teach geriatric patients to be aware of fall hazards—
   rugs, slick floors, similarly colored floors and walls (con-
   trasting colors are better), and stairways.
3. Stress the hazards of drinking alcohol before or during
   driving or swimming. Consider implementing injury
   prevention educational programs (for groups at increased risk).
4. Encourage patients to use helmets when participating in
   recreational and sports activities.

Head Injuries
See Procedure 20.

References

1. Bullock R, Chestnut R, Clifton G, et al: Guidelines for the
   management of severe head injury, *Eur J Emerg Med* 3:109-127,
   1996.
2. Olshaker JS, Whye DW: Head trauma, *Emerg Med Clin North
   Am* 11(1):165-181, 1993.
3. Bullock R, Chestnut R, Clifton G, et al: *Guidelines for the management of severe head injury,* New York, 1996, Brain Trauma
   Foundation.
4. Rudy EB, Turner BS, Baun M, et al: Endotracheal suctioning
   in adults with head injury, *Heart Lung* 20(6):667-674, 1991.
5. March K, Mitchell P, Grady S, et al: Effect of bedrest position
   on cerebral perfusion pressure, *J Neurosci Nurs* 22(6):375-381,
   1990.
6. Bullock R, Chestnut R, Clifton G, et al: Guidelines for the
   management of severe head injury, *J Neurotrauma* 13:639-734,
   1996.
7. Marano-Morrison CA: Brain herniation syndromes, *Crit Care
   Nurse* 7(5):35-51, 1987.
8. Hickey JV: *The clinical practice of neurological and neurosurgical
   nursing,* Philadelphia, 1992, JB Lippincott.
9. Nagani PH, Guze PA: Infectious disease emergencies. In
   Saunders CE, Ho MT, editors: *Current emergency diagnosis and
   treatment,* Norwalk, Conn, 1992, Appleton & Lange, pp 614-
   615.
10. Bartkowski HM: Head trauma. In Saunders CE, Ho MT, edi-
    tors: *Current emergency diagnosis and treatment,* Norwalk, Conn,
    1992, Appleton & Lange, pp 239-249.

Chapter 15

Obstetric and Gynecologic Conditions

Pamela S. Kidd

CLINICAL CONDITIONS
Ovarian Cysts
Dysfunctional Uterine Bleeding
Miscarriage
Ectopic Pregnancy
Preterm Labor
Abruptio Placentae
Placenta Previa
Ruptured Uterus
Trauma in Pregnancy
Pregnancy-Related Hypertensive Disorders
Emergency Delivery
Newborn Resuscitation
Postpartum Bleeding

TRIAGE ASSESSMENT

Gynecologic Conditions

Any source of bleeding is potentially life threatening. Many patients come to the triage area with a chief complaint of vaginal bleeding. The clinician should assess to determine if the bleeding is associated with pregnancy, endocrine changes through the menstrual cycle, or a systemic problem such as a hematologic disorder, use of anticoagulants, or traumatic injury.

The following are questions about the nature of vaginal bleeding that help the nurse determine the type of gynecologic problem.

Vaginal bleeding

Ask the patient to compare present vaginal bleeding with normal menstrual flow. The number of pads or tampons used may be an indicator of the amount of bleeding. Determine if the patient has passed any tissue (hamburger-looking substance) or blood clots. Bleeding that is associated with clotting or that lasts longer than 7 days is suggestive of substantial blood loss.[1]

Previous episode

Ask the patient if she has experienced the same symptoms at other times. Bleeding that occurs at regular intervals and is associated with premenstrual symptoms such as breast tenderness and water weight gain is indicative of ovulatory bleeding.

Last menstrual cycle

Ask the patient the date of her last menstrual cycle. Irregular cycles are associated with uterine dysfunction.

Pain

Ask if the patient is experiencing pain. Uterine dysfunction is usually painless, whereas endometriosis is painful.

Contraceptive and sexual activity history

Determine the type of contraceptives used and the patient's sexual history (see Chapter 17). Vaginal bleeding has been associated with the use of intrauterine devices. It may also occur with some sexually transmitted diseases (STDs).

Pregnancy history

Gravida is the number of pregnancies and *para* is the number of live births. Abortions include spontaneous, therapeutic, and elective abortions.

Medication history

Determine what medications the patient is currently using. Anticoagulants, hormonal supplements, and oral contraceptives may induce vaginal bleeding.

Vaginal discharge

Assess the type and amount of vaginal discharge. Determine if this is different from normal vaginal discharge. Vaginal discharge is associated with some STDs.

Obstetric Conditions

If a pregnant patient has suffered a traumatic injury, establish a patent airway, administer oxygen and effective ventilation, support her circulation with IV fluids as necessary, and stop the source of the bleeding. Complications of traumatic injury in pregnancy are uterine rupture, abruptio placentae, emergency delivery, and neonatal resuscitation (see Collaborative Interventions); liver and splenic lacerations (see Chapter 20); and pelvic fractures (see Chapter 10). To effectively assess abnormal clinical signs in pregnancy, the nurse must be aware of normal physiologic changes in pregnancy as related to airway, breathing, and circulation (ABCs) (See the "Physiologic Changes in Pregnancy" box).

NURSING ALERT

Because of these physiologic changes, the pregnant patient will not demonstrate the classic signs of hypovolemic shock until the shock state is advanced. "Normal vital signs" may indicate a shunting of blood from the uterus to maintain core maternal body functions, causing fetal deterioration.
Changes in fetal activity and heart rate may be the first signs of maternal hypovolemia.

Vaginal bleeding

Ask the patient to compare present vaginal bleeding with normal menstrual flow. Asking for the number of pads or tampons used may be an indicator of the amount of bleeding. Determine if the patient has passed any tissue (hamburger-looking substance) or blood clots. Bleeding that is associated with clotting or that lasts longer than 7 days is suggestive of substantial blood loss.[1] Tissue passing is associated with miscarriage. Bleeding may also be associated with self-induced abortion attempts.

Last menstrual cycle

Ask the patient the date of her last menstrual cycle.

PHYSIOLOGIC CHANGES IN PREGNANCY

1. Increased heart rate
2. Increased cardiac output
3. Increased relative fluid volume
4. Decreased blood supply to the heart (vena cava compression)
5. Decreased blood pressure (BP) during first trimester
6. Increased BP during last 2 months of pregnancy (3 to 5 mm Hg systolic change and 5 to 10 mm Hg diastolic change)
7. Increased oxygen consumption

From Harvey M, Troiano N: *NAACOGS Clin Iss in Perinatal and Women's Health Nurs* 3(3):52-59, 1992.

Pain

Ask the patient if she is experiencing pain. Placenta previa is usually painless, whereas ectopic pregnancy and abruptio placentae are painful. Preterm labor is associated with lower back pain. Term labor contractions are more regular in timing. Abdominal pain after a motor vehicle crash or other traumatic event may indicate a serious injury.

Pregnancy history

Gravida is the number of pregnancies and *para* is the number of live births. Abortions include spontaneous, therapeutic, and elective abortions. Determine the estimated date of confinement. Calculate the week of pregnancy (abruptio placentae and placenta previa are more prevalent in the last trimester).

Medical history

Women with chronic hypertension have a greater risk for poor pregnancy outcomes than do patients with pregnancy-induced hypertension. Diabetes and thyroid disorders may be exacerbated during pregnancy because of hypermetabolism.

Surgical history

Determine if the patient has had any prior cesarean section deliveries.

Medication history

Elicit any history of recreational, prescribed, and over-the-counter drug use. These drugs may precipitate labor or enhance bleeding.

Precipitating event

If the patient has received physical trauma from a motor vehicle crash, ascertain if the crash involved a head-on or broadside impact. Serious injury to the fetus is associated with broadside crashes, although speed and restraint status are important factors.

NURSING ALERT

Fetal heart tones must be assessed, although they may not be audible in the first trimester.

Fetal activity

Fetal activity escalates predictably 24 hours before labor.

Vital Signs (Gynecologic and Obstetric Conditions)

- *Heart rate:* Tachycardia related to hypovolemia and pain
- *Blood pressure:* Hypotension related to hypovolemia; hypertension related to pregnancy-induced vascular changes
- *Respirations:* Tachypnea resulting from acidosis secondary to anaerobic metabolism, related to a decrease in cellular oxygenation (in cases of hypovolemic shock related to abruptio placentae, placenta previa, ruptured ectopic pregnancy)
- *Fever:* Related to infection (STD, ruptured ectopic pregnancy, premature rupture of membranes in pregnancy)

General Observations
Skin

Assess the patient's skin for circulatory changes. Hypovolemia is associated with cool, pale extremities. Pregnancy-related hypertensive disorder (PRHD) may produce facial flushing.

FOCUSED NURSING ASSESSMENT (OBSTETRIC CONDITIONS)

Nursing assessment should focus on ventilation and perfusion.

Ventilation
Breath sounds

Pulmonary edema occurs rapidly in a pregnant patient who has PRHD or in one who receives fluid resuscitation. Coarse or fine crackles may be auscultated.

Perfusion
Blood pressure and pulse

A single systolic blood pressure (BP) reading of 140 mm Hg or greater before 20 weeks' gestation indicates a higher than normal risk of pregnancy-induced hypertension, preeclampsia, and premature delivery.[2] A diastolic BP of 90 mm Hg or more should be the criterion for a diagnosis of hypertension in pregnancy.[3] A systolic BP greater than 169 mm Hg or a diastolic BP greater than 109 mm Hg is considered an emergency, and hydralazine, labetolol, or nifedipine should be administered.[4]

Assess the fetal heart rate (FHR). Hemorrhage may occur and be concealed in cases of ectopic pregnancy, abruptio placentae, or uterine rupture. The FHR may decrease in situations in which fetal hypoxia is occurring, such as placenta previa, abruptio placentae, uterine rupture, and PRHD.

Vaginal discharge and bleeding
Mucoid, watery, or blood-tinged discharge is associated with preterm labor. The passage of tissue is suggestive of spontaneous abortion. Test the discharge for amniotic fluid (turns blue on contact with nitrazine paper). The presence of amniotic fluid indicates the rupture of membranes and an increased risk for maternal infection and fetal deterioration. Meconium staining (green) of the amniotic fluid is associated with fetal problems.

Risk Factors (Obstetric Conditions)
1. Cigarette smoking increases the likelihood of premature labor, abruptio placentae, and placenta previa.
2. Age is a risk factor for hemorrhage in the last trimester of pregnancy. Women 35 years of age or older are at risk for placenta previa. Women less than 20 years of age and more than 30 years of age are at risk for abruptio placentae. Uterine rupture is common with older females.
3. Previous cesarean section ("C-section") is a risk factor for ectopic pregnancy,[6] spontaneous abortion, uterine rupture, and placenta previa.[5]
4. Uterine trauma is associated with placenta previa, abruptio placentae, and uterine rupture.
5. Diabetes is associated with placenta previa and PRHD.
6. Alcohol consumption and cocaine use are associated with abruptio placentae and placenta previa.[7]
7. Hypertension is associated with abruptio placentae.
8. A history of infertility is associated with ectopic pregnancy.
9. A history of bleeding in the first trimester is associated with later development of both abruptio placentae and placenta previa.[5]
10. Nulliparity and young maternal age are risk factors for hypertension in labor.
11. Chinese and Caucasian women have a higher inci-

dence of hemolysis, elevated enzymes, and low platelets (HELLP) syndrome.

Life Span Issues (Gynecologic Conditions)

1. Vaginal bleeding may occur in early adolescence because of irregular menstrual patterns rather than because of a pathologic condition.
2. Vaginal bleeding may occur in middle age as a result of the beginning of menopause rather than because of a pathologic condition.

INITIAL INTERVENTIONS

Gynecologic and Obstetric Conditions

1. Initiate IV access and send a blood specimen to the laboratory for a type and crossmatch and complete blood count (CBC) for all patients with vaginal bleeding and abnormal vital signs.
2. Initiate cardiac and BP monitoring for patients with significant vaginal bleeding.
3. Initiate pulse oximetry to monitor oxygen saturation.

Obstetric Conditions

1. Place all pregnant patients who are in their second trimester or beyond on their left side to facilitate venous return. If the patient is on a backboard because of traumatic injury, elevate the right side of the backboard with a wedge.
2. If the patient is pregnant and hypertensive, anticipate seizure activity. Pad the side rails and keep the bed in a low position. Have suction and airway materials available.
3. If available, initiate external fetal monitoring for pregnant patients with vaginal bleeding.
4. Treat the pregnant patient's fear and anxiety by explaining all procedures and offering support from clergy, family, or significant others.

PRIORITY NURSING DIAGNOSES (GYNECOLOGIC AND OBSTETRIC CONDITIONS)

Risk for fluid volume deficit
Risk for pain
Risk for fear

Risk for anticipatory grieving
Risk for injury
♦ **Fluid volume deficit** related to hemorrhage:
   INTERVENTIONS
   • Initiate IV access.
   • Administer IV crystalloids and blood components as ordered.
   • Anticipate surgical intervention.
♦ **Pain** related to uterine contractions or peritoneal irritation:
   INTERVENTIONS
   • Administer analgesics as ordered.
   • Use imagery techniques and distraction if they are helpful to the patient.
♦ **Fear** related to unknown pregnancy outcome:
   INTERVENTIONS
   • Allow the mother to hear the FHR.
   • Encourage participation in maternal tests and treatments by explaining the benefits to the fetus.
♦ **Anticipatory grieving** related to loss of pregnancy and reproductive abilities:
   INTERVENTIONS
   • Explain treatment options and probable consequences.
   • Maintain a support base as identified by the patient.
♦ **Injury** related to infection from peritoneal contamination or retained placental fragments:
   INTERVENTIONS
   • Administer antibiotics as ordered.
   • Anticipate dilatation and curettage (D&C) or surgery.
   • Monitor fever and leukocytosis.

PRIORITY DIAGNOSTIC TESTS (GYNECOLOGIC AND OBSTETRIC CONDITIONS)

Many of the tests in this section are initiated in the ED, but results may take several days. The information is provided to support patient teaching.

Laboratory Tests
Complete blood count (CBC): A CBC may indicate infection if the white blood cell count is elevated or bleeding if hemoglobin and hematocrit are low.
Iron level: The iron level is low when vaginal bleeding has been excessive or chronic.

Kleihauer-Betke test: A positive test result suggests fetomaternal hemorrhage, usually from abdominal trauma. This is indicative of placental products entering the maternal circulation.

Platelet level: The platelet level may be low if the cause of vaginal bleeding is leukemia, idiopathic thrombocytopenic purpura, or disseminated intravascular coagulation (DIC).

Prothrombin time: This level may be high if vaginal bleeding is associated with von Willebrand's disease and other clotting disorders such as DIC, which is associated with abruptio placentae and uterine rupture.

Human chorionic gonadotropin (hCG) test: Detection of hCG in the blood indicates pregnancy; the higher the level, the longer the gestation period. The level of hCG for a woman with an ectopic pregnancy is lower than for a woman with an intrauterine pregnancy of the same gestation.

Type and crossmatch: A type and crossmatch may be ordered if a blood transfusion is needed as a result of bleeding.

Serum gonadotropins: A follicle-stimulating hormone level >40 IU/L suggests impending ovarian failure (menopause), whereas a luteinizing hormone/follicle-stimulating hormone ratio that is >2 suggests chronic anovulation.

Other Tests

Endometrial biopsy: An endometrial biopsy is used to determine the presence of ovulation by measuring progesterone and estrogen levels in the endometrial lining.

Ultrasound: An ultrasound examination is used for identification of ovarian cysts, for early diagnosis of ovarian tumors, for evaluation of abnormal uterine bleeding, for ectopic pregnancy, and for guidance during aspiration procedures (e.g., pelvic and ovarian abscesses). A transabdominal scan may be performed using a full urinary bladder. The patient then voids, and a transvaginal scan is conducted if indicated.

NURSING ALERT

Determine the type of ultrasound examination to be performed so the patient can be instructed to void if needed. The

Continued

NURSING ALERT—cont'd

patient must have a full bladder for a transabdominal ultrasound examination and an empty bladder for a transvaginal ultrasound examination.

Culdocentesis: Removal of >5 ml of nonclotting blood from the cul-de-sac indicates a ruptured ectopic pregnancy. This test is painful and is not used as frequently as an ultrasound or CT scan to detect ectopic pregnancy.

COLLABORATIVE INTERVENTIONS (GYNECOLOGIC AND OBSTETRIC CONDITIONS)

1. For compromised pregnant patients complaining of vaginal bleeding, administer high-flow oxygen using a nonrebreather mask at 10 to 15 L/min until diagnostic test results are back.
2. If it has not been done earlier, initiate a large-bore IV line for all patients complaining of vaginal bleeding.
3. Prepare the patient for a speculum examination. Obtain culture media, swabs, and specimen containers for conception products examination.

Clinical Conditions (Gynecologic)
Ovarian cysts
Ovarian cysts are difficult to identify on the physical examination. Their clinical presentation is similar to that of ectopic pregnancy and appendicitis. Hormonal changes, endometriosis, or neoplasms may produce ovarian cysts.

SYMPTOMS
- Patients experience a wide range of pain severity with ovarian cysts.
- Generally the pain is worse during the latter half of the menstrual cycle.
- The pain may be localized to the right or left lower abdominal quadrant.
- The pain is increased with motion.
- If the cyst has ruptured, the patient experiences severe pain.

DIAGNOSIS
- A pelvic ultrasound examination is the diagnostic tool of choice.
- A CBC and hCG test may be performed.

- If rupture is suspected, a type and crossmatch and PT level may be ordered.
- Nausea and vomiting (N/V), fever, leukocytosis, and a firm to rigid abdomen without bowel sounds may be present.

TREATMENT

- Hormone supplements may be ordered.
- Pain medication is usually prescribed.
- A follow-up ultrasound examination is essential to detect enlargement.
- A ruptured ovarian cyst necessitates surgery for removal of products and irrigation of the peritoneal cavity.
- One or two large-bore IV catheters should be inserted, and Ringer's lactate or normal saline solution should be infused.
- IV antibiotics should be started in the ED.
- The patient must be monitored for shock (via BP, CVP [if available], base deficit [ABG], and urine output).
- Obtaining oxygen saturation levels is helpful.

Dysfunctional uterine bleeding

Dysfunctional uterine bleeding is usually associated with anovulation (most frequently during puberty and menopause).

SYMPTOMS

- The most common symptom is abnormal uterine bleeding associated with anovulation, either acute (menarche and menopause) or chronic.

DIAGNOSIS

- Diagnosis is based on clinical findings and presentation.
- An endometrial biopsy may be performed.

TREATMENT

- If the bleeding is significant or the patient is hemodynamically unstable, a D&C should be performed in the operating suite. Estrogen and progesterone medications may be administered (Table 15-1).

Clinical Conditions (Obstetric)
Miscarriage (spontaneous abortion)

A spontaneous abortion occurs before the 20th week of pregnancy. It may be threatened or complete.

SYMPTOMS

- Crampy abdominal pain may be present.
- Vaginal bleeding with or without the passage of tissue may occur.

TABLE 15-1 Drug Summary

Drug	Dose and route	Special considerations
Progesterone	100-200 mg IM	Used to treat dysfunctional uterine bleeding
Medroxyprogesterone acetate	10-40 mg qd for 5-10 days PO	Used to treat active uterine bleeding
Estrogen	25 mg q4hr × 3 doses IV	Used in persistent uterine bleeding Progesterone is started after the estrogen is administered
Oxytocin	Comes in 10 U/ml concentration; add 10-40 U to 1000 ml normal saline or Ringer's lactate for IV 10 U IM	Titrate drug to achieve uterine contractions; usually takes 200-500 ml/hr at the described concentration
Ergonovine and methylergonovine maleate	0.2 mg IM, repeat q2-4hr 0.2 mg IV	IV route is used only in life-threatening situations Used to achieve uterine contractions
Terbutaline sulfate	10 µg/min IV titrated up to a maximum of 80 µg/min for 4 hr, then switch to 2.5 mg PO q4-6hr	Used to stop premature labor Cardiac monitoring of both mother and fetus should be instituted because of side effect of tachycardia May cause hyperglycemia

Magnesium sulfate	4 g in 250 ml D_5W IV infused slowly, followed by 4-5 g IM in alternate buttocks q4hr	Used to prevent seizures in HELLP syndrome, preeclampsia, and eclampsia; also used to stop premature labor. Check reflexes and respiratory function before administration and during administration; may cause respiratory depression in mother and newborn
Rh_0 immune globulin	Preferred dose is 1 vial within 3 hr but at least within 72 hr after ectopic pregnancy, abortion, miscarriage, amniocentesis; one vial within 72 hr of delivery in postpartum	Used to prevent hemolytic disease of the newborn in a subsequent pregnancy
Hydralazine	5 to 20 mg IVP q20-30min	Used in PIH, preeclampsia to maintain diastolic BP at 90 mm Hg

HELLP, hemolysis, elevated enzymes, and low platelets syndrome; *PIH*, pregnancy induced hypertension.

DIAGNOSIS
- An hCG test is performed to confirm pregnancy.
- An ultrasound examination is performed to determine if a gestational sac is present and to determine the location of the sac.
- A speculum examination is performed to determine if the cervix is dilated and to determine the source of the bleeding.

TREATMENT
- Oxytocin or Methergine may be administered to promote expulsion of all material.
- Antibiotics and analgesics may be ordered.
- A D&C may be needed.
- The patient should be tested for Rh status, and Rh immunoglobulin administered if the mother is Rh negative.

Ectopic pregnancy

An ectopic pregnancy occurs when the fertilized ovum implants on tissue other than the uterine endometrium, usually because of impaired passage through the fallopian tubes.

SYMPTOMS
- Amenorrhea, pelvic or abdominal pain, and abnormal vaginal bleeding are the most common symptoms.
- A pelvic mass can be palpated in some cases.
- Symptoms most frequently occur at 4 to 6 weeks' gestation.
- An ectopic rupture with intraperitoneal bleeding occurs at 6 to 10 weeks' gestation. Thus symptoms may include hypotension, tachycardia, N/V, a rigid abdomen without bowel sounds, fever, and leukocytosis.

DIAGNOSIS
- An ultrasound examination may detect an ectopic pregnancy before clinical symptoms appear.
- Ultrasound examination findings are compared with hCG levels.
- The presence of nonclotting blood in the cul-de-sac may be present upon culdocentesis.

TREATMENT
- Surgery is usually performed to remove the products of conception and to repair the damaged fallopian tube.
- Rh testing of the mother should be performed and Rh immunoglobulin given if the patient is Rh negative.

Preterm labor

Many women ignore the signs of preterm labor and come to the ED after the membranes have ruptured or cervical dilation has occurred. The gestational age of the fetus may be reflected in the baseline FHR, a pattern of reactivity, and changes in the behavioral state of the fetus.

SYMPTOMS

- The symptoms associated with preterm labor may include an elevated FHR (150 to 160 beats/min).[8]
- If fetal monitoring is available in the ED, preterm fetuses will be seen to have fewer accelerations and less amplitude with acceleration.
- Painless contractions and a change in vaginal discharge (mucoid, watery, or blood-tinged appearance) are the best predictors of preterm labor.

DIAGNOSIS

- Preterm labor is diagnosed by labor pattern and not by FHR alone.
- A speculum examination is conducted to rule out premature rupture of the membranes as the cause of the change in vaginal discharge, followed by a digital examination of the cervix to evaluate cervical dilatation and effacement.

TREATMENT

- Tocolytic agents (e.g., ritodrine, terbutaline, and magnesium sulfate) are administered.
- The patient is placed on bed rest in the left lateral recumbent position.
- Fetal monitoring is used to detect activity and heart rate variability.

Abruptio placentae

Abruptio placentae usually occurs after 20 weeks' gestation. It is a tearing and bleeding into the inner layer of the endometrium that compresses and impairs the functioning of the placenta. Abruptio placentae may be concealed (rarely) because of internal uterine bleeding or revealed or external (in 80% of cases) where bleeding dissects the membrane from the uterine wall[6] (Figure 15-1).

SYMPTOMS

- The patient complains of sharp, sudden generalized pain over the abdomen.
- Rapid, continuous, or intermittent uterine contractions may occur. Vaginal bleeding may be present. If present, it is usually dark in color.

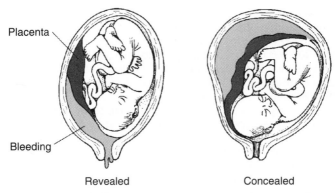

Revealed   Concealed

Figure 15-1 Abruptio placentae. (From Murphy P: *JEMS* 17[9]:48-49, 1992.)

- Fetal activity is less and the FHR may decrease as fetal hypoxia occurs.
- Signs of hypovolemic shock may be present (an increased heart rate and a decreased level of consciousness, urine output, oxygen saturation, and BP).
- DIC is common in cases of abruption.

DIAGNOSIS
- Diagnosis is usually based on clinical presentation.
- DIC may be confirmed by a prolonged PT and the presence of fibrin degradation products.

TREATMENT
- The aim of treatment is to maintain maternal blood volume by fluid resuscitation with crystalloids and blood components (initially two large-bore IV lines infusing Ringer's lactate solution).
- High-flow oxygen (10 to 15 L/min) is administered.
- The fetus is delivered and resuscitated as necessary.

Placenta previa
Placenta previa is a condition in which the placenta is located either close to or over the internal os of the uterus. The placenta may cover the os partially or completely (Figure 15-2). The danger in placenta previa is a separation of the placenta from the uterine wall and subsequent hemorrhage. Perinatal mortality is greater because of decreased fetal perfusion, both from the implanted placenta and from decreased circulating blood volume of the mother.

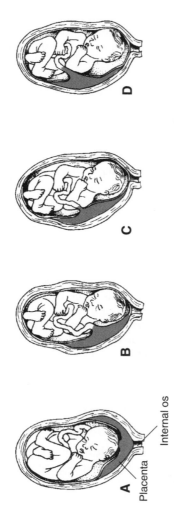

Internal os

Placenta

Figure 15-2 Placenta previa. **A,** Total placenta previa. Internal cervical os is completely covered by the placenta. **B,** Partial previa. Internal os is partially covered by the placenta. **C,** Marginal previa. Edge of the placenta is at the margin of the internal os. **D,** Low-lying previa. Placenta is implanted in the lower uterine section, and the edge is close to the internal os. (From Murphy P: Problem pregnancies, *JEMS* 17[9]:48-49, 1992.)

SYMPTOMS

- Almost half of all placenta previa patients have their first episode of bleeding before 30 weeks' gestation.
- Initial bleeding is usually self-limiting.
- The earlier this episode occurs in the pregnancy, the less likely the pregnancy will reach term.
- Painless, bright red bleeding, not associated with contractions, is the most frequent clinical sign.

DIAGNOSIS

- A speculum examination may be performed, but digital examination is not advisable because of the potential for hemorrhage.
- An ultrasound examination is used to detect placental location.

TREATMENT

- The aim is to postpone labor to promote fetal maturation.
- Bed rest may be initiated.
- If the patient continues to bleed, the baby may be delivered by cesarean section.
- Vaginal delivery is possible if previa is marginal.

Ruptured uterus

A ruptured uterus may be considered complete when a tear occurs through the uterus and peritoneal covering, allowing intrauterine contents to be "spilled" into the peritoneal cavity. An incomplete (occult) tear may also occur. Rupture of the healthy uterus most frequently occurs during labor with oxytocin administration. Rupture of a previously scarred uterus (e.g., by a cesarean section) may occur as pregnancy advances.

SYMPTOMS

- Bleeding may be great if the tear is complete but not visible; thus the patient will have signs of hypovolemia (an increased heart rate and decreased BP and oxygen saturation).
- Parts of the fetus may be palpable in the abdomen.
- If the tear is partial, minor bleeding may occur and seal itself off by hematoma formation.
- Sharp, shooting abdominal pain or a tearing sensation may be present.
- Contractions may stop suddenly.
- Fetal mortality is high (50% to 75%).

DIAGNOSIS

- Diagnosis is based on clinical presentation.

TREATMENT

- Emergency surgical delivery by cesarean section is indicated for delivery of the fetus and repair of the peritoneum and uterus.
- Rapid fluid resuscitation is indicated.
- Two large-bore IV lines are inserted and crystalloids and blood components are administered.
- Administer high-flow oxygen (10 to 15 L/min).

Trauma in pregnancy

SYMPTOMS

- Any event resulting in physical trauma from the release of energy may injure the mother and fetus. Warning symptoms include vaginal bleeding, uterine contractions, and abdominal tenderness. Abruptio placentae and uterine rupture are the most serious complications of trauma in pregnancy.

DIAGNOSIS

- The degree of diagnostic testing used depends on the severity of the precipitating event. At a minimum, external fetal monitoring should be performed for 4 hours.[9] If abdominal trauma is a possibility, a Kleihauer-Betke test may be performed. An ultrasound examination may be used to assess fetal status.

TREATMENT

- Monitor the fetus and uterine contractions.
- Provide hemodynamic stabilization. Two large-bore IV lines are inserted and crystalloids and blood components may be administered.
- Administer high-flow oxygen (10 to 15 L/min).
- Anticipate an emergency cesarean section and surgery.
- The patient can usually be discharged after 4 hours of monitoring if there are no signs of fetal or maternal distress.[9]

Pregnancy-related hypertensive disorders (PRHD)

The four types of PRHD are chronic hypertension (hypertension diagnosed before pregnancy or persisting after the 42nd week [postpartum]), transient hypertension (increased blood pressure after 20 weeks or 24 hours after delivery), preeclampsia superimposed on chronic hypertension, and preeclampsia and eclampsia.[10] Preeclampsia is defined as BP >140/90, a systolic increase of 30 mm Hg or greater, or a diastolic increase of 15 mm Hg or greater at two readings taken 6 or more hours apart. Edema and proteinuria are present. Eclampsia is the development of seizures in a preeclamptic patient.[4] The arterial wall responds differently to angiotensin II and renin, resulting in arterial spasms.

SYMPTOMS
- The patient may exhibit a variety of clinical signs.
- Patients may complain of visual changes, edema, persistent vomiting, or decreased urine output.
- A classic sign is seen in the second trimester; the mean arterial pressure (MAP) does not drop lower than the first-trimester MAP.
- A 30 mm Hg or greater increase in systolic BP or a 15 mm Hg or greater increase in diastolic BP must be present for the diagnosis to be made.
- Papilledema and seizures may occur.
- In cases of eclampsia, epigastric pain (occurring from liver edema) is associated with impending seizure and is a late sign.
- Fetal movement may decrease.
- Reflexes are hyperactive.

DIAGNOSIS
- BP changes occur as described earlier in the section.
- Urine protein levels increase (1+ in mild cases, up to 3+ or greater in severe cases). A urine protein level of more than 0.3 g/day is the criterion for diagnosis of proteinuria.[3]
- Platelet levels may be low, fibrin degradation products may be present, and liver enzyme levels may be elevated if the preeclampsia has progressed into HELLP syndrome.

TREATMENT
- Seizures are treated as outlined in Chapter 14.
- Severe cases are treated with magnesium sulfate to prevent seizures, or Valium, phenytoin, and phenobarbital are given when seizures occur.
- Hydralazine, urapidil, labetalol, or nifedipine may be given to decrease the BP.[4]
- Terbutaline may be given to prevent contractions.
- Milder cases are treated with bed rest, a no-added-salt diet, and home monitoring of BP and urine protein levels.

- Delivery is the last resort, since BP decreases after delivery.

Emergency delivery

The multiparous pregnant patient is at the greatest risk for imminent delivery.

SYMPTOMS

- Ask the patient if she is aware of when her bag of water ruptured. If so, was the fluid green or did it have a greenish tint?
- Green fluid (meconium) indicates infants who may need suctioning and intubation.
- The patient will have bloody show secondary to rapid dilation of the cervix and a bulging anus and perineum indicating fetal descent, and the fetus will display crowning of the head.
- If the baby's head remains visible between contractions, birth is imminent.

DIAGNOSIS

- Diagnosis is based on clinical presentation.

TREATMENT

- Follow the steps in the "Steps in Emergency Delivery" box for emergency delivery.

NURSING ALERT

If the cord prolapses before the baby appears, place the mother in the knee-chest position or Trendelenburg's position. Administer high-flow oxygen (10 to 15 L/min) to the mother.

STEPS IN EMERGENCY DELIVERY

1. Place the mother on her left side to slow fetal descent.
2. Have the mother open her mouth and pant to slow progress.
3. Have a neonatal resuscitation bag and oxygen supply available. Suction equipment is also needed.
4. Wash your hands and put on gloves.
5. Wash the patient's perineum, then reglove.
6. Ease the perineum back until the head emerges.
7. As the baby's head emerges, check for the umbilical cord. If it is around the baby's neck, slip it over the head or back over the shoulders.

Continued

STEPS IN EMERGENCY DELIVERY—cont'd

8. Suction the baby's mouth first, then the nose. Suctioning the nose first may elicit a reflex gasp of fluids in the lungs.
9. Place your hand under the cord as the baby emerges.
10. If the cord is extremely tight, clamp the cord with two clamps and cut between the clamps.
11. Keep the baby's head lower than its trunk during birthing to promote drainage.
12. Do not pull the baby out; allow the baby to advance on its own.
13. Cut the cord after clamping 1½ inches from the infant's umbilicus after the cord stops pulsating. Use two clamps to prevent cord bleeding.
14. Document the time of delivery and the baby's Apgar score.

PERTINENT DATA TO RECORD DURING THE INTRAPARTUM AND POSTPARTUM PERIODS

Intrapartum

1. Gravida, para, abortions, Last menstrual period, estimated date of confinement
2. Fetal heart rate
3. Membranes status
4. Amount of vaginal bleeding
5. Percent effacement, centimeters of dilatation, station
6. Anesthetic agent(s), episiotomy, sutures
7. Amniotic fluid cultures

Postpartum

1. Time fetus delivered
2. Time placenta delivered
3. Cord blood samples obtained
4. Time placenta sent to laboratory for examination
5. Fundal massage and position q15min
6. Lochia color and amount q15min × 1 hr, then q1hr
7. Perineum assessment q15min × 1 hr, then q1hr

TABLE 15-2 Apgar Score

Sign	0	1	2
Heart rate	Absent	Slow—below 100 beats/min	Above 100 beats/min
Respirations	Absent	Slow—irregular	Good crying
Muscle tone	Flaccid	Some flexion of extremities	Active motion
Reflex irritability	None	Grimace	Vigorous cry
Color	Pale blue	Body pink with blue extremities	Completely pink

DOCUMENTATION
1. Record intrapartum and postpartum care. The "Pertinent Data" box includes pertinent information to record.
2. Record neonatal assessment and treatments. Table 15-2 provides information about scoring Apgar at 1 and 5 minutes. Neonatal ophthalmic medications vary according to state law. Beware that the infant is at risk for hypothermia and ineffective airway clearance.

Newborn resuscitation
An Apgar score of 5 or less is frequently a predictor of the need for resuscitation.

SYMPTOMS
- An Apgar score of <5 after 1 minute (because of poor ventilation and circulatory response) is usually present.

DIAGNOSIS
- There is no respiratory effort, and the pulse is irregular, decreased, or absent.

TREATMENT
- After the infant's airway is suctioned, 100% oxygen is administered using a bag-valve mask or blow-by device.
- Intubation should follow immediately.
- Perform cardiac massage if the heart rate is <100 beats/min.
- Epinephrine 0.01 mg/kg of a 1:10,000 solution may be given endotracheally, or through the umbilical cord in cases of cardiac arrest.
- An IV line must be initiated (the umbilical cord may be used).

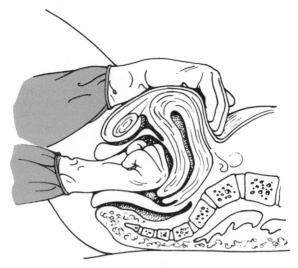

Figure 15-3   Bimanual compression of the uterus and massage with the abdominal hand usually will control hemorrhage from uterine atony. (From Cunningham FG, et al: *Williams obstetrics,* ed 20, Norwalk, Conn, 1998, Appleton & Lange.)

- Warming lights should be placed over the baby to prevent hypothermia.

Postpartum bleeding

Postpartum bleeding is defined as a blood loss >500 ml at delivery or during the first 24 hours after delivery. It is related to uterine atony or cervical and vaginal lacerations. However, in some cases postpartum bleeding may occur 2 to 4 weeks after delivery because of retained placental fragments.

SYMPTOMS

- Vaginal bleeding with clots and a soft uterus indicates atony.
- Tissue may be passed vaginally.
- Fever is present in cases of leukocytosis if bleeding occurs several weeks after delivery.

DIAGNOSIS

- A speculum examination is made to determine the presence of cervical and vaginal lacerations.
- A CBC may be performed.
- Diagnosis is usually based on clinical presentation.

TREATMENT

- If the bleeding occurs early in the postpartum period, the physician may perform uterine massage with one hand externally massaging and the other gloved hand supporting the lower uterine segment through a vaginal approach (Figure 15-3).
- Oxytocic drugs are administered (e.g., Methergine, Ergotrate, and Pitocin).
- Breastfeeding (if appropriate) helps the uterus to contract.
- Fluid resuscitation with two large-bore IV lines infusing crystalloids or blood components may be indicated.
- High-flow oxygen (10 to 15 L/min) may be necessary.

NURSING SURVEILLANCE

1. Trend vital signs and oxygen saturation.
2. Monitor contractions for timing and duration.
3. Monitor the FHR during contractions.
4. Monitor the level of consciousness.
5. Trend pain.
6. Diligent pulmonary assessment is crucial in a pregnant patient who has been receiving IV fluids because of hemodilution and the chance of pulmonary edema occurring.
7. Monitor arterial blood gases and beware of an increased CO_2 level, since respiratory alkalosis is normal for pregnancy.

EXPECTED PATIENT OUTCOMES

1. The patient's level of consciousness improves or remains stable.
2. Vaginal bleeding decreases.
3. Pain decreases or is absent.
4. Urine output is >30 ml/hr.
5. Fever decreases or is absent.
6. Vital signs improve and the systolic BP remains >90 mm Hg but <140 mm Hg.
7. There is no seizure activity.
8. The FHR is normal for gestational age.
9. The newborn infant's Apgar score is >5 at 1 minute and improves at 5 minutes.

DISCHARGE IMPLICATIONS

1. All patients discharged with vaginal bleeding should be told to check their temperature qid and to return if fever occurs.

2. Tampons should not be used until the abnormal vaginal bleeding stops.
3. Patients with a threatened abortion should be told to abstain from sexual intercourse until the bleeding stops. They should save all passed tissue for examination.
4. Pregnant patients with PIH should receive teaching about a low-salt or no-added-salt diet. They should be taught how to take their BP and to perform urine reagent testing for protein content.
5. Patients who are found to be Rh negative should be told to wear a medical alert bracelet with this information.

References

1. Bayer S, DeCherney A: Clinical manifestations and treatment of dysfunctional uterine bleeding, *JAMA* 269:1823-1838, 1993.
2. Broughton-Pipkin F, Sharif J, Lal S: Predicting high blood pressure in pregnancy: a multivariate approach, *J Hypertens* 16:221-229, 1998.
3. Helewa M et al: Report of the Canadian Hypertension Society Consensus Conference: definitions, evaluation and classification of hypertensive disorders in pregnancy, *CMAJ* 157:715-725, 1997.
4. Rey E et al: Report of the Canadian Hypertension Society Consensus Conference: pharmacologic treatment of hypertensive disorders in pregnancy, *CMAJ* 157:1245-1254, 1997.
5. Ananth C, Smulian J, Vintzileos A: The association of placenta previa with history of cesarean delivery and abortion: a meta-analysis, *Am J Obstet Gynecol* 177:1071-1078, 1997.
6. Murphy P: Problem pregnancies, *JEMS* 17(9):44-60, 1992.
7. Macones G et al: The association between maternal cocaine use and placenta previa, *Am J Obstet Gynecol* 177:1097-1100, 1997.
8. Eganhouse D, Burnside JS: Nursing assessment and responsibility in monitoring the preterm pregnancy, *JOGNN* 21:355-363, 1992.
9. Aitokallio-Tallberg A, Halmesmaki E: Motor vehicle accident during the second or third trimester of pregnancy, *Acta Obstet Gynecol Scand* 76:313-317, 1997.
10. Creasy R, Resnik R: *Maternal-fetal medicine, principles, and practice,* Philadelphia, 1999, WB Saunders.

Chapter 16

Respiratory Conditions

Darlene Welsh
Pamela S. Kidd

CLINICAL CONDITIONS
Asthma
Bronchitis
Pulmonary Alveolar Edema
   Noncardiogenic Pulmonary Alveolar Edema
   Cardiogenic Pulmonary Alveolar Edema
Pulmonary Embolism
Pneumonia
Chronic Obstructive Pulmonary Disease
Spontaneous Pneumothorax

TRIAGE ASESSMENT

Acutely ill emergency department (ED) patients may need airway management. Common respiratory conditions treated in the ED include asthma, pulmonary alveolar edema (PAE), pulmonary embolism (PE), pneumonia, spontaneous pneumothorax, and chronic obstructive pulmonary disease (COPD). COPD is usually a combination of two disease processes, chronic bronchitis and emphysema. Documenting patient complaints and medical history at triage helps differentiate these conditions. Obtain the following patient information from transport personnel, patients, or family members:

Precipitating event

Obtain a history of any electrical injury, overdose, paralysis secondary to cerebrovascular attack or spinal cord injury, carbon monoxide poisoning, or smoke inhalation (suspect impending airway obstruction). Triage to the treatment area immediately.

Previous need for intubation

A history of intubation for respiratory failure is highly significant for fatal asthma. Triage to the treatment area immediately.

R

Exercise ability and steroid use

Note any history of exercise limitations, current use of steroids, and prior hospitalization for acute asthma (suspect bronchoconstriction).

Dyspnea

Identify any history of paroxysmal nocturnal dyspnea, orthopnea, dyspnea upon exertion, lower extremity edema, unexplained fatigue, and known cardiovascular disease (suspect cardiogenic PAE). Note progressive dyspnea upon exertion with cough and clear sputum (suspect COPD).

Burn and trauma history, altitude changes, near-drowning

Identify any history of recent trauma, major burn, toxicant inhalation, hemorrhage (secondary to hypoperfusion and stimulation of the inflammatory response), drug overdose, altitude changes, massive infection, or near-drowning (suspect noncardiogenic PAE).

Potential for thrombus or embolus formation

Note any history of venous insufficiency, deep vein thrombosis (DVT), orthopedic trauma or surgery, obesity, recent pregnancy or delivery, prolonged immobility, or estrogen therapy (suspect PE).

Pneumothorax history

Note any history of a spontaneous pneumothorax (suspect underlying pulmonary disease [e.g., COPD or spontaneous pneumothorax reoccurrence, particularly if original pneumothorax was treated with chest tube insertion or aspiration]). The recurrence rate of spontaneous pneumothorax is at least 30%.[1,2]

Infection

Look for a history of the patient's having a recent upper respiratory infection (URI) or living in proximity to others who have a URI (which may cause increased exposure to the respiratory pathogens of others). Also look for a decreased level of consciousness (LOC), fever, leukocytosis, or acquired immunodeficiency syndrome (AIDS) (suspect pneumonia).

Cough

Note any history of productive cough (3 months' duration for 2 to 3 consecutive years), wheezing, dyspnea, smoking, or exposure to environmental pollution (suspect COPD). A cough at night is associated with asthma.

Airway and breathing pattern signs

- A change in respiratory rate or pattern may be an early sign of respiratory insufficiency.
- Inward chest movement is noted on inspiration.
- Outward abdominal movement is noted on inspiration.
- Suprasternal, supraclavicular, and sternocleidomastoid muscle retractions are noted.
- Retraction of intercostal spaces is noted.
- The patient has noisy inspiratory breathing (Table 16-1). Figure 16-1 shows the relationship between anatomy and type of stridor.

TABLE 16-1 Discriminating Source of Airway Obstruction

Origin	Etiology	Symptoms

Nasal
URI
  Allergy
  Foreign bodies and tumors
	Incidence may be increased during certain seasons if related to allergens or infection
	Related to inflammation of nares
		Absence of stridor
		Rarely life threatening
		Patient demonstrates mouth breathing

Pharyngeal Infection Foreign bodies	Regurgitation of gastric contents Dislodged or broken teeth Nasal, oral, and pharyngeal bleeding Occlusion of tongue in unconscious patient	Snoring Inspiratory stridor
Laryngeal Infection Foreign bodies and tumors Trauma	Spasm may occur as a result of foreign material or suctioning Edema may occur as a result of intubation attempts or inhalation of caustic substances	Crowing Inspiratory stridor is equal to expiratory stridor

Continued

TABLE 16-1 Discriminating Source of Airway
Obstruction—cont'd

Origin	Etiology	Symptoms

Tracheal
  External
    pressure
    on trachea
	Hematoma from
	  repeated attempts at
	  internal jugular
	  cannulation
	Compression of neck by
	  hanging or strangling
		Inspiratory stridor
		  is equal to
		  expiratory
		  stridor

Bronchial
  Inflammation
	Exposure to allergens
	Exposure to caustic
	  substances
	Foreign-body inhalation
		Expiratory stridor
		  and wheezing

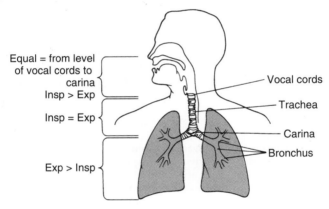

Figure 16-1   The airway. Types of stridor heard with obstruction of
the airway. *Insp,* Inspiratory; *Exp,* expiratory. (Redrawn from
Josephson G et al: *Med Clin North Am* 77[3]:542, 1993.)

- The patient exhibits psychosocial symptoms.
- Ask about a living will, power of attorney, and wishes concerning intubation for patients with known COPD.

NURSING ALERT

When wheezing decreases while the patient is waiting for
treatment, check to see if the patient is improving or if the pa-

tient's condition is worsening because of less airflow. Stridor indicates a life-threatening problem. It occurs when at least 75% of the airway is occluded. Triage immediately to the treatment area.

- Nasal flaring is noted.
- The patient has cyanosis (very late sign).
- The patient demonstrates extreme anxiety.
- The patient has a decreased LOC.

Vital Signs
- *Pulse:* A paradoxical pulse (a fall in systolic BP of at least 12 mm Hg during inspiration) indicates severe asthma related to the negative intrapleural pressure created as an asthmatic patient inspires
- *Tachycardia:* Related to fever, pain, change in cardiac output
- *Bradycardia:* Related to ischemic heart disease
- *Fever:* Related to infection
- *Tachypnea:* Related to hypoxemia and impaired ventilation
- *Blood pressure:* Hypotension related to heart failure, shock hypertension related to fluid volume overload

Pain
- Chest pain that increases on inspiration and respiratory movement and is limited to one side (suspect spontaneous pneumothorax)
- Chest tightness—associated with airway inflammation and bronchoconstriction

Dyspnea
- Continuous dyspnea unrelieved with rest (suspect spontaneous pneumothorax)
- Dyspnea that occurs during eating (suspect partial airway obstruction)
- Nocturnal dyspnea—associated with severe asthma and PAE

R

NURSING ALERT

Most patients visit the ED as a last resort measure after several home strategies have been unsuccessful. Take any complaint of dyspnea seriously.

General Observations

1. Patients in moderate to severe respiratory distress sit in the high Fowler's position and cannot tolerate lying lower than 30 degrees (orthopnea).
2. The presence of jugular vein distention (JVD) suggests right-sided heart failure, a common problem in those with PE, cardiogenic PAE, or severe COPD.
3. Patients with severe dyspnea are often extremely anxious, apprehensive, and afraid.
4. Pursed-lip breathing may be observed in patients who have pneumonia or COPD.
5. An increased anteroposterior diameter of the chest may be noted in patients who have COPD.
6. Patients with emphysema are often thin and exhibit muscle wasting.
7. Patients with asthma tend to have other allergic signs such as dark circles around the eyes, watery eyes, clear nasal discharge, eczema, and dermatitis.

NURSING ALERT

Patients with respiratory conditions can quickly decompensate. Triage those with severe dyspnea, tachypnea, chest pain, or other signs of acute respiratory distress to the ED treatment area immediately. A spontaneous pneumothorax, if it is of significant size, can progress into a tension pneumothorax, which is a medical emergency (see Chapter 20).

FOCUSED NURSING ASSESSMENT

Nursing assessment of patients with respiratory conditions centers on ventilation, perfusion, cognition, and elimination.

Ventilation
Breath sounds

Crackles (rales) or wheezing can be heard with many respiratory conditions. Absent or diminished breath sounds are also significant findings and may indicate a pneumothorax or some form of alveolar consolidation. Crackles that do not clear with coughing may indicate heart failure. Breath sounds may be absent or diminished as a result of bronchoconstriction caused by foreign-body aspiration. The right mainstem bronchus is a common site for foreign-body lodgment or passage because of the lesser angle at which it comes off the trachea in comparison to the left mainstem bronchus. Wheezing is not a reliable indicator of severity.

Respirations

Determine the character of respirations. Patients with COPD frequently use accessory muscles to assist with breathing. Tripod positioning (torso upright with elbows placed on a supporting object) is common for patients with respiratory distress. They may use the triage counter in this manner. Hyperventilation, tachypnea, and orthopnea are additional signs of respiratory distress.

A respiratory rate of >50 breaths/min for infants or >40 breaths/min for children <3 years of age is sensitive and specific for lower respiratory tract infections.

Expiratory flow rate

If the patient has a history of COPD or asthma, obtain the peak expiratory flow rate using a peak flow meter. If this value is <200 L/min, triage to the treatment area immediately.

Oxygen saturation

Determine SpO_2 levels with continuous pulse oximetry. An SpO_2 level of 91% or less is highly predictive of hospital admission.[3]

Sputum

Describe sputum production. Pink, frothy sputum is a sign of cardiogenic PAE. Patients who have pneumonia produce green, yellow, or rust-colored sputum. A change in sputum production or appearance in those with COPD indicates an acute pulmonary infection.

Dyspnea

Assess dyspnea using a standardized scale (Figure 16-2).

Perfusion

Heart sounds

A third heart sound is often noted in cases of heart failure.

Point of maximal impulse

Palpate the point of maximal impulse (PMI). The apex of the heart usually touches the anterior chest wall at or near the fifth left intercostal space, midclavicular line. Lateral displacement of the PMI is a clinical indicator of cardiac hypertrophy and possible heart failure.[4]

Jugular vein distention

Determine the presence of JVD. Place the patient in the semi-Fowler's position with the head turned to the right or

R

Circle the Number That Best Matches Your Shortness of Breath	
0	None at all
0.5	Very, very slight (just noticeable)
1	Very slight
2	Slight
3	Moderate
4	Somewhat severe
5	Severe
6	
7	Very severe
8	
9	Very, very severe (almost maximal)
10	Maximal

Figure 16-2 Dyspnea scale.

the left. Observe the jugular vein at the posterior border of the sternocleidomastoid muscle. Right atrial congestion is suspected when jugular veins distend 2 inches or more above the sternal notch (Figure 16-3). Jugular veins may be distended and the trachea shifted away from midline if a spontaneous pneumothorax has resulted in a tension pneumothorax.

Peripheral pulses and skin

Assess peripheral pulses, edema, skin temperature and color, and capillary refill. Observe for peripheral and central cyanosis. Indicators of venous insufficiency (a risk factor for PE) include pedal edema and brown, leathery extremity skin. Pedal pulses will be palpable. Pedal pulses are diminished or absent in cases of arterial insufficiency.

Cardiac rhythm

Identify the cardiac rhythm. Patients who have atrial fibrillation are at increased risk for congestive heart failure (CHF) and subsequent PE. Suspect atrial fibrillation if

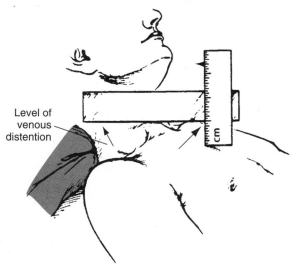

Level of
venous
distention

Figure 16-3 Jugular venous distention. (From Barkauskas V et al: *Health and Physical Assessment,* ed 2, St Louis, 1998, Mosby.)

there is a discrepancy between the radial and apical pulses. In cases of atrial fibrillation, the QRS rhythm is irregular. When in doubt, attach the patient to a cardiac monitor and obtain a rhythm strip. Individuals who have cardiogenic PAE experience tachycardic or bradycardic dysrhythmias.

Weight

Record the weight of hemodynamically stable patients. If the patient is unstable, obtain a baseline weight from the patient or family. The doses for many medications are based on weight.

Cognition

Perform a neurologic assessment and document a Glasgow Coma Scale (GCS) score (Reference Guides 10 and 18). Medications (e.g., theophylline and Alupent) used to treat pulmonary disorders exert central nervous system effects such as nervousness, tachycardia, and agitation.

Hypoxemia and hypercapnia can cause restlessness and a decreased LOC. Thrombolytics used to dissolve blood clots with some forms of PE can cause intracranial bleeding.

Elimination

Monitor the patient's urinary output. Patients who have cardiogenic PAE can experience hypervolemia and a de-

R

creased urine output. Hypovolemia or hypervolemia may occur in cases of noncardiogenic PAE. Renal response to diuresis should be documented.

Risk Factors

1. **Exposure risk:** Homosexuality, multiple partners, and IV drug abuse increase the risk of AIDS and *Pneumocystis carinii* pneumonia (PCP) (Chapter 6). PCP predisposes the patient to the development of spontaneous pneumothoraces. Smoking, air pollution, and occupational dust exposure lead to COPD development. An increased risk of spontaneous pneumothorax is associated with smoking.

2. **Gender:** Pregnancy or estrogen therapy can increase the possibility of PE.

3. **Medical history:** People with a cardiovascular disease such as CHF or atrial fibrillation are prone to cardiogenic PAE and PE. Those with deep vein thrombophlebitis are at high risk for PE.

4. **Environmental:** Institutionalized individuals are prone to pneumonia. Changes in altitude can precipitate noncardiogenic PAE.

5. **Situational:** Patients with prolonged immobility, obesity, or recent orthopedic surgery are at risk for PE. A depressed gag or cough reflex can result in aspiration pneumonia, as encountered in some patients after cerebrovascular accidents or patients with a diminished LOC. Neurologic injury, trauma, and burns are causes of noncardiogenic PAE.

6. **Anthropometric:** An increased height in proportion to decreased weight (tall and thin individuals) predisposes the individual to the development of spontaneous pneumothoraces resulting from a greater negative pleural pressure at the apex of the lung.[2]

Life Span Issues
Pediatric patients

1. Newborns are at risk for a spontaneous pneumothorax related to hyaline membrane disease and meconium aspiration.

2. Young children and adolescents experience noncardiogenic PAE secondary to trauma.

3. The incidence of staphylococcal pneumonia is greatest in children younger than 2 years of age. Respiratory syn-

cytial virus (RSV) is the most common cause of viral pneumonia in children.[5]
4. Children with a history of cystic fibrosis have a higher incidence of spontaneous pneumothorax.
5. Infants and children exposed to passive smoking experience a higher incidence of asthma.

Pregnancy
One third of pregnant women with asthma have increased symptom severity, particularly during the 19 to 36 weeks gestation period.

Geriatric patients
1. COPD occurs mainly among middle-aged and older adults. It is frequently associated with asthma.
2. Geriatric patients are at risk for pneumonia.
3. For patients older than 40 years of age, a spontaneous pneumothorax is associated with a history of COPD or pulmonary tuberculosis.[6]
4. A blunted perception of breathlessness has been found in geriatric patients. Patients may not be dyspneic with respiratory conditions. If a patient complains of dyspnea, the condition may be severe.

INITIAL INTERVENTIONS
Airway Obstruction
1. Perform the Heimlich maneuver if appropriate. Perform the chin-lift/jaw-thrust maneuver to displace the mandible and move the tongue away from the back of the throat. Assume that the patient has a cervical spine injury and do not tilt the head.
2. If the patient is not ventilating, administer two breaths by pocket mask through the patient's mouth. If resistance is met, perform the chin-lift/jaw-thrust maneuver a second time.
3. Insert an artificial airway. Artificial airways decrease gastric inflation. Oral airways are used to help keep an airway open when ventilating an unconscious patient. Have suction equipment available, since placement may stimulate the gag reflex, producing vomitus. The proper size of an oral airway can be estimated by measuring from the external corner of the patient's mouth up to the tragus of the ear (a protrusion above the earlobe). An oral airway can be inserted more easily if it is wet. Do not tape the oral airway. The patient should be able to cough out the airway if the gag reflex returns. If the patient is alert

R

enough to cough out the airway, he or she is alert enough not to need the airway. Ventilate the patient by applying a mask over the mouth and nose with the airway in place (pocket mask with one-way valve for mouth-to-mask ventilation). The most effective way of ventilating the patient is by connecting the mask to a manual resuscitation bag with an oxygen reservoir attached. The bag should be connected to oxygen at a 10- to 15-L rate. Ventilate the patient 12 times a minute. Nasopharyngeal airways may be used if the patient is awake but not alert. The use of a nasopharyngeal airway is contraindicated when the patient is receiving anticoagulants. Apply local anesthetic ointment to the device before insertion. Figure 16-4 shows proper insertion technique. The nasopharyngeal airway can be connected to a manual resuscitation bag via an endotracheal tube adaptor inserted into the nares' end of the airway (Figure 16-5). The mouth and opposite naris must be occluded while squeezing the bag. If the patient's heart rate decreases during passage, suspect that the airway is too long and is compressing the epiglottis against the laryngeal entrance, producing vagal stimulation.[7]

NURSING ALERT

If resistance is encountered during ventilation, suspect that obstruction or the patient's preexisting illness (e.g., CHF, bronchospasm, or pneumothorax) has produced increased pulmonary resistance. The underlying cause must be treated. If no resistance is encountered, suspect a leak in the ventilation system. Check all tubing and connections, the integrity of the manual resuscitation bag, and the fit of the mask, if appropriate.

4. In cases of massive emesis or bleeding associated with facial injuries, upper airway edema, or a known cervical spine fracture, anticipate the performance of a surgical cricothyroidotomy. This procedure is performed at the level of the larynx through the cricothyroid membrane. In the ED, a 1- to 2-cm transverse incision is made through the skin and cricothyroid membrane (Figure 16-6). A no. 4 Shiley tracheostomy tube or a no. 7 or smaller endotracheal tube is inserted and connected to a manual resuscitation bag.[8]

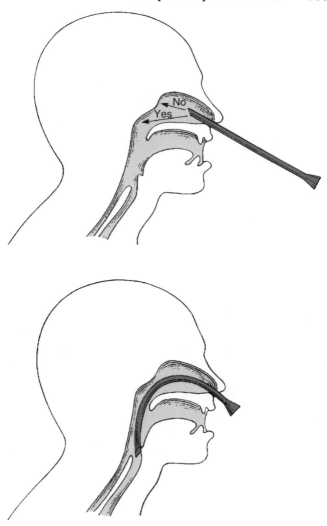

Figure 16-4 To insert a nasal airway. Insert the airway into the nostril and advance it along the floor of the nose *(top)*—not upward toward the frontal sinus, which will increase the risk of epistaxis. Slide it forward to place it in the posterior pharynx *(bottom)*. (Redrawn from Whitten: *Emerg Med* p. 115, March 15, 1990.)

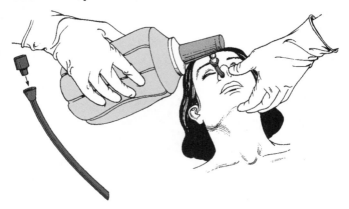

Figure 16-5 Nasal ventilation. When bag-and-mask ventilation is difficult, insert an endotracheal tube connector into a nasal airway *(left)*, place the airway, close the opposite nostril and mouth, attach the bag, and ventilate *(right)*. (Redrawn from Whitten: *Emerg Med*, 1990.)

5. Obstruction below the larynx requires emergency bronchoscopy or surgery for foreign-body removal.
6. Perform an endotracheal intubation.

Blind Nasotracheal Intubation
Blind nasotracheal intubation (BNTI) is used to minimize cervical spine movement and in some cases to avoid placing the patient in the supine position (e.g., a patient with pulmonary edema who cannot tolerate the supine position or a patient who has taken an overdose and is at risk for aspiration). However, the intubation increases blood pressure and pulse and thus may worsen hypoxemia. (See Procedure 15 for additional information.)

Orotracheal Intubation
Orotracheal intubation is the most frequently used method of definitive airway management. The patient may be conscious or unconscious. Conscious patients are usually sedated but still retain the ability to maintain an open airway and spontaneous respiratory effort. Patients are preoxygenated with 100% oxygen for 2-5 minutes. Once the endotracheal tube is in place, correct placement must be confirmed by aus-

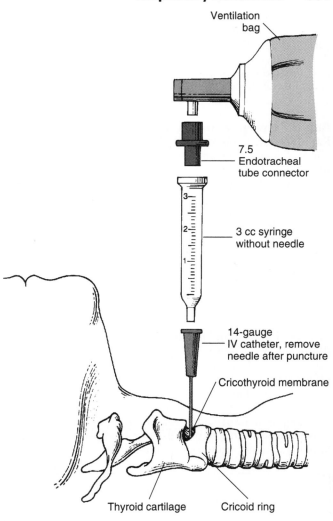

Ventilation
bag

7.5
Endotracheal
tube connector

3 cc syringe
without needle

14-gauge
IV catheter, remove
needle after puncture

Cricothyroid membrane

Thyroid cartilage   Cricoid ring

Figure 16-6   Emergency needle cricothyrotomy. Identify the
cricothyroid membrane, and puncture it with a large intravenous
catheter-over-needle. To attach the ventilation bag, place the connector from a no. 7.5 endotracheal tube into the barrel of a 3-cc syringe
and attach that to the catheter hub. (Redrawn from Whitten:
Management of the airway, *Emerg Med,* 1990.)

cultating equal and bilateral breath sounds, fogging of the endotracheal tube, equal rise and fall of the chest, no epigastric gurgling with ventilations, and improved oxygenation of the patient. The depth of the endotracheal tube should be documented by noting the centimeter mark on the endotracheal tube at the level of the teeth. The tube should be firmly secured. (See Procedure 15 for further information.)

Rapid Sequence Induction

Rapid sequence induction (RSI) is a method of inducing anesthesia and neuromuscular blockade just prior to performing endotracheal intubation. RSI facilitates success of the procedure by producing a fully relaxed state. The patient is preoxygenated with 100% oxygen, then medications are given to provide sedation (e.g., midazolam, fentanyl, etomidate) followed by a short-acting neuromuscular blocking agent (NMBA) (e.g., succinylcholine). Cricoid pressure is applied to occlude the esophagus and endotracheal intubation is performed. If the patient is a child or an adolescent, atropine is administered prior to the NMBA to prevent bradycardia during the procedure.

The use of RSI to facilitate endotracheal intubation is not without risk. Patients who cannot be successfully intubated must be ventilated by bag-valve mask with 100% oxygen until the paralysis resolves. The ability to provide a good seal on the face with the mask is of paramount importance for effective ventilations. This should be determined prior to the initiation of an RSI protocol. A surgical cricothyrotomy is an option should endotracheal intubation be unsuccessful. Additional information can be found in Procedure 15. Table 16-2 lists these steps in greater detail so the nurse can anticipate medications to be administered.

INDICATIONS FOR A DIFFICULT INTUBATION

Immobilized trauma patient	Limited jaw opening
Children, especially small children	Limited cervical mobility
Short neck	Upper airway conditions
Prominent upper incisors	Facial trauma
Receding mandible	Laryngeal trauma

TABLE 16-2 Steps for Rapid Sequence Induction

Preparation	Assess the patient for difficulty of intubation and bag-mask ventilation. Ensure adequate intravenous access. Test suction. Load the endotracheal tube with a stylet, and test the cuff. Assemble all necessary equipment and draw up all drugs. Initiate preoxygenation. Establish cardiac and blood pressure monitoring. Initiate pulse oximetry. Establish a backup plan in case of an unsuccessful intubation.
Preoxygenation	Apply 100% oxygen by mask for 5 minutes of normal tidal volume breathing. This crucial step replaces the nitrogen reserve in the lungs with oxygen and allows for at least 3 minutes of apnea without significant desaturation in a reasonable healthy adult. It is this step that allows the administration of the succinylcholine and sedative to a spontaneously breathing patient, which allows paralysis and unconsciousness to ensue, then intubation without interposed mechanical ventilation. If time does not permit 5 minutes of preoxygenation, approximately 80% of the effect can be achieved by administration of 100% oxygen for three vital capacity breaths (largest breaths that the patient can take).

Continued

Warning: Do not use a paralyzing agent if you are not prepared to surgically manage the patient's airway!

R

TABLE 16-2 Steps for Rapid Sequence Induction—cont'd

Pretreatment	In most cases, no pretreatment medication is necessary. In all children under 10 years of age, administer atropine 0.01 mg/kg IV, which will prevent the bradycardia induced by succinylcholine in this age group. This step is not necessary in adults. In patients with severe reactive airway disease, consider lidocaine 1.5 mg/kg IV, which may reduce the adverse response of the small airways to intubation. Lidocaine 1.5 mg/kg IV is also recommended in patients with proven or presumed elevation in intracranial pressure (ICP). Lidocaine in this setting is thought to reduce the ICP response to intubation that would otherwise occur. Also in cases of elevated ICP, administer a pancuranizing dose of a competitive neuromuscular blocking agent such as pancuronium or vecuronium. The dose is pancuronium 0.01 mg/kg IV or vecuronium 0.01 mg/kg IV. This dose is thought to reduce the ICP response to succinylcholine.
Paralysis	Approximately 2 minutes after the administration of the last pretreatment drug, administer a sedative agent and the succinylcholine. The choice of sedative agents is highly individual and might include thiopental sodium 3 mg/kg IV or midazolam 0.1 to 0.3 mg/kg IV among others. In general, only a single sedative agent should be used, and the agent should be administered rapidly. Immediately following the sedative, administer succinylcholine 1.5 mg/kg IV. This potent, depolarizing neuromuscular blocking agent

induces intubation-level paralysis universally in 45 to 60 seconds. As soon as the patient begins to lose consciousness and ventilation, have an assistant perform the Sellick maneuver, which is firm posterior displacement of the cricoid cartilage to occlude the esophagus and prevent gastric regurgitation. The Sellick maneuver should remain in place until the endotracheal tube has been placed with the cuff inflated and the position confirmed by auscultation and CO_2 detection. Do not ventilate the lungs during this brief phase of paralysis unless the patient was severely hypoxic before the intubation sequence was begun and the benefits of oxygenation are believed to outweigh the risks of aspiration.

Placement

Approximately 45 seconds after administration of the succinylcholine, check the mandible for flaccidity and proceed with intubation. After intubation is achieved, confirm tube placement, release the Sellick maneuver; secure the tube, and obtain a chest radiograph. In addition to auscultation of both lung fields and the epigastric area, a carbon dioxide detection device must be used to confirm tube placement. After intubation is achieved, long-acting neuromuscular blocking agents and sedatives to facilitate ongoing therapy. If the intubation attempt is unsuccessful, continue with the Sellick maneuver and ventilate and oxygenate the lungs with a bag and mask for 30 to 60 seconds before undertaking a second attempt. Continue in this manner until the airway is secured. If neither intubation nor ventilation is successful, a surgical airway or needle cricothyrotomy should be performed immediately.

Warning: Do not use a paralyzing agent if you are not prepared to surgically manage the patient's airway!

General Interventions to Promote Respiration

1. Place the patient in high Fowler's position for maximal lung expansion. If heart failure is suspected, dangle the lower extremities to decrease venous return.

> **NURSING ALERT**
>
> Do not place the patient supine with a pillow under the head, since this can precipitate airway obstruction.

2. Initiate cardiac monitoring.
3. Monitor oxygen saturation with continuous pulse oximetry.
4. Assess vital signs as acuity dictates.
5. Keep the patient NPO until stabilized. In some instances, surgery or invasive tests may be required.
6. Monitor urine output.
7. Save a sputum sample in a sterile container. Sputum cultures may be ordered.
8. Suction the patient's airway if appropriate. Hyperoxygenate and ventilate before suctioning.
9. Reassure the patient. Severe dyspnea frequently produces anxiety.

> **NURSING ALERT**
>
> Oxygen administration is controversial for some respiratory conditions. In situations where diminished breath sounds are auscultated (spontaneous pneumothorax), oxygen can be administered per device tolerated by the patient (e.g., nasal cannula or simple face mask). However, if the patient has a history of pulmonary disease (and the pneumothorax may be a secondary condition), administer a low concentration of oxygen, preferably 2 L or less. Reference Guide 14 lists oxygen devices and their possible oxygen delivery ranges. It is preferable to obtain a blood sample for arterial blood gas analysis before initiating oxygen administration, but patient distress should determine your sequence of actions.

PRIORITY NURSING DIAGNOSES

Risk for impaired gas exchange
Risk for ineffective airway clearance
Risk for altered tissue perfusion

Risk for ineffective breathing pattern
Risk for pain
Risk for infection (pulmonary)
Risk for activity intolerance
Risk for ineffective individual coping
Risk for knowledge deficit

◆ **Impaired gas exchange** related to decreased pulmonary ventilation and perfusion as demonstrated by low Po_2 levels, elevated CO_2 levels, dyspnea, cyanosis, and decreased oxygen saturation:
INTERVENTIONS
- Administer oxygen.
- Monitor arterial oxygen saturation via pulse oximetry.
- Report and treat significant changes in ABGs (pH <7.35 or >7.45, Po_2 <80 mm Hg, Pco_2 <35 or >45 mm Hg, HCO_3^- <22 or >26 mEq/L, and Sao_2 <95).
- Administer bronchodilators as ordered.

◆ **Ineffective airway clearance** related to obstruction, decreased mucociliary function, increased mucus production and viscosity, muscle weakness, and fatigue, as demonstrated by frequent nonproductive cough, adventitious or diminished breath sounds, airway noise, and tachypnea:
INTERVENTIONS
- Assist with coughing and deep breathing exercises.
- Initiate endotracheal suctioning as ordered.
- Administer mucolytic and bronchodilating agents as ordered.
- For airway obstruction, see Initial Interventions in the Triage Assessment section.

◆ **Altered tissue perfusion** related to hypoxemia, as demonstrated by peripheral or central cyanosis, cool extremities, chest pain, and mental status changes:
INTERVENTIONS
- Administer vasodilators and oxygen as ordered.
- Limit activity to decrease myocardial oxygen demands.

R

◆ **Ineffective breathing pattern** related to muscle weakness and alveolar hyperinflation, as demonstrated by tachypnea, hyperventilation, and dyspnea:
INTERVENTIONS
- Assist with breathing by placing the patient in the high Fowler's position.
- Initiate the administration of supplemental oxygen as ordered.

- Coach the patient's breathing (see Discharge Implications for COPD).
- Promote nutritional status by encouraging a high-carbohydrate diet when appropriate.
- Encourage fluid intake.
- Decrease the patient's anxiety by acknowledging the patient's dyspnea.

◆ **Pain** related to pleural irritation as demonstrated by complaints of pleuritic (sharp) pain with respirations, by chest wall tenderness, and by restlessness:
INTERVENTIONS
- Administer analgesics as ordered.
- Teach the patient splinting with cough.

◆ **Pulmonary infection** related to a bacterial or viral invasion of the pulmonary system and by immunosuppression, as demonstrated by fever, positive sputum cultures, productive cough, dyspnea, and tachypnea:
INTERVENTIONS
- Administer antibiotics as ordered.
- Encourage dietary supplements as ordered.
- Administer antipyretics for fever >100° F (38.3° C).

◆ **Activity intolerance** related to decreased pulmonary function, as demonstrated by shortness of breath, fatigue, chest pain, and noncompensatory vital sign changes with activity:
INTERVENTIONS
- Gradually increase activity.
- Monitor the patient for vital sign changes inappropriate for activity.
- Assist the patient with movement, using a wheelchair as appropriate.
- Assess the home environment for breathing demands (e.g., steps and transportation ability).
- Seek appropriate home health referral.

◆ **Ineffective individual coping** related to dyspnea, increased dependence, and changes in body structure:
INTERVENTIONS
- Reassure the patient.
- Include the patient and the patient's family in the treatment plan development when feasible.

◆ **Knowledge deficit** related to lack of information regarding the disease process, as demonstrated by the in-

ability to describe home care, minimal participation in
the treatment plan, and the verbalizing of inaccurate
information:

INTERVENTIONS
- Instruct the patient and the patient's family on the disease process and the treatment plan.
- Determine the patient's and family's understanding with
  nonthreatening questions.

PRIORITY DIAGNOSTIC TESTS

Laboratory Tests

Serum electrolyte levels: Potassium, chloride, and sodium
levels fluctuate with diuresis and impaired renal function. Diuretics are used to treat fluid volume excess in
cases of cardiogenic PAE.

Complete blood count: White blood cell counts are elevated
or decreased in cases of pulmonary inflammation or infection. An elevated hemoglobin level may indicate polycythemia, a clinical indicator of prolonged hypoxemia.

Antibody titers and blood serology: These tests are used to
determine the cause of pulmonary infection.

Arterial blood gases: An ABG test is used to evaluate oxygenation and the acid-base balance. It is useful in most
respiratory conditions. The test is not definitive for PE.
Supplemental oxygen is adjusted according to ABG test
results and clinical symptoms. Respiratory alkalosis is
common in cases of asthma. If the PCO_2 starts to return
to normal, it may indicate respiratory muscle fatigue.
With patients who have chronic conditions, a forced expiratory volume (FEV) of 1 liter in 1 second indicates the
need for ABG analysis.

Activated partial thromboplastin time (aPTT): An aPTT
test is used to evaluate the effectiveness of heparin therapy in cases of pulmonary embolism. The goal is to maintain aPTT at 1.5 to 2 times the control time.

Prothrombin time (PT): A PT test is used to evaluate the effectiveness of oral anticoagulation (e.g., Coumadin). The
goal is to maintain PT at approximately 2.5 times the
control time. Coumadin is used to prevent clot formation with patients who are at risk for PE.

Prealbumin, transferrin levels: These levels are used to
evaluate nutritional status.

R

Blood cultures: Blood cultures are used to diagnose bacteremia and the causative agent for those with pneumonia.

Sputum culture and sensitivity: These are used to determine the causative agent of pneumonia and other respiratory infections. If pneumonia is suspected, broad-spectrum antibiotics are started before culture results return, in most instances. More organism-specific antibiotics are ordered when culture results become available.

Plasma DNA assay: This is used to diagnose a pulmonary embolism in the event of inconclusive lung scans.[9]

Radiographic Tests

Chest x-ray: A chest x-ray examination is used to evaluate heart and lung structures. It is nonspecific for a pulmonary embolus. Infiltrates may be present with cases of pneumonia. Hyperinflation, a flattened diaphragm, and cardiomegaly are present with cases of COPD. Negative lung expansion is present in cases of spontaneous pneumothorax. Some foreign bodies may be radiopaque. Atelectasis of the involved lung may be present in cases of foreign-body aspiration.

Venography: A venography is the injection of dye into the veins to detect DVT, a risk factor for pulmonary embolism. IV access is necessary for this procedure.

Pulmonary angiogram: Dye is injected into the pulmonary vasculature. This is the most definitive test for a pulmonary embolism. Emergency medications may be administered if complications occur during the procedure; therefore IV access is required.

NURSING ALERT

Determine that the patient is not allergic to radiographic dye, iodine, or seafood before dye tests. Premedication with Benadryl or Tylenol or the use of a less allergenic substance may be required.

Other Tests

Ventilation and perfusion scan: A lung scan is performed after the inhalation of xenon-127. The perfusion scan is completed after the IV injection of technetium-97 macroaggregated albumin. Areas of poor ventilation and inadequate perfusion are identified.

Doppler ultrasonography: When Doppler ultrasonography is used, a handheld transducer that produces high-frequency sound waves is moved across the skin of the extremity being examined. Audible tones proportional to blood velocity help with the detection of thrombi.

Electrocardiogram (ECG): An ECG is used to detect heart failure, dysrhythmias, and strain on the right side of the heart.

Echocardiogram: The echocardiogram is used to assess right ventricular function.

Bronchoscopy: A fiberoptic or rigid scope is inserted to examine the internal structures of the airway and lungs. The administration of premedication such as Demerol or atropine may be necessary to decrease secretions and discomfort during the procedure. The patient is NPO after the procedure until the gag reflex returns. Rigid bronchoscopy is performed in the operating room. Bronchoscopy may be used to remove foreign bodies.

Peak expiratory flow rate (PEFR): This is the greatest flow that can be obtained during forced exhalation starting from full-lung inflation. A peak flow meter is used to measure this value. The patient can monitor the PEFR at home. A normal peak flow ranges from 400 to 600 L/min. A peak flow <200 L/min indicates obstruction or respiratory fatigue. PEFR correlates well with forced expiratory volume (FEV_1) obtained by spirometry. The PEFR may not be reliably obtained from children. Oxygen saturation values may be more useful in determining the severity of the situation.

Spirometry (pulmonary function test): Use a spirometer to determine lung capacities, lung volumes, and flow rates. This is useful for determining the severity of airway obstruction in cases of COPD and other respiratory problems. Airway obstruction is confirmed by a reduction in the ratio of FEV_1 to forced vital capacity (FEV_1/FVC).

Bronchoprovocation testing: Airway response to histamine or methacholine is tested. If FEV_1 is <1000 ml or PEFR is <200 L/min after medication administration, a diagnosis of asthma is made.

R

COLLABORATIVE INTERVENTIONS
Overview
1. Administer supplemental oxygen as ordered. The delivery system and amount of oxygen used for enhancing oxygenation outcomes depend on the severity of the disease process. Various types of oxygen delivery systems are described in Reference Guide 14. Be prepared for intubation, since respiratory conditions can rapidly deteriorate.
2. Initiate IV access. Two IV lines are preferable in cases of severe respiratory distress. An intermittent infusion device may be substituted for continuous IV fluids if fluid volume overload is suspected.
3. Place a urinary catheter according to the physician's order. Patients with cardiogenic PAE require diuretics and accurate urinary output measurement.

Clinical Conditions
Asthma
Asthma is characterized by airway inflammation (mucus hypersecretion), increased airway responsiveness to stimuli (airway edema), and reversible airway obstruction. The aim of treatment is decreasing inflammation, thereby decreasing obstruction.
SYMPTOMS
- The patient experiences wheezing, has a paradoxical pulse, and has a PEFR <400 L/min.
- The use of beta-blocking agents (e.g., propranolol, timolol, and pindolol) may precipitate asthma in a geriatric patient.
DIAGNOSIS
- Diagnosis is based on clinical presentation. The "Asthma Classification by Severity" box classifies asthma according to severity.
TREATMENT
- Although medications are addressed in Table 16-3, further discussion is needed about some medications.
- Inhaled beta-agonist (e.g., albuterol) agents in either inhaler or nebulizer form are initially used. Continuous nebulization is more effective than intermittent nebulization for patients with PEFR <200 L/min.[10]
- Beta-adrenergic agonist agents (e.g., subcutaneous epinephrine) are used only for younger asthmatic patients

ASTHMA CLASSIFICATION BY SEVERITY

Mild asthma

More than two exacerbations weekly
Good exercise tolerance
Awakened from sleep with symptoms less than twice monthly

Moderate asthma

More than two exacerbations weekly
Fewer than three severe episodes requiring urgent care annually

Severe asthma

Daily symptoms
More than three episodes requiring urgent care annually
More than two hospitalizations year

(<35 years old) whose airways are so narrowed because of bronchoconstriction that inhaled medication may not penetrate far enough into the lungs. They are not used to treat older patients or patients with a positive cardiac history because of their cardiovascular side effects (e.g., an increased heart rate and contractility). The response to beta-agonists decreases with age.

- Children who are taking steroids on a long-term basis need close monitoring for signs of adrenal suppression and decreased growth.
- Hospitalization is indicated for patients with the following:
  1. A respiratory rate >30 breaths/min
  2. A heart rate >120 beats/min (bradycardia may be present if severely hypoxic)
  3. PEFR <120 L/min
  4. FEV_1 <1000 ml
  5. O_2Sat ≤91%

The best indicator of a good response to treatment is improvement in the PEFR or FEV_1 within 30 minutes of therapy.

R

NURSING ALERT

If an asthmatic patient requires intubation and mechanical ventilation, monitor the patient closely for barotrauma and pneumothorax. High airway pressure may be needed to ventilate the patient.

Text continued on p. 582

TABLE 16-3 Drug Summary

Drug	Classifications	Douse and route	Special considerations
Acetylcysteine (Mucomyst)	Mucolytic	*Inhalation:* Adult: 1-10 ml of 20% solution q4-6h or 2-20 ml of 10% solution q4-6h *Direct instillation:* Adult: 1-2 ml or 10% to 20% solution q1-4h; child same as adult	Cautious use with patients who have asthma or severe respiratory infections and with geriatric patients May be instilled directly into tracheostomy Have suction apparatus available for immediate use
Albuterol (Proventil)	Beta-adrenergic agonist, bronchodilator	*PO:* 2 to 4 mg, three to four times per day *Inhaled:* 1 to 2 inhalations q4-6h *Nebulizer:* 2.5 mg in nebulized form	Side effects include CNS stimulation Proper use of inhaler necessary for therapeutic dosing
Captopril* (Capoten)	Angiotensin-converting enzyme inhibitor, vasodilator	*PO:* 6.25 to 12.5 mg tid up to 50 mg tid	Exaggerated hypertension may occur with first dose
Cromolyn sodium	Nonsteroidal antiinflammatory agent, inhibits release of mediators, prevents degranulation of mast cells	*Metered dose inhaler:* One spray inhaled qid	Not recommended for children less than 6 years of age

Drug	Classification	Dosage	Side Effects/Notes
Digoxin*(Lanoxin)	Cardiac glycoside	Initially, PO 10 to 15 µg/kg in divided doses over 24 to 48 hr; IV: 10 to 15 µg/kg in divided doses over 24 hr	Side effects include AV block; Cautious use with geriatric patients and in cases of hypokalemia, cor pulmonale, and lung disease
Diltiazem*(Cardizem)	Calcium channel blocking agent, vasodilator	PO: 30 mg qid	May cause headache, dizziness, lightheadedness; advise patient to make slow position changes
Epinephrine	Alpha- and beta-adrenergic agonist, bronchodilator	*Asthma:* Adult: *SC*—0.1 to 0.5 ml of 1:1000 q20min to 4 hr; *Inhalation*—1 inhalation q4h prn; Child: *SC*—0.01 ml/kg of 1:1000 q20min to 4 hr; *Inhalation*—1 inhalation q4h prn	Use tuberculin syringe for greater accuracy; May cause CNS stimulations and cardiovascular side effects
Erythromycin (E-Mycin)	Antiinfective, antibiotic	*Moderate to severe infections:* Adult: PO 250-500 mg q6h; Child: PO 30-50 mg/kg/day divided q6h	Do not administer on empty stomach; can cause severe abdominal pain, nausea, and vomiting

Continued

*Data from Wilson BA, Shannon MT: In *Govoni and Hayes nurses' drug guide,* 1993, Norwalk, Conn, 1993, Appleton & Lange.
AV, Atrioventricular; *CNS,* central nervous system; *GI,* gastrointestinal; *MI,* myocardial infarction; *HR,* heart rate; *PFT,* pulmonary function test.

TABLE 16-3 Drug Summary—cont'd

Drug	Classifications	Douse and route	Special considerations
Furosemide*(Lasix)	Loop diuretic	Adult: PO 20-80 mg in one or more divided doses up to 600 mg/day IV/IM: 20-40 mg in one or more divided doses up to 600 mg/day	Cautious use with geriatric patients Cardiogenic shock associated with acute MI Adverse affects: postural hypotension, circulatory collapse, electrolyte imbalance
Heparin	Anticoagulant	IV: 100 U/kg loading dose followed by maintenance or intermittent doses of 25,000-35,000 U/day	Goal: a PTT of 1-2 times control Monitor for bleeding
Hydralazine hydrochloride (Apresoline)	Nonnitrate vasodilator, antihypertensive	Adult: PO—10-50 mg qid; IM—10-50 mg q4-6h; IV—10-20 mg q4-6h Child: PO 3-7.5 mg/kg/day in 4 divided doses	Adverse affects include headache, orthostatic hypotension
Ipratropium bromide (Atrovent)	Bronchodilator, anticholinergic, inhibits bronchoconstricting vagal reflex	Inhalation: 20 µg ipratropium, 2-4 inhalations 4 times/day	Frequent PFTs to determine effectiveness Used in chronic management of COPD, not in acute asthma Side effects include dry mouth

Magnesium sulfate	Bronchial smooth muscle–relaxing agent	1.2 g over 20 min	Still used experimentally in acute asthma Mechanism of action not clear
Methylprednisolone	Corticosteroid	Adult: *PO*—40-60 mg/day; *IM*—240 mg; *IV*—60-80 mg up to 125 mg Inhaler comes in a variety of forms (e.g., beclomethasone); adult: 0.84 mg/day (depending on concentration, about 20 puffs/day); child: 0.42 mg/day (depending on concentration, about 10 puffs/day)	Used in treatment of acute severe asthma in IV form Must be used cautiously with geriatric patients, since side effects may exacerbate conditions of aging (e.g., osteoporosis, hypertension, and diabetes) Side effects include thrush, hoarseness; inhaler use side effects can be prevented by rinsing mouth and throat after using inhaler or by using a spacer device
Minocycline hydrochloride (Minocin)	Antiinfective, tetracycline antibiotic	PO/IV: Adult—200 mg followed by 100 mg q12h	Use with pleural sclerosis: 5 mg/kg in total volume of 50 ml sterile water Extremely painful for patient

Continued

*Data from Wilson BA, Shannon MT: In *Govoni and Hayes nurses' drug guide*, 1993, Norwalk, Conn, 1993, Appleton & Lange.
AV, Atrioventricular; *CNS*, central nervous system; *GI*, gastrointestinal; *MI*, myocardial infarction; *HR*, heart rate; *PFT*, pulmonary function test.

TABLE 16-3 Drug Summary—cont'd

Drug	Classifications	Douse and route	Special considerations
Morphine sulfate*	Narcotic (opiate) agonist	Adult: IV 2.5-15 mg q4h or 0.8-10 mg/hr by continuous infusion	Adverse effects include severe respiratory depression IV push: may dilute in 4-5 ml of sterile water and give slowly over 4-5 min; undiluted: push slowly 1 mg/min
Nitroprusside,* sodium (Nipride)	Antihypertensive, nonnitrate vasodilator	Adult: IV 0.5-10 μg/kg/min	Must be diluted in 250-500 ml D_5W Use infusion pump Constant monitoring of BP indicated with use Protect solution from light
Penicillin G	Antiinfective, beta-lactam antibiotic	Adult: *PO*—1.6-3.2 million U divided q6h; *IV/IM*—1.2-2.4 million U divided q4h Child: *PO*—25,000-100,000 U/kg divided q6hr; *IV/IM*—25,000-300,000 U/kg divided q4h	Contraindicated in hypersensitivity to any penicillin Monitor for signs of sensitivity to drug; allergy is unpredictable

Pneumococcal vaccine (Pneumovax)	—	SC/IM: 0.5 ml in a single SC or IM dose, preferably in deltoid or lateral midthigh	Should not be used with active infections May cause local and systemic reactions, including fever, local soreness, erythema, induration
Prazosin* hydrochloride (Minipress)	Alpha-adrenergic antagonist, vasodilator	PO: 1 mg hs, then 1 mg bid or tid, may increase to 20 mg/day in divided doses	Hypotensive effects increased with diuretics and other hypotensive agents; monitor BP for hypotension
Streptokinase	Thrombolytic enzyme	IV: 250,000 IU over 30 min loading dose, then 100,000 IU/hr for 48-72 hr	Used in cases of severe hemodynamic compromise with pulmonary embolism Avoid punctures, tissue trauma, observe for bleeding
Talc	Sclerosing agent	0.5 g talc in 250 ml isotonic saline for pleural sclerosis	Extremely painful for patient
Terbutaline sulfate (Brethine)	Beta-adrenergic agonist, bronchodilator	Adult: PO—2.5-5 mg tid at 6-hr intervals; SC—0.25 mg q15-30 min up to 0.5 mg in 4 hr; Inhaled—2 inhalations separated by 60 sec q4-6h	May cause CNS stimulation Monitor BP and HR

Continued

*Data from Wilson BA, Shannon MT: In Govoni and Hayes nurses' drug guide, 1993, Norwalk, Conn, 1993, Appleton & Lange.
AV, Atrioventricular; CNS, central nervous system; GI, gastrointestinal; MI, myocardial infarction; HR, heart rate; PFT, pulmonary function test.

R

TABLE 16-3 Drug Summary—cont'd

Drug	Classifications	Douse and route	Special considerations
Theophylline (Theo-Dur)	Bronchodilator	PO/IV: 400-2000 mg/day	Observe for toxicity, GI upset, nervousness, insomnia, palpitations, dysrhythmias, seizures Presence of CHF, cor pulmonale, hepatic disease, use of cimetidine, erythromycin, or ciprofloxacin decreases theophylline clearance and degradation, increasing the likelihood of toxicity
Urokinase	Thrombolytic enzyme	IV: 4400 IU/kg diluted in 0.9% NaCl or D_5W infused over 10 min loading dose, followed by 4400 IU/kg/hr for 12 hr	Special filter required; see streptokinase for additional nursing implications

Verapamil* hydrochloride (Calan)	Calcium channel blocker, vasodilator	Adult: *PO*—40-80 mg tid or 90-240 mg sustained release 1-2 times/day up to 480 mg/day; *IV*—5-10 mg IV push, dilute in 5 ml sterile water, administer no faster than 10 mg/min	Monitor BP and HR Transient hypotension may occur with IV bolus
Warfarin sodium* (Coumadin)	Oral anticoagulant	PO: 10-15 mg/day for 2-5 days, then 2-10 mg once per day to maintain a PT of 1.5-2.5 times control	Observe for minor or major hemorrhage Periodic PTs are measured
Zafirlukast	Leukotriene receptor antagonist (used in asthma)	20 mg PO bid	Not approved for use in children younger than 12 years
Sileuton	Lipooxygenase inhibitor (used in asthma)	600 mg PO qid	Not approved for children

*Data from Wilson BA, Shannon MT: In *Govoni and Hayes nurses' drug guide*, 1993, Norwalk, Conn, 1993, Appleton & Lange.
AV, Atrioventricular; *CNS*, central nervous system; *GI*, gastrointestinal; *MI*, myocardial infarction; *HR*, heart rate; *PFT*, pulmonary function test.

R

Bronchitis
SYMPTOMS
- The patient experiences substernal chest discomfort, dyspnea, wheezing, fatigue, fever, and chills. Scattered wheezes and rhonchi are auscultated. A focal area of crackles, wheezes, or rhonchi is more indicative of PE or pneumonia.

DIAGNOSIS
- Diagnostic tests usually are not necessary unless the symptoms have lasted for 2 weeks or longer or the possibility of CHF exists. In these cases a chest x-ray is obtained. A CBC and chest x-ray may be obtained in cases where a pneumonia could be more serious (e.g., child, elderly, or immunosuppressed patient).

TREATMENT
- Direct the patient to have rest, fluids, and humidification of heat.
- The patient should use cough suppressant only at night.
- Administer acetaminophen.
- Administer albuterol syrup (children) or an inhaler.
- Initiate the use of antibiotics if the sputum of a smoker is purulent of if the mucus has changed from clear to purulent.

Pulmonary alveolar edema
Noncardiogenic pulmonary alveolar edema
Noncardiogenic pulmonary alveolar edema is also known as adult respiratory distress syndrome.

SYMPTOMS
- The patient has respiratory distress with tachypnea, orthopnea, crackles, hypovolemia or hypervolemia, hypotension, low or high pulmonary artery pressures, and faint heart sounds.

DIAGNOSIS
- A chest x-ray examination indicates infiltrates.
- Severe hypoxemia is documented by ABGs.
- Pulmonary artery catheterization reveals low or high pulmonary artery pressures.
- The patient has a history of risk factors for noncardiogenic PAE (e.g., recent trauma, hemorrhage, drug overdose, or infection).
- The patient demonstrates clinical symptoms.

TREATMENT
- Initiate the administration of supplemental oxygen.
- Continuous positive airway pressure (CPAP or BiPAP) by

mask or positive end-expiratory pressure (PEEP) or pressure support for the intubated patient may be necessary to improve alveolar inflation.

- The use of steroids is controversial.
- Initiate inhaled surfactant.
- Careful diuresis or fluid replacement may be used, depending on preload measurements.

Cardiogenic pulmonary alveolar edema

SYMPTOMS

- The patient has or exhibits tachypnea, orthopnea, crackles, wheezes, pink and frothy sputum, high pulmonary artery pressures, hypervolemia, signs of heart failure (e.g., JVD, peripheral edema, and organomegaly), and hypertension.

DIAGNOSIS

- Diagnosis is based on the presence of clinical symptoms.
- An arterial blood analysis reveals hypoxemia and, eventually, hypercarbia secondary to fatigue.
- Infiltrates can be seen on a chest x-ray film.
- Pulmonary artery catheterization reveals high pulmonary artery pressures.
- The patient has a history of cardiovascular disease.

TREATMENT

- Initiate supplemental oxygen, intubation, and mechanical ventilation in cases of severe respiratory distress. CPAP or BiPAP may be used before intubation and mechanical ventilation.
- Provide preload and afterload reduction by diuretics (e.g., furosemide), as well as vasodilators (e.g., nitroprusside or hydralazine [direct acting]), calcium channel blockers (e.g., verapamil or diltiazem), prazosin (an alpha-adrenergic blocking agent), and captopril (an angiotensin-converting enzyme inhibitor). Administer nitroglycerin sublingually, as a paste or IV.
- Use bronchodilators (e.g., albuterol by inhaler) to enhance alveolar ventilation. Use cardiac glycosides (e.g., digoxin) and inotropes to improve cardiac contractility.
- IV morphine sulfate is administered to decrease venous return and alleviate anxiety. Beware of respiratory suppression if the patient is not intubated.
- Dialysis or continuous venous-venous hemofiltration may be indicated.
- In some instances rotating tourniquets are used in cases refractory to medical treatment.[11]

R

Pulmonary embolism
SYMPTOMS
- The patient experiences dyspnea, sudden pleuritic chest pain, cough, hemoptysis, diaphoresis, apprehension, tachypnea, tachycardia, or crackles.
- The triad of petechiae (chest, axilla), dyspnea, and mental confusion is suggestive of fat emboli.

DIAGNOSIS
- Diagnosis is based on a ventilation and perfusion scan, a chest x-ray examination, a pulmonary angiography, hypoxemia by ABG analysis, and the presence of clinical symptoms.
- Diagnostic tests also include those such as a Doppler ultrasound (color duplex ultrasonography) of the lower extremities to assess for DVT.

TREATMENT
- Initiate the administration of supplemental oxygen, and initiate intubation with mechanical ventilation in cases of severe respiratory distress.
- Initiate anticoagulation (e.g., heparin IV or low-molecular-weight heparin, then PO Coumadin).
- Administer thrombolytics (streptokinase, urokinase IV, or intrapulmonary) in cases of severe PE.
- Immobilize as applicable the lower extremity that has DVT.
- Apply antiembolic devices (e.g., elastic, gradient, or intermittent compression stockings) on lower extremities in the absence of DVT.
- Surgical embolectomy is a last resort for massive life-threatening PE.

Pneumonia
SYMPTOMS
- The patient has fever, shaking chills, pleuritic chest pain, tachypnea, diaphoresis, crackles, and a productive cough with purulent or rust-colored sputum.

DIAGNOSIS
- Diagnosis is based on infiltrates on a chest x-ray examination, positive results from sputum cultures, a CBC showing leukocytosis, and the presence of clinical symptoms.

TREATMENT
- Initiate the administration of supplemental oxygen.
- Administer broad-spectrum antibiotics (e.g., penicillin and erythromycin).

- Use bronchodilators and mucolytics such as theophylline and acetylcysteine to mobilize secretions.
- Administer analgesics for pleuritic chest pain.
- Provide chest physiotherapy.
- Provide nutritional support.
- Initiate oral or IV hydration.
- Direct bed rest to decrease oxygen demands.

Chronic obstructive pulmonary disease

SYMPTOMS

- The patient has dyspnea, a productive cough, wheezing, pursed-lip exhalation (see Discharge Implications), tripod positioning, the use of accessory respiratory muscles, increased chest anteroposterior diameter, and diminished breath sounds.

DIAGNOSIS

- Pulmonary function tests show a reduced FEV_1/FVC ratio. ABG test results indicate hypoxemia and hypercapnia.
- A chest x-ray examination reveals hyperinflation.
- Clinical symptoms are present.

TREATMENT

- Initiate supplemental oxygen based on ABG results.
- Administer inhaled anticholinergics (e.g., ipratropium bromide [Atrovent]) to bronchodilate.
- Provide antibiotics for infection.
- The use of steroids is controversial.
- Provide mucolytics to mobilize secretions.
- Administer beta-adrenergic agonists (e.g., albuterol) to bronchodilate.
- Subcutaneous epinephrine or terbutaline is administered in cases of severe airway obstruction for those who are unable to receive aerosol bronchodilating agents.
- Oxygen may be administered using a Venturi mask with an oxygen concentration of 24% to 28%.
- If the patient is using home oxygen, the same dosage is used in the ED. Home oxygen is indicated when PaO_2 is <55 mm Hg or O_2 saturation is <85%.

Spontaneous pneumothorax

Spontaneous pneumothorax may occur as a primary disorder, disassociated with pulmonary disease, or as a secondary condition, usually related to pulmonary fibrosis or the presence of pulmonary bullae and blebs. Symptoms for both types of spontaneous pneumothorax are similar, but

R

severity is greater when the pneumothorax is caused by a preexisting pulmonary condition.

SYMPTOMS

- The patient experiences pain on inspiration on the same side as the pneumothorax.
- Dyspnea is present, depending on the size of the pneumothorax and the remaining pulmonary reserve.
- In cases of secondary spontaneous pneumothorax, the PaO_2 may be <55 mm Hg and the $PaCO_2$ may be >50 mm Hg.
- FEV_1 may be <1000 ml.
- Subcutaneous emphysema may be present.
- Percussion over the affected area produces tympany.

DIAGNOSIS

- The size and location of the pneumothorax are confirmed by chest radiography.

TREATMENT

Observation

If the patient is not dyspneic and the respiratory rate is within normal limits, observation may be preferred. Usually the pneumothorax is $<15\%$ of the hemithorax as confirmed by chest radiography.[2] This type of treatment is used for first occurrences without the presence of preexisting pulmonary disease.

Aspiration (using unidirectional valve device)

Aspiration of air from the pleural space is more successful for patients who have primary spontaneous pneumothorax. A guidewire is inserted over a 16-gauge needle. An 8 Fr aspiration catheter is then inserted over the guidewire, and the guidewire is removed. A 60-ml syringe is attached to the catheter using a three-way stopcock. Before removal the stopcock is closed to the patient and a repeat chest radiograph film is obtained. If no lung expansion occurs, a Heimlich valve is attached to the catheter. If no lung reexpansion is seen on the second radiograph, the Heimlich device is connected to a chest catheter draining system (e.g., Pleurovac) at a negative pressure of 20 cm H_2O.[2,12]

NURSING ALERT

Aspiration is rarely successful in cases of iatrogenic pneumothorax from central venous line placement. Anticipate the need for chest tube insertion.

Chest tube insertion

A 16 to 24 Fr thoracostomy tube may be placed in the 4th
to 6th intercostal space, midaxillary line, for air expulsion.
The patient should be placed in the supine position with
the head of the bed elevated 30 degrees. The patient's arm
nearest the procedure should be placed behind the patient's head. The tube is connected to a closed draining system (see Procedure 7).

NURSING ALERT

If reexpansion is not occurring after placement of the chest
tube, check to see if the connecting tubing is kinked or
clogged. Confirm that the tubing is connected to the suction
apparatus correctly, if appropriate.

Chest tube insertion with instillation of sclerosing agent

A sclerosing agent (such as minocycline) may be injected
through the chest tube. This is a painful procedure. The
patient should be sedated before the instillation, and lidocaine 4 mg/kg in 50 ml saline should be injected intrapleu-
rally before the instillation of the sclerosing agent. The recurrence rate of spontaneous pneumothorax is lower when
this form of treatment is used.

Thoracoscopy

The patient may be admitted, and thoracoscopy may be
performed. After a thoracoscope is inserted, a sclerosing
agent may be administered, bullae ligated, or blebs ablated
by laser or resection.

Thoracotomy

The patient is admitted, and surgical intervention is used.
This treatment is rare and is associated with severe unilateral pneumothorax that is unresponsive to reexpansion by
other modalities. It may also be used for simultaneous bilateral pneumothoraces.

R

NURSING ALERT

The size of the pneumothorax is not related to response to
treatment. The longer the symptoms have been present, the
easier the pneumothorax is to resolve.

NURSING SURVEILLANCE

1. Monitor respiratory function, including breath sounds.
2. Monitor dyspnea.
3. Note the trend of vital signs and oxygenation status (SaO_2, PaO_2, PcO_2).
4. Monitor intake and output.
5. Monitor the patient for cardiac dysrhythmias.
6. Analyze laboratory tests and report significant changes to the physician.
7. Assess the patient for therapeutic response and adverse reactions to medications.
8. Evaluate and support effective coping strategies.
9. Monitor PEFRs (if appropriate).

EXEPECTED PATIENT OUTCOMES

1. Shortness of breath improves from initial assessment.
2. The ABG levels trend toward normal.
3. The heart rate ranges from 60 to 100 beats/min.
4. The mean arterial pressure remains at 70 to 100 mm Hg.
5. Urinary output is >30 ml/hr or >0.5 ml/kg/hr.
6. Life-threatening dysrhythmias are absent.
7. The patient and patient's family use effective coping strategies.
8. Wheezing and stridor are absent, and spontaneous ventilation is present.

DISCHARGE INSTRUCTIONS

General

1. Teach patients who are using oxygen at home about safety. There must be no open flame within 6 feet of the oxygen.
2. Guide the smoker to appropriate resources for smoking cessation. These may include medications, support groups, and relaxation training. Teach the smoker to avoid secondhand smoke.
3. Encourage adequate nutrition to support respiratory function.
4. The geriatric population and those with COPD may benefit from annual influenza vaccines and in some instances from the one-time pneumococcal pneumonia vaccine (Pneumovax). The pneumococcal

vaccine is contraindicated for those with an active pulmonary infection. Assist the patient with an appropriate referral.
5. Environmental pollutants should be avoided for all patients with or without respiratory disease.
6. Infection control can be supported by frequent hand washing, the use of tissues, and masks for those who are immunosuppressed.
7. Instruct patients regarding the home administration of medications.

Asthma
1. Involve children in the management of their asthma.
2. Teach the use of metered dose inhalers (MDIs). MDIs may be difficult to use for persons with impaired mental function, poor motor coordination, or weakened, arthritic hands. The use of spacers attached to the MDI allows the drug to be expelled into a large plastic chamber. The patient can inhale the medication from the chamber so activation of MDI does not have to be coordinated with inhalation. Spacers also decrease the incidence of thrush and hoarseness associated with steroid MDI. The "Proper Metered Dose" box explains proper technique.
3. Stress to pregnant asthma patients that hypoxia is a greater risk to the fetus than are inhaled medications.

PROPER METERED DOSE INHALER TECHNIQUE

- Shake the canister.
- Hold the canister approximately 2 inches (4-5 cm) in front of the mouth.
- Completely exhale.
- Begin to inhale.
- Activate the canister.
- Continue to breathe deeply and hold your breath for 5 sec.
- Wait for response (1 to 10 min) depending on your symptoms.
- Repeat as needed.

R

4. Teach parents about the effect of passive smoking on children with asthma.
5. Teach home monitoring of PEFR. PEFR is best measured with the patient in the standing position. The patient breathes deep and blows out fast and hard through the peak flow meter. This maneuver is performed three times, and the highest value is recorded. Portable peak expiratory flow meters should be calibrated regularly, since accurate readings depend on a spring mechanism that can stretch with time. PEFR should be measured at the same time each day (twice daily up to four times daily during acute exacerbations). Values obtained in the morning are usually lower than those obtained in the evening.
6. Many patients believe that asthma medication is harmful and addictive. Stress that the continuous use of medication is the key to prevention and is required for this chronic illness.
7. Teach patients when to seek urgent care. Classic symptoms are the need for frequent use (>4 times/day) of an inhaler, frequent nocturnal awakening with symptoms, and a drop in PEFR in the morning to 50% of the evening value or a drop in PEFR to 50% or less of the predicted normal value at any time.
8. Teach patients to lower the amount of allergens by removing all carpeting, washing animals weekly, and covering mattresses and pillows with impermeable covers.
9. Teach the patient the use of the inhaler before exposure to known allergens.
10. Teach patients the use of steroid inhalers, the monitoring of their blood sugar, and signs of gastrointestinal bleeding.
11. Warn patients that asthma is associated with sensitivity to aspirin and nonsteroidal inflammatory medication. Acetaminophen should be used for pain and fever relief. Sulfite sensitivity may also be present. Sulfating agents are found in processed potatoes, shrimp, dried fruits, beer, and wine.

Pulmonary Alveolar Edema
1. Teach the patient about home administration of respiratory and cardiac medications.
2. Patients with severe PAE are hospitalized.

Pulmonary Embolism

1. Advise the patient to avoid long periods of immobility.
2. Instruct the patient on home administration of Coumadin when applicable, as follows:
   - Wear a medical alert bracelet indicating anticoagulation.
   - Use an electric razor and a soft toothbrush.
   - Watch for bleeding and report black or maroon stools to a physician.
   - Avoid foods high in vitamin K (e.g., green leafy vegetables, tomatoes, cauliflower, and fish) to maintain anticoagulation.
3. Encourage the patient to wear loose-fitting clothes.
4. Instruct the patient on the use of elastic or gradient stockings.

Pneumonia

1. Pneumonia is often slow to resolve, especially in geriatric patients. Instruct the patient to schedule frequent rest periods to minimize oxygenation needs.
2. Instruct the patient to avoid people known to have URIs.
3. Ensure that the patient understands home administration of antibiotics. Reinforce the importance of finishing antibiotic prescriptions.

Chronic Obstructive Pulmonary Disease

1. Ask the patient to demonstrate use of the inhaler to determine the proper technique.
2. Teach breathing techniques to enhance oxygenation as follows:
   - Pursed-lip breathing. Breathe in slowly through nose, purse the lips (as if to whistle), then breathe out slowly through pursed lips.
   - Diaphragmatic breathing. In an upright position, place one hand on the abdomen just above the waist, place the other hand on the upper chest, and breathe in through the nose. The lower hand should push out and the hand on the chest should not move. Then breathe out through pursed lips and feel the lower hand move in.[5]
3. Avoid alcohol, spicy foods, and dairy products that increase bronchospasm and sputum production.

R

4. Avoid extremes in temperature. Wear a mask when going from warmth indoors to coldness outdoors.
5. Drink 2 to 3 liters of fluid each day for sputum liquefication.

Spontaneous Pneumothorax

1. Symptoms may take up to 10 days to resolve.
2. Instruct the patient to avoid air travel and scuba diving until total lung reexpansion is confirmed by chest radiography. Follow-up is recommended 7 to 10 days after the event.
3. Alert the patient that recurrences are likely and that treatment should be sought if symptoms return.

References

1. Catena E, Pastore V: Spontaneous pneumothorax: medical or surgical treatment? *Monaldi Arch Chest Dis* 48:159-160, 1993.
2. Light R: Management of spontaneous pneumothorax, *Am Rev Respir Dis* 148:245-248, 1993.
3. Fleisher G et al: Management of asthma, *Pediatr Emerg Care* 8:167-170, 1992.
4. Kozier B, Erb G, Olivieri R: *Fundamentals of nursing: concepts, process, and practice,* ed 4, 1991, Addison-Wesley.
5. Dettenmeier PA: *Pulmonary nursing care,* St Louis, 1992, Mosby.
6. Abolnik I et al: Primary spontaneous pneumothorax in men, *Am J Med Sci* 305:297-303, 1993.
7. Somerson S, Sicilia M: Emergency oxygen administration and airway management, *Crit Care Nurse* 12(4):23-29, 1992.
8. Salvino C et al: Emergency cricothyroidotomy in trauma victims, *J Trauma* 34:503-505, 1993.
9. A lab test for pulmonary embolism, *Emerg Med* 22:45-46, 1990.
10. Rudnitsky G et al: Comparison of intermittent and continuously nebulized albuterol for treatment of asthma in an urban emergency department, *Ann Emerg Med* 22:1842-1846, 1993.
11. White BS, Roberts SL: Pulmonary alveolar edema: preventing complications, *Dimensions Crit Care Nurs* 11(2):90-103, 1992.
12. Tomlanovich M: A stepwise approach to a collapsed lung, *Emerg Med* 21:45-48, 116, 1989.

Chapter 17

Sexually Transmitted Diseases

Pamela S. Kidd

CLINICAL CONDITIONS
Candida Infection
Chancroid (Genital Ulcer Disease)
Chlamydia Infection
Gonorrhea
Human Papillomavirus Infection
Pelvic Inflammatory Disease
Syphilis
Herpes Simplex Virus Infection
Hepatitis B Virus Infection
Trichomonas Infection
Vaginosis

TRIAGE ASSESSMENT

Sexually transmitted diseases (STDs) can be divided into four etiologic categories: viral, bacterial, fungal, and protozoal. Bacterial diseases (e.g., syphilis, gonorrhea, *Chlamydia* infection, and chancroid) are easily treatable. The viral STDs (e.g., herpes, human papillomavirus [HPV], hepatitis B virus, and human immunodeficiency virus [HIV] infections) are incurable, and the potential for transmission often remains for life. HIV and hepatitis B infections are discussed in Chapter 6 because of their systemic effects beyond the genitalia. The usual chief complaints associated with STDs are abdominal pain, genital discharge or lesions, and vaginal itching. Patients may exhibit rashes and joint pain. The most frequently encountered STDs in the ED are gonorrhea, syphilis, and infections with *Chlamydia,* hepatitis B virus, herpes simplex, HIV, human papillomavirus, *Trichomonas,* and *Candida.* At triage, determining the causative agent of the problem is not important. The focus should be on determining if the disease is localized to the genital area or if it has ascended to the pelvic region. Patients with pelvic involvement have

S

a higher incidence of ectopic pregnancy and ruptured ovarian cyst, both of which are considered life threatening. At triage it is important to elicit the following data.

Pain

Determine the type and location of the pain. The onset of low, bilateral abdominal pain is the first sign of ascending infection. The pain may be associated with menses and sexual intercourse (especially if gonorrhea is the causative agent).

Last menstrual period

Determine the date of the last menstrual period, the present point in the menstrual cycle, and the degree of normality of menses. Protective properties of the cervical mucus against ascending infection are at their lowest during ovulation and menstruation and immediately after abortion or childbirth. An abnormal menstrual flow and cycle are associated with many STDs.

Genital discharge

Purulent vaginal discharge that may be blood stained is associated with pelvic inflammatory disease (PID). Males may have purulent urethral discharge.

Initial or recurrent problem

Once the genital tract is infected, it may fail to recover its protective mechanisms and STDs may recur frequently. PID is more common after an initial vaginal infection. Forty percent of adolescent females treated for *Chlamydia* infection will become reinfected within 14 months. If herpes is suspected, ask about exposure to reactivating factors: menses, stress, and sunlight and tanning beds.

Medication history

Several medications may increase a person's risk for STDs. Hormonal supplements such as progesterone and estrogen may alter the cervical area. Progesterone makes the cervical mucus more hostile to ascending microorganisms. Estrogen increases the cervical epithelium surface area, increasing the likelihood of gonorrhea and *Chlamydia* infection, since these organisms adhere to the epithelium. Thus women who are using estrogen replacement after a hysterectomy are at greater risk for PID.[1] Current antibiotic use may mask STD symptoms or alter diagnostic results of cultures. Conversely, contraceptive pill use is a protective mechanism against PID.

Surgical history

Women who have had a hysterectomy are still vulnerable to STDs. The urethra is the usual site of infection.

Birth control method

Birth control methods may increase susceptibility to some STDs while decreasing risk for others. Barrier methods (e.g., condoms and diaphragms) and oral contraceptives protect against ascending genital infection.[2] The use of oral contraceptives increases the risk of HPV infection. The intrauterine device (IUD) increases the risk for PID.

Smoking

Smoking decreases the density of Langerhans cells in the cervix. Thinner cells are more susceptible to STDs.

Dysuria

Males with STDs commonly complain of dysuria and frequency.

Systemic symptoms

Many STDs do not present with vaginal, penile, or abdominal symptoms. Patients may complain of a sore throat, anal discomfort, or systemic symptoms (e.g., rash and fever).

General Observations

Gait

- Observe how the patient walks. Patients with PID may shuffle and walk in a bent-over position as a result of cervical and ovarian tenderness.

Skin

- Look for obvious lesions. Patients with syphilis may have a diffuse papular rash on their palms and the soles of their feet and a facial rash that resembles acne.

FOCUSED NURSING ASSESSMENT

Nursing assessment should center on pain, elimination, metabolic changes, and sexuality.

Pain

Where is the pain located? What are the characteristics of the pain? Auscultate bowel sounds, then palpate the abdomen for rigidity and tenderness. A rigid abdomen and absent bowel sounds may indicate PID, a ruptured ectopic pregnancy (see Chapter 15), or a ruptured ovarian cyst. Alert the physician to the urgency of evaluating this patient.

S

Elimination

1. When was the last time the patient voided? A urinalysis can detect nonspecific urethritis in men if they have not voided for 1 hour.
2. If the patient needs to void while waiting for evaluation and treatment, provide a sterile container and instructions on clean-catch urine collection. Advise menstruating women that they may need to be catheterized to obtain a specimen.
3. Does the patient have constipation or rectal drainage? Advise the patient that a stool specimen may be needed, and provide a proper container.

Metabolic and Vital Signs

A full set of vital signs, including temperature, should be obtained. Blood pressure (BP) may be decreased, and the patient's pulse may be elevated in cases of hemorrhage (rigid abdomen). Fever is common when the disease has progressed to salpingitis, particularly if the causative agent is gonorrhea. When genital infection has progressed to systemic sepsis, fever may be present, depending on the causative organism and the patient's immune status.

Sexuality

Depending on the privacy of the triage area, several of these questions may have been explored at triage. If the information has not been collected, ask about the following:

- The date of the onset of sexual activity and of the last sexual activity
- The number of partners and number of the significant other's partners
- The type of sexual activity (e.g., oral or anal)
- The type of protection used to prevent STDs and pregnancy
- The date of the last menstrual period and the type of product used; tampons, perfumed panty liners, and pads may increase susceptibility to *Candida*
- Any symptoms associated with the sexual activity

Risk Factors

1. Vaginal douching has been associated with PID, *Candida* infection, and bacterial vaginosis.[2]
2. Smoking has been associated with PID and other STDs.[2]

3. Having multiple sexual partners (defined as more than three in a lifetime[3]) increases the risk for PID.
4. Diabetes is associated with a higher incidence of *Candida* infection.
5. The use of tight undergarments or feminine hygiene sprays is associated with vaginitis and *Candida*, as are hyperglycemia and increased sugar intake.
6. The early onset of sexual activity is associated with HPV.
7. Pregnancy may activate HPV and herpes.

Life Span Issues

It is not typical for children to experience genital problems or vaginal discharge. Always obtain information about day care or any person who is with the child alone. Ask about a change in the child's behaviors. Suspect sexual abuse.

Females between the ages of 15 and 19 have the highest incidence of gonorrhea and *Chlamydia*.[4] This is because gonorrhea preferentially infects columnar epithelial cells. In adolescence these cells are everted over part of the ectocervix, increasing the amount of susceptible tissue exposed during intercourse. For this same reason HPV incidence is greatest among 15- to 24-year-old women.[5,6] Pregnancy increases the incidence of STDs because of metaplasia and relative immunosuppression.

INITIAL INTERVENTIONS

1. If the patient has a fever and a rigid, painful abdomen, anticipate the need for a large-bore IV catheter. Normal saline or Ringer's lactate solution may be administered at a keep-vein-open rate (e.g., 30 ml/hr). While starting the IV, obtain two large red-top tubes and a purple-top tube for possible type and crossmatch, Rapid plasma reagin/Venereal Disease Research Laboratory testing, and a complete blood count. Monitor vital signs closely.
2. Anticipate a pelvic examination, and communicate this possibility to the patient. Find out if the patient prefers to have certain individuals remain in the room during the examination. Prepare the patient by having the patient undress. Note any discharge on the undergarments. Next, prepare the equipment (e.g., speculum; slide; slide cover; fixative; KOH; culture media and DNA probe for *Chlamydia* and gonorrhea; viral culturette; bacterial culturette; gauze sponges; swabs; wooden spatula

S

or brush, if a Pap smear is to be completed; lubrication for bimanual examination; Hemoccult testing for stool). Make sure the bed allows for performing a pelvic examination (i.e., breaks down with stirrups). Have a high-powered light source available.
3. Obtain a urine specimen. If the patient is menstruating, obtain a catheter specimen. Otherwise, a clean-catch specimen is usually adequate. Test the specimen using a urinary reagent strip for blood, protein, pH, and glucose. Split the specimen into two containers using sterile technique in anticipation of microscopic analysis and culture.

PRIORITY NURSING DIAGNOSES

Risk for pain
Risk for fluid volume deficit
Risk for impaired body image and self-concept
Risk for knowledge deficit

◆ **Pain** related to infection and inflammation:
  INTERVENTIONS
  • Administer analgesics by PO or IV route.
  • Apply warm compresses to genital lesions after diagnostic procedures are performed.

◆ **Fluid volume deficit** related to fluid shifts from infection and intraperitoneal hemorrhage:
  INTERVENTIONS
  • Administer IV fluid resuscitation (as indicated by vital signs and perfusion status) and antibiotics.
  • Prepare the patient for surgery, if indicated.

◆ **Impaired body image and self-concept** related to alteration in sexual function or reproductive abilities:
  INTERVENTIONS
  • Listen to the patient's concerns.
  • Explain measures to protect the patient and partners.
  • Offer suggestions for alternative sexual activities during exacerbations.
  • In cases of decreased fertility from STD sequelae, initiate a referral to infertility services.

◆ **Knowledge deficit** related to contraception and prevention of STDs:
  INTERVENTIONS
  • See Table 17-1.

TABLE 17-1 The Relationship Between
Contraceptive Method, STD Protection,
and Patient Education

Disease	Contraceptive method that provides protection	Information for follow-up
Chlamydia infection	Contraceptive sponge Spermicide Condom (male and female) Diaphragm	Refer partner(s) for evaluation
HPV	Condom (female better than male)	Have annual Pap smear Examine partner(s) for warts Weekly treatment until lesions resolve Use condoms or abstain during treatment Stress relationship between HPV and cervical cancer; no evidence that treatment of visible warts affects the development of cervical cancer
Gonorrhea	Condom (male and female) Spermicide Contraceptive sponge	Abstain until cured Return for evaluation 2-3 days after treatment Have partner(s) treated
Herpes	Condom (female better than male)	Abstain when lesions are present Have an annual Pap smear May transmit virus when asymptomatic, use condoms during sexual activity
Syphilis	Condom (male and female)	Return for follow-up at 3-, 6-, 12-, and 24-month intervals Refer partner(s) for evaluation

Oral contraceptives and IUDs may increase risk of some STDs.

PRIORITY DIAGNOSTIC TESTS

Laboratory Tests

Gram stain: Gram staining of cervical and urethral specimens (with men) is conducted to determine the presence of gonorrhea. This test has a low sensitivity and is followed by a culture. It is also used to determine the source of the organism in cases of vaginitis.

Wet Prep: This test is a microscopic examination with normal saline and KOH. This will show the presence of clue cells, yeast, and trichomoniasis.

Blood cultures: Cultures may be conducted in cases of suspected PID and disseminated gonorrhea.

DNA probe: A DNA probe may be used to identify *Chlamydia* and gonorrhea. DNA probes tend to have false positive results with children. Nonculture tests (Gram stain smear and DNA probe) should not be used alone in diagnosing gonorrhea in children.[8]

Genital cultures: Vaginal, cervical, rectal, and urethral drainage may be cultured.

1. **Gonorrhea:** Thayer-Martin or Martin-Lewis culture media are commonly used and contain antibiotics against other organisms that commonly invade genital sites. Discharge is obtained on a swab and applied directly to the culture medium using a back-and-forth motion. The inoculated culture should be sent to the laboratory as soon as possible to be placed in a CO_2-rich environment or incubator. With children, specimens from the vagina, urethra, pharynx, and rectum should be obtained.

2. *Chlamydia:* A special culture media is used for this organism. A cytologic swab is used to obtain the specimen. The swab is placed in the test tube of medium. This specimen should be obtained last during the pelvic examination because epithelial cells are needed and all discharge must be swabbed away. The specimen must be refrigerated quickly. Place the specimen in cup of ice until it is taken to the lab.

Throat culture: A throat culture is indicated with symptoms of pharyngitis in sexually active patients who engage in oral sex.

Rapid plasma reagin (RPR): This test is used to detect syphilis. Results yield a nonreactive or reactive state. A

Sexually Transmitted Diseases 601

nonreactive reading does not rule out an incubating disease. If the disease is suspected, the RPR should be repeated at 1-week, 1-month, and 3-month intervals. A reactive test may indicate a past infection inadequately treated or a new infection. Treated individuals should be retested at 3-month intervals for 1 year or until a nonreactive test occurs. If the RPR test result is positive, a VDRL test is performed because of its increased specificity for syphilis.

Venereal Disease Research Laboratory: A VDRL test is used to detect syphilis.

Erythrocyte sedimentation rate (ESR): The erythrocyte sedimentation rate is obtained in cases of suspected PID. The value is elevated with any inflammatory condition.

Complete blood count (CBC): In cases of systemic symptoms (e.g., fever), a CBC is obtained to detect leukocytosis. The WBC count is elevated in cases of PID.

Blood glucose level: The blood glucose level may be obtained if the woman complains of several episodes of *Candida* infection.

Serum pregnancy (Human chorionic gonadotropin) test: A pregnancy test should be completed for all females with suspected STDs, since some treatments differ during pregnancy.

Direct fluorescent antibody test: Monoclonal antibodies are used to detect *Chlamydia* and herpes.

Urinalysis and urine culture: Several STDs may infect the urethra, as well as other genital areas. Urethral leukocytosis with pyuria may be present in male patients who have *Chlamydia* infection or gonorrhea.

Other

Joint aspiration: Joint aspiration is indicated in cases of suspected disseminated gonorrhea with symptoms of joint pain and swelling, fever, and rash (gonorrheal arthritis).

Lumbar puncture: A lumbar puncture may be performed to obtain a cerebrospinal fluid specimen to test for syphilis if neurologic symptoms are present.

COLLABORATIVE INTERVENTIONS
Overview

1. Perform or assist with a pelvic examination and obtaining specimens. If a Pap smear is being performed,

follow the procedure listed in the "Pap Smear Procedure" box.

2. Perform or assist with obtaining a wet smear using the technique listed in the "Wet Smear Procedure" box.

3. Obtain necessary cultures using appropriate technique. Refer to the Priority Diagnostic Tests section for more information.

Clinical Conditions

Some STDs produce enlarged inguinal lymph nodes and genital lesions. Table 17-2 compares several STDs on these symptoms.

The treatment of STDs involves medication administration. Drugs used to treat common STDs are summarized in Table 17-3.

PAP SMEAR PROCEDURE

Nursing action

1. Warm the speculum or wet it with warm tap water. Do not use lubricants.

Physician actions

2. Use a cotton swab to remove excess discharge.
3. With a cytobrush or a wooden spatula, scrape the cervix.
4. Use the cytobrush to brush the endocervical canal.
5. Smear the brush or spatula on a slide.

Nursing action

6. Spray the slide with a fixative (95% alcohol may be used).

WET SMEAR PROCEDURE

1. Place one drop of vaginal discharge on each end of a plain, unfrosted microscope slide, or use two slides.
2. Add one drop of 10% KOH. Note the odor when KOH is applied. (A fishy smell is present in cases of vaginitis.)
3. Cover the KOH drop with a coverslip.
4. Add enough saline to the remaining drop of vaginal secretion to dilute the specimen.
5. Place a coverslip over the saline specimen.

Candida **infection (considered a sexually associated but not sexually transmitted disease)**

SYMPTOMS

- A thick, white, curdy vaginal discharge is present, accompanied by vaginal itching and burning.

DIAGNOSIS

- Diagnosis is based on a microscopic examination of a discharge with 10% KOH on a wet mount slide.

TREATMENT

- Miconazole nitrate or clotrimazole vaginal suppositories or cream may be prescribed.
- Diflucan, fluconazole 150 mg PO × 1 can be prescribed.
- Recurrence is common.

Chancroid and genital ulcer disease

Chancroid has been associated as a cofactor in HIV transmission. Serologic testing for HIV should be conducted. Ten percent of individuals infected also have syphilis or herpes. Serologic testing and a DNA probe or culture should be obtained.[7]

SYMPTOMS

- Symptoms include the presence of lesions on external genitalia. The lesions begin as small papules and break down into painful exudative ulcers with ragged edges.
- Inguinal lymph nodes may be painful when palpated.

TABLE 17-2 Differential Diagnosis of STDs

Diagnosis	Nodes	Lesion
Syphilis	Firm, painless, usually not enlarged	Single, painless lesion
Herpes	Tender, bilateral inguinal node enlargement	Multiple, tender vesicles that ulcerate
Chancroid	Tender, unilateral, or bilateral nodes that may not be enlarged	Multiple painful, leaking lesions with ragged edges
HPV (genital warts)	Possible enlarged inguinal lymph nodes	Pinhead papules to cauliflower-like masses that are flesh colored, pink, or red and that may cluster

604   **Chapter Seventeen**

TABLE 17-3 Drug Summary[7]

Condition	Drug	Dose/route	Special considerations
Pelvic inflammatory disease	Inpatient: cefoxitin or doxycycline Outpatient: cefoxitin, doxycycline, ofloxacin	Inpatient: cefoxitin 2 g IV q6h; doxycycline 100 mg IV or PO q12h Outpatient: 1. Cefoxitin 2 g IM plus probenecid 1 g PO plus doxycycline 100 mg PO bid 14 days 2. Ofloxacin 400 mg PO bid 14 days plus metronidazole 500 mg PO bid × 14 days 3. Ceftriaxone 250 mg IM plus doxycycline 100 mg bid × 14 days 4. Trovafloxacin 200 mg qd × 10 to 14 days	Trovafloxacin can be given IM or PO; not recommended for pregnancy
Syphilis	Penicillin G benzathine; if allergic, give doxycycline, tetracycline, or erythromycin	Penicillin G benzathine 2.4 million U IM Doxycycline 100 mg PO × 14 days Tetracycline 500 mg PO × 14 days Erythromycin 500 mg PO × 14 days	Dosage and route may vary according to stage of syphilis

Continued

Gonorrhea	Ciprofloxacin
	Norfloxacin
	Ofloxacin
	Cefixime
	Ceftriaxone
		Ciprofloxacin 500 mg PO × 1 dose
		Norfloxacin 800 mg PO × 1 dose
		Ofloxacin 400 mg PO × 1 dose
		Ceftriaxone 125 mg IM plus
		  azithromycin 1 g PO or tetracy-
		  cline 100 mg PO bid × 7 days
			Ciprofloxacin is not recommended for
			  persons under 17 years of age because
			  it inhibits cartilage development; it is
			  not approved for use in pregnancy;
			  tetracycline is not approved for
			  pregnancy; use a cephalosporin or
			  spectinomycin IM if patient is preg-
			  nant; ceftriaxone is very painful and
			  may be mixed with a 1% lidocaine
			  solution for administration

Chlamydia	Azithromycin
	Doxycycline
	Erythromycin
	Ofloxacin
		Azithromycin 1 g PO × 1 dose
		Doxycycline 100 mg PO bid ×
		  7 days
		Erythromycin 500 mg qid × 7 days
		Ofloxacin 300 mg PO bid × 7 days
			Use erythromycin or amoxicillin (500 mg
			  PO tid × 7 days) in pregnancy

Herpes	Acyclovir	First occurrence: Acyclovir 400 mg
		  PO tid for 7 to 10 days or 200
		  mg PO 5 times/day for 7 to
		  10 days
		Repeat occurrence: Acyclovir 200
		  mg PO 5 times/day for 5 days or
		  400 mg tid × 5 days, or
		  800 mg PO bid × 5 days	

S

TABLE 17-3 Drug Summary—cont'd

Condition	Drug	Dose/route	Special Considerations
HPV	Podophyllum (provider applies) Imiquimod[12] 5% (patient applies)	Podophyllum 0.5% solution applied bid × 3 days, withheld for 4 days, and then may be reapplied weekly Apply cream qd × week for as long as 16 weeks	May wash off 1 to 4 hours post application to reduce local irritation Wash with mild soap and water 8 to 10 hours after application. Do NOT use for urethral, intravaginal, cervical, or rectal lesions
Candida infection	Miconazole Clotrimazole	Miconazole vaginal suppository 200 mg qd × 3 days or 100 mg × 7 days	Recommended for bedtime use Creams and suppositories are oil based and may weaken latex condoms and diaphragms
Vaginosis Chancroid	Metronidazole Erythromycin Ceftriaxone Azithromycin	Metronidazole 2 g PO × 1 dose Erythromycin 500 mg PO qid × 7 days or ceftriaxone 250 mg IM × 1 dose or azithromycin 1 g PO × 1 dose Ciprofloxacin 500 mg bid × 3 days	Contraindicated in pregnancy Contraindicated in pregnancy
Trichomoniasis	Metronidazole	Metronidazole 2 g PO × 1 dose	Contraindicated in pregnancy

- Rectal bleeding may be present.
- Dyspareunia is common.

DIAGNOSIS
- Diagnosis is based on clinical presentation. A culture may be obtained, but sensitivity is poor (80%).
- Usually four or fewer lesions are present.
- The condition may be diagnosed by default, when a herpes culture or probe result is negative.

TREATMENT
- Treatment involves administration of ceftriaxone, azithromycin, ciprofloxacin, or erythromycin.

Chlamydia infection
Chlamydia infection is the most common STD in the United States.

SYMPTOMS
- The majority of cases are asymptomatic and are detected by routine screening. If the condition is left untreated, a female patient may complain of abdominal pain, vaginal pain and dysuria, and postcoital pain and bleeding.[7] Male patients complain of a thick, cloudy penile discharge with dysuria.

DIAGNOSIS
- Diagnosis is based on a culture and DNA probe.

TREATMENT
- Sexual partners should be screened and treated.
- Drugs of choice include azithromycin 1 g PO in a single dose or doxycycline 100 mg PO bid × 7 days. Erythromycin 500 mg PO qid × 7 days or amoxicillin 500 mg PO tid × 7 days may be used for pregnant patients.

Gonorrhea
Males have a higher transmission rate of gonorrhea than females do because of the high organism load in the ejaculate of an infected male.

SYMPTOMS
- Gonorrhea may be asymptomatic.
- Males may have urethral discharge, dysuria, and testicular tenderness. Men should be warned not to ignore a drop of urethral exudate seen on arising before urination.
- Females may have vaginal discharge, dysuria, abnormal menses, dyspareunia, and abdominal pain.
- Rectal pain and discharge may be present in males or females if anorectal gonorrhea is present.

- Gonococcal pharyngitis is possible after oral sexual exposure.
- Disseminated gonococcal infection may be present in untreated cases.
- Symptoms of fever and joint pain are common.
- A sparse pustular or blister-type rash may be present on the extremities.

DIAGNOSIS

- Diagnosis is based on a Gram stain smear, culture, and DNA probe.

TREATMENT

- Cultures should be taken from sexual partners, and the partners should be treated.
- Cephalosporins (cefixime), ciprofloxacin (quinolones), or tetracycline is administered. Pregnant women should be treated only with cephalosporins or spectinomycin IM. Children weighing less than 45 kg should be treated with ceftriaxone 125 mg IM.
- Gonorrhea is commonly resistant to penicillin.

Human papillomavirus

Human papillomavirus (HPV) is commonly referred to as genital warts. The period from exposure to disease development varies from 1½ to 8 months. There is a positive relationship between HPV and the occurrence of cervical cancer. HPV also occurs in conjunction with HIV.

SYMPTOMS

- Warty growths (condylomata, cauliflower-like appearance) appear in moist genital areas where coital friction occurs. These growths are painless.

DIAGNOSIS

- Diagnosis is based on clinical presentation.
- No culture method is available.
- Cervical HPV infections are usually detected by Pap smear.
- Because of the possibility of neoplasia, biopsy should be performed on all warts with atypical appearance and warts that are pigmented or located on the cervix.

TREATMENT

- This virus is difficult to treat, and recurrences are frequent.
- Liquid nitrogen may be applied.
- Imiquimod 5% (Aldara) may be prescribed.
- Podophyllum (podofilox [Condylox]) or trichloracetic acid may also be used by the provider.

- Lesions are removed by laser therapy in severe cases.
- Consider concurrent STDs as well.

Pelvic inflammatory disease

Pelvic inflammatory disease refers to an infection of the uterus, fallopian tubes, and adjacent pelvic structures. It may be called salpingitis. It ranges in severity from mild to life threatening. Infertility or ectopic pregnancy may occur because of tubal scarring and occlusion.

SYMPTOMS

- Symptoms are not always apparent.
- The most common symptom is bilateral lower abdominal pain. Bleeding or pain with intercourse and spotting between periods may also occur.
- Pain is also present with manipulation of the cervix and bimanual examination of the ovaries.
- Abnormal vaginal discharge is present and varies depending on the type of organism(s) involved.
- *Neisseria gonorrhoeae* and *Chlamydia trachomatis* are most common.
- Fever and an elevated WBC count, ESR, and C-reactive protein level may be present if the disease is severe.

DIAGNOSIS

- Diagnosis is based on clinical presentation.
- Fever (greater than 102.2° F [39° C] is considered severe), abnormal vaginal discharge, and an elevated ESR may be present, and an ultrasound examination may reveal a mass.
- Because of the severity of possible sequelae, the diagnosis is made without a confirming endovaginal ultrasound or endometrial biopsy.
- Treatment is initiated on suspicion of the condition.
- A pregnancy test should be performed to minimize the possibility of missing an ectopic pregnancy.[2]
- Hospitalization is indicated when the possibility of a surgical emergency cannot be excluded, when a pelvic abscess is suspected, when the patient is pregnant, when an adolescent is unable to follow outpatient therapy or return for follow-up, or when a patient is HIV positive. Outpatient therapy is used for mild cases (WBC <11,000/mm^3 with no evidence of peritonitis).[9]

TREATMENT

- Antibiotics are the drug of choice (cefoxitin, doxycycline, clindamycin, and ofloxacin are most commonly used).

S

Syphilis

Syphilis, caused by *Treponema pallidum*, has four stages. Symptoms vary according to stage. When the syphilis is associated with HIV, serologic testing is indicated. All patients with an STD are at risk for asymptomatic syphilis. Syphilis can be contracted through blood and body fluids.

SYMPTOMS

- **Stage One:** Painless, indurated chancres are present.
- **Stage Two:** This stage occurs 2 to 8 weeks after the appearance of chancres. A skin rash and infectious lesions on mucous membranes are present in the early days of stage two. Flulike symptoms may be present.
- **Stage three:** This is a latent, symptom-free stage in which the disease is usually detected through routine laboratory screening procedures (e.g., prenatal and premarital).
- **Stage four:** Neurologic and cardiovascular symptoms occur.

DIAGNOSIS

- In stages one and two, genital scrapings are viewed under darkfield microscopy, or fluorescent antibody techniques are used.
- RPR and VDRL titers detect the organism.

TREATMENT

- Penicillin remains the treatment of choice.
- For penicillin-allergic individuals, doxycycline, tetracycline, or erythromycin is recommended.
- Certain antibiotics prescribed for other STDs (antibiotics with beta-lactam resistance and tetracycline) are also effective against syphilis.
- Patients treated for an STD with antibiotics other than beta-lactams or tetracycline should be tested for syphilis 1 month later.

Herpes simplex virus

Herpes occurs from direct physical contact with infected secretions. Rectal herpes can occur from anorectal sex. During oral sex, fever blisters of the mouth can be transmitted to the genital area and vice versa. Although unlikely, transmission can occur through wet clothing and towels. These items should not be used by others during an outbreak. Contact lens wearers should cleanse their hands thoroughly before applying lenses, since the virus can multiply under the lens.

SYMPTOMS
- Single or multiple vesicles appear on the genitalia. These rupture and cause ulcers. They may be located on the buttocks and thighs as well.
- Recurrent infections vary but are usually milder and of shorter duration.
- Prodromal signs of tenderness, burning, tingling, and itching may occur.
- Inguinal lymph nodes may be enlarged.
- Females have a higher incidence of systemic symptoms during their first occurrence.
- Fever, headache, and malaise may be present.
- Dysuria may result in urinary retention.

DIAGNOSIS
- Diagnosis is usually based on clinical presentation or viral culture. Herpes simplex antigen by direct fluorescent antibody technique is now available and may replace culture as the test of choice.[9]

TREATMENT
- Acyclovir accelerates healing, particularly in first occurrences and particularly when it is started within 48 hours of the outbreak, but its efficacy decreases with recurrent episodes. Suppressive therapy with lower, daily doses of acyclovir reduces recurrence in patients who have greater than six recurrences a year.[10,11]
- Warm compresses, sitz baths, and aspirin may help during outbreaks.

Hepatitis B virus
Sexual contact is the most frequently reported method of hepatitis B viral transmission and is especially prevalent among homosexuals (see Chapter 6).

SYMPTOMS
- Malaise, fatigue, jaundice, and abdominal pain are frequent complaints.

DIAGNOSIS
- Diagnosis is based on the results of serologic testing.

TREATMENT
- Prevention is the key to treating hepatitis B.
- A single dose of hepatitis B vaccine can be administered if treatment occurs within 24 hours of exposure, but a full series of three IM injections is still needed for protection.
- An HIV screen should be drawn before the administration of vaccine.

S

Trichomoniasis (considered a sexually associated but not a sexually transmitted disease)

Trichomoniasis is caused by protozoa.

SYMPTOMS

- An odorous, frothy, yellow-green discharge is present and associated with vulvar irritation.

DIAGNOSIS

- Motile organisms are identified on a normal saline smear of the discharge.

TREATMENT

- Metronidazole is the drug of choice.
- Sexual partners should be treated simultaneously.

Vaginosis

Vaginosis is caused by a change in the natural ecology of the vagina resulting in overgrowth of anaerobic organisms.

SYMPTOMS

- Patients have a malodorous, gray-white, thin, adherent vaginal discharge associated with vulvar itching.

DIAGNOSIS

- Diagnosis is based on the presence of an amine odor to the vaginal discharge when mixed with 10% KOH.
- Vaginal pH is >4.5.

TREATMENT

- Treatment is initiated with metronidazole.
- Clindamycin may be used if the patient is pregnant.

NURSING SURVEILLANCE

1. Monitor the pain level and changes.
2. Monitor the trend of fever, vital signs, and urine output if the abdomen is rigid.

EXPECTED PATIENT OUTCOMES

1. Pain decreases in intensity.
2. The patient understands the differences in contraceptive methods and methods for preventing STDs.

DISCHARGE IMPLICATIONS

NURSING ALERT

Avoid using terms that assume marital status and sexual preference when conducting patient teaching. The term "partner" is preferred.

1. Sexual partners within the previous 60 days should be examined.
2. Follow-up cultures (test of cure) should be obtained from infected sites. The time at which this follow-up test is performed varies from 3 to 7 days after the completion of therapy, to 2 weeks after the initial diagnosis, to 4 to 6 weeks after therapy.
3. Remind the patient to avoid intercourse until he or she is cured or adequately treated.
4. When discussing birth control options and STD prevention, warn patients that some diseases are not prevented by proper and consistent use of male condoms. Herpes, syphilis, HPV, and chancroid may be transmitted, despite condom use, depending on the site of the lesions. Hepatitis B virus can be transmitted through natural skin condoms.
5. To encourage the use of condoms, instruct the patient on how to use the condom to increase excitement during the sexual act, for example, by having the partner place the condom. The value of anticipating orgasm, relief from an STD, and contraception protection may increase the involvement of both partners.
6. Teach the female patient about the need for Pap smears to detect dysplasia. All women, beginning with the onset of sexual activity or at age 21, should have regular Pap smears. Pap smears should be performed annually if the woman is sexually active. Two consecutive annual Pap smears should be obtained, and thereafter a Pap smear should be obtained every 3 years unless the patient has multiple partners.[3] In cases where the woman has multiple partners, annual Pap smears are suggested. If the patient has known HPV disease, more frequent Pap smears are recommended because of the high risk for cervical cancer. Table 17-1 summarizes information related to contraception and partner and patient protection against STDs.

Candida

Treatment of male partners is not recommended unless the man has balanitis or the woman has recurrent infections. Balanitis may be treated with topical antifungal agents.

Chancroid

Sex partners who have contact with a patient who has a case of chancroid (genital ulcer disease) diagnosed within the last 10 days should be treated. All patients should be tested at the time of the initial diagnosis and three months later for HIV and syphilis. Uncircumcised and HIV-infected patients may not respond to initial treatment and may require retreatment.

Chlamydia
Pregnant women should be retested for cure because erythromycin and amoxicillin are not as effective against the organism.

Gonorrhea
Sex partners who have contact with a patient who has had a case of gonorrhea diagnosed within the last 60 days should be treated.

Herpes
Barrier methods should be used during sexual activity at all times. The condom must cover all infected places. Female condoms cover more genital area than male condoms. Sexual contact should be avoided during prodromal and symptomatic stages of the disease. Warn the patient about cross-transmittal between oral and genital lesions if the patient engages in oral sex.

Pelvic Inflammatory Disease
Coitus should be avoided until inflammation and pain subside. Intrauterine devices should be removed. Follow-up should be arranged 24 to 48 hours after ED discharge.

Vaginosis
Treatment of male partners is not recommended. The consumption of larger amounts of complex carbohydrates and less simple sugars has been helpful in some cases.[11]

References
1. Williams D, Riddle J: Understanding salpingitis. A pelvic inflammatory infection, *Prof Nurse* 6(4):217-219, 1991.
2. McCormick W: Pelvic inflammatory disease, *N Engl J Med* 330:115-119, 1994.
3. Matthews W: The ubiquitous human papilloma virus, *J Am Acad Physic Assist* 5:500-505, 1992.
4. Alexander L: Sexually transmitted diseases: perspectives on this growing epidemic, *Nurse Pract* 17(10):31, 34, 37, 38, 41-42, 1992.

5. Bonny A, Biro F: Recognizing and treating STDs in the adolescent, *Contemporary Nurse Practitioner* 3(1):15-24, 1998.

6. Beutner K, Tyring S: Human papilloma virus and human disease, *Am J Med* 102(5a):9-15, 1997.

7. DiCarlo R, Martin D: The clinical diagnosis of genital ulcer disease in men, *Clin Infect Dis* 25(2):292-298, 1997.

8. Reddy S, Yetura S, Sleepik R: *Chlamydia trachomatis* in adolescence: a review, *J Pediatr Adolesc Gynecol* 10(2):59-72, 1998.

9. Mackay T, Soper D, Sweet R: PID: suspect more, treat more, hospitalize less, *Patient Care* 31:109-129, 1997.

10. Centers for Disease Control and Prevention: Guidelines for treatment of sexually transmitted diseases, *MMWR* 47(No. RR-1):88-94, 1998.

11. Beutner K, Ferenczy A: Therapeutic approaches to genital warts, *Am J Med* 102(5A):28-37, 1997.

12. Crook W: Diet changes may aid vaginitis prophylaxis, *Nurse Pract* 18:13, 1993.

S

Chapter 18

Surface Trauma

Julia Fultz
Patty Sturt
Chris Lindsey
Kimberly Short

CLINICAL CONDITIONS
Abrasions
Avulsions
Lacerations
Contusions
Puncture Wounds
Mammalian Bites

TRIAGE ASSESSMENT

Nearly 10 million patients with surface trauma are seen annually in emergency departments (EDs) throughout the United States. Surface trauma is any disruption or damage that causes open wounds or closed contused areas in the continuity of the skin layers. Surface trauma can occur with any major trauma or medical conditions (e.g., seizures or syncope) or can be an isolated injury. Mechanisms of injury include mechanical forces of shearing, tension, and compression. Victims of surface trauma may have associated life-threatening injuries. Airway, breathing, and circulation (ABCs) must be assessed, and appropriate interventions must be implemented. For this reason many surface trauma injuries are low priority upon admission to the emergency department.

The goals of wound care are to relieve discomfort, minimize the risk of infection, restore function, and repair tissue integrity with optimum cosmetic appearance. The risk of infection can be significant. Wound infection generally causes delayed healing, decreased tissue strength, and a poor cosmetic result. Considerations of wound assessment, potential complications, and nursing care are important to ensure positive outcomes for the patient.

Vital Signs

Tachycardia: Related to pain and blood loss
Hypotension: Related to hemorrhagic blood loss from wound
Fever: Related to infection in an older wound

General Observations

- What is the location of the wound? Wounds involving the foot, lower extremity, hand, or face have a higher rate of infection.
- Is the wound open or closed? Open wounds include lacerations, avulsions, punctures, or mammalian bites. Contusions are closed wounds.
- Is there bleeding from the wound? Assess the amount of bleeding to determine if there is uncontrolled bleeding or oozing from the site.

History

Injury information and a medical history should be obtained from the patient, family, and prehospital personnel. A high index of suspicion must be maintained for surface trauma that may have been caused by abuse, assault, or self-inflicted injury.

- *Time of injury:* The greater the time between the injury and delivery of care, the greater the risk of wound complications such as infection.
- *Blood loss before arrival at the ED:* Wounds to the head and face may result in profuse bleeding.
- *Tetanus immunization status: Clostridium tetani* is found in soil and in the gastrointestinal tracts of many domesticated animals. The incubation period for tetanus is 7 to 21 days but can range from 3 to 56 days.[1]
- *Allergies:* Determine if the patient has an allergy to local anesthetics. It is uncommon to find an allergy to a local anesthetic; however, a good history is essential to determine allergy status.[1]
- *Medical conditions:* Patients with a history of cardiac or respiratory disease, diabetes mellitus, or peripheral vascular disease may be at greater risk for infection and delayed healing.
- *Medications:* Patients using anticoagulant (e.g., Coumadin or Persantine) or antiplatelet (e.g., aspirin) medications may have prolonged bleeding times and greater blood loss. Individuals using immunosuppressive medication

S

(e.g., cyclosporine), corticosteroids, or chemotherapy are at greater risk for infection.

- *Alcohol dependence:* Alcohol dependence is associated with nutritional deficits and delayed healing.

Mechanism of injury

- *What was the wounding object?* The mass and velocity of the object should be considered. Increases in mass and velocity result in greater amounts of kinetic energy that must dissipate within the tissue, thereby increasing the amount of injury.
- *What was the environment in which the injury occurred?* Knowledge of the environment in which the injury occurred can provide information on possible wound contamination. Wounds contaminated by foreign matter are at increased risk for infection. Saliva and feces contain a concentration of bacteria in excess of the numbers needed to produce infection. The presence of soil particles with organic components or inorganic clay particles markedly raises the infective potential of bacteria.

FOCUSED NURSING ASSESSMENT

Tissue Integrity

Assess and document characteristics of the wound. A ruler may be helpful for measuring the wound. Document the color and shape and whether the wound is open or closed.

Perfusion

Assess neurovascular status distal to the wound if an extremity is involved. Monitor the trend of peripheral pulses, skin color, skin temperature, capillary refill, sensation, movement, and the degree and character of pain. A weak or absent pulse, pale, cool skin, capillary refill of greater than 2 to 3 seconds, decreased or absent sensation, or a decreased ability to move the area indicates decreased perfusion. Perfusion may be altered if there is damage or compression to underlying neurovascular structures.

Risk factors

1. **Drugs and substance abuse:** Cognition may be impaired and increase the risk for trauma.
2. **Abuse:** Suspect abuse when the surface trauma present does not correlate with the history given by the patient and family or caregiver (see Chapter 2).

3. **Nutritional status:** Malnourished states, regardless of the cause, may result in impaired wound healing.[2]

Life Span Issues
Geriatric

1. Wound healing may be delayed because of age-related diseases and skin changes associated with healing. Aging skin becomes less vascular and thinner and contains fewer elastin fibers.[3]
2. The geriatric patient may have decreased mobility and sensation, thus increasing susceptibility to injury.
3. Many geriatric patients have limited financial resources. Access to dressing supplies and medications may be limited. A social services consultation should be considered.

Youth

School-aged children are frequently involved in recreational and sports activities that increase the risk of surface trauma.

Infants and toddlers

1. Infants and toddlers have a greater head size relative to the overall body size. Wounds to the head and face may bleed vigorously.
2. Toddlers are at increased risk for surface trauma because of lack of coordination during ambulation.

INITIAL INTERVENTIONS

1. Control bleeding.
2. Obtain vital signs.
3. Flush the wound with normal saline, and cover the wound with gauze.
4. Elevate the affected extremity.
5. Apply an ice pack to the area if it is edematous. Place a thin cloth between the ice pack and the skin to protect the skin from cold injury.
6. Remove all constrictive clothing and jewelry.
7. Assess and document neurovascular status in the affected extremity.

PRIORITY NURSING DIAGNOSES

Risk for fluid volume deficit
Risk for impaired skin integrity
Risk for infection
Risk for alteration in tissue perfusion

S

Risk for pain
Risk for anxiety
Risk for impaired mobility

♦ **Fluid volume deficit** related to bleeding:

INTERVENTION

- Apply pressure to the site and pressure points (see Figure 10-1 in Chapter 10).
- Insert a large-bore IV (16-gauge or larger) and administer Ringer's lactate or normal saline solution as needed for hypovolemia secondary to blood loss from the wound. Obtain blood specimens for a type and crossmatch.
- Elevate the affected extremity

♦ **Impaired skin integrity** related to disruption of skin:

INTERVENTION

- Prepare the patient and equipment for skin closure by sutures, stapling, tape closures, or tissue adhesive (Table 18-1).

♦ **Infection** related to contamination of wounds and preexisting medical conditions (e.g., diabetes, peripheral vascular disease, and alcohol abuse):

INTERVENTION

- Cleanse the wound (Procedure 32). Irrigation with 7 lb psi decreases the number of bacteria and the incidence of infection.[1]
- Assist with debridement. Debridement is the removal of foreign matter and devitalized tissue from the wound. The presence of devitalized tissue in the wound significantly increases the risk of infection.

♦ **Alteration in tissue perfusion** related to damage or compression of underlying neurovascular structures:

INTERVENTION

- Elevate the affected extremity to the level of the heart.
- Provide supplemental oxygen.

♦ **Pain** related to surface trauma and treatment:

INTERVENTION

- Immobilize the injured extremity.
- Apply an ice pack to the area if it is edematous.
- Prepare the patient for infiltration of a local anesthetic agent or nerve block. (see Table 18-2)
- Consider the use of EMLA. EMLA is a topical cream that contains lidocaine and prilocaine. EMLA should be applied to the site with an occlusive dressing 30 to 60 minutes before the wound is closed.

TABLE 18-1 Wound Closure Methods

Method and use	Advantages	Disadvantages
Steri-Strips		
May be used for partial-thickness lacerations or small superficial lacerations without signs of adjacent tension	Eliminate the need for anesthetic	Potential for wound edge inversion
Approximate the wound edges, applying Steri-Strips uniformly; use benzoin or Mastisol on adjacent skin to secure adhesiveness of Steri-Strips	Decreases tissue trauma	Less strength than sutures
	Decreases risk for infection	
Sutures		
May be used for simple and more involved lacerations; closure of deep wounds is done in layers; suture selection is a matter of individual choice	Definite closure of wound edges	Local anesthetic used
• Absorbable suture is used for deeper layers; examples are plain or chromic catgut and the synthetics Dexon and Vicryl	Patient able to shower, and dressing is not always needed after 24 hr	Follow-up appointment needed for suture removal
• Nonabsorbable suture is used for skin closure and must be removed; examples are silk or synthetics (nylon, polypropylene)		
NOTE: Synthetics have a decreased wicking action that decreases scarring potential		

Data from Markovchick V: Suture materials and mechanical after care, *Emerg Med Clin North Am* 10:673-689, 1992; Simon B: Principles of wound management. In Rosen P et al, editors: *Emergency medicine*, ed 4, St Louis, 1998, Mosby.

Continued

TABLE 18-1 Wound Closure Methods—cont'd

Method and use	Advantages	Disadvantages
Staples		
May be used for linear lacerations to scalp, trunk, and extremities	Less painful Eliminates exposure to sharp needles Time to closure is less More acceptable to some patients for cosmetic reasons	Provides less precise approximation Should not be used when magnetic resonance imaging of the affected part may be conducted
Tissue adhesive (e.g., Dermabond) Used for closure of traumatic laceration; may be used in closure of clean, simple facial laceration; thin film of adhesive is applied to the edges, and manual approximation is maintained for 30 seconds to 2 minutes	Less painful Eliminates exposure to sharp needles Time to closure is less More acceptable to some patients for cosmetic reasons	Cannot be used near the eyes Cannot be used close to wounds under tension, or across joints

Data from Markovchick V: Suture materials and mechanical after care, *Emerg Med Clin North Am* 10:673-689, 1992; Simon B: Principles of wound management. In Rosen P et al, editors: *Emergency medicine*, ed 4, St Louis, 1998, Mosby.

- Apply LET as prescribed by the physician. LET is a topical anesthetic solution of lidocaine, epinephrine, and tetracaine. LET is considered safer than and as effective as TAC, which contains tetracaine, adrenalin, and cocaine. Application of TAC near or to the mucous membranes has resulted in serious complications, including seizures and death.
- Consider the use of distraction techniques to relieve discomfort. Music and visual imagery may be helpful.
- Obtain a physician order for analgesics as needed.

◆ **Anxiety** related to the precipitating event, pain, and the potential for disfigurement:

INTERVENTION

- Offer support and explain all procedures.

◆ **Impaired mobility** related to muscle, tendon, or ligament damage:

INTERVENTION

- Splint and elevate the injured area.
- Continue to monitor neurovascular status because edema may progress and impinge on neurovascular structures.

PRIORITY DIAGNOSTIC TESTS

Radiographs: A radiograph aids in assessment of bony structures and in identification of foreign objects. Pieces of glass greater than 1 mm thick are visible with appropriate views.[1] Organic substances such as wood are not easily seen on radiographs.

Xerograms: A xerogram will identify most organic substances (e.g., wood, seeds, and beans). This test will miss some plastics.[1]

Computed tomography scan: A CT scan is useful in identifying all foreign substances; however, the test is expensive.[1]

Ultrasonograms: This test is useful in identifying almost all substances. Air, pus, and edema may cause puzzling echoes.[1]

Complete blood count (CBC): A CBC may be obtained to monitor blood loss. An elevated WBC count may be present if an infection is present, especially with old or contaminated wounds.

PT and PTT: Obtain this for patients who have multiple injuries that are associated with blood loss or patients who have a history of anticoagulant use or blood dyscrasia.

s

Type and crossmatch: A type and crossmatch is obtained if multiple injuries exist with hypovolemia, or if there is a possible need for surgical intervention.

Compartment pressure readings: Record readings in severe cases of surface trauma with associated edema that is limb threatening (see Chapter 10).

Culture and sensitivity: Obtain these on the wound exudate if the wound is infected.

COLLABORATIVE INTERVENTIONS

1. *Wound care:* Assist with wound debridement, wound irrigation, and wound closure. Closing wounds within 8 to 12 hours of the injury can reduce the risk of infectious complications. Lacerations more than 8 to 12 hours old may not be sutured, but instead allowed to heal by secondary intention and dressing changes.[1] Fine linear facial lacerations may be sutured 24 hours after the injury because of the greater disfigurement potential and the good vascularity of the face.[1]

2. *Oxygen:* Supply supplemental oxygen to patients who have indicators of hypovolemia secondary to blood loss.

3. *Hypovolemia:* Initiate crystalloid infusion (Ringer's lactate or normal saline) by large-bore IVs.

4. *Tetanus toxoid:* Administer tetanus toxoid as ordered (Reference Guide 24).

5. *Pain medication:* Administer pain medication as ordered.

6. *Diagnostic tests:* Facilitate steps necessary to obtain diagnostic tests.

7. *Dressings:* Obtain supplies and apply an appropriate dressing to the wound.

Clinical Conditions
Abrasions

An abrasion is a wearing, grinding, or rubbing away of the outer layer of the skin, leaving the underlying dermis exposed (e.g., "road rash" from falls on pavement or rug or rope burns).

SYMPTOMS

- The patient experiences minimal bleeding. The wound may be moist from an oozing of the capillary.
- Pain is usually localized to the injured area.
- Localized edema may be present as a result of capillary vasodilation.
- Erythema is related to the inflammatory response.

DIAGNOSIS
- Diagnosis is based on a clinical examination.

TREATMENT
- Anesthetize the area. Use a topical anesthetic for small abrasions. Anesthetic injections may be necessary to achieve pain control for large areas of abrasion.
- Clean the abrasion using aseptic technique. All foreign bodies must be removed (rock, grit, or fibers will frequently be embedded in the wound). High-pressure irrigation with saline is suggested[1] using an 18-gauge IV catheter (with the needle removed) connected to a 25- to 35-cc syringe. If debris is not removed from an abrasion by high-pressure irrigation, it may be necessary to cleanse the abrasion with saline and a fine pore–sized sponge[1] or a soft sterile brush in a circular motion. Care must be taken not to increase tissue damage with a sponge or soft brush. Failure to remove dirt and debris from the wound will result in a permanent tattooing once the wound has healed (Procedure 32).
- Cover the abrasion with a topical antibiotic. This will prevent the wound exudate from becoming dry and crusted and from thereby interfering with wound healing.
- Leave the wound open or consider applying either a dry, sterile dressing or a vapor-permeable membrane.

Avulsions

An avulsion is a forcible separation or detachment. An avulsion may be as significant as an amputation (Chapter 10), or it may be a piece of skin and possibly the underlying tissue torn away from the body in varying degrees (e.g., eyelid, nose, ear, or a degloving injury).

SYMPTOMS
- Bleeding is usually present.
- The patient feels pain.
- Underlying structures are exposed (e.g., subcutaneous tissue, muscle, tendons, and bone).
- The patient may have a loss of function.

DIAGNOSIS
- An examination reveals obvious tissue loss. Tissue may be partially attached.

TREATMENT
- Apply direct pressure to control bleeding and use pressure points if bleeding continues.
- Evaluate the patient for fluid loss and the need for fluid replacement if the injury is large.

S

- A local anesthetic or IV conscious sedation (Procedure 8) for wound care may be administered before cleansing and irrigating the wound.
- Cleanse the wound with high-pressure irrigation with saline as described in the section on "Abrasions." Cleansing of the avulsed tissue is necessary if it is to be reattached. Ensure that all debris has been removed. When a person's head strikes a vehicle windshield, multiple small avulsions in which glass is embedded may result. Careful evaluation is necessary to ensure that all of the glass has been removed.
- Debridement of damaged tissue from the injury by the physician may be necessary.
- Closure of the wound will depend on the wound's severity. A skin flap still attached is cleaned and debrided and then undergoes primary closure. If the tissue loss is extensive, cleaning and irrigating may be done in the operating room and skin grafting may be required.

Lacerations

A laceration is a cut or tear into the dermal layer of the skin that may involve the underlying structures. A laceration may be the result of either sharp or dull forces. The wound edges may be smooth and even or jagged.

SYMPTOMS

- The amount of bleeding depends on the depth, location, and involvement of structures.
- Edema, erythema, crusting, and purulent drainage may be present, depending on the length of time since the injury.
- The patient may exhibit sensory or motor deficits.

DIAGNOSIS

- Diagnosis is based on a clinical examination.

TREATMENT

- Bleeding is controlled by direct pressure and by use of pressure points if bleeding continues.
- Premedicate the patient with anesthetics or analgesics for wound care, cleansing, and closure.
- Clean the wound with a high-pressure saline irrigation described in the section "Abrasions."
- Once the wound has been debrided, wound closure can be done in one of three ways—primary closure, delayed closure, and "open."[1] If primary closure is used, the wound is debrided, cleaned, irrigated, and closed imme-

diately with sutures, tape, staples, or a tissue adhesive.[1] If delayed closure is used, the wound is cleaned, debrided, irrigated, and packed to prevent it from closing on its own. The patient has wound checks and a packing change in 24 hours, and in 48 hours definitive repair occurs.[1] If the wound is to be left open to heal on its own, it is debrided, cleaned, irrigated, and dressed.

- Lacerations that have been closed are dressed with an antibiotic ointment and covered with a microporous polypropylene dressing for the first 24 hours.[1] The wound will be sealed by then and a dressing will no longer be necessary.[1]
- If the laceration is over a joint, immobilize the extremity to prevent stress on the wound.

Contusions

Contusions are characterized by bleeding within the dermis and epidermis from the disruption of small blood vessels, usually caused by blunt trauma.

SYMPTOMS

- Swelling is apparent.
- There is discoloration from blood leaking into the tissue.
- The patient experiences pain.
- In children the most common sites are bony prominences such as the knees, elbows, and shins.
- There is potential damage to underlying structures (e.g., swelling may cause vascular compromise; a left upper quadrant contusion may involve a splenic injury; a right upper quadrant contusion may involve a liver injury; a lower leg contusion may involve compartment syndrome).

DIAGNOSIS

- Diagnosis is based on a clinical examination.

TREATMENT

- Treatment is aimed at providing comfort and preventing further edema and tissue damage.
- Ice is applied for the first 24 to 48 hours.
- The injured area may be elevated at or above the level of the heart.
- The affected extremity may be immobilized for 24 to 48 hours after the injury, depending on the location and severity of the injury (e.g., Ace, splint, or sling).

Puncture wounds

Puncture wounds are penetrating wounds from an object forced through the skin and into the underlying tissue.

S

Most puncture wounds occur to the extremities and involve such substances as nails, glass, or wood.

SYMPTOMS

- Bleeding may be present.
- The patient experiences pain.
- Signs and symptoms of infection (e.g., erythema, warmth, edema, and drainage) may be present, depending on the age of the puncture wound.
- The wound may have an embedded foreign body (pain on deep palpation over the wound is indicative of an embedded foreign body).
- Superficially, the wound may seem minor; evaluate the patient for signs of underlying tissue damage.

DIAGNOSIS

- Diagnosis is based on clinical examination and on history.

TREATMENT

- Bleeding should be controlled with pressure and the use of pressure points if bleeding continues.
- If a foreign body is suspected, obtain appropriate diagnostic studies as described in Priority Diagnostic Tests.
- Analgesics or anesthetics may be administered for wound care, cleansing, and possible exploration.
- The infection rate for puncture wounds is high, so the wound must be well irrigated. Anesthesia and excision of the area may be necessary for an adequate cleaning and exploration of the wound.
- A dressing is applied as indicated after wound exploration and closure.

Mammalian bites

Mammalian bites are bites from humans or animals that cause puncture wounds but that may have associated abrasions, avulsions, contusions, and lacerations. Dog bites are the most commonly seen and tend to be lacerations, avulsions, or crush-type injuries. Cats have sharp, pointed teeth, so the bite tends to be a deep puncture wound that may penetrate deeper structures, including joints and bones.[4]

SYMPTOMS

- Bleeding and ecchymosis may be present.
- Edema, erythema, and pain usually occur.
- Signs and symptoms of infection may be present. Many patients bitten by their own animals do not seek treat-

ment immediately. The age, type, and location of the wound, in addition to the health of the individual, contribute to the potential for infection.[4]

- Fever may be present.
- The patient may have a decreased range of motion if a joint is involved.

DIAGNOSIS
- Diagnosis is based on the patient's history and on a clinical examination.

TREATMENT
- Control the patient's bleeding.
- Analgesics or anesthetics may be administered for wound care, cleansing, and possible closure.
- If an infection is present, cultures of the wound and exudate should be obtained.
- Infection is of significant concern because bite wounds are contaminated with oral flora.[4,5] Meticulous cleansing and irrigation are needed. Cat bites have a significantly higher infection rate than dog bites,[4] and human bites are considered more serious than dog or cat bites. The wound should be evaluated for injuries to underlying structures and for foreign bodies. High-pressure saline irrigation should be performed (as described in the section on "Abrasions").
- Closure is controversial because of the high incidence of infection.
- If the wound is sutured, a wound check within 24 hours should be scheduled.
- Ice and elevation may be necessary for treating edema until improvement is noted.
- Notify the health department to report animal bites according to local policy.
- Rabies vaccination may be required, as well as a tetanus shot.

NURSING SURVEILLANCE
Patient Observation
1. Monitor the wound for continued bleeding or drainage. Monitor dressings for occult bleeding.
2. Evaluate contusions for expansion.
3. Monitor skin color, temperature, and capillary refill.
4. Evaluate sensory function distal to the injury.
5. Evaluate the effectiveness of pain control measures.

6. Evaluate the wound for signs and symptoms of infection (e.g., erythema, edema, warmth at the wound site, purulent drainage, or unexplained temperature elevation).

Family or Significant Other Support

1. Inform family members of the procedure. Place a chair by the patient's bed so the family members may sit down if desired.
2. Involve the family members in learning wound care instructions and discharge instructions.

EXPECTED PATIENT OUTCOMES

1. The bleeding is controlled, and neurovascular status remains intact.
2. The patient reports relief from pain.
3. No further tissue damage occurs from cleansing or irrigating.
4. The patient demonstrates an understanding of wound cleansing and closure.
5. The wound is approximated or protected by dressing before discharge.
6. The patient understands the signs and symptoms of infection and the need to return to the ED or a primary care physician should infection occur.
7. The patient or significant other understands the care of the wound.
8. The patient or significant other demonstrates knowledge of medications (e.g., analgesics, antibiotics, and immunizations) and potential side effects (Table 18-2).
9. The patient understands follow-up instructions for wound checks and suture or staple removal.

DISCHARGE INSTRUCTIONS

Socioeconomic factors that may affect compliance with wound care at home and follow-up care should be assessed. Money for supplies and medications, the existence of running water or electricity in the home, the availability of follow-up care, and transportation to receive care should be discussed before discharge.

Wound care instructions vary according to the type of wound, the location of the wound, and the type of closure (if any) used. The following are general instructions and must be adapted according to the type of wound:

TABLE 18-2 Drug Summary

Agent	Dose/route (maximum recommended doses)	Special considerations
Lidocaine		
With epinephrine*	7 mg/kg SC	Used as local anesthetic before wound procedure
Without epinephrine	4 mg/kg SC	Administered to wound edges only
Procain		
With epinephrine*	14 mg/kg SC	Used as local anesthetic before wound procedure
Without epinephrine	8 mg/kg SC	Administered to wound edges only
Bupivacaine		
With epinephrine*	4 mg/kg SC	Used as local anesthetic before wound procedure
Without epinephrine	1 mg/kg SC	Administered to wound edges only

*Do not use agents with epinephrine in areas with decreased blood flow (e.g., digits).

1. Keep the dressing clean and dry for 24 hours.
2. Keep the area elevated for 24 to 48 hours with an ice pack application, if needed, to decrease edema or pain. If a laceration is over a joint, immobilization should be maintained until the sutures are removed.[1]
3. Wash hands thoroughly with soap and water before and after wound care.
4. After the first 24 hours, remove the dressing. Cleanse the wound gently of medication residue and wound exudate with soap and water. (The patient must have his or her own bar of soap in the home designated for wound care). Half-strength hydrogen peroxide may be used to clean the wound debris and clots that form between the

S

sutured edges of the wound until the scab separates.[1]
(Hydrogen peroxide should not be used once the scab
has separated, because it is toxic to the epithelium.)[1]

5. Advise the patient that it is safe to get the wound wet
   after 24 hours; however, prolonged immersion of the
   wound in water (e.g., tub bath, swimming pool, or long
   showers) should be avoided.

6. The wound may be redressed or left open to the air as
   appropriate. Factors to consider for redressing are the
   location of the wound (e.g., joints, hands, or feet), the
   severity of the wound, wound drainage, and the potential for contamination.

7. Reapply a thin layer of antibiotic ointment if necessary.
   Antibiotic ointment protects the wounded area and decreases scarring.

8. Describe the signs of infection—increased pain, redness, swelling, pus (thick white or yellow liquid as opposed to serous drainage), fever, and the presence of
   red streaks moving up an extremity. High-risk injuries
   (e.g., animal and human bites or highly contaminated
   wounds) should be rechecked in 24 to 48 hours regardless of their appearance.[1]

9. Take the complete dose of antibiotics as prescribed. If
   a rabies vaccination is indicated, the patient should be
   instructed to return for follow-up injections.

10. Return for wound check and suture removal as appro-
    priate. Sutures are usually removed in 5 to 14 days
    (Procedure 29).

11. Cover the affected area with a dressing or sunscreen
    for 1 year to minimize discoloration and scarring.

References

1. Simon B: Principles of wound management. In Rosen P et al,
   editors: *Emergency medicine,* ed 4, St Louis, 1998, Mosby.
2. Hackley LV: Surface trauma. In Kett S et al, editors: *Emergency
   nursing: a clinical and physiologic perspective,* ed 2, Philadelphia,
   1995, WB Saunders.
3. Emergency Nurses Association: *Emergency nursing pediatric course
   manual,* ed 2, Chicago, 1998, the Association.
4. Weber EJ, Callaham M: Animal bites and rabies. In Rosen P et
   al, editors: *Emergency medicine concepts and clinical practice,* ed 4,
   St Louis, 1998, Mosby.
5. Bunzli WF, Wright DH, Hoang AD, et al: Current management
   of human bites, *Pharmacotherapy* 18(2):227-234, 1998.

Chapter 19

Toxicologic Conditions

Pamela S. Kidd
Patty Sturt

SPECIFIC OVERDOSES
Acetaminophen (Tylenol)
Salicylates (Aspirin)
Alcohol
Specific Alcohol Agents (Methanol and Ethylene Glycol)
Benzodiazepines
Tricyclic Antidepressants
Opioid (Codeine, Heroin)
Cocaine
Hydrocarbons
Organophosphates
Iron
Lead
Anticholinergic and Antihistamine Drugs
Calcium Channel Blockers and Beta-Blockers
Cardiac Glycosides

TRIAGE ASSESSMENT

The most common agents involved in overdoses encountered in the emergency department (ED) are acetaminophen, alcohol, antihistamines, aspirin, tricyclic antidepressants (TCAs), and benzodiazepines. Calcium channel blockers and beta-blockers are increasingly being abused. It is important at triage not to determine what agent was abused, but to determine if the patient's airway, breathing, and circulation (ABCs) are intact. Suspect an overdose with anyone who arrives with an abrupt onset of multiple symptoms. Assuming that immediate lifesaving interventions are not necessary, the following data should be elicited.

Route of exposure (skin, IV, or PO)
The route of exposure determines where the patient is placed in the ED (e.g., decontamination versus resuscitation room). If exposure is through the skin (e.g.,

organophosphates), the patient's skin requires flushing
and the health care providers are at risk for exposure.

Drugs ingested

Determine the name of the drugs ingested. Some drugs
are slowly absorbed (e.g., digoxin, aspirin, and phenytoin).
Slow-release forms of drugs are treated differently.

Ingestion history

Determine how much earlier and over what period drug
ingestion occurred. Preferably, emptying should be initiated within 2 hours of ingestion.[1]

Determine if the medication container or bottle is available. Calculate the number of pills or amount of fluid missing from the initial amount prescribed.

Determine whether the patient's occupation involves possible exposure to chemicals (e.g., lead or organophosphates).

Medical history

Determine the patient's age, weight, height, medical history, and current medications. This information helps in
drug calculations and with anticipating the patient's ability
to metabolize drugs. Current medication history also helps
determine the treatment modality (e.g., if the patient takes
furosemide, he or she may be potassium depleted before
ingestion, and the use of a cathartic may further decrease
the potassium level).

Determine if there is a history of depression, schizophrenia, or suicide attempts. Patients with these conditions will
need to be placed in a room where they can be closely
monitored.

Patient's last meal

Determine the amount and time of the patient's last meal.
The presence of food in the stomach may delay absorption.

Treatment before arrival

If ipecac has been given, emesis should occur within
30 minutes. The administration of ipecac may delay the administration of oral antidotes and may alter the amount
given. Vomiting may produce a vagal response and further
decrease the heart rate of a patient who has ingested cardiotoxic drugs.

Vital Signs

- *Tachycardia:* Related to sympathetic nervous system
  (SNS) stimulation (e.g., cocaine)
- *Bradycardia:* Related to myocardial depression or interfer-

ence with calcium channels, the SNS (e.g., beta-blocking and calcium channel-blocking agents), or excessive acetylcholine at receptor sites (e.g., organophosphates)

- *Hypotension:* Related to peripheral vasodilation or direct myocardial depression (e.g., opiates and tricyclic antidepressants)
- *Hypertension:* Related to SNS stimulation (e.g., cocaine and PCP)
- *Tachypnea:* Related to metabolic acidosis (e.g., salicylates)
- *Bradypnea:* Related to respiratory depression (e.g., narcotics, sedatives, and tranquilizers)
- *Fever:* Related to the anticholinergic effect or hypermetabolism (e.g., cocaine)
- *Hypothermia:* Related to hypometabolism (e.g., changes in the glucose level)

General Observations
Pupil size and reaction
Constricted pupils may indicate the use of organophosphates, opiates, or cocaine. Dilated pupils may indicate tricyclics, anticholinergic drugs, alcohol, amphetamines, cocaine, sympathomimetics, and mushrooms.
Skin
Inspect the skin for needle track marks indicating IV drug use or a multidrug overdose.

NURSING ALERT

All overdoses are potentially life threatening and should be treated as such. Patients should be triaged immediately to the ED treatment area. Symptoms occur later in patients who have ingested acetaminophen, sustained release drugs, and methanol and ethylene glycol. These are considered acute agents. Do not be fooled by a patient who is asymptomatic but may deteriorate in the ED waiting area.

The primary nurse should call the poison control center to determine definitive treatment.

FOCUSED NURSING ASSESSMENT

Nursing assessment should center on ventilation, perfusion, cognition, and elimination. The following should be assessed even if they were assessed at triage, because changes occur rapidly.

Ventilation
Breath sounds
Pulmonary edema (PE) occurs frequently with hydrocarbon and opiate ingestion. Acute alcohol intoxication may also produce PE as a result of chronic alcohol abuse and its resulting congestive heart failure (CHF). Coarse or fine rales (crackles) may be auscultated. Wheezing may occur with inhalation of organophosphate insecticides.

Breathing pattern
Opiate overdoses produce respiratory depression and PE. Respirations may be slow, shallow, and wet. Hydrocarbons vaporize at low temperatures. They enter the pulmonary tree easily, producing bronchospasm, PE, and aspiration pneumonitis. Salicylates, methanol, and ethylene glycol (antifreeze) produce metabolic acidosis. In cases of salicylate overdose, respirations are deep and slow, related to direct stimulation of the respiratory center in the brainstem.

Perfusion
Apical heart rate
Obtain an apical heart rate for 1 minute and compare this rate and rhythm with a peripheral pulse. Many of the commonly ingested drugs produce cardiovascular effects. Calcium channel-blocking and beta-blocking agents decrease the heart rate and increase the susceptibility for conduction blocks and ectopy. Anticholinergic drugs and cocaine produce tachydysrhythmia.

Blood pressure
Peripheral vasodilation and myocardial depression increase as more of the ingested drug is absorbed.

Skin
Check skin color, temperature, capillary refill, and peripheral pulses. Iron ingestion can produce gastric hemorrhage and hypovolemic shock. Anticholinergic agents produce hyperthermia, but the skin will be dry because the patient is unable to sweat. A cocaine overdose may produce diaphoresis.

Cognition
Mental status
Perform a neurologic assessment. Seizures and an altered level of consciousness (LOC) ranging from lethargy to confusion to coma may occur at any time if the ingested

amount of any agent is great enough. The Glasgow Coma
Scale (GCS) (Reference Guides 10 and 18) should be used
to document eye, motor, and verbal response.

Hallucinations

You can hold up an imaginary piece of string and ask the
patient to tell you the color of the string. A patient who
tells you a color is having visual hallucinations. Hallucinations are common with cocaine and lead poisoning.

Unresponsive patient

If the patient is unresponsive, a coexisting traumatic injury
(e.g., a fall) may be present (see Chapter 20). Assess the patient for evidence of trauma such as abrasions, bleeding,
ecchymoses, edema, and deformity. Keep the patient flat
with the spine immobilized until cervical spine injury is
ruled out.

Elimination

Bowel sounds

The absence of bowel sounds is a good sign. This allows the
drug to sit in the gut, slowing absorption.

Urinary output

Assess and measure urinary output. Has the patient voided
since the ingestion? Some drugs may produce acute tubular necrosis (ATN) (e.g., methanol and ethylene glycol).
Organophosphates overstimulate the parasympathetic nervous system, causing urination and defecation.

Bowel movement

Assess the patient's stools. As noted previously, organophosphates produce defecation. Bloody stools may result from
iron ingestion.

Emesis

Assess and measure emesis. Are there pill fragments?
Bloody emesis may occur with iron ingestion. If the patient
has received ipecac, it is important to note the amount of
emesis that occurs after administration.

Risk Factors

1. Young children who have access to medicine
2. Geriatric patients with failing eyesight or memory
3. People who are in pain or who have chronic illness and
   are using drugs that may impair judgment
4. Previous suicide attempts

Life Span Issues
Adolescent issues
Adolescents tend to overdose on over-the-counter drugs instead of prescribed drugs.
Geriatric issues
1. The majority of overdoses among geriatric patients who are not depressed are the result of confusion, improper use of the product, improper storage in a container other than the original, or mistaken identity. This has discharge teaching implications.
2. Hemodialysis or hemoperfusion may be required at lower serum concentrations for a geriatric patient.
3. Geriatric patients are more likely to have chronic intoxication secondary to daily or multiple use of agents for other disorders (e.g., aspirin).
4. Suicide attempts by geriatric patients are more likely to be successful because the patients are more determined and their ability to recover is decreased. Decreased hepatic and renal blood flow associated with aging decreases drug metabolism and excretion.

INITIAL INTERVENTIONS
Regardless of the drug ingested, the following interventions will not harm the patient and may be beneficial:
1. Implement measures to protect the patient's airway. If the patient is awake and a spine injury has been ruled out, place the patient in the semi-Fowler's position. Remove pillows if the patient has decreased responsiveness. Insert a nasopharyngeal airway. If the patient is unresponsive or has no gag reflex, insert an oral airway until the patient is intubated with an endotracheal or nasotracheal tube.
2. Anticipate aspiration and have suction available. If the patient is unresponsive, place the patient in the left lateral recumbent position. This position allows the drug to remain in the curvature of the stomach and decreases drug absorption. It is easier to hear posterior breath sounds and to obtain a rectal temperature reading when the patient is in this position.
3. Initiate pulse oximetry to monitor the degree of oxygen saturation.
4. Initiate cardiac and blood pressure (BP) monitoring.
5. Protect the patient from injury. Seizures are common

because of the drug overdose, hypoxia, and hypoglycemia. Pad the side rails. Keep the bed in a low position. As noted previously, have airway and suction materials available.

6. Do not punish the patient. Use a nonjudgmental approach. Remember to ask why the patient took the overdose, not just what he or she took. The patient would
not be in the ED if he or she knew a better way to manage problems.

PRIORITY NURSING DIAGNOSIS

Risk for aspiration
Risk for impaired gas exchange
Risk for injury
Risk for altered tissue perfusion
Risk for decreased cardiac output
Risk for altered bowel elimination
Risk for fluid volume deficit
Risk for ineffective individual coping
Risk for knowledge deficit

◆ **Aspiration** related to a depressed LOC and nausea and
vomiting:
INTERVENTIONS
• Place the patient in the semi-Fowler's position if the pa-
tient is alert, and in the left lateral recumbent position if
the patient is unresponsive.
• Insert an airway adjunct as necessary.
• Suction prn.
• Administer the following agents as ordered: antiemetics,
naloxone, thiamine, glucose, and flumazenil.

◆ **Impaired gas exchange** related to altered serum pH,
breathing pattern (salicylate), or bronchospasm (beta-
blocking agents):
INTERVENTIONS
• Apply a pulse oximeter.
• Administer oxygen.
• Monitor the respiratory effort and anticipate fatigue.

◆ **Injury** related to seizures (TCAs, flumazenil) and a change
in body temperature (cocaine):
INTERVENTIONS
• Pad the side rails of the bed and keep the stretcher in a
low position.
• Suction prn.

T

- Administer anticonvulsant medications prophylactically as ordered.
- Administer the following agents as ordered: flumazenil (slowly), dantrolene IV (as appropriate), and antipyretics (as appropriate).
- Apply a warming or cooling blanket (as appropriate).
- Use an ice lavage (as appropriate).
- Administer warm, IV fluids (as appropriate).

◆ **Altered tissue perfusion** related to vasodilation and hypotension:
INTERVENTIONS
- Administer IV fluid cautiously.
- Administer vasopressors and diuretics as ordered.
- Assess the skin color and temperature, capillary refill (for children), and pulse oximetry readings.

◆ **Decreased cardiac output** related to dysrhythmia, altered contractility, and increased afterload (cocaine):
INTERVENTIONS
- Administer the following agents as ordered: calcium, sodium bicarbonate, glucagon, atropine, esmolol (cocaine), and vasodilators (cocaine).
- Anticipate external and internal pacing (calcium channel blockers).

◆ **Altered bowel elimination** related to cathartic use and decreased motility (anticholinergic drugs):
INTERVENTIONS
- Administer sorbitol and magnesium citrate as ordered.
- Monitor intake and output.
- Monitor electrolytes.
- Administer whole bowel irrigation for removal of drug packets, lithium, heavy metals, and sustained release medications.

◆ **Fluid volume deficit** related to forced diuresis, alkalinization of urine (salicylates), and acute renal failure (ARF):
INTERVENTIONS
- Monitor vital signs.
- Monitor intake and output.

◆ **Ineffective individual coping** related to lack of perceived resources:
INTERVENTIONS
- Initiate a psychologic or spiritual referral system.
- Ask why the overdose was taken.
- Treat the patient humanistically.

♦ **Knowledge deficit** related to the improper use of medication:
INTERVENTIONS
• Clarify the area of misunderstanding.
• Initiate patient teaching once the patient is stable.

PRIORITY DIAGNOSTIC TESTS

Laboratory Tests
General considerations
Toxicology screening may be necessary to identify the ingested drug(s).
   Obtain a coagulation profile if hemodialysis is necessary.
Serum toxicology screening: Toxicology screening may be performed, since acetaminophen, salicylate, lithium, theophylline, digoxin, and mercury levels may alter the treatment plan.[2]
Arterial blood gases: ABGs may be analyzed to check for anion gap acidosis associated with salicylate, ethylene glycol, and methanol ingestion.
Electrolyte levels: Baseline potassium, chloride, and sodium levels are usually obtained because treatments may produce electrolyte abnormalities.
Glucose level: A check of the glucose level may be ordered to rule out hypoglycemia as an associated factor in unresponsiveness.
Liver enzymes and amylase level: Liver enzyme and amylase levels may be elevated in acetaminophen overdoses as a result of hepatic necrosis.
Blood ethanol level: The blood ethanol level is elevated in cases of acute alcohol intoxication.
Cardiac enzyme and isoenzyme levels: Enzyme levels may be elevated with amphetamine, TCA, and cocaine overdoses.
Blood urea nitrogen and creatinine: BUN and creatinine levels may be obtained to confirm normal renal function cases in which forced diuresis is a treatment modality.
Urinalysis: A baseline urinalysis level may be obtained to confirm normal renal function in cases where forced diuresis is used as treatment modality.
Urine toxicology screen: This may be ordered to help confirm the type of drug(s) ingested.
Gastric lavage screen: This may be ordered to help confirm the type of drug(s) ingested.

NURSING ALERT

> If metabolic acidosis is present, anticipate the administration of IV sodium bicarbonate. Metabolic acidosis is common with overdoses of TCAs, salicylates, and cocaine. An initial bolus is given, followed by a continuous infusion.

Radiographic Examination

Abdominal films: Undissolved tablets (e.g., enteric-coated aspirin) may accumulate in the stomach, particularly if the patient has a gastric outlet disorder. This may be detected on film. Iron is radiopaque. Its presence can be detected by abdominal radiographs.

COLLABORATIVE INTERVENTIONS

1. Provide oxygen. Most ingested drugs induce acidosis.
2. Initiate IV access. Antidotes, antiemetics, fluids, and vasopressors may need to be administered.
3. Treat unresponsiveness. Dextrose is administered as 0.5 to 1 g/kg, usually in $D_{25}W$ solution for the child and $D_{50}W$ solution for the adult for hypoglycemia. Glucagon 1 mg IM may be used if IV access is not possible.[3] Naloxone 2 mg IV push is administered in case the unresponsiveness is related to an opiate overdose.
4. Maintain perfusion by promoting normal BP. Fluid is administered carefully (250- to 500-ml boluses) to avoid PE. In children, fluid is administered in doses of 1 ml/kg. PE is a common complication after opiate, salicylate, pesticide, and hydrocarbon overdoses. Vasopressors are used as a last choice for hypotension, since they increase susceptibility for dysrhythmia in addition to the overdosed drug.[4]
5. Impair drug absorption, modify drug metabolism, and enhance drug excretion.

Ipecac: Suggested doses are 30 ml for an adult, 15 ml for a child 2 to 12 years of age, and 10 ml for a child 6 months to 2 years of age. Ipecac is contraindicated for children younger than 6 months.[3] Infants 6 to 12 months of age should receive ipecac only in the hospital setting. Ipecac may be used more successfully for children because they usually do not ingest substances that produce sedation. Ipecac directly stimulates the brain to induce emesis and irritates the gastric mucosa. Drinking water immediately after administration dilutes the ipecac and allows it to cover a larger surface area in the gut, producing greater emesis. Large items (e.g., iron pills) and heavy metals are best removed through emesis. It is contraindicated with hydrocarbon, TCA, and multidrug ingestion. At best, ipecac can remove only 30% of gastric contents. It takes 20 to 30 minutes to work. If emesis does not occur within 20 minutes the dose should be repeated. Oral antidote administration may need to be delayed after ipecac use due to continued emesis. If a cardiotoxic drug (beta-blocker or calcium channel blocker) was ingested, the act of vomiting may cause a vagal response and further decrease the heart rate. If overdose occurred more than 1½ hours before the patient is treated, ipecac or lavage is not helpful with most drugs. Ipecac is believed to have little value in the ED.[5]

Milk: If a corrosive substance has been ingested, 4 to 6 oz may be given PO or via gastric tube.[6]

Charcoal: Charcoal is administered in a 10:1 ratio (10 parts charcoal to 1 part drug). It may be used after emesis or lavage. A 50- to 100-g dose is used for adults. The suggested dose for a child is 10 to 30 g or 1 g/kg. Charcoal may not be tolerated for 1 to 6 hours after ipecac administration. Combined therapy (charcoal after ipecac or charcoal after lavage) does not produce greater benefits and increases the risk of complications. The use of charcoal alone has been found to be effective.[7] ED stays are longer for patients receiving combined therapy.[2] A large dose may be given before whole bowel irrigation. Soak the bottle in hot water for 10 to 15 minutes to make it easier to swallow or push. Water may be added to the charcoal and the solution shaken before administration.

Charcoal is not used to treat ingestion of corrosive substances, since it makes endoscopy impossible. Charcoal produces diarrhea and increases the chance of aspiration. Charcoal aspiration produces prolonged, severe bronchospasm. If the charcoal splatters in the eye, a corneal abrasion may occur. Charcoal does not absorb ethanol, hydrocarbons, or iron.

NURSING ALERT

Activated charcoal is often mixed in sorbitol (a cathartic agent). When multiple doses of activated charcoal are given, make sure they are not administered in a sorbitol solution to prevent electrolyte abnormalities and hypovolemia.

Gastric lavage: There is controversy over using gastric lavage without first inserting a cuffed endotracheal (ET) tube, because of potential aspiration. Lavage must be performed within 2 hours of ingestion of most drugs to be effective. After 1 hour, there is no difference in drug retrieval between use of lavage and charcoal and use of charcoal alone. If vomiting occurs before ED admission, lavage may not remove any additional drug and it may force the gastric contents into the small intestine. The procedure is to administer tap water or normal saline until returns through the orogastric tube are clear (1.5 to 2 liters for adults, 10 ml/kg for children). A large orogastric tube (36 to 42 Fr for adults, 26 to 28 Fr for children) should be inserted. A double-lumen tube allows for simultaneous delivery and aspiration.

Cathartics: Cathartics are frequently used to help remove drug packets and iron. They should be used only with the first dose of charcoal. This is especially true with children and geriatric patients because of potential electrolyte abnormalities.

- **Sorbitol:** Sorbitol is an oral cathartic available as a 70% solution that is diluted to 35% with water. A 0.5 to 1 g/kg dose (usually 2 to 3 cc/kg) is given to a maximum dose of 50 g.[3] Sorbitol produces fewer electrolyte abnormalities and has the shortest gastrointestinal (GI) transit time of all cathartics. It works faster than magnesium citrate. Sorbitol gives charcoal a sweet taste and decreases the grittiness, so charcoal is more palatable.
- **Magnesium sulfate and citrate:** Magnesium sulfate and citrate are cathartic agents. They should not be used with patients who have CHF secondary to increased saline load. Magnesium cathartics are contraindicated for patients with impaired renal function.[8]

Cation exchange resins: Sodium polystyrene sulfonate is a cation exchange resin used to bind lithium. A side effect of this treatment is hypokalemia. Cation exchange resins may be used until dialysis is available.

Forced diuresis: Forced diuresis is used if an agent is distributed mainly within the extracellular fluid with minimal protein binding, and the agent is excreted in the urine. This treatment is controversial because of potential dehydration and electrolyte imbalances.

Altering urine and serum pH: The aim of this intervention is to change the agent into a less absorbable ionized form.

Acidic agents (e.g., salicylate and phenobarbital) clear more rapidly in alkaline urine. A pH level of 7.45 is desired. It is true that basic agents (PCP and amphetamines) clear more rapidly in acidic urine, but acidic urine may result in acute tubular necrosis. Thus treatment to make urine more acidic is usually not initiated. If it is initiated, ascorbic acid is administered.

Hemodialysis: Hemodialysis is used if the ingested drug is distributed primarily within the extracellular fluid, and it is able to penetrate the dialysis membrane. This intervention is preferred for drugs distributed in extracellular water.[2] Lithium, ethylene glycol, methanol, theophylline, and salicylate may be removed using dialysis. Dialysis can reverse metabolic acidosis if it is used early, before the drug diffuses into the tissue. It can correct electrolyte problems. Hemodialysis necessitates anticoagulation.

Hemoperfusion: This intervention is used in overdoses of digoxin, paraquat, TCAs, glutethimide, barbiturates, and acetaminophen. Hemoperfusion is used to remove lipid-soluble drugs. Charcoal and ionic exchange resins serve as filters that blood passes through. The filter adsorbs the drug. Acetaminophen may be removed by hemoperfusion, decreasing the degree of hepatic toxicity associated with the drug. Hemoperfusion causes greater hemolysis than does hemodialysis. It is preferred for drugs that are highly protein bound. The method uses direct exposure of blood to adsorbent particles.

Continuous arteriovenous hemofiltration (CAVH): CAVH may be used in cases involving lithium toxicity. An advantage of this procedure is that hemodialysis facilities are not needed. It is a very slow process and it is used to remove agents that remain in the blood for a long time.

Exchange transfusion: Exchange transfusions may be used for children with lead poisoning and drugs that produce hemolytic anemia. A series of three complete transfusions may be needed to exchange and remove drugs.

Whole bowel irrigation: The aim of whole bowel irrigation is to flush pill fragments through the GI tract. Opponents argue that this procedure may distribute pills throughout the GI tract, enhancing absorption. Polyethylene glycol-electrolyte solution (PEG-ELS, Go-Lytely) is infused via a nasogastric or orogastric tube at rates varying from 200 to 2000 ml/hr for 5 hours. Up to 40 liters has been administered. This intervention can cause electrolyte abnormalities. It is good for treating overdoses of sustained-release drugs, (e.g., theophylline), metals (iron, zinc, and lead), foreign bodies, "body packers" who smuggle cocaine, and lithium. If administered with charcoal, the solution may bind with the charcoal, decreasing the charcoal's ability to bind with the overdosed drug.[9]

Antidotes are summarized in Table 19-1.

Specific Overdoses
Acetaminophen (Tylenol)

Acetaminophen is one of the most common pharmaceutical agents involved in overdoses in the United States.[10]

SYMPTOMS

- Patients with acetaminophen overdose look good in the ED, and symptoms do not occur until later (up to 12 hours after ingestion).[4]
- Initial symptoms of acetaminophen overdose are nausea and vomiting, pallor, and diaphoresis.
- Patients may arrive at the ED 24 to 48 hours after ingestion with right upper quadrant pain related to liver failure. Prothrombin time (PT) begins to increase 24 hours after ingestion.

DIAGNOSIS

- A serum level of 140 mg/kg or greater is toxic.
- It takes at least 4 hours after ingestion for the level to be dependable.
- The risk of hepatotoxicity can be determined with the Rumack-Matthew nomogram (Figure 19-1).

TREATMENT

- A loading dose of acetylcysteine (Mucomyst) at 140 mg/kg PO is indicated if more than 140 mg/kg of acetaminophen has been ingested or if the level is within toxic range. Acetylcysteine may be of benefit up to 24 hours after an acetaminophen overdose. Subsequent doses of 70 mg/kg are repeated at 4-hour intervals for 17 doses or until the acetaminophen assay reveals a nontoxic level. Acetylcysteine is used to prevent hepatic failure (defined as AST/AAT; SGPT/SGOT >1000 IU/L). Acetylcysteine protects the liver by enhancing glutathione synthesis. Hepatic enzymes should be monitored. When acetylcysteine is given PO, it can make the patient vomit because of its smell. It may be mixed with cola or orange juice to enhance palatability.

TABLE 19-1 Common Overdoses in the Emergency Department

Drug	Symptoms	Treatment
Acetaminophen	None initially; right upper quadrant pain, N/V, pallor, diaphoresis 48-72 hr later	Acetylcysteine, antiemetic, cimetidine, activated charcoal
Salicylate	N/V, rapid, deep respirations, tinnitus	Sodium bicarbonate, hemodialysis, whole bowel irrigation
Alcohol	Tachycardia, hypoventilation, confusion, diplopia	Benzodiazepine, hemodialysis, lavage
Benzodiazepines	Hypotension, tachycardia, respiratory depression	Flumazenil
Tricyclic antidepressants	Bradycardia conduction blocks, hypotension, seizures	Lavage, activated charcoal, sodium bicarbonate, physostigmine
Opiates	Constricted pupils, hypotension, PE, bradycardia	Naloxone
Hydrocarbons	Bronchospasm, PE	Lavage
Methanol and ethylene glycol	Delayed symptoms (coma, acute rheumatic fever), tachycardia, confusion	Ethanol IV, hemodialysis
Organophosphates	Salivation, lacrimation, urination, defecation, N/V, constricted pupils, muscle weakness	Pralidoxime chloride IV, atropine, skin and eye irrigation

Continued

ACE, Angiotensin-converting enzyme; *PE,* pulmonary edema; *N/V,* nausea and vomiting.

TABLE 19-1 Common Overdoses in the Emergency Department—cont'd

Drug	Symptoms	Treatment
Iron	Bloody vomit and stools	Deferoxamine chelating agent
Anticholinergic drugs (antihistamines, decongestants, sleeping pills)	Blurred and double vision, nonreactive dilated pupils, unable to sweat, hyperthermia, tachycardia	Physostigmine in cases of cardiac instability, lavage, activated charcoal
Calcium channel blockers	Bradycardia conduction blocks	Calcium, dopamine, pacemaker
Lead	Confusion, anemia	2,3-Dimercaptosuccinic acid (DMSA)
Cocaine	Tachycardia, hypertension, dilated pupils, dyspnea, chest pain, thrombosis, hyperthermia, hallucinations	Whole bowel irrigation for body packets, sodium bicarbonate, alpha- and beta-blocking agents, vasodilators, ACE inhibitors, calcium channel blockers, activated charcoal, lavage
Beta-blocking agents	Bradycardia, blocks	Atropine, glucagon, whole bowel irrigation

ACE, Angiotensin-converting enzyme; *PE,* pulmonary edema; *N/V,* nausea and vomiting.

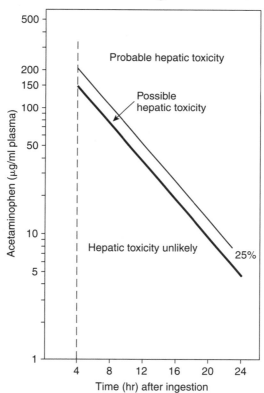

Figure 19-1 Rumack-Matthew nomogram for acetaminophen poisoning. (Reproduced with permission from Rumack BH, Matthew H: *Pediatrics* 55:871, 1975.)

- Antiemetics may be administered.
- Patients may also be treated with activated charcoal, since it is highly effective in binding the drug. Activated charcoal may bind acetylcysteine, but there is no evidence that it makes acetylcysteine ineffective.[3,11]
- Administration of acetylcysteine has priority over administration of charcoal. The administration of both agents (if multiple doses of charcoal are used) can be alternated every 2 hours.
- If the patient arrives at the ED >2 hours after ingestion, activated charcoal is not helpful.

- Beware if the patient has preexisting liver disease, because toxicity occurs at a lower level.
- The patient should not be discharged until the serum acetaminophen level is determined.
- A liver transplant is indicated if there is early metabolic acidosis, renal failure, and prolonged PT (>100 seconds).

Salicylates (aspirin)

Salicylates are used regularly by many people; therefore, chronic as well as acute overdosage is possible, especially if the patient has a gastric outlet problem or uses an antacid.

SYMPTOMS

- Nausea and vomiting, tinnitus, rapid, deep respirations (secondary to metabolic acidosis and direct stimulation of the respiratory center in the brainstem), and hyperthermia occur in cases of salicylate overdose.

DIAGNOSIS

- Diagnosis is based on serum level, using a Done nomogram (Figure 19-2). This nomogram does not apply with long-term ingestion of salicylates or an overdose of enteric-coated tablets.

TREATMENT

- Treatment depends on the salicylate level. If the level is >30 mg/dl but <60 mg/dl, multiple doses of charcoal are administered.
- Urinary alkalinization should be considered for patients with salicylate levels >35 mg/dl or rapidly increasing salicylate levels. Alkalinizing the urine traps ionized salicylate and increases excretion.
- Maintain urine output at 2 to 3 ml/kg/hr.
- Hemodialysis is used in cases in which the salicylate level exceeds 100 mg/dl and with a coma, a severe acid-base imbalance, and a failure to respond to multiple doses of charcoal and urinary alkalinization.
- Salicylates can form large clumps (bezoars) that clog orogastric tubes. These clumps may be dialyzed. Alkalinization of the urine and serum with the use of IV sodium bicarbonate enhances excretion.
- In cases of an overdose of enteric-coated aspirin, absorption may be delayed.
- Whole bowel irrigation may be considered when enteric-coated aspirin has been ingested.
- D_5LR or D_5NS IV solutions are given to correct dehydration.

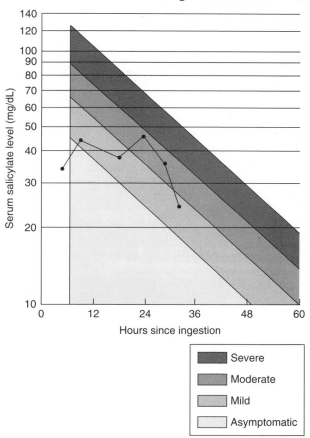

Figure 19-2 The Done nomogram showing sequential serum salicylate levels in patient who ingested toxic dose of enteric-coated aspirin. (From Pierce R, Gazewood J, Blake R: *Postgrad Med* 89[5]:62, 1982.)

- Glucose is administered to correct ketosis and hypoglycemia.
- Vitamin K may be administered to treat hypoprothrombinemia and bleeding tendencies.
- Monitor potassium levels. Significant potassium loss occurs because of vomiting and increased renal excretion of potassium.

Alcohol
Symptoms
- Alcohol intoxication produces tachycardia, hypoventilation, confusion, and seizures related to hypoglycemia.
- Diplopia is the first sign of thiamine deficiency.

Diagnosis
- Diagnosis is based on the serum ethanol level. Alcohol is eliminated at a rate of 10 to 20 mg/dl/hr in the nonalcoholic.

Treatment
- Ethanol is rapidly absorbed from the stomach and small intestine. An alcohol overdose is usually treated with lavage. Lavage is most effective if the patient arrives at the ED <1 hour after ingestion.
- Benzodiazepine may be given to prevent withdrawal side effects.
- In cases of alcohol intoxication, thiamine is administered before glucose. Thiamine is used as a cofactor to make adenosine triphosphate (ATP). If glucose is given, the only available thiamine (which is already deficient) is depleted to break down the glucose. Wernicke-Korsakoff encephalopathy and permanent psychosis can occur. Chronic alcohol abusers may also have gastritis, pancreatitis, and liver disease.

Specific alcohol agent (methanol and ethylene glycol)
Methanol is found in antifreeze, windshield wiper fluid, paint thinner, and "bootleg" whiskey. Ethylene glycol is found in antifreeze, cosmetics, solvents, and paint. Methanol is rapidly absorbed from the gastrointestinal tract, and blood levels peak 30 to 90 minutes after ingestion. Methanol metabolites produce toxicity with symptoms appearing anywhere from 40 minutes to 72 hours after ingestion. Ethylene glycol blood levels peak 1 to 4 hours after ingestion.

Symptoms
- Symptoms are similar to alcohol intoxication.
- Slurred speech, ataxia, confusion, and tremors may be present.
- The toxic metabolites of methanol produce visual disturbances such as cloudy or blurred vision.
- These substances may produce renal damage and metabolic coma.

DIAGNOSIS

- Diagnosis is confirmed by a specific test for the serum methanol and ethylene glycol level.

TREATMENT

- Gastric lavage is indicated if the patient arrives in the ED within 1 to 2 hours of ingestion.
- Ethanol may be given IV to block the conversion of methanol into more toxic substances (e.g., formaldehyde).
- Hemodialysis is indicated for patients with metabolic acidosis, renal compromise, or visual symptoms (methanol).

Benzodiazepines

Benzodiazepines include diazepam, lorazepam, and midazolam.

SYMPTOMS

- Hypotension, tachycardia, ataxia, slurred speech, respiratory depression, and hypothermia are frequently associated with benzodiazepine overdoses.

DIAGNOSIS

- Positive benzodiazepine serum levels confirm the overdose.

TREATMENT

- Flumazenil (Romazicon) reverses benzodiazepines. An initial dose of 0.2 mg over 60 seconds is given. Repeat with 0.3 mg IV every 60 seconds up to a maximum dose of 3 mg, depending on the patient's condition.
- Before flumazenil is administered, life-support equipment should be at the bedside. After 30 to 45 minutes, patients become resedated.
- Seizure activity may be related to quick withdrawal from chronically used benzodiazepines and not to flumazenil administration.[16] Controversy exists regarding flumazenil administration for a patient with a positive seizure history or for a mixed overdose involving TCAs because of dysrhythmia associated with TCA overdose.
- Because benzodiazepines may have a therapeutic effect with mixed overdoses involving convulsive agents (e.g., cocaine), flumazenil may not be administered to reverse sedation. Flumazenil may be used as a diagnostic aid for cases of unexplained coma.

Tricyclic antidepressants

The TCAs (e.g., amitriptyline, doxepin, and imipramine) vary in dose, creating toxic effects and varying in absorption. An individual's response to an overdose is difficult to predict.

SYMPTOMS

- An overdose of a TCA has an anticholinergic effect and produces respiratory depression, a decreased level of consciousness, ventricular tachycardia, atrial and ventricular blocks, hypotension, seizures, agitation, hyperreflexia, cardiac arrest, and rapid deterioration without notice.
- Seizures usually occur right before cardiac arrest.

DIAGNOSIS

- Diagnosis is based on clinical symptoms and blood plasma and urine analysis.

TREATMENT

- TCAs are highly bound to plasma proteins, so dialysis and forced diuresis are not helpful.[12]
- Initiate orogastric lavage followed with charcoal and cathartics. The patient may need to be intubated first to prevent aspiration.
- Begin alkalinizing the blood with sodium bicarbonate. Serum alkalinization (pH 7.5-7.55) is the mainstay of treatment for cardiac side effects due to TCA overdose.
- Ipecac is contraindicated as a result of the patient's rapidly deteriorating LOC.
- Physostigmine is contraindicated. This medicine can produce seizures, bronchospasm, and cardiac arrest.
- Seizures are treated with benzodiazepines. Phenobarbital may be administered if benzodiazepines fail to terminate seizures.
- Treat hypovolemia with isotonic crystalloids such as Ringer's lactate. Norepinephrine and dopamine may be given if hypotension persists after volume repletion.

Opioid (codeine and heroin)

SYMPTOMS

- The patient exhibits constricted pupils, vomiting, seizures, hypotension, bradycardia, PE, respiratory depression, and coma.
- Complications arising from a heroin overdose are usually evident on arrival in the ED.
- Heroin is rapidly metabolized to morphine with an action of 4 to 5 hours.
- If the patient is awake, alert, and without pulmonary

complications in the ED, he or she probably does not require hospitalization.[13]

DIAGNOSIS
- A urine toxicology screen is the most sensitive detecting device.
- A positive response to naloxone administration is confirmatory.

TREATMENT
- Naloxone 2 mg IV push is used initially. It can be administered SC, IM, or through an ET if necessary. The amount of naloxone given varies.
- Some agents (e.g., codeine and fentanyl) require large doses (approximately 35 mg) of naloxone to reverse. This should be given in 2- to 5-mg boluses.
- Naloxone drips can be used (as in methadone overdoses). Watch the patient for potential agitation.
- In some opiate overdoses, poisoning occurs again 12 to 18 hours after the naloxone drip is discontinued.

Cocaine
- Cocaine may be administered nasally (snorted), orally, or through smoking or IV injection. Cocaine produces central and autonomic stimulation by blocking neurotransmitter uptake.

SYMPTOMS
- Cocaine increases serum catecholamines; thus it has SNS effects. In the brain, cocaine blocks the uptake of dopamine and norepinephrine. This excessive dopamine produces hyperstimulation. With long-term use of cocaine, dopamine and norepinephrine are depleted in the cells because of lack of cellular uptake.[14]
- Cocaine produces increased systemic vascular resistance (hypertension) and, subsequently, myocardial ischemia resulting from increased afterload.
- Chest pain is a common complaint of cocaine users.
- The patient may experience supraventricular arrhythmias (e.g., atrial fibrillation atrial flutter) and ventricular arrhythmias (e.g., ventricular ectopy ventricular tachycardia).
- The patient's pupils dilate.
- Hyperthermia may result.
- Coronary vasospasm and thrombosis may result from increased platelet aggregability secondary to epinephrine release and increased thromboxane production.

T

- The patient may have pulmonary symptoms (such as respiratory depression and PE) related to an inhalation injury (freebasing) or long-term use.
- A hypermetabolic state results in weight loss, insomnia, and fatigue.
- The patient experiences confusion, tremors, hallucinations, and paranoia.

DIAGNOSIS
- Diagnosis is based on results of a urine drug screen and clinical findings.

TREATMENT
- Administer diazepam or lorazepam for sedation or as needed for seizure activity.
- Beta-blocking agents (e.g., propranolol) are not used, since the beta-blockers may result in unopposed alpha stimulation and worsening of BP.
- Arrhythmias that are not self-limiting can be treated with benzodiazepines (5-20 mg IV over 5-20 minutes) in the hemodynamically stable patient.
- Mixed alpha- and beta-blocking agents (e.g., esmolol and labetalol), ACE inhibitors, calcium channel blockers, and vasodilators may be used.
- Cooling blankets, a tepid water spray, and fans are the treatment of choice for cocaine-induced hyperthermia. Dantrolene administered IV has been used in some cases to treat hyperthermia.[15]
- Cocaine is metabolized to a less acute form in an alkaline medium. Whole-bowel irrigation with PEG-ELS and sodium bicarbonate promotes rapid transit of cocaine into the small intestine, decreasing the risk of toxicity.
- Activated charcoal adsorbs cocaine in the stomach and small intestines well.
- Gastric lavage can be used if the patient arrives quickly after ingestion or use (as with body packets). Paper packets are rapidly broken down. Condom packets liberate less cocaine.

Hydrocarbons
Hydrocarbons (e.g., methane, propane, gasoline, kerosene, and turpentine) vaporize at low temperatures. They enter the pulmonary tree easily.

SYMPTOMS
- Vomiting
- Wheezing from bronchospasms

- Crackles from PE pulmonary edema
- Coughing
- Noisy respirations
- Tachypnea

DIAGNOSIS
- A hydrocarbon overdose is diagnosed on the basis of history and symptom presentation.

TREATMENT
- Remove any contaminated clothing. Wash skin with soap and copious amounts of water.
- The patient must be lavaged with an endotracheal tube in place because of the aspiration potential.
- Oxygen and mechanical ventilation are often needed.
- Activated charcoal poorly absorbs hydrocarbons.

Organophosphates

Organophosphate exposure (e.g., commercial sprays, bug bombs, insect repellents, and flea collars) can occur by inhalation or ingestion or through the skin.[6]

SYMPTOMS
- Organophosphates overstimulate the parasympathetic nervous system.
- An overdose produces SLUDGE (salivation, lacrimation, urination, defecation, gastrointestinal manifestations, nausea and vomiting, and emesis) syndrome, or oversecretion.
- Pinpoint pupils and muscle weakness occur.

DIAGNOSIS
- Diagnosis is based on history and the presence of symptoms.

TREATMENT
- Remove contaminated clothing and jewelry. Flush contaminated skin with water.
- Overdose and exposure are treated with IV atropine. Large doses may be required, such as 2 to 5 mg every 5 minutes until control of mucous membrane hypersecretion is attained.
- Pralidoxime chloride (Protopam) is administered as an IV drip of 1 to 2 g over 30 minutes. This medicine reactivates cholinesterase. It is most useful when administered within 24 hours of exposure. Indications for use include muscle weakness and fasciculations. The dose is not based on heart rate or pupil size.

T

NURSING ALERT

The patient and family should not be given their removed clothing or any leather items. These articles absorb the pesticides for an indefinite period. Health care providers must avoid contact with patient secretions, since they may be contaminated.

Iron

SYMPTOMS

- Iron poisoning produces corrosive effects on the GI mucosa.
- Patients may vomit blood or have bloody stools.
- Hypovolemia may occur with children.
- Patients may not have any real ill effects for the first 6 to 8 hours.
- Patients may be inappropriately discharged from the ED after vomiting.
- Severe effects (e.g., acute renal failure, GI bleeding, coma, and coagulopathy) may occur later at home.
- An overdose produces anion gap acidosis and shock.

DIAGNOSIS

- Diagnosis is based on results of abdominal radiographs and on the serum level.

TREATMENT

- The iron is removed by using chelation therapy with deferoxamine.
- Approximately 100 mg of deferoxamine binds 8.5 mg of elemental iron.
- Deferoxamine is administered either IV (15 mg/kg/hr) or IM (90 mg/kg q8hr) until urine returns to yellow or the serum iron level is normal. Rapid IV administration of large doses can lead to hypotension.

Lead

SYMPTOMS

- Lethargy, decreased responsiveness, and confusion are symptoms of lead poisoning.
- Seizure activity may occur.

DIAGNOSIS

- The Centers for Disease Control and Prevention has defined toxic blood levels in children as greater than 10 μg/dl.[16] Lead toxicity with adults is usually from inhalation.

TREATMENT
- Lead poisoning is treated by administering a chelating agent, 2,3-DMSA. It is given orally. DMSA does not cause elimination of body stores of iron, copper, or zinc.

Anticholinergic and antihistamine drugs

These are over-the-counter drugs (e.g., sleeping pills, decongestants, and antihistamines). Jimson weed also has anticholinergic properties.

SYMPTOMS
- An overdose produces an altered mental status (e.g., delirium or hallucinations), blurred and double vision, hyperreflexia, seizures, and coma.
- The patient may have dilated pupils that do not react to light because of the paralysis of ciliary muscles.
- The patient is unable to sweat and may die of hyperthermia.
- Usually, ileus and supraventricular tachycardia are present.

DIAGNOSIS
- Urine and serum toxicology screening detects these drugs.

TREATMENT
- An overdose is treated with physostigmine if the patient has tachycardia and cardiovascular instability.
- Gastric emptying and activated charcoal may be useful for several hours after ingestion as a result of slowed gastric motility.

Calcium channel blockers and beta-blockers

These drugs (verapamil, nifedipine, diltiazem amlodipine, felodipine, atenolol and propranolol) decrease cardiac output and systemic vascular resistance. Individuals with preexisting pulmonary disease or asthma are at higher risk for serious complications as a result of the unopposed bronchoconstriction that occurs.

SYMPTOMS
- Bradycardia, atrio-ventricular blocks, respiratory depression, seizures, coma, and hypotension occur from an overdose of these agents.

DIAGNOSIS
- A serum drug level test confirms the diagnosis.

TREATMENT
- Administer activated charcoal if the patient is awake and alert.
- Calcium and dopamine may be administered for an over-

dose of calcium channel blockers.[17,18] The exact dose is individualized.

- Administer crystallized fluids IV for hypotension.
- Many of these agents are sustained-release formulations. Patients who have taken the sustained-release forms should be monitored overnight, since effects may take 6 to 12 hours to manifest.
- External pacing and pacemaker insertion may be required.
- An intraaortic balloon pump may be used to increase cardiac output.
- Atropine may be administered for overdoses of beta-blocker and calcium channel blockers.
- Glucagon is given to increase the availability of adenosine monophosphate, which increases intracellular calcium. The increased calcium improves contractility and increases the heart rate. A dose of 3 mg or 0.05 mg/kg to be given over 30 seconds followed by continuous infusion at 0.07 mg/kg/hr is administered.

Cardiac glycosides

These drugs include digoxin and digitalis.

SYMPTOMS

- Anorexia and nausea may occur.
- Visual disturbances are a common complaint.
- Life-threatening dysrhythmias (e.g., bradydysrhythmias, conduction blocks, and multifocal premature ventricular contractions) and hyperkalemia may occur.

DIAGNOSIS

- A serum drug level test confirms the overdose.

TREATMENT

- Emesis may enhance vagal tone and produce bradycardia. Activated charcoal may be used to absorb and to promote elimination.
- Digibind (digoxin-specific Fab antibody fragments) is used to counteract digoxin overdoses. These antibodies remove therapeutic, as well as toxic, amounts of the drug.
- Be aware that the underlying condition that required digoxin use may be exacerbated (e.g., CHF).
- Electrolyte imbalances such as hyperkalemia and hypomagnesemia must be corrected.

NURSING ALERT

Table 19-2 summarizes overdoses commonly encountered in the ED.

TABLE 19-2 Common Antidotes in the ED Setting

Antidote	Common dosage	Use
Acetylcysteine	17 doses at 70 mg/kg or until acetaminophen level is 0	Acetaminophen overdose
2,3-Dimercapto-succinic acid (DMSA)	30 mg/kg/day in 3 divided doses for 5 days followed by 20 mg/kg/day in 2 divided doses for 14 days*	Lead poisoning
Digoxin-specific Fab antibody fragments	Administered in equimolar dose to the digoxin load; 40 mg binds 0.6 mg of digoxin*	Cardiac glycoside overdose
Glucagon	3-5 mg up to 10 mg IVP; a continuous IV infusion may be used	Beta-blocker and calcium channel blocker overdose
Naloxone	2 mg IVP initially; can be repeated; a continuous IV infusion may be used	Opioid overdose
Flumazenil	0.2 mg IVP over 60 sec initially; if needed, 0.1 mg IVP over 60 sec can be repeated until a total dose of 1 mg is given	Benzodiazepines
Deferoxamine	1-2 g IM	Iron poisoning
Physostigmine	0.5-1 mg IVP over 60 sec	TCAs
Pralidoxime chloride	2 g IV infusion over 30 min	Organophosphates

*Data from Fine J, Goldfrank L: *Pediatr Emerg Med* 39:1031-1051, 1992.
IVP, Intravenous push.

NURSING SURVEILLANCE

1. Monitor the patient's consciousness level.
2. Monitor the trend of the vital signs and oxygen saturation.
3. Monitor intake and output to assess fluid balance and effects of interventions.
4. Monitor the patient for cardiac dysrhythmia.

EXPECTED PATIENT OUTCOMES

1. The patient's level of consciousness improves from the time of arrival.
2. The mean arterial pressure is maintained between 70 and 105 mm Hg.
3. The airway remains patent without aspiration.
4. Drug absorption is inhibited.
5. ABG levels trend toward normal limits.

DISCHARGE IMPLICATIONS

1. Check the serum level before discharge if possible.
2. Teach the family seizure precautions.
3. Teach the family the need for follow-up to rule out complications that may occur later.
4. Teach the family about aspiration prevention, since the patient may vomit at home.
5. Beware of discharging a patient with a known overdose of acetaminophen or sustained-release medications, since symptoms may occur later.
6. Teach the family to have the poison control center phone number immediately available.
7. Teach the family the importance of the proper storage of medications and poisonous substances.

References

1. Zull D: Poisoning and drug overdose. In Kitt S: *Emergency nursing,* ed 2, Philadelphia, 1995, WB Saunders.
2. Platt D: Pharmacokinetics of drug overdose, *Clin Lab Med* 10:261-269, 1990.
3. Fine J, Goldfrank L: Update in medical toxicology, *Pediatr Emerg Med* 39:1031-1051, 1992.
4. Pruchnicki S: Just say know: recognizing the dangers of commonplace drugs, *JEMS* 16(2):26-41, 1991.
5. ACEP: Clinical policy for the initial approach to patients presenting with toxic ingestion or dermal or inhalation exposure, *Ann Emerg Med* 25:570-585, 1996.
6. Kirk M, Bowers L: Clueing in on the acutely poisoned patient, *JEMS* 16(5):64-78, 1991.
7. Kulig K: General management principles. In Rosen P, Barkin R: *Emergency medicine,* ed 4, St Louis, 1998, Mosby.
8. Cuddy P, Hamburger S: Poisoning: responding to the crisis, *Physic Assist* 12:77-86, 1988.
9. Burkhart K, Wuerz R, Donovan J: Whole bowel irrigation as adjunctive treatment for sustained release theophylline overdose, *Ann Emerg Med* 21:1316-1320, 1992.

10. Smilkstein M, Bronstein A, Linden C, et al: Acetaminophen overdose: a 48 hour intravenous *N*-acetylcysteine treatment protocol, *Ann Emerg Med* 20:1058-1063, 1991.
11. Spiller H, Krenzelok E, Grande G, et al: A prospective evaluation of the effect of activated charcoal before oral *N*-acetylcysteine in acetaminophen overdose, *Ann Emerg Med* 23:519-523, 1994.
12. Johnson R, Steiner J: Tricyclic antidepressant overdose: a toxicologic emergency, *J Am Acad Physic Assist* 2(1):16-22, 1989.
13. Smith D, Leake L, Loflin J, et al: Is admission after intravenous heroin overdose necessary? *Ann Emerg Med* 21:1326-1330, 1992.
14. House M: Cardiovascular effects of cocaine, *J Cardiovas Nurs* 6:1-11, 1992.
15. McMullen M: Cocaine, amphetamines and other sympathomimetics. In Rosen P, Barkin R: *Emergency medicine,* ed 4, St Louis, 1998, Mosby.
16. Centers for Disease Control and Prevention: *Preventing lead poisoning in young children,* Atlanta, 1991, Department of Health and Human Services.
17. Boisvert S: A 27-year-old woman with verapamil overdose, *J Emerg Nurs* 16:317-320, 1990.
18. Ramoska E, Spiller H, Winter M, et al: A one year evaluation of calcium channel blocker overdoses: toxicity and treatment, *Ann Emerg Med* 22:196-200, 1993.

T

Chapter 20

Trauma

Colleen Swartz
Steve Talbert

CLINICAL CONDITIONS
Chest Trauma
Sentinel Injuries
Blunt Cardiac Injury
Cardiac Tamponade
Aortic Transection
Flail Chest
Pneumothorax and Tension Pneumothorax
Hemothorax and Tension Hemothorax
Pulmonary Contusion
Ruptured Diaphragm (Hemidiaphragm)
Ruptured Bronchus and Trachea
Abdominal Trauma
Pelvic Fractures

TRIAGE ASSESSMENT

Although most trauma patients are transported to the emergency department (ED) by prehospital personnel, occasionally a patient walks in or is brought to the ED by a friend or family member. Triage personnel must recognize the potential severity of the trauma and escort the patient immediately to the treatment area where the initial assessment can be made.

Care of the trauma patient begins with the primary survey. The purpose of the primary survey is to identify and correct any life-threatening conditions.[1,2] This includes assessing the airway (while taking cervical spine precautions), breathing, and circulation and performing a brief neurologic examination (to examine for deficit). Once the primary survey is complete, the patient is completely exposed, then covered to maintain body temperature, and a full set of vital signs is obtained. Finally, a thorough head-to-toe examination is performed to identify all potential injuries. The "Trauma Assessment" box summarizes the trauma assessment and provides a simple acronym to help remember the proper sequence.[2]

Primary Survey
Airway with cervical spine precautions
1. Inspect for an actual or potential airway obstruction.
   - Foreign body
   - Blood
   - Vomitus
   - Tongue
   - Swelling
2. Listen for air movement.
   - If the patient's airway is not patent, steps must be taken immediately to open the airway. Table 20-1 lists life-threatening airway problems, their signs and symptoms, and immediate interventions.

NURSING ALERT

A talking patient has a patent airway.

NURSING ALERT

Any patients who have blunt trauma or who have penetrating trauma above the nipple line must have the cervical spine immobilized simultaneously with airway assessment.

TRAUMA ASSESSMENT

Primary assessment

Airway with cervical spine precautions
Breathing
Circulation
Deficit (brief neurologic examination)

Secondary assessment

Expose (remove all clothing) and **E**vacuate (if necessary)
Fahrenheit (maintain body temperature)
Get full set of vital signs
Head-to-toe examination
Inspect the back

TABLE 20-1 Life-Threatening Airway Problems

Problem	Signs and symptoms	Interventions
Airway obstruction (complete or partial)	Dyspnea, labored respirations Decreased or no air movement Cyanosis Presence of foreign body in airway Trauma to face or neck	Airway opening maneuvers • Jaw thrust • Chin lift • Suction Airway adjuncts • Nasal airway • Oral airway • Endotracheal tube Surgical airway • Cricothyrotomy • Tracheostomy
Inhalation injury	History of enclosed-space fire, unconsciousness, or exposure to heavy smoke Dyspnea Wheezing, rhonchi, and crackles Hoarseness Singed facial or nasal hairs Carbonaceous sputum Burns to face or neck	Provide high-flow oxygen (100%) via nonrebreather mask or bag-valve device Prepare for endotracheal intubation as soon as possible

NURSING ALERT

Intubation of the trauma patient may be difficult. Use of rapid sequence induction for intubation may be helpful; however, application of this procedure should be reserved for practitioners with excellent airway skills.

Breathing
1. Inspect for rise and fall of the chest.
   • Asymmetry may indicate a pneumothorax or hemothorax.
   • Paradoxical movement indicates a flail chest.

2. Inspect for open chest trauma.
   - Assume that a pneumothorax is present in the case of a sucking chest wound.
3. Inspect for work of breathing.
   - Increased work of breathing is a sign of potential breathing problems.
   - Nasal flaring and the use of accessory muscles are classic signs of dyspnea.
4. Inspect and palpate for tracheal position.
   - The trachea may deviate away from a tension pneumothorax (usually a late sign).
5. Auscultate lung fields for the presence of breath sounds.
   - Unequal, diminished, or absent sounds may indicate a pneumothorax, hemothorax, or viscerothorax.
6. Palpate the chest for instability and subcutaneous air.
   - The presence of either crepitus or subcutaneous air indicates an underlying chest injury and a probable pneumothorax.

Initially, trauma patients should receive 100% oxygen by a nonrebreather mask or bag-valve device. Table 20-2 lists life-threatening breathing problems, their signs and symptoms, and immediate interventions.

Circulation

1. Inspect for an obvious external hemorrhage.
2. Inspect skin color, temperature, and moisture.
   - Skin that is pale, cool, or moist indicates a poor perfusion state.
3. Palpate for central and peripheral pulse presence, rate, and symmetry.
   - Weak, thready, or absent pulses indicate a poor perfusion state.
   - Early manifestations of shock include tachycardia and cutaneous vasoconstriction.
   - Weak peripheral pulses relative to central pulses indicate a poor perfusion state.

Initially, trauma patients should receive warm isotonic crystalloid solution (Ringer's lactate or 0.9% NaCl) through two large-bore IV lines. A large-bore IV is a 14- or 16-gauge for adults and a 22-gauge or greater for pediatric patients.[1,2] Table 20-3 lists life-threatening circulation problems, their signs and symptoms, and immediate interventions.

T

TABLE 20-2 Life-Threatening Breathing Problems

Problem	Signs and symptoms	Interventions
Tension pneumothorax (tension pneumothorax is a clinical diagnosis)	Dyspnea, labored respirations Decreased or absent breath sounds on affected side Unilateral chest rise and fall Tracheal deviation away from affected side Cyanosis Jugular venous distention Tachycardia and hypotension History of chest trauma or mechanical ventilation	Provide high-flow oxygen (100%) via nonrebreather mask or bag-valve device Rapid chest decompression by needle thoracostomy on affected side Chest tube placement on affected side
Pneumothorax	Dyspnea, labored respirations Decreased or absent breath sounds on affected side May have unilateral chest rise and fall May have visible wound to chest or back History of chest trauma	Provide high-flow oxygen (100%) via nonrebreather mask or bag-valve device Chest tube placement on affected side Place occlusive dressing over any open chest wound and secure on three sides with tape

Condition	Signs/Symptoms	Interventions
Hemothorax	Dyspnea, labored respirations; Decreased or absent breath sounds on affected side; May have unilateral chest rise and fall; Tachycardia and hypotension; May have visible wound to chest or back; History of chest trauma (usually penetrating)	Provide high-flow oxygen (100%) via nonrebreather mask or bag-valve device; Chest tube placement on affected side; Consider autotransfusion (Procedure 4)
Sucking chest wound	Dyspnea, labored respirations; Visible, sucking wound to chest or back; Decreased or absent breath sounds on affected side	Provide high-flow oxygen (100%) via nonrebreather mask or bag-valve device; Cover wound with occlusive dressing and secure on 3 sides with tape; Watch for signs of tension pneumothorax and remove dressing during exhalation if they are noted
Flail chest	Dyspnea, labored respirations; Paradoxical chest wall movement; Chest pain; Tachycardia	Provide high-flow oxygen (100%) via nonrebreather mask or bag-valve device; Prepare for intubation and mechanical ventilation
Full-thickness circumferential burn of thorax	Dyspnea, labored respirations; Shallow respirations; Obvious circumferential burns to thorax	Provide high-flow oxygen (100%) via nonrebreather mask or bag-valve device; Prepare for immediate escharotomy (Chapter 4)

T

TABLE 20-3 Life-Threatening Circulation Problems

Problem	Signs and symptoms	Interventions
External hemorrhage	Obvious bleeding site	Direct pressure Elevation (see box below)
Shock	Tachycardia Weak, thready pulses Cool, pale clammy skin Tachypnea Altered mental status Delayed capillary refill Oliguria or anuria	Provide high-flow oxygen (100%) via non-rebreather mask or bag-valve device Place two large-bore IV lines with warm isotonic crystalloid solution infusing (Ringer's lactate or 0.9% NaCl) Administer fluid bolus (2 liters in adults or 20 ml/kg in children) Prepare to administer blood

NURSING ALERT

Most hemorrhaging can be controlled with direct pressure. Clamping bleeding vessels or placing a tourniquet is a measure of last resort. Direct pressure may be best applied by direct fingertip pressure to the bleeding vessel. This may involve the removal of pressure dressings so that hemorrhage control can be obtained.

Deficit (brief neurologic assessment)

The brief neurologic assessment consists of assessing the best eye opening, best motor response, best verbal response, and pupil size and reactivity. The Glasgow Coma Scale (GCS) assigns a number to the eye opening, motor response, and verbal response, then combines the numbers for a total score (Table 20-4).

1. Check for the best eye opening.
   • The eye opening may be spontaneous or in response to voice or to pain, or there may be no eye opening.

TABLE 20-4 Glasgow Coma Scale

Clinical finding	Score	Clinical application
Best eye opening		
Spontaneous	4	Be sure to give the patient the best score for demonstrated eye opening
Voice	3	
Pain	2	
None	1	
Best motor response		
Follows commands	6	Localization should be tested and be present in both upper and lower extremities
		Be sure to give the patient the best score for demonstrated motor response
Purposeful to pain	5	
Withdraws to pain	4	
Flexes to pain	3	
Extends to pain	2	
None	1	
Best verbal response		
Oriented	5	If the patient is intubated, the score is "1" with a notation of intubation (e.g., "1T")
		Be sure to give the patient the best score for verbal response
Confused	4	
Inappropriate words	3	
Incomprehensible sounds	2	
None	1	

2. Check for the best motor response.
   - The patient may obey commands, demonstrate purposeful movement (localize to pain), withdraw in response to pain, demonstrate abnormal flexion (decorticate) or extension (decerebrate), or not respond at all.

3. Check for the best verbal response.
   - The patient may be oriented or confused, use inappropriate words or incomprehensible sounds, or demonstrate no verbal response.
4. Check for pupil size and reactivity.
   - Fixed, dilated pupils are consistent with a severe closed-head injury.
   - Unilateral dilation may indicate transtentorial herniation.
   - Constricted pupils may indicate a drug overdose.

The GCS evaluation should include an evaluation of motor responsiveness for all four extremities. Lateralizing motor findings are important to report and should be handled with a sense of urgency because transtentorial herniation may be imminent. When a physical examination reveals an unequal motor response, the *best* motor score should be assigned, with appropriate notation of inequality in the narrative description of the physical examination.

Trauma patients who have a head injury and a GCS score <13 should be evaluated by a neurosurgeon. Patients who have a GCS score <8 should be intubated. For patients who have severe head injuries (a GCS score <8), treatment goals are to maintain a systolic blood pressure (BP) >90 mm Hg and a PaO_2 >60 mm Hg (Chapter 14), and avoid secondary injury exacerbated by hypoxemia or hypotension.

FOCUSED NURSING ASSESSMENT
Secondary Survey
Once the primary assessment is complete and all life-threatening conditions are corrected, the secondary examination can be performed. The secondary survey involves a thorough head-to-toe examination and a history of the events surrounding the injury.
Expose and evacuate
Expose the patient by removing all articles of clothing. If the patient is immobilized, it is usually necessary to cut off the clothes. Exposing the patient is necessary to identify injuries rapidly. Make plans to evacuate the patient to a definitive care facility if necessary.

Optimal care for the critically injured trauma patient is frequently time dependent. Outcomes can be improved if the patient receives rapid, definitive care. The trauma nurse should compare the needs of the patient with resources available at the facility. If the necessary resources are not available at the facility in which the trauma patient is receiving care, arrangements for transfer should be made as quickly as possible. Do not delay a transfer for diagnostic studies.

Fahrenheit (maintain body temperature)

The patient should not be left uncovered. Hypothermia is common with the trauma patient and has detrimental effects. Measures should be taken to preserve body heat and prevent hypothermia. These measures include warm blankets, special warming blankets, an increase in the temperature of the resuscitation room, the use of warming lights, and the use of warm IV fluids. If continuous core temperature monitoring (e.g., a temperature-sensing indwelling urinary catheter) is available, it should be used to ensure prevention of hypothermia.

Get vital signs

A full set of vital signs should be obtained as quickly as possible. These include the heart rate, respiratory rate, blood pressure, and core body temperature. Heart monitoring and pulse oximetry should be initiated if possible. End-tidal CO_2 monitoring may be instituted with intubated patients to measure the effectiveness of ventilation.

Head-to-toe examination

The head-to-toe examination is a thorough and systematic assessment of the entire body. It includes auscultation, inspection, palpation, and percussion.

- *Head and neck:* The head should be inspected for obvious wounds (e.g., lacerations, contusions, abrasions, or burns), external hemorrhage, deformities, impaled objects, or drainage from the nose (rhinorrhea) or ears (otorrhea). The head also should be palpated for deformities, areas of tenderness, or subcutaneous air. Furthermore, the stability of the midface and alignment of the teeth should be assessed.

  The neck should be assessed for any obvious wounds, external hemorrhage, or impaled objects. The presence or absence of jugular venous distention (JVD) should be noted. The tracheal position should be palpated. Any areas of tenderness should be noted. Auscultation of bruits over major vessels may indicate vascular injury. The quality of the patient's voice should be evaluated for hoarseness. The patient also should be evaluated for the inability to manage his or her secretions because of pain with swallowing, which may be indicative of direct airway trauma.

NURSING ALERT

Alignment of the cervical spine must be maintained during assessment of the neck.

- *Chest:* The chest should be inspected for signs of obvious injury, including the presence of a sucking chest wound, external hemorrhage, or impaled objects. The rise and fall of the chest wall should be observed for symmetry and equality. Palpate the chest wall for tenderness, crepitus, and the presence of subcutaneous air. Finally, auscultate for the depth, quality, and equality of breath sounds. The presence or absence of bowel sounds in the chest should be noted as well.
- *Abdomen:* An abdominal assessment begins with an inspection of the abdomen for signs of obvious trauma, external hemorrhage, or impaled objects. Next, auscultate for bowel sounds or bruits in all quadrants. The abdomen should be palpated for areas of tenderness, firmness, and distention. Rigidity, distention, and pain are indicators of possible internal injury and ongoing hemorrhage or peritonitis. With any abnormal findings during the abdominal examination, a surgical abdomen should be assumed and accordingly treated with a sense of urgency.
- *Pelvis:* The pelvis should be inspected for signs of obvious trauma, external hemorrhage, or impaled objects. Next, it should be palpated for tenderness and stability. This is accomplished by first pushing downward simultaneously on the anterior aspect of the iliac crests, then pushing inward simultaneously on the lateral aspect of the iliac crests. Finally, gentle pressure should be applied to the symphysis pubis. As a general rule, this assessment elicits pain or reveals instability if the pelvis is fractured. In cases of pelvic instability, repeated bony pelvic examination should be deferred to prevent additional blood loss caused by repeated manipulation of the pelvis.
- *Genitourinary:* The genitourinary and gynecologic assessment begins with an inspection for signs of obvious

trauma, external hemorrhage, impaled objects, blood at the urethral meatus, vaginal bleeding, or a scrotal hematoma. If blood is present at the urethral meatus, insertion of an indwelling urinary catheter should be postponed until the patency of the urethra is confirmed. All women should receive a vaginal examination to rule out internal injuries.

- *Extremities:* Finally, the extremities should be assessed. Inspect for signs of obvious trauma, external hemorrhage, impaled objects, or deformities. Palpate each extremity for areas of tenderness or deformity, determine capillary refill time, and assess pulse presence and quality. Pulse quality should be compared bilaterally simultaneously for equality. Likewise, sensation should be checked in each extremity and compared bilaterally for equality. Lastly, the range of motion may be checked unless contraindicated.

Inspect the back

NURSING ALERT

Cervical spine immobilization must be maintained while the patient is logrolled and the back assessed. Neurologic checks for movement and sensation of extremities should be performed before and immediately after the logroll.

The patient should be carefully logrolled onto either side. Inspect the back, buttocks, and dorsal side of lower extremities for signs of obvious trauma, external hemorrhage, or impaled objects. The spine should be palpated for areas of tenderness, muscle spasms, stepoffs, or deformity. A rectal examination should be performed to determine rectal tone, the presence of blood, and direct rectal trauma. The position of the prostate should also be established for male trauma patients before insertion of an indwelling urinary catheter. The patient should be carefully rolled back into the supine position when the back assessment is complete.

T

NURSING ALERT

Before performing the rectal examination, the practitioner should put on a new glove. This minimizes the risk of a false positive reading for rectal bleeding.

History

Another component of the secondary assessment is obtaining a rapid, focused history that provides important data for anticipating injuries and guiding patient care. This history includes an AMPLE data set: *A*llergies, *M*edications, *P*ast medical history, *L*ast oral intake, and *E*vents surrounding the traumatic event (e.g., mechanism of injury, seat belt or helmet use, type of weapon used, and loss of consciousness after the injury). The acronym AMPLE can serve as a reminder for the information needed. The history should include the mechanism of injury, the extent of injuries (based on prehospital assessment), vital signs in the field, and interventions in the field (MIVI).[2]

Risk Factors

Age

Trauma is the leading cause of death during the first four decades of life. Although historically the young are trauma patients, trauma is a growing problem for the geriatric population. The mechanisms of injury differ for these age groups. Younger patients are frequently involved in motor vehicle crashes (driver, passenger, and pedestrian or bicyclist) or violence. Falling is the leading cause of injury for the geriatric population.

Preexisting medical conditions

Certain medical conditions can predispose patients to injury. These diseases create one of several conditions that increase the risk of injury, such as an altered level of consciousness, altered sensory input, or altered thought processes. Table 20-5 lists common chronic medical conditions and their mechanism for predisposing patients to traumatic injury. Also, intercurrent illnesses may alter the normal physiologic response to injury. The patient's past medical history should be carefully reviewed to determine the "expected" response to the stress of trauma.

Medications

As with preexisting medical conditions, certain medications can predispose patients to injury. Drugs that directly or indirectly alter the mental status are the prime contributors. Table 20-6 lists classes of medications and their mechanism for predisposing patients to traumatic injury.

TABLE 20-5 Common Medical Conditions That Increase Risk for Injury

Medical condition	Mechanism of increased risk	Etiology of increased risk
Diabetes mellitus	Altered level of consciousness	Hypoglycemia Hyperglycemia
Seizures	Altered level of consciousness	Hitting head or face Fractured extremity Falling into path of vehicle
Cardiovascular disease	Altered level of consciousness	Syncope
Peripheral vascular disease	Altered sensory input	Orthostatic hypotension Dysrhythmias Myocardial infarction Cerebral vascular accident Transient ischemic attack Neuropathies
Substance abuse	Altered level of consciousness Altered sensory input Altered thought process	Altered judgment Altered reflexes Unconsciousness
Psychiatric illness	Altered thought process	Depression Suicidal ideation Self-destructive behavior

Life Span Issues

NURSING ALERT

Assessment and intervention priorities are the same for all patients, regardless of age.

Pediatric considerations
General considerations

1. Blunt trauma is the leading cause of injury, accounting for up to 80% of pediatric traumas.
2. Deterioration of the child's clinical condition may be insidious–frequent systems reassessment is critical.

TABLE 20-6 Common Medication Classes That Increase Risk of Injury

Medication class	Etiology of increased risk of injury
Antidiabetic	Hypoglycemia
Antiseizure	Depressed level of consciousness
Antihypertensives	Syncope
	Orthostatic hypotension
Antidysrhythmias	Hypotension
	Bradycardia
	Dysrhythmias
Antihistamines	CNS depression
Antineoplastics	Anemia
Antipsychotics	Extrapyramidal symptoms
	Hypotension
	Dysrhythmias
Barbiturates	CNS depression
Benzodiazepines	CNS depression
Diuretics	Hypovolemia
	Hypotension
	Electrolyte imbalances
Narcotics	CNS depression
Thyroid hormone	Thyroid storm

CNS, Central Nervous System.

3. Children have higher metabolic rates and require increased amounts of oxygen and substrates.
4. The skeletal system of a child is immature and flexible. It provides little protection for underlying structures. Consequently, a serious underlying injury may be present in the absence of fractures.
5. Children, especially young children, have immature or inadequate thermoregulation. The prevention of heat loss through the use of warmed fluids, blankets, and management of the environment is critical.
6. Children have immature immune systems. The prevention of infection through the use of strict sterile technique is important.
7. The presence of the primary caregiver is important to help the child cope with the stress of a traumatic injury.
8. When assessing the child and intervening, keep the child's developmental level in mind.

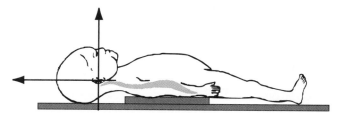

Figure 20-1 Proper spinal immobilization for children younger than 8 years of age. (Modified from Nypaver M, Treloar T: *Ann Emerg Med* 23:209, 1994.)

Airway and breathing

1. Children <12 months of age are obligatory nose breathers. Nasal passages must remain clear unless an artificial airway (e.g., an endotracheal tube [ET]) is provided.
2. The trachea is shorter and more anterior in children. Intubation may be difficult.
3. Uncuffed ET use in smaller children necessitates frequent respiratory assessments to confirm placement. Securing these tubes and providing frequent ongoing assessment of tube position are critical.
4. Provide high-flow oxygen (100%) via nonrebreather mask, bag-valve device, or mechanical ventilator.

Cervical spine

1. Children <8 years of age should have padding placed under the back and shoulders to alleviate flexion of the cervical spine. Figure 20-1 illustrates proper spinal immobilization for children.

Circulation

1. Children compensate well for hypovolemia, and clinical shock symptoms (especially hypotension) may be masked for a prolonged period.
2. The peripheral IV selected should be as large as possible.
   - Infant: 20- to 24-gauge
   - Young child: 16- to 20-gauge
   - Older child: 18-gauge or larger
3. Intraosseous fluid and drug administration is an option if peripheral access cannot be obtained (Procedure 22).
4. Fluid volume replacement is as follows:
   - Initiate 20 ml/kg of isotonic crystalloid solution by rapid IV push.

T

- If there is no response, repeat 20 ml/kg bolus of isotonic crystalloid solution by IV push.
- If a shock state persists, administer 10 ml/kg packed red blood cells by IV push.
- Repeat blood administration as necessary.

NURSING ALERT

Hypothermia has severe detrimental effects on the pediatric trauma patient. All fluids should be warmed before administration if possible. Blood should be mixed with warm saline or given via blood warmer.

A general rule of thumb to guide volume replacement is the "3 for 1" rule: for each milliliter of blood loss, replacement should occur with 3 ml of crystalloid. Ongoing evaluation of the patient's response to fluid resuscitation is essential to ensure a good patient outcome and maintenance of end organ perfusion status.

Deficit
1. When assessing mental status, keep the patient's development level in mind.
2. Table 20-7 shows the pediatric GCS.

Geriatric considerations
General considerations
1. A diminished ability to compensate (loss of physiologic reserve) is a hallmark of aging.
2. Mortality is higher among the geriatric population for every body region.
3. Mortality increases with age up to 85 years.
4. Falling is the leading cause of injury for the geriatric population.
5. Geriatric patients have an increased mortality from motor vehicle crashes and burns.
6. Physiologic changes are seen in every system and vary with lifestyle and preexisting medical conditions.
7. The patient's response to medication can change with age because of altered body tissue (e.g., decreased lean body mass and increased adipose tissue), altered receptor response, altered absorption (e.g., decreased GI blood flow), or altered metabolism (e.g., decreased renal clearance).
8. The immune response is diminished. Careful attention to the prevention of infection is important.

TABLE 20-7 Pediatric Glasgow Coma Scale (Children Ages 3 and Under)

Clinical finding	Score
Eye opening	
Spontaneous	4
Reaction to speech	3
Reaction to pain	2
No Response	1
Motor response	
Spontaneous (obeys commands)	6
Localizes to pain	5
Withdraws to pain	4
Abnormal flexion to pain	3
Abnormal extension to pain	2
No response	1
Verbal response	
Smiles, coos, babbles, appropriate phrases of talking	5
Irritable, appropriate crying, consolable	4
Persistent/inappropriate crying, screaming	3
Grunts/moans, agitated, restless	2
No verbal response	1

9. Thermoregulation, especially the ability to generate heat, is also diminished. Take immediate steps to prevent hypothermia. If possible, continuously monitor the core temperature.
10. Medication use may further reduce the ability to compensate and may mask clinical signs of shock. Medication use also may affect the success of interventions.
11. Traditional "norms" that are used to guide resuscitation must be adjusted for the geriatric population. A high index of suspicion should be maintained, even with minor injuries, because of the effect of aging on physiologic reserve and ability to mount the response needed to recover from the injury sustained.

Airway and breathing
1. There is a generalized reduction in pulmonary function.
2. Preexisting diseases (e.g., chronic obstructive pulmonary disease) may have a significant effect on compensatory mechanisms for shock.

Cervical spine

1. Arthritic changes may complicate assessment and immobilization.
2. Composition changes (e.g., osteoporosis) increase the likelihood of injury.

Circulation

1. If arteriosclerosis or peripheral vascular disease is present, higher arterial pressures (hypertension) may be necessary to perfuse organs and extremities. *"Normal" BP may be present even though a state of inadequate tissue perfusion exists.*
2. Fluids should be administered with caution. Do not withhold needed volume, but perform frequent reassessment of the cardiovascular and respiratory systems. Watch closely for signs of fluid overload.
3. Many geriatric patients are candidates for early invasive monitoring, and the monitoring should be used to guide resuscitation efforts if indicated.

Deficit

Cognitive skills may be slowed or diminished with increasing age and certain degenerative diseases (e.g., Alzheimer's and dementia). Make an early effort to determine a baseline neurologic status from reliable sources.

Obstetric Considerations

General considerations

1. Motor vehicle crashes are the leading cause of maternal injury.
2. Intravascular fluid volume, cardiac output, minute ventilation, and oxygen consumption increase during pregnancy.
3. Normal WBC counts may be as high as $25,000/mm^3$.
4. Normal hematocrit and hemoglobin levels are decreased.
5. Gastric emptying and peristalsis are slowed.
6. Maternal concern may be focused on the well-being of the fetus. Reassurance is important.

Airway and breathing

Increased oxygen consumption requires an increase in oxygen delivery. Provide pregnant trauma patients with high-flow oxygen.

Cervical spine

Fully immobilize the pregnant patient.

Circulation

1. Increased plasma volume allows for maternal compensation, but harm may come to the fetus because of a decreased oxygen and substrate supply.

2. Pregnant women may compensate for a prolonged period with only minimal clinical signs.
3. The supine position, especially in later gestation, causes the uterus to rest on the inferior vena cava, causing diminished venous return, which in turn decreases cardiac output. The pregnant patient should be rolled slightly to the left side while immobilization is maintained.

INITIAL INTERVENTIONS

Once the primary and secondary assessments are complete and all life-threatening conditions are corrected, other initial interventions may be necessary.
1. Gastric distention poses two potential problems for the trauma patient. First, distention pushes a full stomach upward into the diaphragm, decreasing pulmonary capacity and, consequently, gas exchange. Furthermore, gastric distention increases the risk of vomiting and aspiration. Decompression of the stomach should be accomplished via a nasogastric tube as early in the resuscitation as possible. Evacuation of the stomach contents early may also minimize the degree of contamination in cases of direct trauma to the gastrointestinal tract.

NURSING ALERT

If a basilar skull fracture is suspected or if the midface is unstable, the gastric tube should be passed orally, not nasally.

2. Bladder distention also poses a unique set of problems. Not only is it uncomfortable for the patient, but it can increase anxiety, BP, and heart rate as well. An indwelling urinary catheter should be placed as early in the resuscitation as possible.

NURSING ALERT

Before an indwelling urinary catheter can be inserted, the meatus should be assessed for bleeding or signs of trauma. With males, assessment for a scrotal hematoma and prostate size and position must be done before catheter placement.

T

3. Other interventions include tetanus prophylaxis, dressing wounds, and immobilization of any known or suspected fractures.

4. The psychosocial interventions are an important part of the resuscitation. Trauma patients are under extreme stress and usually in a state of crisis. It is natural for them to mobilize usual coping mechanisms in order to adapt. However, normal coping mechanisms may be quickly overwhelmed by fear, pain, and loss of control. The nurse should facilitate the use of normal coping mechanisms, reduce anxiety and pain, and give the patient as much control as possible. Interventions such as informing the patient of procedures before they are done, maintaining eye contact, holding a hand, or taking time to listen can facilitate coping. Allowing a significant other to remain at or near the bedside may improve adaptation as well.

5. Significant others (e.g., family and friends) may also be experiencing feelings of anxiety, fear, anger, and guilt. Taking the time to keep them informed of the patient's condition and prognosis is critical for their coping. Allowing them to see the patient as quickly as possible and reassuring them that the trauma team truly cares about the patient also helps them deal with the crisis.

PRIORITY NURSING DIAGNOSES

Risk for altered tissue perfusion
Risk for pain
Risk for alteration in gas exchange

♦ **Altered tissue perfusion** related to hypoperfusion and shunting of blood:

INTERVENTIONS
- Initiate two large-bore IVs for fluid resuscitation.
- Administer warmed Ringer's lactate or 0.9% NaCl solution as indicated to maintain systolic BP ≥90 mm Hg and urine output 1 ml/kg/hr.
- Apply direct pressure to external sources of bleeding.
- Monitor the patient for internal bleeding, abdominal rigidity, expanding hematomas, a decreasing level of consciousness, diminishing breath sounds, or dullness on lung percussion.

♦ **Pain** related to stimulation of nerve endings:

INTERVENTIONS
- Administer IM or IV nonsteroidal antiinflammatory agents per physician order.

- Place the patient in a position of comfort after clearance for spinal injuries.
- Use imagery to help the patient cope with the pain.
- Use distraction to help the patient cope with the pain.
- Allow the presence of support systems.

◆ **Alteration in gas exchange** related to an occluded or partially occluded airway, chest and lung injury, and hypoperfusion:

INTERVENTIONS
- Maintain a patent airway and suction as necessary.
- Administer high flow O_2 per mask or bag-valve device and ET.
- Monitor breath sounds and chest wall excursion and movement.
- Prepare for chest tube insertion if appropriate.
- Monitor ABGs, blood lactate levels, and SpO_2 readings.

PRIORITY DIAGNOSTIC TESTS

During the initial resuscitation of the trauma patient, priority diagnostic tests should be individualized based on the mechanism of injury and clinical findings. However, there are a number of laboratory tests, radiographic examinations, and special procedures that may be anticipated. Tables 20-8 to 20-10 list common diagnostic tests and special procedures, their clinical indications, and clinical implications.

TABLE 20-8 Common Laboratory Tests

Laboratory test	Clinical implications
Complete blood count (CBC)	Hematocrit and hemoglobin levels may be normal or above normal despite acute hemorrhage
	Normal values do not exclude hemorrhagic shock
Electrolytes	Baseline data
	Rule out electrolyte imbalance
Prothrombin time	Baseline data
Partial thromboplastin time	Rule out coagulopathies
Amylase	Baseline data
	Elevated value may indicate possible intra-abdominal injury

Continued

TABLE 20-8 Common Laboratory Tests—cont'd

Laboratory test	Clinical implications
Lipase	Baseline data
	Elevated value may indicate possible intra-abdominal injury
Lactate	Baseline data
	Elevated level correlates with acute hemorrhage, shock, and increased anaerobic metabolism
Arterial blood gas	Assess ventilatory and respiratory status
	Acidosis, especially in the presence of normal or decreased $PaCO_2$ level, correlates with shock
	Base deficit of -6 or greater correlates with acute hemorrhage and shock
	Decreased PaO_2 and SaO_2 and an elevated $PaCO_2$ may indicate an airway or breathing emergency
Liver function tests	Baseline data
	Elevated values may indicate liver damage
Type and crossmatch	Prepare for administration of blood and blood products

TABLE 20-9 Common Radiographic Examinations

Radiographic examination	Indication	Clinical implications
Chest x-ray	Chest trauma or pain	Anteroposterior examination with patient in supine position if immobilized
	Shortness of breath	Should be taken immediately upon arrival if possible
		Do not delay treatment of a suspected tension pneumothorax for a chest x-ray

CT, Computed tomography.

TABLE 20-9 Common Radiographic Examinations—cont'd

Radiographic examination	Indication	Clinical implications
Pelvis x-ray	Blunt trauma Pelvic pain or instability Blood at urethral meatus	Anteroposterior examination with patient in supine position Should be taken early in the resuscitation
Cervical spine x-ray	Blunt trauma Trauma above nipple line Neck tenderness Neurologic deficit	Cross-table lateral film usually obtained early in resuscitation Immobilization should be maintained until the spine is radiographically and clinically cleared
Thoracic and lumbar spine x-ray	Blunt trauma Back pain or trauma Neurologic deficit	Patient should be logrolled until spine is cleared radiographically and clinically
Extremity x-ray examinations	Extremity trauma, deformity, or pain	Suspected fractures should be immobilized before radiographs
Head CT scan	Head trauma Loss of consciousness Focal neurologic findings Altered level of consciousness	Transfer to a definitive care facility should not be delayed to obtain a head CT scan
Abdominal CT scan	Abdominal trauma or pain Altered level of consciousness Unreliable clinical examination	Transfer to a definitive care facility should not be delayed to obtain an abdominal CT scan
Abdominal ultrasound	Abdominal trauma or pain	Interference in imaging may occur with obesity, bowel gas, and subcutaneous emphysema

T

TABLE 20-10 Common Special Procedures

Procedure	Indication	Clinical implications
Angiography	Suspected vessel injury Cerebral blood flow study	Be prepared to assess and intervene in the event of an anaphylactic reaction Insertion site must be watched closely for bleeding after procedure
Diagnostic peritoneal lavage	Abdominal trauma or pain, especially in a hemodynamically unstable patient	Gastric and bladder decompression must be done before performing a diagnostic peritoneal lavage This procedure does not evaluate the retroperitoneal space
Transesophageal echocardiogram	Widened mediastinum Significant chest trauma	Patient is usually rolled on side for procedure Patient may be sedated during procedure

COLLABORATIVE INTERVENTIONS

Although trauma may affect every body region and system, this chapter focuses on injuries to the chest, abdomen, and pelvis. Trauma to other regions is discussed in the appropriate chapters.

Clinical Conditions
Chest trauma

Of all patients admitted with a chest injury, only 15% require a thoracotomy for definitive management. Thus, 85% of patients with chest injuries can be managed with general resuscitative techniques, including ventilatory support, a tube thoracostomy, or other interventions for management of chest injuries.

Sentinel injuries

Some injury patterns are not particularly life threatening by themselves but should raise suspicion of other potentially life-threatening injuries. These injuries are termed

SENTINEL INJURY AND ASSOCIATED INJURY PATTERN

- First rib fracture: heart or great vessel injury (subclavian vein and artery), CNS injury (head and neck)
- Scapula fracture: brachial plexus, pulmonary contusion, great vessel, CNS injury
- Sternal fracture: blunt cardiac injury, great vessel, pulmonary contusion
- Right lower rib fractures: liver lacerations
- Left lower rib fractures: spleen lacerations

CNS, Central nervous system.

"sentinel" injuries and should prompt the emergency nurse to watch for the more life-threatening associated injuries. The sentinel injuries of particular importance are outlined in the "Sentinel Injury" box.

Blunt cardiac injury

Symptoms

- Anginal chest pain, dyspnea, hypoperfusion, and hypotension may be present.
- Symptoms vary depending on the extent of the injury.
- The patient may arrive in frank left ventricular failure with crackles on auscultation and with the presence of S_3 and JVD.
- A 12-lead ECG may reveal conduction or rhythm disturbances.
- Premature atrial contractions, premature ventricular contractions, atrial fibrillation and flutter, ventricular tachycardia, and bundle branch block may occur. This is especially true of the right bundle branch block, since the right ventricle is situated to the right of the sternum, positioned anteriorly, leaving it virtually unprotected against a high-energy impact.

Diagnosis

- A 12-lead ECG and transthoracic or transesophageal imaging may be used for diagnosis.
- Some institutions use creatinine phosphokinase and lactate dehydrogenase with isoenzymes to evaluate blunt cardiac injury; however, these fail to detect injury with one third to one half of patients who have actual myocardial damage detected via transthoracic imaging and who

have been removed from most initial protocols for evaluation of blunt cardiac injury.

Review your institutional blunt cardiac injury evaluation protocol.

TREATMENT

- Evaluate and intervene during the primary assessment and evaluation of airway, breathing, and circulation (ABCs).
- Oxygen should be applied and vigilant ECG monitoring should ensue with early recognition and treatment of dysrhythmias.
- Potential pump failure with large contusional patterns may occur, and interventions should be initiated accordingly to maximize contractility (addition of inotropes, maximizing filling pressures), reduce afterload (addition of vasodilators), and optimize preload (optimizing volume status via volume infusion or diuresis, infusion of vasoactives).
- Central venous pressures should be monitored closely to guide volume resuscitation.
- Intensive-care unit or telemetry admission is likely and should be anticipated early during the patient's resuscitation if the initial ECG reveals a pattern consistent with blunt cardiac injury.

Cardiac tamponade

Cardiac tamponade is actually an expression of the injury (blunt or penetrating); however, it occurs most frequently with the patient experiencing penetrating chest trauma. The manifestation is denoted by a rapid accumulation of blood in the pericardial sac, causing a restriction of myocardial pump motion and chamber filling. Diminished stroke volume occurs along with a noticeable increase in chamber pressures.

SYMPTOMS

- The patient has anxiety, dyspnea, and duskiness or cyanosis.
- The patient demonstrates Beck's triad: hypotension, muffled heart tones, and JVD. Beck's triad manifests all three facets in only 35% to 65% of cases.
- Kussmaul's sign (a paradoxical rise in venous pressure with inspiration when breathing spontaneously) may occur when the patient inspires deeply.
- A progression of JVD occurs with deep inspiration, instead of the normal flattening of the jugular vein.

DIAGNOSIS

- Because cardiac tamponade and tension pneumothorax have similar symptoms, auscultation of breath sounds is crucial to a diagnosis.
- The patient with cardiac tamponade will have adequate, equilateral breath sounds.
- The patient with a tension pneumothorax, tension hemothorax, or tension viscerothorax will not have clear, equal breath sounds.
- Transthoracic or transesophageal imaging should be anticipated if the patient's condition is amenable to further diagnostic evaluation.
- With acute deterioration, prepare for pericardiocentesis.

TREATMENT

- Administer high-flow oxygen to maximize DO_2 (oxygen delivery).
- Prepare for pericardiocentesis. Have a basin available to evaluate the aspirated blood for coagulability and send a specimen to the laboratory to analyze the hematocrit level.
- Inherent to the procedure is the possibility of the puncture of an uninjured chamber.
- Ongoing evaluation for the recurrence of tamponade or creating an environment conducive to the development of tamponade (by puncturing an uninjured chamber) must be considered and remain in the decision tree for ongoing assessment.
- Should the patient experience acute deterioration, prepare for an open, resuscitative thoracotomy to decompress the pericardial effusion.
- Adequate technique and equipment is essential to the success of this procedure and should be done in centers where surgical backup is readily available (Procedure 25).

Aortic transection

Eighty-five percent of patients who have acute aortic transection die before reaching the hospital. The 15% who live to make it to the hospital are usually experiencing aortic dissection. Remember, the vessel has three layers of tissue—the intima, the media, and the adventitia. With dissection, the intimal and possibly the medial walls are torn. However, the adventitial layer is intact, containing a ballooning pseudoaneurysm or allowing for dissection down into the layers of the vessel. Patients with this condition are extremely fragile, and the condition must be diagnosed quickly and the patients transferred to where cardiothoracic surgical services are immediately available. The usual site of injury is just distal to the subclavian artery at the ligamentum arteriosum that tethers the aorta posteriorly, creating a focal point for the dissipation of the shear forces in blunt injury.

SYMPTOMS

- A conscious patient typically complains of intense and severe midscapular or low back pain, possibly referred down into the pelvic area and lower extremities.
- Dyspnea, tachycardia, and anxiety are often evident.
- Pulse amplitude is commonly magnified in upper extremities and diminished in lower extremities.
- Acute coarctation syndrome (e.g., hypertension in upper extremities and hypotension in lower extremities) may manifest itself.
- During auscultation, a harsh systolic parascapular murmur may be heard.
- Patients typically demonstrate an impressive variability in hemodynamic parameters, especially BP variability.
- Patients' BPs commonly vary from 40 to 60 mm Hg diastolic to 150 to 170 mm Hg systolic. Such wide swings in hemodynamic parameters may be caused by the stretching phenomenon on the baroreceptors contained within the walls of the injured aorta and should encourage consideration of aortic dissection in the differential diagnosis.

DIAGNOSIS

- Diagnosis is based on a radiographic evaluation of the chest, specifically the mediastinum, with the following findings: a widened mediastinum, a loss of aortic knob shadow (may be hazy or obscured), deviation of the trachea to the right (if the patient is nasogastrically intubated, the nasogastric tube will also deviate to the right), a left apical pleural cap, and depressed or downward displacement of the left mainstem bronchus.

    The diagnosis of the aortic dissection has traditionally been confirmed via aortography; however, more studies are validating the role of transesophageal imaging for the detection of acute aortic dissection. A transesophageal echo circumvents the need for dye load, transportation off-site for special procedures, and arterial access. Nationally, aortography remains the gold standard for the confirmation of a diagnosis. Dynamic CT scanning is also being used in many institutions to confirm the diagnosis of aortic dissection.

- Consult your hospital's individual protocol for evaluation of an aortic injury.

TREATMENT

- Hypervolemia should be prevented to minimize additional wall stress on the already stressed or injured vessel.
- Intensive BP monitoring must be done to evaluate hypotension, as well as to treat hypertension as necessary, to avoid additional dissection and possible rupture of the aorta.
- Beta-blockers and other pharmacologics are given to reduce afterload, thereby minimizing vessel wall stress and turbulent flow.
- A tube thoracostomy with autotransfusion may be performed for excessive blood loss.
- A resuscitative, open thoracotomy may be conducted to facilitate emergent surgical control of the aorta (Procedure 14).
- Once the diagnosis is confirmed, anticipate hasty transport to the operating room with an armamentarium of blood products to minimize the potential for acute and excessive blood loss.

Flail chest and multiple rib fractures

SYMPTOMS

- Bony crepitus over fracture sites may be palpated, the patient experiences pain, and the expression of concomitant tissue injury may be evident (e.g., pulmonary contusion, pneumothorax, and hemothorax).
- Paradoxical chest wall movement with inspiration or expiration is indicative of a flail segment.
- The patient may also experience acute oxygen desaturation because of the contusional pattern that may create a shunt.

The concept of shunt implies adequate perfusion to nonventilated alveoli. Some degree of physiologic shunt (2% to 5%) occurs in healthy individuals; however, shunt resulting from conditions such as a pulmonary contusion, atelectasis, or right mainstem intubation may result in shunt as high as 40% to 50%. This will tremendously affect gas exchange (both onloading oxygen to hemoglobin and offloading CO_2 for exhalation).

T

DIAGNOSIS

- A chest radiograph remains the hallmark in the diagnosis of rib fractures and flail segment (two or more rib fractures at two or more adjacent sites).
- The diagnosis of flail chest can also be a clinical diagnosis without the use of a chest radiograph.
- A clinical evaluation of the chest wall movement may lead the clinician to the diagnosis of flail chest.

TREATMENT

- Tube thoracostomy is performed for pneumothoraces and hemothoraces.
- Intubation and positive pressure ventilation may be used for a pulmonary contusion with flail segment.
- Pain management is critical for these patients to maximize respiratory effort and gaseous exchange and to minimize atelectasis and pneumonia.
- Alternative methods for adequate pain management include IV analgesic administration, an epidural anesthetic for pain management, and traditional approaches to pain control, as well as other pain management techniques such as imagery and therapeutic touch.
- Vigilant monitoring of oxygen saturation, respiratory effort, work of breathing, and CO_2 is critical in the ongoing evaluation of respiratory function.
- An arterial line may be placed to facilitate serial ABG measurement and real-time BP monitoring.

Pneumothorax and tension pneumothorax

A pneumothorax is manifested by the entry of air into the pleural space, with the loss of negative pressure causing partial or total collapse of the lung parenchyma on the affected side. A pneumothorax may progress to a tension pneumothorax if air continues to enter the pleural space with no mechanism for escape on exhalation. Pressure continues to rise within the thoracic cavity resulting in the collapse of lung parenchyma on the affected side. Unrelieved, the pressure shifts the heart, great vessels, and trachea and eventually collapses the contralateral lung. Detection and treatment of a tension pneumothorax should be conducted within the context of the primary assessment.

NURSING ALERT

Particular concern should be given to the development of a pneumothorax or tension pneumothorax if the patient needs intubation and positive pressure ventilation for the injuries sustained. Positive pressure ventilation can quickly convert a simple pneumothorax to a tension pneumothorax; thus a high index of suspicion must be maintained after intubation.

SYMPTOMS
- The patient demonstrates dyspnea, tachypnea, hyperpnea, diminished or absent breath sounds ipsilaterally, and, possibly, diminished sounds bilaterally if a tension pneumothorax has progressed and is compressing contralateral lung parenchyma.
- Subcutaneous emphysema is possible with the development of a tension pneumothorax, as is tracheal deviation away from the involved hemithorax.
- JVD may occur, as may hypotension if severe compression of the thoracic mediastinal structures ensues.

DIAGNOSIS
- A clinical diagnosis is more than adequate. A radiograph is not and should not be necessary to make a diagnosis.

TREATMENT
- Immediate decompression using needle or tube thoracostomy is indicated (Procedure 7).
- Typically, a rush of air with either decompressive technique is heard or felt.
- An immediate improvement in the patient's condition and clinical appearance usually occurs within minutes after the decompression of a tension pneumothorax.

NURSING ALERT

REMEMBER: Once a needle thoracostomy has been performed, a chest tube must follow to ensure adequate and ongoing, definitive chest management. The chest drainage system should be monitored closely for output and air leak (Procedure 7).

Hemothorax and tension hemothorax
The presence of blood in the pleural space represents a hemothorax. Each hemithorax can contain up to 2.5 liters of blood. The capacity of the hemithorax makes acute or ongoing blood loss a possibility, a condition that would precipitate hemorrhagic shock.

SYMPTOMS

- The patient exhibits dyspnea, hyperpnea, dullness on percussion, oxygen desaturation, diminished or absent breath sounds on the side of the injury, and, possibly, symptoms of a shock state if blood loss is excessive.
- In the case of a tension hemothorax, the clinical presentation is the same as a tension pneumothorax, except that the causative agent is blood instead of air.

DIAGNOSIS

- The condition is usually detected via a clinical examination.
- If the hemothorax is small (<250 ml), a chest radiograph may be necessary to definitively diagnose the hemothorax.
- An anteroposterior film may not delineate the hemothorax if it is small, and an upright chest film may be necessary to allow the blood to collect and be visible radiographically.

TREATMENT

- Perform a tube thoracostomy (Procedure 7).
- Prepare for autotransfusion if the hemothorax is known or is suspected to be large (Procedure 4).
- Monitor chest drainage closely.
- If the patient has lost >1000 ml of blood initially or demonstrates an ongoing blood loss of >200 ml/hr for 3 to 4 hours, elective surgical thoracotomy may be pursued (for children, >5 ml/kg/hr).

Pulmonary contusion

Approximately 75% of patients with blunt chest trauma have some degree of underlying pulmonary contusion. Signs and symptoms of the contusion may take as long as 48 hours to manifest themselves, allowing time for the contusion to blossom and create an environment of physiologic derangement, especially in children. A high index of suspicion is critical for evaluation and management of these patients. Initial lung hemorrhage occurs with interstitial and alveolar edema at the site of the contusion, followed by general inflammation. Ventilation and perfusion mismatching (shunt) develops, resulting in systemic hypoxia and hypercapnia.

SYMPTOMS

- Surface ecchymosis over the chest wall may be present, as may hyperpnea (without subsequent auscultation of breath sounds that would be expected with the degree of hyperpnea).

- Diminished respiratory excursion, hemoptysis, and oxygen desaturation usually occur in cases of pulmonary contusion.

DIAGNOSIS

- A chest radiograph initially may reveal a contusional pattern, and this may "fluff out" in 48 to 72 hours.

TREATMENT

- Supportive therapy is indicated as dictated by the patient's condition.
- Intubation and positive pressure ventilation may be necessary to minimize shunting.
- Pain control is essential to maximize alveolar insufflation for the patient with a pulmonary contusion.
- Vigilant monitoring of oxygen saturation is required.
- The judicious administration of IV fluids (crystalloid and colloid), to prevent the exacerbation of tissue edema, should be the rule of thumb.
- Simultaneous independent lung ventilation may be considered to minimize barotrauma sustained by the "good" lung. Intubation with a double-lumen ET is necessary to achieve this.

Ruptured diaphragm (hemidiaphragm)

A ruptured diaphragm usually results from a rapid deceleration injury. A ruptured diaphragm is more common on the left than the right. This may be because the liver protects the diaphragm on the right or because of the pattern of the kinetic energy dissipated with certain types of injuries. The diaphragm rupture allows herniation of the abdominal contents into the chest, compressing the lungs and possibly the mediastinum. If this condition is left untreated, a tension viscerothorax may result.

SYMPTOMS

- The patient exhibits dyspnea, Kerr's sign (sharp, relentless left shoulder pain as a result of irritation of the phrenic nerve), and diminished breath sounds.
- Bowel sounds may be auscultated in the thoracic cavity in an extreme case with severe herniation.
- Hamman's crunch may be appreciated with mediastinal emphysema. This is a crunching sound heard best over the anterior chest wall at the apex. The crunching sound appreciated is synchronous with the cardiac cycle and

can be auscultated in conditions leading to the presence of mediastinal air.

DIAGNOSIS

- A chest radiograph may reveal the herniation.
- Nasogastric intubation with the radiopaque nasogastric tube supports the diagnosis by the tubes presence in the thoracic cavity on radiograph.
- A diagnostic peritoneal lavage may also be performed to evaluate for additional intraabdominal injury.

NURSING ALERT

With a ruptured diaphragm, a communication exists between the abdominal and the thoracic cavity. When lavage fluid is instilled, monitor for lavage fluid drainage from the chest tube; a chest tube may need to be inserted if the fluid extravasates from the abdominal cavity to the thoracic cavity.

TREATMENT

- Nasogastric intubation and gastric decompression may lessen the effects of the herniation on chest structures.
- Inadvertent esophageal intubation and positive pressure ventilation would be lethal because the herniated contents would then be insufflated, compounding the effects of the herniation.
- Prepare for immediate surgical intervention.

Ruptured bronchus and trachea

The most common site of injury is at the distal trachea or proximal mainstem bronchus. This injury usually occurs as a result of compressive or shear forces or a penetrating injury. The left mainstem bronchus is affected more often than the right mainstem bronchus. This is because the left bronchus is longer and more horizontal, predisposing it to the effects of shear force.

SYMPTOMS

- Respiratory distress, forceful coughing, subcutaneous emphysema, and hemoptysis are frequently present.
- With placement of a tube thoracostomy, a persistent large air leak is usually present.

DIAGNOSIS

- Diagnosis is determined by bronchoscopy and clinical examination.

TREATMENT

- Begin resuscitation initially per primary assessment.
- A tube thoracostomy is usually necessary to optimize ventilation.
- Again, monitor for a persistent air leak and troubleshoot accordingly.
- The ET cuff must be distal to the injury to maximize ventilation.
- Aggressive management and surgical intervention should be anticipated.

NURSING ALERT

In cases of laryngeal injuries, the patient may often exhibit hoarseness, dysphagia, and the inability to tolerate the supine position as a result of a collapsing airway lumen with fracture. When the patient assumes the supine position, the usual airway lumen collapses on itself because of a fracture of the structure itself. Thus, when patients are forced to lie supine, as they normally are to ensure adequate spinal immobilization, the false lumen achieved with a more upright position is collapsed and airway obstruction occurs. Laryngeal injuries are exceedingly difficult to manage, and finding a position of comfort and maintaining immobilization should be the approach taken until management in a controlled environment (e.g., the operating room) can be achieved.

Abdominal trauma

Unrecognized injuries to the abdomen are major factors contributing to preventable mortality and morbidity in trauma patients. As many as 20% of patients with acute hemoperitoneum have benign abdominal findings when first examined in the ED. The peritoneal cavity is a major reservoir for significant occult blood loss.[1]

A high index of suspicion must be maintained with patients who have a suspected abdominal injury, especially when the suspected injury is related to occult vascular and retroperitoneal injuries. Serial abdominal examinations must be approached in a systematic and meticulous fashion, with thorough documentation of findings and changes in findings. The patient with peritoneal signs or signs of ongoing blood loss must be approached with a vigorous

T

and aggressive posture in terms of discovery of injury and appropriate management.

NURSING ALERT

The following is an outline for the approach to the abdominal evaluation. It is not essential to identify a specific type of injury, but it is most essential to determine that an abdominal injury exists. The liver, spleen, and kidneys are the organs predominantly involved after a blunt injury. Essentially the patient should be evaluated for blood loss following major solid organ injury (liver, spleen, or kidney) or hollow viscus injury to the small or large bowel. The initial systematic evaluation of the abdomen using inspection, auscultation, percussion, and palpation are outlined under Secondary Assessment. Refer to this section in the chapter to review the initial approach to the abdominal examination.

DIAGNOSIS
- A definitive evaluation of abdominal injuries is conducted in different ways, based on the philosophy and resources of the institution. A protocol for evaluation of blunt abdominal trauma should be developed and followed for cases in the ED.
- Penetrating abdominal trauma is usually more straightforward in terms of evaluation.

NURSING ALERT

The diaphragm rises to the 4th intercostal space during exhalation and extends to the 6th or 7th intercostal space, midclavicular line, or the 8th or 9th intercostal space, midaxillary line, on inspiration. This must be a consideration, especially when evaluating penetrating thoracic or abdominal trauma, because the adjacent cavity must also be closely evaluated to ascertain the extent of the injury. With lower-chest injuries the possibility of an abdominal injury must be entertained, and chest injuries must be suspected in cases of upper abdominal injuries.

- Nasogastric intubation and urinary catheterization are both diagnostic and therapeutic.
- The nasogastric tube decompresses the stomach, re-

moves gastric contents and reduces gastric volume and pressure, and thus reduces the risk of aspiration.
• The urinary catheter permits bladder decompression and evaluation for hematuria. The catheter also allows for the monitoring of urinary output that serves as a solid guide to the efficacy of fluid resuscitation.

NURSING ALERT

Inspection of the meatus and the rectal examination should be performed before the insertion of the urinary catheter. Contraindications to urinary catheter placement such as blood at the meatus, an inability to palpate the prostate, a high-riding prostate, or a boggy prostate may be discovered during the examination.

Laboratory screening
Laboratory screening should be conducted per the abdominal evaluation protocol for your facility. Baseline studies typically include a CBC with differential, an amylase test, a urinalysis, and a urine pregnancy test. Alcohol and other drug screening is generally performed, based on individual facility protocol and clinical relevance to the patient's care. Routine screening for alcohol and other drugs is no longer performed in some institutions unless clinical relevance is established.

Diagnostic studies
For evaluation of genitourinary trauma, see Chapter 12. The three major mechanisms for definitive abdominal evaluation are diagnostic peritoneal lavage (DPL), CT scanning of the abdomen, and the focused abdominal sonogram for trauma. Determination of the approach taken is usually related to the hemodynamic stability of the patient and the time available to determine the presence or absence of intraabdominal injury, as well as to the individual facility's approach based on blunt abdominal trauma protocol.

1. *DPL:* The DPL is usually conducted to evaluate patients with hemodynamic instability. The DPL is considered 98% sensitive for intraperitoneal bleeding. The only absolute contraindication to the DPL is an existing indication for celiotomy. Relative contraindications include morbid obesity, previous abdominal operations,

T

advanced cirrhosis, and preexisting coagulopathy. The
DPL may be approached with an open or closed
(percutaneous) technique. This is dictated by the
general philosophy of the department of surgery. See
Procedure 11.

NURSING ALERT

Before a DPL, patients should have a nasogastric tube and
urinary catheter in place. During a DPL a catheter is inserted
and initially aspirated. If gross bloody aspirate is obtained,
this is an immediate indication for surgical intervention. If aspiration yields no blood, the patient should be lavaged with
1 liter of warmed isotonic fluid. Lavage fluid drained from the
abdomen should then be sent to the laboratory. Microscopic
evaluation leading to celiotomy usually yields results of
>100,000 RBCs or 500 WBCs per cubic millimeter for patients
with a blunt injury. A more sensitive indicator of bleeding
(the presence of fewer RBCs) may be used as a surgical indicator for patients with a penetrating injury.[1]

2. *CT scan:* The CT scan is more specific, but less sensitive
than a DPL. Usually both IV and oral contrast media are
administered to heighten specificity of the examination.
The CT scan provides information relative to specific organ injury and its extent and can also give information
related to the pelvis and retroperitoneum. If the CT
scan reveals free fluid, a DPL may be performed to evaluate the nature of the fluid. The advantages of CT scanning versus DPL must be weighed carefully to provide
optimal care for the injured patient. Even patients with
hemodynamic stability but with an impressive abdominal examination indicative of peritoneal signs may be
candidates for a DPL. Another consideration is the availability of resources in the facility and the time needed to
marshal those resources for the patient instead of transferring the patient to a higher level of care. These decisions must be made collaboratively with the attending
physician, receiving physician, and attending nurse
based on the patient's condition and the facility with
the resources available that best match the needs of the
patient.

NURSING ALERT

Be cautious regarding the timing of administration of oral contrast to allow for a long enough dwell time to ensure an adequate study. Examination of the lower thoracic or upper lumbar vertebrae via plain films may be obscured or equivocal with the contrast dye.

3. *Abdominal ultrasound:* The abdominal ultrasound has recently been gaining more acceptance in many centers as another adjunct to the evaluation of both blunt and penetrating abdominal trauma. Ultrasonography equipment must be readily available, as well as a trained operator to perform the examination. The abdominal ultrasound has many advantages in that it is portable and can be done at the patient's bedside, it is noninvasive and relatively time efficient, and it is relatively inexpensive. Disadvantages include diminished specificity for organ injury when compared with CT scanning, poor yield with obese patients or those who have extensive subcutaneous emphysema, and a learning curve for the equipment operator. Abdominal ultrasound can be repeated easily, mitigating some of the aforementioned weaknesses. The sensitivity of ultrasound ranges from 80% to 100%, the specificity from 89% to 100%, and the accuracy from 86% to 99%.

Pelvic fractures
Pelvic fractures, especially those involving the posterior columns, can bleed vigorously, leading to exsanguination and the formation of a retroperitoneal hematoma. The hematoma can become so enlarged that it extends from the pelvis into the lower anterior abdominal wall. The DPL may be performed with an approach above the umbilicus to avoid the hematoma and prevent a false positive finding for intraabdominal bleeding. (*NOTE:* Orthopedic consultation should be obtained quickly for these patients to facilitate definitive care of the pelvic fracture.)

The blood loss from the pelvic fracture should be addressed as would any source of blood loss precipitating a shock state. After alternative sources of blood loss have been ruled out, the pelvis should be stabilized (either by external fixation or possibly with a pneumatic antishock

T

garment). This stabilization allows the retroperitoneal space to tamponade the bleeding and control ongoing blood loss.

In some instances (<10%), stabilization does not control blood loss from the fracture. Arteriography may be indicated to embolize ongoing arterial bleeding.

The patient's underlying renal function and physiologic condition must be considered before transport to arteriography. Management of the patient with ongoing blood loss from a pelvic fracture often requires aggressive colloid resuscitation with attention to potential coagulopathy and hypothermia.

NURSING SURVEILLANCE

The ongoing assessment of the trauma patient is a repeated primary and secondary assessment. Airway patency, adequacy of breathing and circulation, and neurologic status should be reassessed as frequently as needed and anytime patient's condition changes. The secondary assessment may be more limited to identified injuries and known system involvement. Frequent reassessment should be done to rapidly identify any deterioration and, consequently, to direct appropriate intervention.

EXPECTED PATIENT OUTCOMES

Expected patient outcomes vary widely from patient to patient. Generally speaking, ABCs and neurologic status should be maintained or improved. If spinal trauma is suspected or present, the preservation of function is an expected outcome. Preventing infection is important for patients with open wounds or burns. Immobilizing fractures and maintaining adequate peripheral tissue perfusion are appropriate for patients with extremity injuries.

DISCHARGE IMPLICATIONS

Trauma patients present the clinician with a unique set of challenges, both clinically and from a systems approach. Although most patients suffering from an injury are admitted to the receiving hospital, a relatively small percentage of injured patients require timely triage and transfer to a higher level of care. Certain categories of trauma patients require transfer to a higher level of care based on the referring and receiving hospitals' capabilities. One set of guidelines for consideration of early transfer of patients has been proposed by the American College of Surgeons Committee on Trauma and is represented in the box, "High-Risk Criteria for Consideration of Early Transfer."

Specific issues arise with interhospital transfer to a higher level of care. Among these are the following:

1. There must be adequate communication between the referring and receiving facilities, including both written and oral communication, and between physicians and nursing personnel.
2. Interhospital transfer forms must be adequate.

HIGH-RISK CRITERIA FOR CONSIDERATION OF EARLY TRANSFER

(These guidelines are not intended to be hospital specific.)

Central nervous system

- Head injury
- Penetrating injury or open fracture (with or without cerebrospinal fluid leak)
- Depressed skull fracture
- Glasgow Coma Scale (GCS) score <14 or GCS score deterioration
- Lateralizing signs
- Spinal cord injury
- Spinal column injury or major vertebral injury

Chest

- Major chest wall injury
- Wide mediastinum or other signs suggesting great vessel injury
- Cardiac injury
- Patients who may require prolonged ventilation

Pelvis

- Unstable pelvic ring disruption
- Unstable pelvic fracture with shock or other evidence of continuing hemorrhage
- Open pelvic injury

T

Continued

HIGH-RISK CRITERIA FOR CONSIDERATION OF EARLY TRANSFER—cont'd

Major extremity injuries

- Fracture or dislocation with loss of distal pulses
- Open long-bone fractures
- Extremity ischemia

Multiple-system injury

- Head injury combined with face, chest, abdominal, or pelvic injury
- Burns with associated injuries
- Multiple long-bone fractures
- Injury to more than two body regions

Comorbid factors

- Age >55 years
- Children
- Cardiac or respiratory disease
- Insulin-dependent diabetics, morbid obesity
- Pregnancy
- Immunosuppression

Secondary deterioration (late sequelae)

- Mechanical ventilation required
- Sepsis
- Single or multiple organ system failure (deterioration in central nervous, cardiac, pulmonary, hepatic, renal, or coagulation systems)
- Major tissue necrosis

3. Decisions must be made regarding transport mode (ground or air), medical evacuation, and the level of care of personnel attending the patient while in transit.
4. The patient's needs must be matched with the resources offered by the receiving facility. This "match" must be done and the patient transferred in a timely fashion.
5. Optimal and maximal stabilization of the patient must occur before transport, within the capabilities of the referring institution. Often physicians from the receiving facility offer guidance regarding stabilization and transport procedures.

Most injured patients can be adequately cared for in the initial receiving hospital. However, patients requiring a higher level of care must be promptly recognized based on the limitations and capabilities of the receiving hospital, and appropriate transfer to the appropriate higher level of care must ensue.

References

1. American College of Surgeons Committee on Trauma: *Advanced trauma life support: course for physicians,* ed 6, Chicago, 1997, The College.
2. Emergency Nurses' Association: *Trauma nursing core course,* ed 4, Chicago, 1995, The Association.

T

Chapter 21

The Unresponsive Patient

Steve Talbert

CLINICAL CONDITIONS
Alcohol
Electrolyte Abnormalities
Encephalopathy
Endocrine
Insulin
Intracranial Lesion
Overdose
Uremia
Trauma
Infection
Psychogenic Disorders
Seizure
Hypovolemic Shock
Cardiogenic Shock
Neurogenic Shock
Anaphylactic Shock
Hypoxia and Hypoxemia
Acid-Base Imbalance
Thermoregulation

TRIAGE ASSESSMENT

Regardless of etiology, the unresponsive patient constitutes a medical emergency and should be taken immediately to an appropriate treatment area. The initial triage assessment focuses on the airway, breathing, and circulation (ABCs), a brief neurologic examination, and a critical history. It is followed by a detailed secondary assessment centered on the risk factors for unresponsiveness.

Airway and Cervical Spine

First, the patient's airway must be examined for patency. A method of checking patency is to apply a modified jaw-thrust maneuver, then observe the airway for any source of potential or actual obstruction, listen for breath sounds, and feel for air movement. If the airway is compromised, the establishment of a stable, patent airway through the removal of any obstruction or the placement of an artificial airway is essential before continuing the assessment. Care must be taken to protect the cervical spine if the etiology of the patient's unresponsiveness is either unknown or known to be traumatic.

Breathing

Assessment of breathing includes the respiratory rate, depth, pattern, and work. Respiratory rates vary with age, anxiety, acid-base balance, and other physiologic and psychologic factors. Tachypnea or bradypnea, especially when prolonged, are signs of respiratory distress and metabolic problems. Assess respiration depth by auscultating lung sounds and inspecting chest rise and fall. Unequal chest rise and fall may indicate a pneumothorax. Paradoxical chest wall movement suggests a flail chest segment. Respirations that are continuously deep or shallow may be symptoms of an underlying respiratory or metabolic disorder. Diminished, absent, or abnormal breath sounds (e.g., wheezing, rales, or rhonchi) are symptoms of breathing problems that impair gas exchange and must be addressed. These conditions include a pneumothorax or hemothorax, pulmonary edema, and airway constriction. Respiratory patterns are also part of the breathing assessment. Abnormal respiratory patterns such as Biot's, Cheyne-Stokes, and Kussmaul's are classically associated with various medical conditions (Table 21-1). Work of breathing or respiratory effort should be assessed. Signs of increased work of breathing include nasal flaring, retractions, and the use of accessory muscles. Initially, unresponsive patients should receive 100% oxygen via an appropriate route (e.g., nonrebreather mask, bag-valve device, or ventilator) until deemed unnecessary based on the history and physical examination.

Circulation

Circulation or perfusion is assessed by noting pulse rate and quality, skin color, temperature, moisture, and capillary refill. The presence or absence of a pulse must be established quickly during the triage assessment. Palpation for the pres-

TABLE 21-1 Respiratory Patterns and Associated Clinical Conditions

Respiratory pattern	Description	Associated clinical conditions
Biot's	Fast, deep inspirations interrupted by sudden periods of apnea	Increased intracranial pressure (late sign)
Cheyne-Stokes	Gradual rhythmic transition, going from hyperventilation to apnea and repeating the cycle over and over	Increased intracranial pressure Encephalopathy Overdose of narcotics, barbiturates, or hypnotics
Kussmaul's	Fast, deep respirations that may be labored	Metabolic acidosis Ketoacidosis Renal failure

ence and quality of carotid, femoral, brachial, or radial pulses is the first step. In the absence of extremity trauma or in the presence of weak, thready pulses, a failure to palpate distal pulses is indicative of poor perfusion and hypotension. Other significant assessment findings consistent with poor perfusion are cool and pale or mottled and clammy skin. Capillary refill time may increase with aging and hypothermia. As a general rule, a prolonged capillary refill time (>3 seconds) is associated with poor perfusion. If perfusion is compromised, steps should be taken to augment circulatory volume. Current recommendations are the placement of two large-bore (e.g., 18-gauge or larger) IV lines and administration of an isotonic crystalloid solution (Ringer's lactate or 0.9% NaCl). Unresponsive patients should have at least one IV line inserted during the initial assessment.

Deficit
The fourth step in the triage assessment is a brief neurologic examination consisting of pupil size and reactivity, best motor response, best verbal response, and best eye-opening response (Reference Guides 10 and 18 list coma scores). This initial examination provides critical baseline data for

TABLE 21-2 Neurologic Findings and Associated Clinical Conditions

Neurologic finding	Associated clinical condition
Dilated, nonreactive pupils, unilateral or bilateral	Increased intracranial pressure
	Overdose of barbiturates
	Anticholinergic drugs (e.g., atropine sulfate)
Constricted pupils	Overdose of narcotics
	Cholinergic activity
Sluggish pupil reactivity	Metabolic process (e.g., drug ingestion)
	Structural problem (e.g., closed-head injury)
Flaccid extremities	Spinal cord injury
	Closed-head injury
Spasticity of muscles	Seizure disorder
	Electrolyte imbalance
Abnormal flexion or extension of extremities	Closed-head injury
	Increased intracranial pressure
Unilateral flaccidity or weakness	Closed-head injury
	Intracranial lesion (bleed, mass, ischemia)

later comparison. Table 21-2 lists some common neurologic findings and their associated clinical conditions.

Other Interventions
Other early interventions include the administration of reversal agents such as naloxone (Narcan) and flumazenil (Romazicon). Recently the universal administration of $D_{50}W$ to the unresponsive patient has been questioned. If a bedside glucose level is readily available, it should be checked before the administration of $D_{50}W$.

History
To complete the triage assessment, the a focused history as quickly as possible. Since the unresponsive patient is un-

U

TABLE 21-3 Patient History and Clinical Implications

Question	Clinical implication
Events surrounding the unresponsive episode	If traumatic, suspect closed-head injury or shock
	If ingestion, suspect overdose and alcohol
	Note any patient complaints before unresponsiveness occurred (e.g., chest pain, nausea, and headache)
When the unresponsiveness occurred	If after trauma, suspect closed-head injury or shock
	If after medication (e.g., insulin), suspect adverse drug reaction or overdose
Associated symptoms	Patient complaints such as dizziness, chest pain, shortness of breath, or headache may indicate a cardiovascular or neurologic etiology
	Symptoms like vomiting, diarrhea, or bleeding point toward hypovolemia
	Fever may indicate an infectious process

CVA, Cerebrovascular Accident; *TIA*, transient ischemic attack.

able to provide this information, it must be obtained from EMS personnel, family, friends, bystanders, or medical alert devices. Searching through pockets, wallets, purses, and bags may provide valuable information regarding medications, regular physicians, and preexisting medical conditions. Table 21-3 lists the questions asked during a focused history and their clinical application.

FOCUSED NURSING ASSESSMENT

Once the initial survey is complete and life-threatening conditions are corrected, the nurse should begin a systematic, head-to-toe examination focusing on the risk factors associated with unresponsiveness. This secondary assessment should begin with exposing the patient, taking measures to maintain the body temperature, and obtaining a complete set of vital signs, including a rectal temperature.

TABLE 21-3 Patient History and Clinical Implications—cont'd

Question	Clinical implication
Regular medications	Insulin use may lead to hypoglycemia
	Diuretics may cause hypovolemia or electrolyte imbalances
	Patients taking antihypertensive medication are prone to intracranial problems such as CVA and bleeding
Medical history	Endocrine disorders may cause unresponsiveness
	Renal failure may cause uremia
	Liver failure may cause encephalopathy
	Patients with a history of CVA, TIA, cerebral aneurysm, or hypertension are more prone to intracranial problems
	Patients with cardiovascular disease are prone to cardiogenic shock
	Immunocompromised patients are more susceptible to infections
Allergies	Exposure to a known antigen may result in anaphylaxis

Risk Factors

The mnemonic "AEIOU TIPS HAT" can be used to help remember risk factors leading to unresponsiveness (see the "Risk Factors for Unresponsiveness" box).

Life Span Issues

NURSING ALERT

Regardless of the patient's age, priorities of care begin with airway, breathing, and circulation (ABCs) and reduction of the neurological deficit. The mnemonic "AEIOU TIPS HAT" is valid for patients of all ages.

Pediatric patients

1. Remember that the priorities of care are the ABCs and any neurological deficit.

RISK FACTORS FOR UNRESPONSIVENESS

A alcohol
E electrolytes, encephalopathy, endocrine
I insulin, intracranial lesion
O overdose
U uremia
T trauma
I infection
P psychogenic
S seizure, shock
H hypoxia
A acidosis, alkalosis
T thermoregulation

2. Intraosseous infusion may be used for children if the nurse is unable to obtain peripheral IV access.
3. Common etiologies of unresponsiveness include the following:
   • Infection
   • Trauma
   • Seizure
   • Overdose
4. Reye's syndrome must also be considered with children. Look for the following signs:
   • A history of recent viral illness (e.g., cold or flu symptoms)
   • A progression from confusion and lethargy to unresponsiveness
   • Abnormal liver enzyme studies
   • Exhibition of abnormal posturing or respiratory arrest

Geriatric patients

1. Remember that the priorities of care are ABCs and any neurological deficit.
2. Common etiologies of unresponsiveness include the following:
   • Trauma
   • Overdose or medication interaction
   • Infection
   • Endocrine
   • Acidosis or alkalosis

- An intracranial lesion (cerebrovascular attack [CVA], subdural hematoma [SDH], mass)
- Hypoxia

Obstetrics

1. Remember that the priorities of care are ABCs and any neurological deficit.
2. Common causes of unresponsiveness include the following:
   - Infection (e.g., sepsis)
   - Shock (etiologies: ruptured uterus or abruptio placentae)
   - Overdose (suicide attempt or attention-seeking behavior; takes available medication [iron pills are common])
   - Seizure
   - Endocrine abnormalities
   - Trauma

INITIAL INTERVENTIONS

Immediate interventions involve the ABCs and any neurological deficit. A patent airway should be established and maintained throughout the resuscitation. Breathing and ventilation should be supported through the administration of 100% oxygen. If the patient is breathing adequately, a nonrebreather mask may be applied. However, if ventilation is inadequate or there are no spontaneous respirations, the patient should be ventilated via a bag-valve mask device. Circulation is supported through the establishment of two large-bore IV lines (14- or 16-gauge for adults) with warm crystalloid solution (0.9% NaCl or Ringer's lactate). Neurological deficit should be addressed through proper positioning of the patient (e.g., do not occlude venous return from the head), special precautions (e.g., padded side rails), and repeated neurologic assessments to rapidly identify any changes.

PRIORITY NURSING DIAGNOSES

Risk for injury
Risk for altered cerebral perfusion
◆ **Injury** related to the etiology of the unresponsiveness:
   INTERVENTIONS
   - Keep the bed in a low position with side rails up.
   - Maintain a patent airway.

U

COMMON DIAGNOSTIC TESTS

Common radiographic tests

Chest x-ray examination
Cervical spine x-ray examination
Computed tomography (CT) scan of head (without contrast first, then with contrast if needed)
Other radiographic tests as indicated by assessment and history

Common laboratory diagnostic tests

Complete blood count (CBC)
Electrolytes (Na, K, Cl, Ca, Mg, PO_4)
Blood urea nitrogen (BUN)
Creatinine
Glucose
Anion gap
Arterial blood gas (ABG)
Alcohols
Drug (toxicology) screen
Hepatic enzymes
Medication levels

Other diagnostic tests

Electrocardiogram (ECG)
Lumbar puncture

- Administer high-flow oxygen (as previously stated).
- Administer neuromuscular blocking agents and anticonvulsants per physician order.
- ♦ **Altered cerebral perfusion** related to the etiology of the unresponsiveness:
  INTERVENTIONS
  - Avoid increases in intracranial pressure.
  - Suction only as necessary.
  - Elevate the head of the bed.
  - Avoid hip flexion.
  - Avoid neck flexion.
  - Administer IV fluids at keep-vein-open rates (30 ml/hr) unless hypovolemia coexists.

PRIORITY DIAGNOSTIC TESTS

As a general rule, diagnostic testing for the unresponsive patient may be referred to as the "safety net" approach, which provides screening for a multitude of potential etiologies in the shortest time. The "Common Diagnostic Tests" box lists common diagnostic tests.

COLLABORATIVE INTERVENTIONS
Overview
Supportive measures for ABCs and any neurological deficit should be continued until a specific cause for unresponsiveness is known and the patient's condition is stabilized. Once known, the underlying cause can be addressed.

Clinical Conditions
Alcohol
See Chapter 19.
SYMPTOMS
- The smell of ethanol on the breath of the unresponsive patient is a good indicator that alcohol may be involved.
- Other findings include an enlarged liver (hepatitis and cirrhosis), ascites, spider angiomas, and signs of malnutrition.
- Family, friends, or bystanders may also confirm ingestion of alcohol.

DIAGNOSIS
- Confirmation of alcohol toxicity is made through blood sample testing. It should be noted that the level of ethanol needed to induce unresponsiveness varies considerably.
- Chronic drinkers may have high blood alcohol levels and still be conscious.

TREATMENT
- Initial treatment focuses on supporting ABCs.
- Oxygen may be administered, and IV fluids (usually isotonic crystalloid solutions) should be given to reverse dehydration and assist with clearing the alcohol from the body.
- It is common to administer thiamine, multivitamins, folic acid, and magnesium IV to reverse electrolyte imbalances and malnutrition.
- Many patients go home after their blood alcohol has returned to an acceptable level.
- Discharge teaching regarding alcohol abuse and detoxification facilities should be provided.

U

Electrolyte abnormalities
SYMPTOMS
- The symptoms associated with electrolyte imbalances are specific for the specific anion (negatively charged particle) or cation (positively charged particle) involved.
- The neurologic, cardiovascular, respiratory, and endocrine systems are the systems most commonly affected by electrolyte imbalances.

DIAGNOSIS
- Clinical signs and symptoms of an electrolyte imbalance are confirmed through blood sample testing.

TREATMENT
- Treatment revolves around correcting the imbalance through supplemental administration of the electrolyte (e.g., potassium chloride infusion) or measures to decrease the concentration of the electrolyte (e.g., dialysis).
- Support of ABCs must be continued until the patient's condition is stabilized.

Encephalopathy
SYMPTOMS
- Encephalopathy is usually associated with conditions causing hepatic or renal failure.
- When either of these systems fails, toxins (e.g., ammonia and urea) can build up in the blood, causing neurotoxicity that is manifested by an altered level of consciousness.
- A history of cirrhosis, liver failure, renal failure, or alcohol abuse should heighten suspicion for encephalopathy.

DIAGNOSIS
- Diagnosis is based on laboratory values, coupled with a history consistent with liver or renal failure.
- Elevations of levels on the following tests are significant: blood urea nitrogen, creatinine, ammonia, and liver enzymes.
- It is also common to see elevated potassium and phosphate levels.

TREATMENT
- Until the underlying cause is resolved, ABCs must be fully supported.
- Treatment is focused on removing the offending toxin(s) as quickly as possible.
- Toxin removal may include the administration of lactulose for ammonia toxicity.

- The patient may also be a candidate for emergency dialysis.

Endocrine

See Chapter 8.

SYMPTOMS

- Endocrine etiologies for unresponsiveness typically involve one of the following glands: pancreas, thyroid, or adrenal.
- Symptoms associated with pancreatic problems (ketoacidosis) are tachycardia, Kussmaul's respirations, and a ketone odor to the breath.
- Symptoms associated with hyperthyroidism (thyroid storm) are tachycardia, hypertension, congestive heart failure, and extreme hyperthermia.
- Hypothyroidism (myxedema coma) is characterized by shock, hypothermia, generalized edema, and hypoventilation and is usually seen in people over the age of 50 years.
- Symptoms associated with acute adrenal crisis are shock, hypotension, and dehydration.

DIAGNOSIS

- Diagnosis of all endocrine disorders is made by combining history, clinical findings, and laboratory tests.
- Ketoacidosis is characterized by acidosis, excessive ketones, hyperglycemia, and hyperosmolarity.
- Thyroid storm may be associated with electrolyte imbalances and hypoglycemia.
- Myxedema coma can be differentiated by the presence of hyponatremia, hypoglycemia, and lactic acidosis.
- Hyponatremia and hypoglycemia are also found in cases of acute adrenal crisis.

TREATMENT

- Treatment begins with the support of ABCs simultaneous with correction of the underlying cause.
- Ketoacidosis is corrected with IV hydration and insulin.
- Thyroid storm is treated by cooling, IV hydration, and glucose. It is not uncommon for a beta-blocker to be administered to protect the cardiovascular system from the excess thyroxine. Glucocorticoids may also be necessary.
- Myxedema coma is usually managed by intubation, IV hydration, and hormone replacement.
- An acute adrenal crisis is treated with IV glucocorticoid therapy, saline infusion, and the administration of glucose.

U

Insulin

See Chapter 8.

SYMPTOMS

- Clinical symptoms associated with insulin shock (hypoglycemia) are hypotension, diaphoresis, tachycardia, seizures, and pale, clammy skin.
- Usually, patients using insulin are known diabetics who have missed meals, have an acute illness (e.g., infection), or have recently exercised.

DIAGNOSIS

- Diagnosis of insulin shock is confirmed by laboratory or bedside blood tests that demonstrate hypoglycemia.

TREATMENT

- Immediate treatment is support for ABCs.
- In the presence of documented hypoglycemia, IV dextrose should be administered.
- Once consciousness has returned, the patient should be able to eat a meal before being discharged from the ED.
- Discharge teaching includes insulin and diet instructions, an explanation of the reason for hypoglycemia, symptoms, and strategies.
- Patient compliance with medications, diet, and follow-up should be assessed.

Intracranial lesion (hemorrhage or mass)

See Chapter 14.

SYMPTOMS

- Regardless of the specific lesion, the unresponsive patient with an acute intracranial mass may manifest a variety of symptoms.
- Symptoms include seizures, focal neurologic findings (e.g., hemiplegia), elevated mean arterial pressure, tachypnea, and bradycardia.
- The patient may have obvious head trauma.
- Significant history includes recent trauma, previous intracranial lesions, known mass, old CVA or transient ischemic attack, history of a cerebral aneurysm, sudden onset of headache, or behavioral changes.

DIAGNOSIS

- Diagnosis of an intracranial lesion is usually confirmed by visualization of the lesion on a CT scan or magnetic resonance image (MRI).

TREATMENT

- The initial management of intracranial lesions is centered on maximizing cerebral perfusion.
- The management of perfusion begins by supporting the ABCs.
- It is common to intubate patients who have intracranial lesions.
- A neurosurgery or neurologic consultation should be obtained as quickly as possible.

Overdose

See Chapter 19.

NOTE: Specific assessment findings vary with different agents.

SYMPTOMS

- Symptoms associated with overdoses vary, depending on the agents ingested.
- Frequently a description of the scene where the patient was found or a recent history by family or friends is the best clue.
- Drugs, medications, or pill bottles at the scene could indicate an ingestion and should be brought to the ED.
- The patient may have a history of overdoses or suicide attempts.
- A family member or friend may have witnessed the overdose.
- Systems commonly affected by overdoses are the cardiovascular system (tachycardia or bradycardia, hypertension or hypotension), the respiratory system (tachypnea or bradypnea), and the neurologic system (abnormal pupil size or reaction or seizures).

DIAGNOSIS

- The diagnosis of overdose is confirmed by results of a drug screen (blood or urine).
- A clinical diagnosis may also be supported by a response to reversal agents such as naloxone (Narcan) and flumazenil (Romazicon).

TREATMENT

- Treatment begins with support of the ABCs.
- Symptomatic support should be continued until the specific agent is identified.
- The regional poison control center is an excellent resource regarding treatment.

U

Uremia
SYMPTOMS
- Uremic patients are usually those with acute or chronic renal failure.
- Symptoms include edema, crackles (Pulmonary edema [PE]), hypertension, and seizures.
- The presence of dialysis access devices (e.g., shunts and central lines) may also be a clue.

DIAGNOSIS
- Laboratory values consistent with uremia are elevated levels of blood urea nitrogen and creatinine, hyperkalemia, metabolic acidosis, and anemia.

TREATMENT
- Unless the patient is a known dialysis patient, initial management is usually conservative (e.g., diuretics).
- If conservative measures do not resolve the uremia, or if the patient normally undergoes dialysis, hemodialysis is the treatment of choice.

Trauma
See Chapter 20. *NOTE:* Three common causes for unresponsiveness associated with trauma are head injuries, hypoxia, and shock.

SYMPTOMS
- Common signs and symptoms associated with trauma are tachycardia, tachypnea, signs of poor perfusion (e.g., weak pulses, clammy skin, and diaphoresis), delayed capillary refill, and focal neurologic findings.
- Trauma patients usually exhibit visible external trauma (e.g., ecchymosis, hematoma, lacerations, deformities, or edema) that provides clues to the etiology of their unresponsiveness.

DIAGNOSIS
- Diagnosis of a traumatic etiology is based on a combination of history, physical findings, and diagnostic testing.
- Common laboratory findings consistent with traumatic injury are acidosis, hypoxemia, hypercapnia, an elevated base deficit, decreased hematocrit, decreased hemoglobin levels, an elevated lactic acid level, hematuria, hyperglycemia, and an elevated WBC count.
- Radiographic studies include x-ray examinations of all suspected injury sites, a CT scan, and possible angiography.
- Other diagnostic tools include diagnostic peritoneal lavage, ultrasound, and MRI.

TREATMENT
- Initial management focuses on supporting ABCs and any neurologic deficits.
- All traumatic injuries should be treated in the following order: life-threatening injuries first, limb-threatening injuries second, and all other injuries.

Infection (sepsis, central nervous system, respiratory)
SYMPTOMS
- Symptoms vary with the severity of the infection, the system(s) involved, and the individual response to the infectious process.
- General symptoms include tachycardia, tachypnea, and fever.
- Respiratory symptoms include abnormal breath sounds (e.g., wheezing, crackles, or rhonchi), diminished breath sounds, cough, and excessive respiratory secretions.
- Neurologic symptoms include seizures, focal neurologic findings, bulging fontanel, and nuchal rigidity.
- Systemic symptoms (sepsis) include hypotension; cool, mottled, clammy skin; petechiae and purpura; and weak, thready pulses.
- Patients with a history of immunosuppression (e.g., AIDS or chemotherapy) and cancer patients are at increased risk for infections.

DIAGNOSIS
- Diagnosis is based on a combination of clinical symptoms and laboratory results.
- Blood test findings include an elevated or decreased WBC count, acidosis, hyperglycemia, hypoxemia, and hypercapnia.
- Gram stains may provide rapid identification of potential sources of infection.
- Positive cultures (e.g., respiratory, cerebrospinal fluid [CSF], blood, urine, or wound) are definitive diagnostic adjuncts but may require several days for results.

TREATMENT
- Treatment begins with support of ABCs and correction of any neurological deficit.
- A high priority for the treatment of a patient who is unresponsive because of an infection is the rapid administration of broad-spectrum antibiotics.
- The use of isolation precautions should also be considered.

U

Psychogenic disorders

> **NURSING ALERT**
>
> Most psychiatric patients eventually die of an organic disease or process (except in cases of suicide). Other life-threatening problems must be identified or ruled out in the presence of a psychiatric history and medication. Assessment findings vary widely from patient to patient.

SYMPTOMS

- Symptoms consistent with a psychiatric cause for unresponsiveness vary widely. However, these symptoms are usually inconsistent with medical conditions.
- A psychiatric history and known psychiatric medication use should raise the index of suspicion for this etiology.
- Other life-threatening causes for unresponsiveness must be ruled out.

DIAGNOSIS

- Psychiatric cause for unresponsiveness is a diagnosis of exclusion.
- After other medical and traumatic causes are ruled out, a psychiatric etiology should be considered.
- A history of similar behavior, depression, and mental illness increases the likelihood of a psychiatric cause.
- Drug levels for specific psychotropic medications also may be found.

TREATMENT

- As with other causes of unresponsiveness, treatment begins with supporting ABCs and correcting any neurological deficit until the underlying cause is determined.
- Treating the unresponsive psychiatric patient can be difficult and dangerous.
- The focus should be addressing the underlying cause, and this may require the intervention of specialists.
- Care must be taken to protect the patient, family members, and other health care workers from injury.

Seizure

See Chapter 14.

SYMPTOMS

- An unresponsive patient may arrive in a seizure or a postictal state.
- Seizure activity could be localized (focal) or involve the entire body (generalized).

- The postictal patient may have been witnessed having a seizure or may have a seizure history.
- Associated symptoms with seizures are tachycardia and warm, flushed, moist skin.
- The patient may also be hyperthermic.
- Incontinence of both bladder and bowel is common.
- Identification of certain traumatic injuries such as lacerations to the tongue, mouth, or head and abrasions or fractures in the extremities, face, or skull may also suggest a seizure etiology.

DIAGNOSIS

- Diagnosis is usually confirmed by the physical findings, medical history, and witnessed seizure activity. However, the etiology of unresponsiveness may remain unknown until levels of an antiseizure drug are confirmed and the patient is lucid enough to provide an adequate medical history.
- Other common laboratory findings include hyperglycemia and an elevated WBC count.

TREATMENT

- Treatment begins with support of the ABCs and correction of the neurological deficit.
- If the patient is having a seizure, antiseizure medication (e.g., diazepam or lorazepam) should be administered IV until the seizure has ceased.
- If the patient is postictal, seizure precautions (e.g., padded side rails) should be instituted to protect the patient from further harm.
- ABCs and neurologic status should be carefully assessed and documented.
- Anticonvulsants may be given if blood levels of antiseizure drugs are subtherapeutic.
- Discharge instructions should include education regarding medication regimen, follow-up instructions, and wound care.

Shock

NOTE: There are five shock states—hypovolemic, cardiogenic, neurogenic, anaphylactic, and septic. Sepsis is discussed in the "Infection" section.

Hypovolemic shock

SYMPTOMS

- Hypovolemic shock is a condition caused by intravascular fluid loss (internal or external).

- A history of traumatic injury, vomiting, or diarrhea is significant and should raise suspicion of hypovolemia.
- Symptoms associated with hypovolemic shock are a manifestation of the body's compensatory mechanisms (e.g., catecholamine release) and inadequate tissue perfusion.
- Tachycardia, tachypnea, delayed capillary refill, narrowed pulse pressure, and pale, cool, clammy, diaphoretic skin are hallmark signs of catecholamine release.
- Inadequate tissue perfusion is manifested by the unresponsiveness and by cyanosis, weak and thready peripheral pulses, and oliguria or anuria.
- Hypotension is associated with hypovolemia, but it is a late sign.

DIAGNOSIS

- A diagnosis of hypovolemic shock is clinically based.
- If a history consistent with hypovolemia is present and coupled with the physical correlates of catecholamine release and inadequate tissue perfusion, the diagnosis is made.
- Obvious internal or external fluid loss (e.g., internal or external bleeding) confirms the diagnosis.
- Laboratory values in cases of hypovolemia include normal, elevated, or decreased hematocrit and hemoglobin, acidosis, moderate or severe base deficit (e.g., ≥ -6), hyperglycemia, an elevated WBC count, and elevated lactate levels.

TREATMENT

- Treatment begins with support of ABCs and reduction of deficit.
- The overall goal of managing shock is to maximize oxygen delivery to the tissues. This is accomplished through two primary mechanisms: stopping the fluid loss and replenishing the intravascular volume.
- Stopping the fluid loss involves a combination of direct pressure (external loss) and surgical intervention (internal loss).
- Replenishing the intravascular volume begins with establishing two large-bore IV lines and rapidly infusing warm isotonic crystalloid solution.
- Administration of blood and blood products should be considered.
- Patients with traumatic injuries require immediate surgical consult or transfer to the closest appropriate trauma center.

Cardiogenic shock

Cardiogenic shock has two primary causes—coronary (e.g., acute myocardial infarction [AMI]) and noncoronary (e.g., cardiomyopathy or valve disease). Regardless of the etiology, the underlying pathophysiology is the impaired pumping ability of the left ventricle.

SYMPTOMS

- Cardiogenic shock is characterized by poor cardiac output and inadequate ventricular emptying.
- Symptoms include hypotension, delayed capillary refill, and pale, cool, moist skin.
- Other assessment findings include cyanosis and pulmonary edema.
- If the origin of shock is coronary, ECG findings may be consistent with acute myocardial infarction.
- As cardiac output and, subsequently, tissue perfusion decrease, oliguria or anuria also may be noted.

DIAGNOSIS

- Diagnosing cardiogenic shock involves a combination of history, physical findings, and other diagnostic tools.
- Twelve- or fifteen-lead ECG findings consistent with AMI, elevated cardiac enzyme levels, and coronary artery occlusion noted on catheterization confirm a coronary origin for cardiogenic shock.
- Other tests such as an echocardiogram and chest x-ray examination can confirm a noncoronary origin.
- Troponin levels may be positive for AMI.

TREATMENT

- As with other forms of shock, treatment begins with support of ABCs and correction of any neurological deficit.
- Therapies specific to cardiogenic shock are directed at correcting the underlying cause and improving cardiac output. These include pharmacologic therapy to augment contractility (e.g., dobutamine) and mechanical adjuncts such as intraaortic balloon pumps or ventricular assist devices.
- Thrombolytic therapy and angioplasty are probable interventions if the shock is coronary in nature.
- Emergency cardiopulmonary bypass or extracorporeal membrane oxygenation is also a possible modality of treatment.
- Both coronary and noncoronary causes may require surgical intervention.

Neurogenic shock

SYMPTOMS

- Neurogenic shock is caused by a blocked sympathetic response secondary to neuron damage.
- The underlying cause is massive vasodilation resulting in a relative hypovolemia and poor venous return.
- Symptoms include warm, flushed skin, bradycardia, and hypotension.
- The patient may exhibit oliguria or anuria.
- Motor and sensory deficits may be present.

DIAGNOSIS

- Diagnosis of neurogenic shock is clinical, based on a history consistent with a spinal cord injury coupled with the previously mentioned clinical findings.
- Confirmation of spinal cord injury is accomplished through the use of a CT scan and MRI.

TREATMENT

- Treatment begins with support of ABCs and correction of the neurological deficit.
- A fluid challenge should be given initially to rule out a hypovolemic source and to augment circulating volume.
- Vasoconstriction can be promoted through the use of vasopressors (e.g., dopamine).
- The injured vertebrae are frequently stabilized with a brace (e.g., halo), surgery, or traction.
- High-dose methylprednisolone is being used in an effort to decrease spinal cord edema and minimize secondary cellular damage.

Anaphylactic shock

SYMPTOMS

- Anaphylactic shock is a life-threatening situation caused by an antigen-antibody reaction, in which chemical mediators (e.g., histamine and kinins) are released in great quantity and produce systemic effects.
- Tachycardia, tachypnea, respiratory distress, wheezing, hypotension, and cyanosis are classic symptoms.

DIAGNOSIS

- As with other forms of shock, anaphylaxis is a clinical diagnosis.
- A history of antigen exposure is a critical part of the diagnosis.
- The WBC count, especially eosinophils, is elevated.

TREATMENT
- As with the other forms of shock, treatment begins with support of ABCs and reduction of the neurological deficit.
- Interventions specific to anaphylaxis include removing the offending antigen if possible and administering pharmacologic agents that inhibit chemical mediator activity and the detrimental effects of the acute inflammatory response.
- Drugs administered include epinephrine, antihistamines, steroids, and bronchodilators.

Hypoxia/hypoxemia
See Chapter 16.

SYMPTOMS
- Hypoxia and the resultant hypoxemia can manifest themselves in a variety of ways. The underlying cause is usually related to inadequate gas exchange at the alveolar capillary membrane or to decreased minute ventilation.
- Patients may have a respiratory rate ranging from apnea or agonal respirations to tachypnea.
- Auscultation of the lungs may reveal adventitious sounds such as stridor, wheezing, crackles, or rhonchi.
- Breath sounds may be diminished or absent unilaterally or bilaterally.
- The heart rate may vary from asystole to tachycardia, and almost any electrophysiologic rhythm may be seen on ECG.
- A complete or partial obstruction of the airway may be observed on inspection.
- Inspection of the chest wall may reveal a mechanical defect (e.g., flail chest segment) or a structural deformity (e.g., sucking chest wound).
- Cyanosis may also be noted.

DIAGNOSIS
- Diagnosis of hypoxia and hypoxemia is confirmed through arterial blood gas analysis that confirms a decreased PaO_2 and SaO_2.
- Other findings may include hypercapnia and acidosis.
- The patient may have a known exposure to toxins such as smoke, chemicals, or vapors.

TREATMENT
- Treatment is targeted at correcting the underlying problem and resolving the hypoxia and hypoxemia.

U

- Treatment begins with ensuring a patent airway through the use of manual manipulation (e.g., jaw thrust or chin lift), clearing techniques (e.g., suctioning), and airway adjuncts (e.g., oral and nasal airway or endotracheal tube).
- Once an airway has been secured, the patient should be given 100% oxygen via nonrebreather mask, bag-valve mask, or ventilator.
- Any life-threatening breathing problems (e.g., tension pneumothorax) should be corrected immediately before moving on to support of the circulation.
- Serial blood gas analysis and ongoing respiratory assessments should be performed to evaluate the effectiveness of any interventions.

Acid-base imbalance

SYMPTOMS

- Conditions leading to an acid-base imbalance are either respiratory or metabolic.
- Regardless of the etiology, the underlying pathologic condition is an excess of either acid or base. The resulting symptoms may vary widely.
- Respiratory acidosis is associated with poor gas exchange that results in hypercapnia.
- The patient may have a partial or complete airway obstruction in either the upper or lower airways or may have a history of inadequate minute ventilation.
- In contrast, respiratory alkalosis is associated with hypocapnia, usually resulting from hyperventilation.
- Metabolic acid-base imbalances are caused by inadequate tissue perfusion (shock and lactic acidosis), renal failure, and drug ingestion.
- Symptoms associated with acid-base imbalance are usually associated with the cardiovascular, respiratory, and neurologic systems.
- Cardiovascular manifestations include dysrhythmias.
- Respiratory symptoms range from tachypnea to apnea.
- Neurologic manifestations are an altered level of consciousness, seizures, and hyperreflexia.

DIAGNOSIS

- Diagnosis of an acid-base imbalance is seen through blood analysis.
- A pH >7.45 is classified as alkalosis.
- A pH <7.35 is classified as acidosis.

- The determination of a respiratory or metabolic etiology may be established through blood gas analysis.
- Other laboratory findings associated with acid-base imbalance include alterations of the following: bicarbonate, potassium, and urine ammonia levels.

TREATMENT

- Treatment begins with support of ABCs and reduction of any neurological deficit.
- Therapy must then be targeted at correcting the underlying cause and resolving the acid-base imbalance through the use of ventilation techniques and administration of buffer solutions.

Thermoregulation

See Chapter 9.

SYMPTOMS

- The patient who is unresponsive because of thermoregulation problems has either extreme hyperthermia or hypothermia. Symptoms are different for each condition.
- Early hyperthermia is characterized by hot, dry skin and by hypertension.
- Late hyperthermia is characterized by cool skin, hypotension, dysrhythmias, and seizures.
- In either case the core body temperature exceeds 40° C (104° F).
- Hypothermia is associated with a core body temperature <35° C (95° F).
- The skin is cool or cold to the touch.
- Cardiac manifestations include hypotension, dysrhythmias, and weak, thready pulses.
- Bradypnea and dilated pupils are also common findings.

DIAGNOSIS

- Diagnosis of hypothermia or hyperthermia is confirmed through core body temperature readings and clinical findings.
- Electrolyte imbalances, hyperglycemia, and an elevated WBC count also may be present.

TREATMENT

- Treatment begins with support of ABCs and reduction of neurological deficit.
- If the patient is hyperthermic, interventions include the provision of a cool environment, IV hydration, and possibly active cooling by special blanket or water.

U

- The treatment of hypothermia is to rewarm the patient safely. Techniques include warm, humidified air, a warming blanket, heat lamps, blankets, and warmed IV fluids.
- If hypothermia is severe enough, warm fluid may be circulated into the peritoneal cavity or passed through a nasogastric tube.

NURSING SURVEILLANCE

In general, ongoing surveillance of the unresponsive patient is a continuation of the primary assessment combined with the safety net approach to diagnosis. Regardless of etiology, every unresponsive patient should have his or her ABCs and any neurological deficit reassessed and documented on a regular basis. If a significant change is noted in the patient's condition, the primary assessment should be repeated, noting any changes from the initial assessment.

Components of Primary Assessment

1. Airway patency and cervical spine control
2. Effectiveness of breathing and ventilation
3. Adequacy of perfusion
4. Mental status and neurologic checks
5. Exposure of all body surface areas, including extremities and back
6. Vital signs, including core body temperature

Focused Assessments

Each specific cause of unresponsiveness is associated with characteristic assessment and diagnostic findings. Once an etiology has been determined, those specific parameters should be reassessed for any improvement or worsening of the patient's condition.

EXPECTED PATIENT OUTCOMES

1. The airway remains patent.
2. Breathing and ventilation are effective.
3. Circulation and perfusion are adequate.
4. Mental status improves or remains the same.
5. Known underlying causes are corrected.

DISCHARGE IMPLICATIONS

Few patients treated for unresponsiveness in the ED are discharged home. from the ED. Exceptions may include patients who have had an alcohol overdose, patients with chronic seizures, hypoglycemic patients who are holding down orally ingested food, and psychiatric patients. Such patients should be going to a safe environment when they leave the ED. When they are discharged, the reason for their unresponsiveness must be clearly explained to them. Timely follow-up with a primary care provider or clinic is essential.

References

1. American College of Surgeons, Committee on Trauma: *Advanced trauma life support: course for physicians,* ed 6, Chicago, 1997, The College.
2. Emergency Nurses' Association: *Trauma nursing core course,* ed 4, Chicago, 1995, The Association.
3. Holleran RS, editor: *Flight nursing: principles and practice,* St Louis, 1996, Mosby.

Procedures

Ace Wrap Application

Betty Gaudet Nolan

DESCRIPTION

An Ace wrap is an elastic bandage that is available in widths ranging from 2 to 6 inches. An Ace wrap can provide or help with support, pressure, and immobilization.

INDICATIONS

1. Support the injured area and help decrease swelling in soft tissue and ligamentous injuries of the extremities.
2. Anchor dressings.
3. Secure and maintain pressure dressings to stop bleeding.
4. Secure splints for the purpose of immobilization.

EQUIPMENT

- Ace wrap (elastic bandage)
- Tape or pins or clips
- Dressings as indicated
- Splints as indicated
- 3- to 6-inch-wide Ace wrap for lower extremities
- 2- to 4-inch-wide Ace wrap for upper extremities

INITIAL NURSING ACTIONS

1. Assess distal pulses, skin color, temperature, capillary re-fill, sensation, and amount of edema in the extremity before applying the Ace wrap.
2. Start at the distal portion of the extremity when applying the wrap. Anchor the wrap by circling around the extremity twice.
3. Unroll the bandage and gently stretch the bandage as you wrap the body part. Overlap each layer of the bandage. Avoid wrinkling.
4. Avoid pressure over the antecubital and popliteal spaces.
5. Use a figure-eight wrap on joints.

A. Wrist or hand application
   - Anchor the bandage on the hand first, then cross over the wrist. Cross back and forth in a figure-eight maneuver until the part is adequately covered.
B. Elbow application
   - Anchor the bandage below the elbow, then cross under the antecubital space and wrap above the elbow. Cross back and forth in a figure-eight maneuver until the part is adequately covered.
C. Knee application
   - Anchor the bandage below the knee, cross over the knee diagonally, and wrap above the knee. Cross back and forth over the knee in a figure-eight maneuver until the part is adequately covered. Avoid pressure on the popliteal space because of the vasculature in the area.
D. Ankle application
   - Anchor the bandage around the foot. Cross over the top of the foot and around the back of the ankle, then bring the wrap back over the foot and under the arch. Cross back and forth in a figure-eight maneuver until the foot (not the toes) and ankle are adequately covered (Figure P1-1).

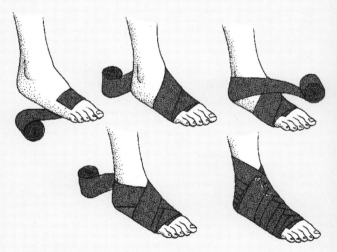

Figure P1-1 Figure-eight ace bandage application to ankle.

NURSING ALERT

The Ace wrap bandage should be loose enough to insert one finger under the bandage comfortably. Check the distal pulses, color, temperature, sensation, and capillary refill of the distal digits.

PATIENT CARE MANAGEMENT

1. Elevate the extremity and apply ice or cold packs as directed to prevent and decrease swelling.
2. If appropriate, instruct the patient to remove and reapply the bandage if it is too loose or tight or for bathing.
3. Teach the patient how to apply the Ace wrap correctly.
4. Instruct the patient to check for changes in sensation, temperature, swelling, and color of distal digits. If any of these changes are present, the patient should remove or loosen the bandage and elevate the extremity. If there is no improvement, call a physician promptly.

Arterial Blood Gas Evaluation

Janet Coyle

DESCRIPTION

Arterial blood gas levels (ABGs) are obtained by direct aspiration of blood from an artery. This may be done by aspiration of blood from an indwelling arterial line or by percutaneous arterial puncture. This procedure focuses on percutaneous arterial puncture.

INDICATIONS

ABGs are useful for the evaluation of oxygenation, ventilation and perfusion, and acid-base disturbances. Often ABGs are obtained to document a baseline for future reference.

EQUIPMENT

- Povidone-iodine swab
- Alcohol swab
- 2 × 2 gauze pads
- Gloves
- Heparinized syringe (usually available in a prepackaged kit): 1 ml for pediatrics, 3 ml for adults
- 25-gauge, ⅝-inch needle
- 20- to 22-gauge, 1½-inch needle (for deeper arteries)
- Butterfly catheter
- Adhesive tape
- Specimen label
- Container of ice

INITIAL NURSING ACTIONS

1. Explain the procedure to the patient.
2. Select the arterial puncture site. Any accessible artery may be used; however, the radial, brachial, and femoral arteries are the most commonly used. Hospital policy may dictate sites from which arterial samples may be taken. When the site for an arterial

puncture is chosen, the following four factors are considered:

- The site must be easily accessible.
- The pulse must be easily palpable.
- The artery must be easily compressible.
- There should be no associated injuries or alterations in skin integrity that would increase the risk of circulatory compromise or infection.

In the absence of palpable peripheral pulses the femoral artery is the recommended site for an arterial puncture. The location of the femoral artery may be estimated by drawing an imaginary line between the anterosuperior iliac spine and the symphysis pubis. The midpoint of that line over the inguinal area should be the femoral artery. The puncture should be made distal to the inguinal ligament.

Before selecting the radial artery as the puncture site, perform the Allen's test to evaluate collateral circulation to the hand. Ask the patient to make a fist, and compress the patient's ulnar and radial arteries with your fingers. After a few seconds, ask the patient to open his or her hand. The hand should appear pale and blanched. Release the ulnar artery and observe the palm or hand for flushing. Rapid flushing indicates good collateral circulation through the ulnar artery. If the hand remains blanched, collateral circulation may be compromised; select another site if this is the case. If the patient is unable to make a fist (e.g., if the patient is unconscious), tightly close the patient's hand manually until blanching occurs.

3. Cleanse the area with povidone-iodine and allow the area to dry.
4. Wipe the area with an alcohol swab. Povidone-iodine leaves a sticky residue on the skin and may interfere with subtle finger movements.
5. Palpate the pulse with the middle and index finger or the index finger only of the nondominant hand. An arterial puncture may then be performed by inserting the needle between the two fingers or by inserting the needle just distal to the index finger.
6. The angle of insertion varies depending on the site selected. For a radial artery puncture the syringe should be held at a 45-degree angle with the bevel of the needle turned upward. A brachial artery puncture may be performed at a 45- to 60-degree angle.

A femoral artery puncture should be performed at a 90-degree angle.

7. Slowly insert the needle over the point of maximal pulsation. Observe closely for the appearance of blood within the needle hub. Arterial pressure should be sufficient to fill the syringe without manual aspiration. However, with patients who have decreased peripheral perfusion or hypotension, gentle aspiration may be necessary. The amount of blood required for ABG analysis may vary between institutions; 0.5 to 1 ml is usually sufficient.

8. During insertion the needle may inadvertently puncture both sides of the artery, resulting in a small flash of blood into the needle hub but no further flow into the syringe. If this occurs, slowly withdraw the needle until blood return is noted. If no blood return occurs and the pulse remains palpable, withdraw the needle until the bevel is visible and redirect it toward the point of maximal pulsation.

9. Loss of arterial pulsation during puncture attempts may indicate arterial spasm or hematoma formation. If this occurs, withdraw the needle, apply manual pressure for 5 to 10 minutes, and select another site.

10. After the arterial blood sample is obtained, withdraw the needle and apply manual pressure for 5 to 10 minutes.

11. Remove air bubbles from the specimen and cap the syringe as soon as possible. Air can be removed from the specimen by holding the syringe upright, tapping the sides of the syringe to direct air bubbles upward, and expelling the air by gently pushing upward on the plunger.

12. Apply a dressing to the site.

13. Label the specimen. Be sure to include the patient's temperature and the type and concentration of supplemental oxygen.

14. Place the specimen in a sealed container and then place the container on ice. Zip-locking bags work well. Place one bag inside another. Put the labeled specimen in the inner bag and seal it. Pour ice into the outer bag around the specimen and seal it. Pushing the specimen into a prefilled ice container may result in inadvertent expulsion of the syringe contents.

NURSING ALERT

All arterial puncture sites require manual pressure for a minimum of 5 minutes. Larger, higher pressure arteries such as the femoral artery may require 10 minutes of manual pressure to establish hemostasis. Clotting times vary depending on the presence of preexisting diseases that alter clotting factors, medical and surgical interventions that deplete clotting factors, the reduction of clotting factors resulting from hemorrhage and multiple blood transfusions, and the use of anticoagulants. The length of application of manual pressure should be increased accordingly. Patients receiving IV thrombolytics require the application of manual pressure followed by a pressure dressing.

NURSING ALERT

To obtain accurate blood gas results, wait 30 minutes after suctioning, respiratory treatments, and ventilator and oxygen concentration changes.

PATIENT CARE MANAGEMENT

1. Assess the puncture site for bleeding after manual pressure is released.
2. If the patient is alert and oriented, instruct him or her to notify you if bloody drainage is noted on or around the dressing or if visible bruising occurs around the puncture site.
3. If the patient is disoriented or unconscious, frequently assess the site for bleeding and hematoma formation for approximately 30 minutes.
4. Assess the circulatory status distal to the puncture site by evaluating skin color and temperature, capillary refill, and distal pulses.
5. Document the arterial puncture site on the nursing record.

Arterial Line Monitoring

Theresa M. Glessner

DESCRIPTION

Indwelling arterial pressure lines are cannulas inserted into peripheral arteries. These lines allow continuous monitoring of the patient's pulse and blood pressure and frequent arterial blood draws.

INDICATIONS

1. Continuous hemodynamic monitoring and frequent assessment of arterial blood gases
2. Significant respiratory compromise
3. Diabetic ketoacidosis
4. Shock
5. Adult respiratory distress syndrome
6. Titration of vasopressor agents
7. Determination of the mean arterial pressure and cerebral perfusion pressure in patients with a ventricular catheter device

EQUIPMENT

- 500-ml IV bag of normal saline (flush solution)
- Pressure bag
- 20-gauge, 1½- or 2-inch angiocatheter
- Antiseptic solution
- Tincture of benzoin
- 2-0 silk sutures
- Lidocaine 1%, 10-ml vial
- Needles (25-gauge for skin, and 18-gauge to withdraw solution from vials) and syringes of different sizes
- Sterile towels
- Sterile scissors
- Sterile needle holder
- Sterile gauze
- Sterile gown
- Sterile gloves
- Male Luer-Lok cap

- Pressure tubing with flush device, transducer, stopcock, and extension set
- Central or deep-line dressing kit, or Tegaderm
- Armboard
- Monitor with hemodynamic capabilities
- Transducer cable

INITIAL NURSING ACTIONS

1. Explain the procedure to the patient.
2. Gather equipment.
3. Determine from the physician which site is to be cannulated. Preferred sites of cannulation are the radial, femoral, dorsalis pedis, and axillary arteries. The radial artery is commonly used because it usually has good collateral circulation and is easily accessible. If the radial artery is to be used, perform Allen's test (Procedure 2).
4. Position the extremity properly. Expose the ventral surface of the forearm, dorsiflex the wrist, and place a rolled washcloth underneath the dorsal surface of the wrist. The hand can be taped to an armboard or other firm surface to maintain this position.
5. Prepare a flush solution. Heparin (500 to 1000 U of a 1:1000 heparin solution) may be added to the 500-ml bag of normal saline according to hospital protocol.
6. Attach the flush solution to the pressure tubing. If the tubing is not fully assembled, connect the transducer to the pressure tubing proximal to the flush device. Attach a stopcock to the end of the pressure tubing and add a pressure extension set.
7. Place the flush solution into the pressure bag and hang the bag on an IV pole.
8. Clear all air from the pressure tubing and transducer by opening the roller clamp and activating the flush device according to the manufacturer's directions.
9. Pump the pressure bag to 300 mm Hg and clamp the bag to maintain the pressure.
10. Connect the transducer to the transducer cable. Attach the cable to the monitor.
11. Place the transducer at the level of the catheter tip.[1]
12. Turn the stopcock off to the patient side. Open the transducer to air and zero the system. The exact mechanism used to zero the system depends on the manu-

facturer. Once the system is zeroed, close it to air.
Zeroing the system negates other pressure influences.

13. When the physician has cannulated the artery, firmly
attach the pressure tubing to the catheter.

14. Activate the flush device to clear the line and catheter
of any blood.

15. Once the catheter is sutured in place by the physician,
clean the site with antiseptic solution. Apply benzoin
around the area. Place sterile gauze over the site. Tape
the gauze securely.

PATIENT CARE MANAGEMENT

1. Apply pressure on the site for 10 to 15 minutes if the
catheter is accidentally dislodged.

2. Monitor the color, temperature, sensation, and movement of the area distal to the catheter. Complications
include hematoma formation, intraluminal clotting,
arterial spasm, thrombosis, and nerve injury. Report all
complications to the appropriate physician because limb
loss can result from long-standing ischemic problems.

3. Withdraw blood for arterial blood gas analysis and
other laboratory tests as ordered by the physician and
based on the patient's clinical condition.
   - Attach a 5-ml syringe to the stopcock port closest to
   the catheter.
   - Turn the stopcock off to the monitor and on to the
   patient. For an adult-sized patient, withdraw 3 to 5 ml
   of blood to clear the line of heparinized solution and
   blood. Turn the stopcock off to the port and discard
   the syringe.
   - Coagulation studies are usually drawn last to ensure
   the use of a nonheparinized specimen.
   - Attach another syringe to obtain needed blood specimens. Use a heparinized syringe to obtain blood for
   an ABG. Turn the stopcock off to the monitor and
   on to the patient. Withdraw the necessary blood.
   Turn the stopcock on to the monitor and patient
   (off to the port). Remove the syringe.
   - Flush the line to the patient. Turn the stopcock off
   to the patient and flush the access port. Turn the
   stopcock on to the patient and monitor. Recap
   the stopcock port with a Luer-Lok cap.

4. Dampening of the waveform is often caused by air in the tubing or transducer, by clot formation, or by a kink in the catheter.
5. The transducer should be zeroed every 4 to 8 hours and each time the patient is repositioned.
6. Change the arterial line site dressing every 48 hours or per hospital protocol.

References

1. Hudak C, Gallo B: *Critical care nursing—a holistic approach,* Philadelphia, 1994, JB Lippincott.

Autotransfusion

Patty Sturt

DESCRIPTION

Autotransfusion is used for the collection and reinfusion of autologous blood. The benefits of autotransfusion include the immediate availability of blood and the diminished incidence of transfusion reactions. Shed blood collected from posttraumatic patients should be transfused or discarded within 4 to 6 hours from the time collection begins. Autotransfusion of >25% of estimated blood volume has been associated with a reduction in platelets, fibrinogen, and clotting factors. For this reason the amount of blood autotransfused should not exceed 2000 ml.[1] Hyperkalemia may result from red blood cell destruction by mechanical forces during collection and reinfusion.

INDICATIONS

Massive hemothorax (see Chapter 20)

CONTRAINDICATIONS

- Suspected thoracoabdominal injury. The risk of sepsis is significant when blood contaminated with gastric or intestinal contents is autotransfused. Thoracoabdominal communication may occur from injuries that disrupt or tear the diaphragm.
- Pulmonary or systemic infections
- Coagulopathies
- Malignant neoplasms
- Blood from injuries more than 4 hours old should not be autotransfused.

ATRIUM SYSTEM*

Equipment

- Atrium 2050 blood recovery system

*Atrium 2050 blood recovery system instruction sheet, Hudson, NH, 1997, Atrium Medical Corp.

- Atrium ATS blood recovery bag
- Y-type blood administration set with 500- to 1000-ml bag of normal saline (NS)
- Microaggregate blood filter
- Alcohol swab
- Citrate phosphate dextrose (CPD) solution (if ordered by the physician)
- 60-ml syringe
- 18-gauge needle

Initial Nursing Actions

1. Prepare 2050 blood recovery chest drainage unit and assist physician with chest tube insertion (see Procedure 7). Flush Y-type blood administration set with NS.
2. Cleanse the collection chamber anticoagulant injection site with an alcohol swab.
3. With an 18-gauge needle and syringe, add the CPD directly to the ATS collection chamber through the anticoagulant injection site on top of the drain. CPD can be added at the discretion of a physician at a control dosage of 14 ml CPD per 100 ml of collected blood.[2]
4. Remove the ATS blood recovery bag from the sterile wrap. Place a label on the bag to include the patient's name, identification number, date, and time of collection.
5. Close the ATS blood bag clamp and the ATS access line clamp on the drainage system.
6. Remove the access line cap, and insert the ATS blood recovery bag spike into the chest drainage access line using a firm, twisting motion. Maintain aseptic technique (Figure P4-1).

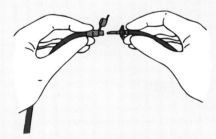

Figure P4-1   Insertion of ATS blood recovery bag spike into the chest drainage access line.

7. Once the blood bag is connected, open the blood bag clamp and the access line clamp.
8. For optimal blood transfer results, hold the ATS blood recovery bag 2 to 4 inches below the chest drain.
9. To activate the blood transfer, bend the bottom of ATS blood bag upward where indicated. The ATS bag will begin to fill and expand as blood enters from the chest drain (Figure P4-2).
10. Once the ATS blood bag is full, displace any residual air into the chest drain by gently squeezing the bag.
11. When blood evacuation is complete, close the access line clamp and blood bag clamp.
12. Remove the bag spike from the access line, and place the spike into the ATS bag spike holder.
13. Replace the access line cap, and place the access line in the holder located on top of the chest drain.

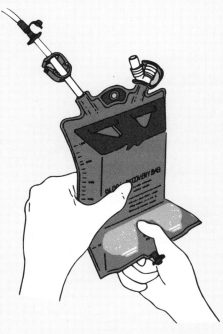

Figure P4-2 Activation of blood transfer by bending bottom of ATS blood bag upward.

14. A microaggregate (microemboli) filter must be used for each new ATS bag. Remove the blood filter cap and spike the microaggregate filter into the blood bag. Spike the Y-type blood administration set (the Y portion not connected to NS) into the microaggregate filter.

15. Prime the blood filter by gently squeezing the blood bag before opening the air vent. Filling the microaggregate filter with NS before squeezing the bag may facilitate the flow of blood through the filter.

16. Open the air vent if the blood is to infuse by gravity. Leave the air vent closed if the blood bag is squeezed by hand or placed on a pressure infuser. Maximum ATS blood bag infusion pressure is 150 mm Hg.

17. When the infusion is complete, close the air vent (if open) by replacing the tethered vent plug. Remove the microaggregate blood filter from the blood bag and replace the tethered cap on the blood filter port. Turn on the Y portion of the blood administration set leading to the NS. Infuse the NS as needed for volume replacement and to maintain a patent line for further blood administration.

THORA-KLEX SYSTEM*

Equipment

- Thora-Klex autotransfusion kit 7756
- Thora-Klex chest drainage unit
- Y-type blood administration set with 500- to 1000-ml bag of NS
- Microaggregate blood filter
- (CPD)
- 60-ml syringe
- 18-gauge needle

Initial Nursing Actions

A. Preparing the autotransfusion unit
  1. Prepare the Thora-Klex chest drainage system according to the manufacturer's instructions. Assist the physician with chest tube insertion.
  2. Connect the chest tube to the Thora-Klex chest drainage unit.

*Thora-Klex autotransfusion quick reference guide, Cranston, RI, 1990, CR Bard.

3. Remove the protective seal from the quick disconnect locking connector located midway on the patient tube of the Thora-Klex chest drainage unit.

4. Separate the connector by twisting the quick disconnect locking connector counterclockwise and pulling apart. Clamp or pinch the chest tube to prevent outflow of blood (Figure P4-3).

5. Using aseptic technique, remove the red cover from the filter of the autotransfusion unit and insert the corresponding red color-coded quick disconnect locking connector of the patient tube to the filter. The connector is locked into place by twisting clockwise. Insert and lock the blue color-coded connector into the bottlecap (Figure P4-4).

6. Release the clamp from the patient's chest tube.

7. The Thora-Klex unit should be positioned below the patient's chest and in an upright position.

8. Place the Thora-Klex unit on suction. The wall or machine suction should be between 80 and 120 mm Hg. The suction control on the chest drainage unit is usually set to -20 cm H_2O.

9. Inject CPD or anticoagulant (as ordered by physician) through the anticoagulant port on the filter. The ratio of CPD to blood is 1:7.[1] Add the anticoagulant by inserting a needle through the latex injection port of the filter housing (Figure P4-5).

B. Steps for Reinfusion

1. Disconnect the Thora-Klex chest drainage unit from suction.

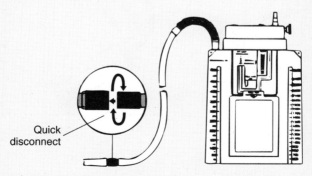

Quick
disconnect

Figure P4-3 Location of quick disconnect on the Thora-Klex chest drainage unit.

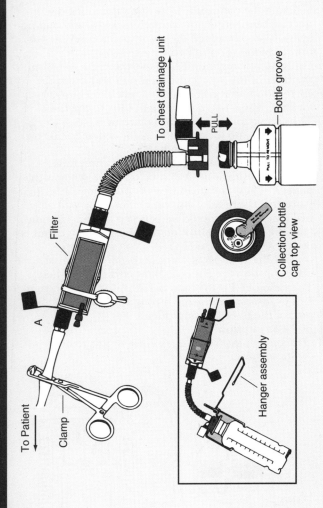

Figure P4-4 Red-color-coded quick disconnect locking connector (A) of the patient tube connected to the filter.

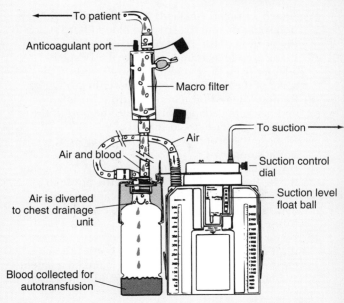

Figure P4-5 Fluid flow into the drainage collection bottle for auto-transfusion. Anticoagulant may be added at the anticoagulant port of the filter.

2. Clamp the patient tube above the filter.
3. Separate the patient tube from the filter connector by rotating the quick disconnect locking connector counterclockwise and pulling it apart.
4. Similarly, separate the Thora-Klex chest drainage patient tube at the bottle cap by rotating the locking connector counterclockwise.
5. Join the patient tubes together at the quick disconnect locking connector.
6. Release the clamp from the patient tube.
7. Reconnect to suction.
8. Remove the spike adapter package from the side of the bottle.
9. Remove the bottle from its hanger.
10. Grasp the bottle cap and pull away from the bottle, exposing the rubber stopper.
11. Discard the bottle cap and filter.

12. Attach a primed (flushed) Y-type blood administration set to the microaggregate blood filter (attach to the portion of the Y not connected to NS).

13. Using aseptic technique, remove the IV spike adapter from the package and insert it onto the spike of the microaggregate blood filter.

14. Remove the red protective cap from the adapter, and insert the adapter firmly into the port of the rubber stopper marked "FLUID."

15. Remove the protective seal from the air vent on the bottle stopper.

16. Invert the bottle and hang it from an IV pole using the hanger loop. Place a label on the bottle to include the patient's name, identification number, date, and time of infusion (Figure P4-6).

17. Infuse blood using gravity.

18. When the autologous blood has infused, turn off the Y-clamp leading to the blood bottle. Turn on the Y-clamp leading to the NS to maintain a patent IV line for further blood and fluid administration.

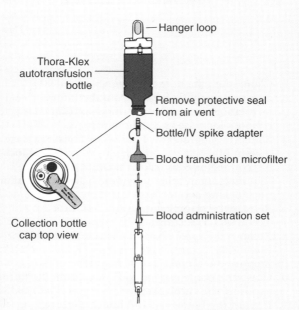

Figure P4-6   Preparation for gravity infusion.

PLEUR-EVAC SYSTEM*

Equipment
- Pleur-Evac chest drainage unit
- Pleur-Evac A-1500 autotransfusion replacement bag
- Y-type blood administration set with 500- to 1000-ml bag of NS
- Microaggregate blood filter
- CPD or heparin
- 60-ml syringe
- 18-gauge needle

Initial Nursing Actions
1. Prepare a Pleur-Evac chest drainage unit according to the manufacturer's instructions. Assist the physician with chest tube insertion.
2. Unwrap the A-1500 replacement bag. Close the two clamps on top of the replacement bag (Figure P4-7).

*Pleur-Evac Autotransfusion Replacement Bag Instruction Sheet, Fall River, Mass, 1992, DeKnatel.

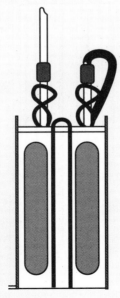

Figure P4-7   A-1500 Autotransfusion bag.

3. Close the clamp on the Pleur-Evac patient tubing, and milk blood from the tubing into the Pleur-Evac.
4. Disconnect red and blue connectors on the patient tubing.
5. Remove the red protective cap from the collection tubing on the autotransfusion bag, and connect the tubing to the patient chest drainage tubing using red connectors.
6. Remove the blue protective cap from the tubing on the A-1500 autotransfusion bag and connect the tubing to the 6-inch Pleur-Evac tube using blue connectors.
7. Open all clamps. Make sure connections are tight.
8. Anticoagulants may be used at the discretion of the physician. Add anticoagulant into the collection bag through the injection site in the autotransfusion system connector.
9. Attach the bag to the Pleur-Evac using the foot hook and hanger on the side of the unit (Figure P4-8).

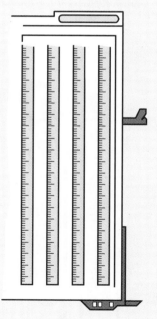

Figure P4-8 Attach the A-1500 Autotransfusion bag to the Pleur-Evac using foot hook and ATS hanger on side of unit.

10. After blood is collected, close the clamp on the patient tubing and on top of the autotransfusion bag.
11. Disconnect all red and blue connectors.
12. Attach red and blue connectors on top of the auto-transfusion bag.
13. Securely attach red and blue connectors joining the patient tube (red) to the 6-inch Pleur-Evac tube (blue).
14. Open the clamp on the patient tube. Patient drainage is collected in the Pleur-Evac.
15. Remove the autotransfusion bag from the hanger on the side of the unit.
16. Invert the bag so the spike port points upward. Place a label on the bag to include the patient's name and identification number and the date and time of infusion.
17. Remove the protective cap, and insert the microaggregate filter into the spike port.
18. Attach one end of the Y-blood administration set to the microaggregate blood filter. The other end of the Y is connected to a bag of NS. Prime the microaggregate filter and blood set with NS. Turn off the Y portion leading to the NS.
19. Invert the autotransfusion bag, and suspend it from an IV pole using the plastic strap. Turn on the Y portion leading to the autotransfusion bag.

PATIENT CARE MANAGEMENT (FOR ALL AUTOTRANSFUSION SYSTEMS)

1. Use a new microaggregate filter for each new autotransfusion bag or bottle.
2. Monitor the patient for coagulopathies and air embolism.
3. Prepare the patient for surgery as indicated.

References

1. Kitt S: Autotransfusion using the Thora-Klex system. In Proehl JA, editor: *Adult emergency nursing procedures,* Boston, 1993, Jones & Bartlett.
2. *Atrium 2050 blood recovery system instruction sheet,* Hudson, NH, 1994, Atrium Medical Corp.

Burn Dressing

Julia Fultz

DESCRIPTION

Burn dressings are applied to accomplish the following:
1. Provide an optimal environment for healing
2. Help prevent infection
3. Absorb exudate
4. Assist in debridement of burned tissue
5. Protect uninjured skin from excretions and secretions

There are two types of burn dressings, open and closed. Open dressings are used on areas that are hard to dress such as the head, neck, or perineum. An antibacterial cream is applied to the wound. After the cream is applied, the wound may be covered with a layer of fine mesh gauze. Leaving the wound without a dressing diminishes the proliferation of bacteria because of the decreased moisture. The application of a closed dressing involves placing a layer of antibacterial cream or a nonstick layer of gauze over the wound and covering it with a bulky dressing. Closed dressings are most frequently used on patients treated on an outpatient basis, ambulatory patients, those who must work specifically with their hands, children, and burns in areas that will be covered with clothing.

INDICATIONS

Burn injuries that interrupt skin integrity

EQUIPMENT

- Pain medication
- Sterile gloves, hats, masks, gowns, and eye protection
- Tongue blades
- Mild soap or antiseptic solution
- Sterile 4×4 gauze sponges
- Semielastic coarse mesh gauze such as Kerlex
- Nonadherent porous mesh gauze saturated with a water-soluble lubricant
- Antibacterial agent

- 35-ml syringe attached to an 18-gauge IV catheter (needle removed) for irrigation
- Sterile saline solution with a sterile basin
- Sterile, curved scissors
- Sterile forceps
- Good light source

INITIAL NURSING ACTIONS

1. Administer pain medication in enough time before procedure, so effective analgesia is obtained.
2. Wear sterile hats, gowns, masks, and eye protection during irrigation of the burn (to prevent splash back into eyes), and sterile gloves before initiation of care.
3. Fill a sterile basin with sterile saline. Using the 35-ml syringe and the 18-gauge catheter, irrigate the burn to remove gross debris.
4. Gently cleanse the burned area with mild soap or antiseptic solution and rinse again with sterile saline.
5. If permitted by your institution's nursing policies and procedures, remove any loose skin, debris, and blisters (broken, tense, or infected) using sterile forceps and scissors. If you are not permitted to debride tissue, notify the physician to perform the debridement.
6. If the patient is to be transferred to a burn unit within 1 to 2 hours, burns can be cleansed with saline and a mild soap or antiseptic solution, grossly debrided, and wrapped in sterile sheets or dry dressings for the transfer.
7. Cotton-tipped applicators dipped in sterile saline can be used to gently remove loose skin from the lips and from around the eyes, ears, and nose. Do not vigorously debride the eyelids because the skin is very thin. Cotton-tipped applicators should be used only on the outer ear, never in the ear canal.
8. Apply neomycin or bacitracin ointment to burns of the face, and do not cover the area.
9. If ordered, apply antibacterial cream using a sterile tongue blade or a sterile gloved hand. (If using a jar of antibacterial cream, do not dip the tongue blade or gloved hand back into the jar after it has come into contact with the wound. Contamination of the cream will occur.)

10. Dress the wound. (Dressings are not usually applied to the head, neck, and perineum because of difficulty securing them.)

   a. Describe the procedure to the patient. (If the patient is to be discharged home and is expected to do dressing changes, explain each step as it is done.)

   b. Apply mesh gauze that contains a water-soluble lubricant to prevent sticking if no antibacterial cream is used.

   c. Cover mesh gauze or antibacterial cream with a bulky dressing such as 4×4 gauze sponges about 1 to 2 inches thick to absorb drainage.

   d. Secure the bulky dressing with semielastic mesh gauze (e.g., Kerlex), wrapping extremities distal to proximal.

   e. Hands must be wrapped in a functional position (fingers slightly flexed with the thumb abducted away from the palm with a roll of gauze such as Kling or Kerlex in the patient's palm to support the position).

   f. Wrap fingers and toes individually to allow for range of motion. Leave the tips of the fingers and toes exposed to evaluate circulation.

COMPLICATIONS

1. Infection
2. Diminished perfusion distal to a circumferential dressing

PATIENT CARE MANAGEMENT

1. Check circulation distal to any circumferential dressing.
2. Administer tetanus toxoid as ordered.
3. Elevate the extremity to minimize swelling.
4. If the patient is to be discharged, teaching about dressing changes and signs of infection must be reinforced and written instructions must be given to the patient. If the wound is infected, ensure that the patient receives a prescription for antibiotics. Plans for follow-up care (with a private physician or with the emergency department) must be made before discharging the patient.

EXAMPLE OF DISCHARGE INSTRUCTIONS

1. How to change your dressing:
   - Assemble your supplies, and keep the area around the supplies clean.
   - Wash your hands. Do not touch anything (e.g., hair, face, clothes, and pets) other than the dressing supplies.
   - Remove the old dressing. If the dressing sticks to the burn, soak it off with cool, clean water.
   - Clean the burn with soap and water, then pat it dry with a clean, dry cloth such as a washcloth or dish towel.
   - Look for one or more of these signs and symptoms of infection:
     a. Increased redness around the burn
     b. Swelling
     c. Red streaks extending away from the burn
     d. Pus
     e. Elevated temperature
     f. Increased pain
   - Apply a thin layer of the antibacterial cream, and cover with a gauze dressing as was done in the hospital.
2. If you think your burn has become infected, call your private physician or the ED.
3. Take your pain medicine as prescribed.
4. Elevate the extremity for 24 hours if possible.
5. Keep the dressing clean and dry.
6. It is very important for you to have your burn checked in about 24 hours. Please comply with the follow-up directions given to you before leaving the ED.
   Follow-up directions:
7. If you have any questions, call your private physician or the ED at _____

Central Venous Pressure Management

Patty Sturt

DESCRIPTION

Central venous pressure (CVP) monitoring refers to the measurement of pressure within the right atrium. "Right atrial pressure" is synonymous with CVP. The CVP can provide an estimate of the volume status of the right heart. The normal range is 3 to 10 cm H_2O.

INDICATIONS

1. Alteration in fluid volume status (A low CVP often occurs in hypovolemic patients. An elevated CVP occurs in cases of fluid overload or retention.)
2. To guide fluid replacement in hypovolemia
3. To assess the effectiveness of diuretic administration
4. To assess right heart function (The CVP may be increased in right-sided heart failure.)

NURSING ALERT

The CVP is not a reliable indicator of left ventricular failure. Left ventricular failure increases filling pressure of the left side of the heart. Eventually this increased pressure results in the backup of blood into the pulmonary vasculature. Pulmonary edema is present by the time the CVP becomes elevated.

EQUIPMENT

1. For catheter placement:
   - Single-, double-, or triple-lumen infusion catheter
   - 1% lidocaine
   - 5- and 10-ml syringes and different-sized needles for injection of lidocaine
   - Antiseptic skin solution such as povidone-iodine solution

- Sterile towels
- Needle introducer
- 10- to 20-ml syringe
- Guidewire

NOTE: These are available in commercially prepackaged kits often referred to as CVP kits or venous pressure trays.

2. For CVP monitoring:
   - CVP water manometer with three-way stopcock
   - Extension tubing
   - IV fluid and administration set
   - Indelible marker
   - A transducer connected to pressure tubing with a flush device may be used in place of a manometer. The transducer must be connected to a monitoring system to obtain the CVP reading. The CVP reading will be recorded in mm HG if a transducer is used.

INITIAL NURSING ACTIONS

1. Attach the stopcock to the end of the manometer. Attach the extension tubing to one port and the IV administration set to the other port. Turn the stopcock off to the manometer, and flush the entire length of tubing with IV solution.
2. Explain the procedure to the patient and obtain informed consent.
3. Prep the catheter insertion site with antiseptic solution.
4. Position the patient supine and in a slight Trendelenburg position (if the patient will tolerate this).
5. After injecting the patient with a local anesthetic and draping the area, the physician usually inserts the infusion catheter into the subclavian or internal jugular vein. A needle is inserted, and a guidewire is placed through the needle. The needle is removed and a catheter is placed over the guidewire. The guidewire is removed, and the catheter is sutured in place. The catheter tip is usually placed into the superior vena cava just above the right atrium.

NURSING ALERT

Monitor for arrhythmias during catheter insertion. Inform the physician immediately if this occurs.

6. Obtain an order for a chest x-ray examination to confirm accurate placement.
7. Connect the end of the extension tubing to the catheter.
8. Adjust the IV rate as prescribed by the physician.
9. For CVP measurement the patient should be supine or the head of bed should be elevated 30 to 45 degrees.
10. Position the zero mark of the water manometer (or the transducer) at the phlebostatic axis. This is located at the junction of the midaxillary line and 4th intercostal space. This point approximates the level of the atria.
11. Mark the point with an indelible marker. This site becomes the zero reference point-the location to be used for all subsequent readings.
12. Turn the stopcock off to the patient (catheter) and open to the IV solution and manometer. Allow IV solution to slowly fill the manometer to the 25-cm level. Do not let fluid overflow from the top of the manometer.
13. Turn the stopcock off to the IV solution, and open it to the patient (catheter) and manometer. The fluid level will fall and fluctuate with respirations.
14. Take the reading when the fluid level stabilizes. The CVP reading should be taken at the end of expiration. The measurement should be recorded at the lowest point of the water meniscus.
15. Turn the stopcock off to the manometer and on to the patient (catheter) and IV solution.
16. Infuse IV solution through the central venous line as prescribed.
17. Document the CVP reading.

PATIENT CARE MANAGEMENT

1. Note the trend of the CVP readings.
2. Instruct the patient to report any tubing disconnections.

Chest Tubes

Patty Sturt

DESCRIPTION

Chest tubes are used to remove air and fluid from the pleural cavity, to restore normal negative intrapleural pressure, and to achieve full reexpansion of a lung.

INDICATIONS

1. Hemothorax
2. Pneumothorax
3. Empyema
4. Large pleural effusion

EQUIPMENT

- Povidone-iodine solution
- 4 × 4 gauze sponges
- Local anesthetic
- Needles of various sizes
- 5- and 10-ml syringes
- Sterile gloves
- Sterile drapes
- Scalpels
- Large clamps and hemostats
- Suture material
- Needle holders
- Occlusive gauze
- 3- to 4-inch tape
- Chest drainage systems
- Chest tube of appropriate size as follows:

Age	Chest tube sizes
Newborn	12-18 Fr
6 months	14-20 Fr
1 year	14-24 Fr
3 years	16-28 Fr

Continued

765

Age	Chest tube sizes
5 years	20-32 Fr
8 years	24-32 Fr
12 years	28-36 Fr
Adult	28-40 Fr

Smaller sizes can be used for removal of air and larger sizes for removal of fluid. Anticipate the need for a 36 to 40 Fr tube in an adult trauma patient.

INITIAL NURSING ACTIONS

1. Assemble the chest drainage system. Fill the water seal and suction control chambers as specified by instructions with the system.
2. If the patient is being monitored by a cardiac monitor, move the electrodes on the involved side of the chest to the shoulder and lateroposterior chest wall.
3. Monitor the patient throughout the procedure. Provide verbal support and comfort measures.
4. The 5th intercostal space in the midaxillary line is often used as the insertion site. The physician cleanses the area with a povidone-iodine solution. The area is draped and locally infiltrated with an anesthetic solution. An incision is made with a scalpel along the rib. A curved clamp is inserted into the incision. A small tunnel is formed by separating the clamp. The clamp is closed and then placed further into the thoracic cage through the intercostal muscles and parietal pleura. The clamp is opened and closed again to enlarge the puncture site. At this point the physician removes the clamp and inserts a gloved finger into the pleural space to ensure a clear passage for the chest tube. The chest tube is inserted into the opening with a curved clamp. The tube is sutured in place.
5. After insertion, connect the chest tube to the tubing from the collection chamber. Connect the tubing from the suction control chamber to the suction source.
6. After the chest tube is sutured in place, apply a dressing with occlusive gauze, 4 × 4 sponges, and 3- to 4-inch tape.
7. Wrap tubing connections with adhesive tape to ensure they are airtight.
8. Coil extra tubing from the drainage system and place it flat on the bed.

9. Confirm correct tube placement with an x-ray examination.

PATIENT CARE MANAGEMENT

1. Assess and note the trend of the patient's vital signs, skin color, and breath sounds.
2. Monitor for blood or fluid in the collection chamber. Mark the level of drainage hourly on the drainage system. Notify the physician if drainage is >100 ml/hr.
3. Observe for fluctuation ("tidaling") of the fluid level in the water seal chamber. The fluid level rises when the patient inhales and drops when the patient exhales. If the patient is using a ventilator, the opposite occurs. The fluid level drops on inspiration (because intrapleural pressure becomes more positive) and rises on expiration. Fluctuation indicates patency of the system. Lack of fluctuation may be indicative of an obstruction or kink in the system.
4. Milk the tubing by gently kneading a small piece of tubing between your fingers if blood clots or tissue obstruct the tubing.
5. Do not clamp the chest tube. Clamping may lead to an accumulation of air in the pleural space and result in a tension pneumothorax.
6. If the patient is to be transported, or if suction is not being used, leave the suction tubing connector open to air. Do not clamp it off.
7. If the chest tube is accidentally pulled out, cover the site with a dressing taped on three sides. Immediately notify the physician.

NURSING ALERT

It may be difficult to assess tidaling and breath sounds when suction is in use. Suction may be turned off. The purpose of the suction control chamber is to facilitate the removal of air and fluid. The water seal remains intact when suction is not in use.

Conscious Sedation

Patty Sturt

DESCRIPTION

IV conscious sedation (IVCS) is produced by the administration of pharmacologic agents. A patient under conscious sedation has a depressed level of consciousness but retains the ability to independently and continuously maintain a patent airway and respond appropriately to physical stimulation and verbal command. The objectives of IVCS include the following:

1. Alteration of mood
2. Maintenance of consciousness
3. Cooperative patient
4. Increase in pain threshold
5. Stable vital signs
6. Some degree of amnesia

INDICATIONS

IVCS may be used in ED patients requiring the following:

1. Closed manipulation or reduction of dislocations and fractures
2. Suction curettage
3. Extensive laceration repairs
4. Incision and drainage
5. Foreign body removal
6. Endoscopic procedures
7. Diagnostic procedures

CONTRAINDICATIONS

IVCS should be used cautiously with patients who have a history of recent alcohol ingestion. Alcohol can compound the actions of many of the medications used for IVCS. Other contraindications include the following:

1. Pregnancy
2. Thyroid, adrenal, or renal dysfunction

3. Patients receiving Monoamine oxidase (MAO) inhibitors or tricyclic antidepressants
4. Hemodynamic instability
5. Significant respiratory distress

EQUIPMENT

- IV fluid, tubing, and catheter
- IVCS medications and their antidotes (Table P8-1)
- Pulse oximeter
- Code cart with airway equipment, bag-valve mask device, resuscitation drugs, and a monitor and defibrillator
- Oxygen and oxygen delivery devices such as a nasal cannula and nonrebreather mask
- Suction
- Automatic blood pressure (BP) device or BP cuff and stethoscope

INITIAL NURSING ACTIONS

1. Obtain a history and baseline assessment data to include the following:
   - Current medications and drug allergies
   - Medical and surgical history-should include information regarding previous adverse experiences with sedation and analgesia
   - History of substance abuse
   - Physical parameters such as blood pressure, heart rate, respiratory rate, level of consciousness, skin color, oxygen saturation, and an Aldrete score (Table P8-2)
   - Planned method of transport home
   - Food or fluid intake within the past 8 hours
2. Establish IV access. Use an 18-gauge or larger if significant blood loss is a possibility.
3. Initiate pulse oximetry.
4. Administer and titrate the medications in small incremental doses (Box P8-1) based on the attending physician's order and the individual's response. The desired effects of conscious sedation include the following:
   - Relaxed and cooperative patient
   - Diminished verbal communication
   - Initiation of slurred speech
   - Arousable sleep

TABLE P8-1 Drug Summary

Drug	Dose and route	Special considerations	Half-life
Flumazenil (Romazicon) (benzodiazepine antagonist)	0.2 mg May be repeated at 1-min intervals until desired level of consciousness is achieved or a total dose of 1 mg has been given IV over 15 sec	Used to reverse the effects of benzodiazepines in adults Not recommended for use in children Some side effects include nausea and vomiting, headache, dizziness, sweating, and flushing	41-79 min
Meperidine (Demerol) (narcotic)	Initial dose of 10-25 mg IV over 30 sec-2 min into an infusing IV May repeat every 10-15 min	Monitor the patient for weakness, nausea and vomiting, respiratory depression, and hypotension	3-4 hr
Lorazepam (Ativan) (benzodiazepine)	1-2 mg or 0.05 mg/kg 2 mg IV over 1 min	Potentiates narcotics, MAOIs, and TCA Effective in 15-20 min	14 hr
Diazepam (Valium) (benzodiazepine)	2-5 mg Slow IV push over 1 min; repeat every 5-10 min; onset is within 1-5 min	Monitor patient for hypotension and respiratory depression	20-50 hr

Drug	Dosage	Comments	Duration
Midazolam (Versed) (benzodiazepine)	0.5-2.5 mg IV push over 2 min into an infusing IV line	Do not give to patients on MAOIs or TCAs	1.2-12.3 hr
Morphine (narcotic)	Initial dose of 2-5 mg Slow IV push over 5 min into an infusing IV line	Reduced doses would be used in those with renal or hepatic dysfunctions	2.5-3 hr
Sublimaze (Fentanyl) (narcotic)	2 µg/kg 0.1 mg over 1-2 min	Respiratory depressant effects outlast analgesics effect; 80 times more potent than morphine; usually under the direct observation of an anesthesiologist	2.5-4 hr
Naloxone (Narcan) (narcotic antagonist)	0.1-0.2 IV at 2-3 min intervals into an infusing IV line	Antagonist for narcotic-induced hypotension and respiratory depression	1 hr

MAOIs, Monoamine oxidase inhibitors; *TCA,* tricyclic antidepressants.

TABLE P8-2 The Aldrete Scoring System

Physical parameters	Score
Activity	
Voluntary movement of all limbs to command	2
Voluntary movement of two extremities to command	1
Unable to move	0
Respiration	
Breathe deeply and cough	2
Dyspnea, hypoventilation	1
Apneic	0
Circulation	
Blood pressure 20% of preanesthetic level	2
Blood pressure 20% to 50% of preanesthetic level	1
Blood pressure 50% of preanesthetic level	0
Consciousness	
Fully awake	2
Arousable	1
Unresponsive	0
Color	
Pink	2
Pale, blotch	1
Cyanotic	0

COMMONLY ADMINISTERED MEDICATIONS FOR IVCS

Benzodiazepines

Midazolam (Versed)
Diazepam (Valium)
Lorazepam (Ativan)

Narcotics

Meperidine (Demerol)
Morphine
Sublimaze (Fentanyl)

Antagonists

Naloxone (Narcan)
Flumazenil (Romazicon)

PATIENT CARE MANAGEMENT

1. A patent IV must be continuously maintained during the procedure.
2. The RN managing the care of the patient receiving IVCS should not leave the patient unattended.
3. Oxygen saturation must be continuously monitored during the procedure. Supplemental oxygen should be given if there is a decrease in the oxygen saturation from the patient's baseline.
4. Anticipate the need to administer oxygen for any patient with a baseline SpO_2 equal to or <90 mm Hg.
5. The blood pressure, heart rate, respiratory rate, level of consciousness, and pulse oximeter values should be obtained and recorded every 5 to 15 minutes during the procedure.
6. Anticipate the need to continuously monitor cardiac rhythm and rate of patients with a history of cardiac or respiratory disease.
7. Vital signs and an Aldrete score should be evaluated and documented at the completion of the procedure and at least every 15 minutes until the patient's values return to baseline. The Aldrete score provides objective, measurable information regarding the degree of sedation. Other sedation scoring systems are available.
8. Before discharge from the ED, the patient and significant others should receive verbal and written instructions to include signs and symptoms of complications, restrictions on diet and activity, and a follow-up appointment as needed. Documentation should reflect that the patient and significant others received, repeated, and understood the instructions.
9. Never allow the patient to drive himself or herself home.

Crutch Walking

Lee Garner

DESCRIPTION

Crutches may be needed for emergency department (ED) patients to facilitate unilateral, non–weight-bearing ambulation. The most frequently used crutches are the underarm or axillary crutches with hand bars.[1]

INDICATIONS

Lower extremity injuries such as sprains, contusions, or fractures

EQUIPMENT

Adjustable crutches with axilla pads, hand bar pads, and crutch tips

INITIAL NURSING ACTIONS

1. Measuring for crutches
   A. Place axilla pads, hand bar pads, and crutch tips on the crutches.
   B. Have the patient stand and bear weight on the unaffected extremity. Place crutches 2.5 to 5 cm (1 to 2 in) or 2 to 3 fingerbreadths below axilla. Adjust the crutches so they extend 5 cm (2 in) in front of and 15 cm (6 in) to the side of the feet. The crutches can be adjusted by removing the screws in the lower portion and shortening or lengthening the inner lower piece. Replace the screws and bolts and tighten firmly.
   C. With the patient standing upright and erect, adjust the hand bars to the point where there is approximately a 30-degree elbow flexion. The hand grips can be adjusted by removing the screws and sliding the hand grips to the appropriate level. Slide screws back into the crutches. Replace the bolts and tighten

firmly. The patient's arms should never be straight (Figure P9-1).

2. Ambulating with crutches
   A. Place weight on palms of the hands and not the axilla.

NURSING ALERT

Continual pressure on the axilla can injure the radial nerve, resulting in weakness to the forearm, wrist, and hand.

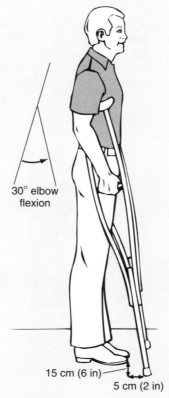

30° elbow flexion

15 cm (6 in)
5 cm (2 in)

Figure P9-1 The standing position to measure the correct length of crutches. (From Kozier B, et al: *Fundamentals of Nursing: Concepts, Process, and Practice*, 6/e, Multimedia. Reprinted by permission of Prentice-Hall, Inc., Upper Saddle River, NJ.)

B. Use the proper standing position, called the tripod position. In this position, the crutch tips are placed about 5 cm (2 in) in front of the feet and out laterally about 15 cm (6 in). This creates a wide and stable base of support.

C. Look forward (not at the feet) and advance the crutches and affected leg forward at the same time.

D. Move the unaffected leg forward and through to a position slightly ahead of the crutches.[2]

3. Going up stairs (Figure P9-2)

A. Assume the tripod position at the bottom of the stairs.

B. While balancing weight on the hands, move the unaffected leg onto the step.

C. Shift body weight to the unaffected leg and move the affected leg and crutches up onto the step. Keep the affected leg slightly bent during this move.

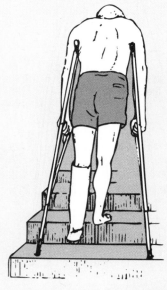

Figure P9-2 When climbing stairs, the patient places weight on the crutches while first moving the unaffected leg onto a step. (From Barber J, Stokes L, Billings D: *Adult and child care*, ed 2, St Louis, 1977, Mosby).

4. Going down stairs (Figure P9-3)
   A. Shift body weight to the unaffected leg. Move the crutches and the affected leg onto the step. Keep the affected leg slightly in front of the body during the move.
   B. Transfer body weight to the crutches and move the unaffected leg to that step. When moving the unaffected leg to the step, land on the heel and not the toes.

NURSING ALERT

A simple way to remind patients of these steps is that the "good" (unaffected leg) goes up first toward heaven when traveling up stairs. Thus the bad (affected) leg goes down first when moving down the stairs.

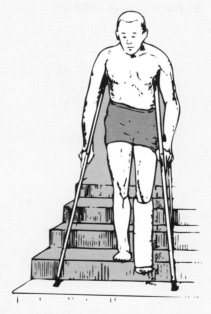

Figure P9-3   When descending stairs the client first moves the crutches and affected leg down to the next step. (From Barber J, Stokes L, Billings D: *Adult and child care,* ed 2, St Louis, 1977, Mosby).

5. Sitting on the chair or bed
    A. Slowly turn around and back up until the back of the unaffected leg touches the chair or bed.
    B. Transfer both crutches to the hand on the same side as the affected leg. Hold onto the crutches with the hand bars. Grasp the arm of the chair with the other hand.
    C. Hold the affected leg slightly forward, and slowly lower self into a sitting position.
6. Getting out of chair or bed
    A. Move forward to the edge of the chair or bed.
    B. Grasp the crutches by the hand bars in the hand on the affected side. Grasp the arm of the chair by the hand on the unaffected side.
    C. Push self up.
    D. Assume the tripod position before moving.

PATIENT CARE MANAGEMENT

Instruct the patient to do the following:
1. Remove loose rugs and small objects on the floor at home.
2. Stay off wet or waxed floors, ice, and grass. These can be slick.
3. Wipe off wet crutch tips.
4. Avoid escalators.
5. Wear sturdy, low-heeled shoes.
6. Avoid alcohol or medications that may impair balance, perception, and judgment.

References

1. Kozier E, Erb G, Olivier R: *Fundamentals of nursing: concepts, process, and practice*, Redwood City, Calif, 1991, Addison-Wesley.
2. Swimm DM: Measuring for crutches/teaching crutch walking. In Proehl JA, editor: *Adult emergency nursing procedures*, Boston, 1993, Jones & Bartlett.

Defibrillation

Darlene Welsh
George P. Glessner III

Defibrillation is the treatment of choice for ventricular fibrillation and pulseless ventricular tachycardia. Until recently, this procedure has been performed only in settings equipped for advanced cardiac life support with the use of complex defibrillators. With the advent of automated external defibrillators (AEDs), defibrillation can now be executed in a variety of settings by emergency cardiac care providers and laypersons. The emergency nurse will be dealing with the prehospital use of AEDs more frequently and therefore must have an understanding of their use and integration into the emergency department (ED) resuscitation of the cardiac arrest patient. AEDs are classified as "fully automatic" or "semiautomatic." Fully automatic AEDs require no intervention beyond the application and initial activation of the device. Semiautomatic AEDs require the operator to initiate the "analyze" feature of the device and then press the appropriate button to deliver the shocks after being advised to do so by the AED. Both devices are considered safe and effective.[1] The semiautomatic AEDs applied in the prehospital setting can be used to continue defibrillation in the ED while other definitive cardiac care measures such as intubation, IV cannulation, and initial resuscitation drug administration are instituted. It is important for the ED nurse to be competent with defibrillation, since the survival of the patient with serious cardiac complications often depends on the successful completion of this procedure.

DESCRIPTION

Defibrillation can be accomplished by delivering nonsynchronized electrical energy (joules) to the myocardium to depolarize the pacemaker cells. With successful defibrillation, a brief period of asystole is followed by an effective cardiac rhythm, eliminating ventricular fibrillation or pulseless ventricular tachycardia.

INDICATIONS

1. Ventricular fibrillation
2. Pulseless ventricular tachycardia

EQUIPMENT

- Automatic external defibrillator or standard defibrillator with cardiac monitor
- ECG electrodes
- Conductive gel, two gel pads, or two self-adhesive disposable defibrillator electrodes

INITIAL NURSING ACTIONS

Defibrillation with Standard Defibrillator

1. Turn on the ECG monitor. Hook the patient up to the ECG monitor in lead II while someone else performs CPR. Turn on the continuous ECG recorder. Confirm ventricular fibrillation and pulseless tachycardia.
2. Apply a conductive gel to the defibrillator paddles. Gel pads designed specifically for defibrillation can be substituted for the defibrillator gel. Do not use ECG gel. Some institutions use pregelled, self-adhesive, disposable defibrillator electrodes in place of paddles for repeated defibrillation.[1] Many defibrillators have the capacity for cardiac monitoring through the defibrillator paddles, omitting the need for ECG electrodes.
3. Charge the defibrillator to 200 joules. Make sure the defibrillator is in the "unsynchronized" mode.
4. Place the paddles on the chest wall for defibrillation or to monitor without ECG cables. The sternal or posterior paddle is placed on the right upper sternum below the clavicle (right atrial area). The apex or anterior paddle is placed near and lateral to the left nipple at the midaxillary line (apex). See Figure P10-1 for standard paddle placement. Infants who weigh <10 kg require 4.5-cm pediatric paddles. Children who weigh >10 kg and are approximately 1 year of age can be defibrillated with 8- to 10-cm paddles.[2,3] Adults require 13-cm paddles.[4] Paddle placement for children is similar to placement for adults, with one paddle over the right side of the upper chest and the other over the apex of the heart to the left of the nipple.
5. Press the paddles on the chest wall with approximately 25 lbs of pressure.

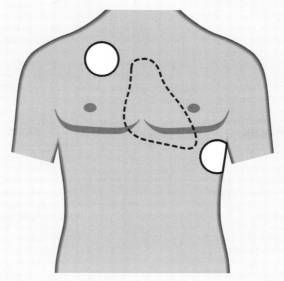

Figure P10-1   Recommended anterior-apex position for defibrillation. The anterior electrode should be to the right of the upper sternum below the clavicle. The apex electrode should be placed to the left of the nipple with the center of the electrode in the midaxillary line. (Reproduced with permission © *Advanced Life Support,* 1997. Copyright American Heart Association.)

6. Determine that everyone in the room is not in contact with the patient or equipment touching the patient. Verify verbally that all rescuers are not in contact by stating, "All clear" before delivering the shock. This reminds everyone to check his or her position and move to a safe location.
7. Deliver the electrical current by simultaneously pressing the appropriate buttons. Defibrillators vary; therefore, it is recommended that nurses seek appropriate training for equipment used in their clinical area.
8. For adults, three consecutive shocks are delivered at 200, 200 to 300, and 360 joules if resolution of ventricular fibrillation and tachycardia does not occur after each attempt.[1] Remember to confirm ventricular fibrillation and tachycardia by cardiac monitor before each

countershock. It is important to deliver the initial three consecutive shocks with little time in between in order to increase the probability of successful defibrillation; therefore, CPR between the three consecutive shocks is not recommended. Pediatric patients require 2 joules/kg initially, followed by successive shocks of 4 joules/kg.

NURSING ALERT

Do not defibrillate over nitroglycerin patches or permanent pacemaker pulse generators. Avoid pulse generators by placing one paddle opposite the insertion site below the clavicle and the other lateral to the sternum at least 5 inches from the pulse generator. See Figure P10-2 for alternate paddle placement.[4] Do not allow gel to form a path between the paddles. A burn injury to the patient could occur under these circumstances.

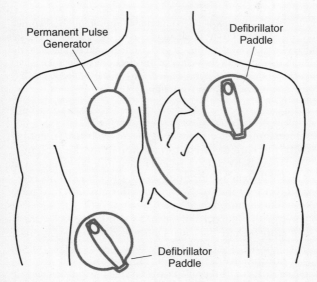

Figure P10-2 Alternate paddle placement for synchronized cardioversion and defibrillation in the patient with a permanent pulse generator. (From Boggs R, Wooldridge-King, M: *AACN procedure manual for critical care,* ed 3, Philadelphia, 1993, WB Saunders.)

9. If the patient does not convert to a pulse generating rhythm after the third attempt, initiate ACLS.

PATIENT CARE MANAGEMENT

1. Continue CPR if delays in defibrillation occur. Do not perform CPR between the three initial consecutive shocks.
2. Continue monitoring and assessing cardiopulmonary status after defibrillation.
3. Other interventions before and after defibrillation may include airway and ventilation management by intubation or cricothyrotomy, IV medication administration, and, in some instances, endotracheal medication instillation if rapid IV access cannot be achieved.
4. Routine care of the defibrillation equipment includes inspection of the equipment every shift. Determine that ECG paper, monitoring electrodes, and defibrillator gel or pads are available. Examine the cables, connectors, paddles, and defibrillator for damage. Test the adequacy of the battery power supply and the ECG display by turning on the equipment and charging the paddles. For most models, the paddles can be safely discharged into the equipment. Clean the equipment and restock supplies after each use.

Defibrillation with AED

1. Turn the power on.
2. Attach the device and "hands off" defibrillation pads to the patient.
3. Initiate analysis of the rhythm if the machine is not "fully" automatic.
4. Deliver the shock if needed (if not fully automatic).
5. If the device is already in place and can be used to continue defibrillation in the ED, skip steps one through four because they have already been done and continue defibrillation without delay by using the "manual" feature of the AED.

NURSING ALERT

Some models of AEDs lack a rhythm interpretation monitor. These monitors should be removed immediately and a standard defibrillator should be used upon arrival at the ED.[1]

References

1. American Heart Association: *Textbook of advanced cardiac life support,* Dallas, 1997, The Association.
2. American Heart Association Emergency Cardiac Care Committee and Subcommittee: Pediatric advanced life support (part 6), *JAMA* 268(16):2262-2275, 1992.
3. Suddaby EC, Rider SL: Defibrillation and cardioversion in children, *Pediatr Nurs* 17(5):477-481, 1991.
4. Walker CB: Precordial shock. In Boggs RL, Wooldridge-King MW, editors: *AACN procedure manual for critical care,* Philadelphia, 1993, WB Saunders.

Diagnostic Peritoneal Lavage

Patty Sturt
Barbara Blake

DESCRIPTION

Diagnostic peritoneal lavage (DPL) is a procedure used to detect intraabdominal bleeding or viscus perforation after abdominal trauma. The accuracy of peritoneal lavage is approximately 95% to 98%. It is less useful with children than with adults. An abdominal computed tomography scan is commonly used for children to assess internal abdominal injuries.[1] DPL is neither organ nor injury specific. It is also unable to detect retroperitoneal bleeding. DPL is usually performed using either the closed or the semiopen approach. In the closed technique the catheter is inserted percutaneously. The semiopen approach involves a small incision and dissection to the rectus fascia. The catheter is then inserted through the peritoneum into the peritoneal cavity.

INDICATIONS

1. Blunt trauma
   - Unreliable examination because of an altered level of consciousness, central nervous system or spinal cord injury, or alcohol or drug intoxication
   - Unexplained history of hypotension in the field or ED[2]
   - Major thoracic or multisystem injuries
   - Patients with multiple trauma requiring general anesthetic for nonabdominal surgical procedures
2. Penetrating trauma
   - Gunshot or stab wound with questionable peritoneal penetration (Depending on the size and shape of the instrument used, stab wounds at or below the nipple line may involve the abdominal or peritoneal cavity.)

CONTRAINDICATIONS

1. The patient has had previous intraabdominal surgery (relative contraindication). Multiple previous abdominal surgeries increase the risk of adhesions. Adhesions may cause the intestines to adhere to the abdominal wall. Intestinal perforation may occur when the catheter is introduced.
2. Morbid obesity (relative contraindications).
3. The patient is pregnant, and the fetus is more than 12 weeks of gestation (relative contraindication).[3]
4. The patient has penetrating abdominal trauma from a gunshot wound. Gunshot wounds to the abdomen require surgical exploration; therefore, a DLP is unnecessary.
5. The patient is hemodynamically unstable, and immediate abdominal surgery is indicated based on the physical examination (see Chapter 20).
6. There is radiographic evidence of free air in the abdomen.
7. Advanced cirrhosis (relative contraindications).
8. Preexisting coagulopathy (relative contraindications).

EQUIPMENT

*   Gastric tube
*   Urinary catheter
*   Antiseptic solution (povidone-iodine solution commonly used)
*   Sterile gloves
*   Mask
*   Gown
*   Razor
*   5-, 10-, and 20-ml syringes
*   Needles of various sizes
*   Sterile drapes (Four sterile towels are usually used.)
*   Gauze sponge
*   Local anesthetic (Lidocaine 1% with or without epinephrine is frequently used.)
*   Peritoneal lavage catheter and introducing stylet (commercially available in preassembled kits)
*   1000 ml warmed ($36.6°$ to $37.7°$ C) normal saline (NS) or Ringer's lactate solution[4]
*   IV tubing: maxidrip solution set
*   Needle holder and straight scissors
*   Suture material (4-0 nylon on a cutting needle)

- Blood collection tubes and sterile specimen container
- Antibiotic ointment
- Small dressing for covering catheter entrance site (*NOTE:* Preassembled kits containing much of this equipment are available.)

INITIAL NURSING ACTIONS

1. If possible, diagnostic abdominal x-rays should be taken before DPL is performed. The procedure may produce artifacts such as intraperitoneal air on the x-ray films.
2. Explain the procedure to the conscious patient.
3. Insert an indwelling urinary catheter before the procedure.

NURSING ALERT

This is extremely important, since a full bladder may be punctured during the advancement of the catheter toward the pelvis.

---

4. Pass a nasogastric or orogastric tube to decompress the stomach and prevent stomach perforation during peritoneal catheter insertion.
5. Spike the IV bag with the maxidrip IV tubing set. Flush the IV tubing. Keep the end of the tubing capped and sterile.
6. Place the patient in a supine position. Provide verbal support for the conscious patient.
7. The nurse or physician should shave the abdomen at and around the insertion site if necessary.
8. The nurse or physician should prep the abdomen with antiseptic solution from the umbilicus to the symphysis pubis.
   NOTE: At this point the physician drapes the abdomen and injects the area with lidocaine. A small transverse incision through the skin and fascia may be performed to allow easy passage of the catheter and stylet (semi-open approach). For adults, the usual site for catheter insertion is midline and 2 to 3 cm below the umbilicus or one third of the distance between the umbilicus and symphysis pubis. For young children an infraumbilical

or supraumbilical approach may be used. The catheter is directed through the peritoneum toward the pelvis. Once the catheter is in place, a 10- or 20- syringe is attached to aspirate peritoneal fluid. If 5 to 10 ml of blood or any gastric or bowel contents are aspirated, the lavage is considered positive, and it is not necessary to infuse the NS or Ringer's lactate into the peritoneal space. The specimen should be sent to the laboratory for confirmation of contents.

9. If no blood or gastric contents are aspirated, attach the IV tubing to the catheter. Open the IV tubing clamp, and infuse 1 liter. For children, infuse 15 to 20 ml/kg. The physician may gently massage the abdomen to distribute the fluid.

10. When the infusion is complete, lower the IV bag and allow the fluid to return by gravity. As much of the fluid as possible should be removed from the peritoneal cavity. A reasonable return is 75% to 80% of the fluid instilled.[4] If the patient's condition permits, turning the patient may facilitate removal of the fluid.

11. Laboratory specimens of the peritoneal fluid should be obtained as ordered by the physician. Commonly ordered laboratory tests include a red blood cell (RBC) count, white blood cell (WBC) count, and measurements of hematocrit (Hct) and levels of bilirubin, amylase, alkaline phosphatase, and serum glutamic-oxaloacetic transaminase. The fluid should be placed in a sterile specimen container or the same laboratory tubes that would be used if the tests were being performed on blood. The following findings (based on 1000 ml infused) are associated with a positive lavage:
    - RBC count >100,000/mm^3
    - WBC count >500/mm^3
    - Hct >2% within the first hour after trauma
    - Amylase level >200 Somogyi units
    - Presence of bile, bacteria, or fecal material (indicates viscus injury)[5]

    NOTE: The ability to read newspaper print through the fluid in the IV bag is not a reliable indicator of a negative lavage.

12. Once the catheter is removed and the wound is sutured (if applicable), place a thin layer of antibiotic ointment and a sterile dressing over the site.

PATIENT CARE MANAGEMENT

1. Monitor for bleeding or signs of infection at the site.
2. Continue to assess the abdomen for pain, distention, rigidity, and tenderness.
3. Prepare the patient for surgery as indicated.

References

1. Clemence B: Procedures involving the gastrointestinal and genitourinary systems. In Bernardo LM, Bove M, editors: *Pediatric emergency nursing procedures,* Boston, 1993, Jones & Bartlett.
2. Marx JA: Abdominal trauma. In Barkin RM, Rosen P, editors: *Emergency pediatrics,* St Louis, 1990, Mosby.
3. Proehl JA: Peritoneal lavage. In Proehl JA, editor: *Adult emergency nursing procedures,* Boston, 1993, Jones & Bartlett.
4. Knighton D, Locksley RM, Mills J: Emergency procedures. In Saunders CF, Ho MT, editors: *Current emergency diagnosis and treatment,* Norwalk, Conn, 1992, Appleton & Lange.
5. Emergency Nurses Association: *Trauma nurse core course,* Chicago, 1995, The Association.

Procedure 12

Diarrhea

Mary Phillips

DESCRIPTION

Diarrhea is a frequently encountered complaint in the emergency department (ED) among adults and children. It is defined as an increase in frequency, fluid content, and volume of stool. There are many causes of diarrhea, including viral infections such as rotaviruses, bacterial infections such as *Shigella* and *Salmonella,* and parasitic invasion such as *Giardia lamblia.* Other noninfectious causes include immune deficiencies, hepatic and pancreatic disorders, and the use of antibiotics. If persistent, diarrhea can lead to dehydration, shock, and subsequent electrolyte imbalances, as well as to a breakdown in skin integrity. When caring for the patient with diarrhea, the nurse will be concerned with identifying the cause, treating dehydration and electrolyte imbalances if they exist, and relieving discomfort.

INITIAL NURSING ACTIONS

1. Triage assessment and history
   - General appearance and level of consciousness
   - Symptoms and their duration
   - Diet and oral intake
   - Number and appearance of stools
   - Estimated urine output
   - Recent exposure to illness
   - Presence of fever
   - Age of patient
   - Preexisting medical conditions
   - Present medications
   - Vital signs including temperature, pulse, blood pressure, and respirations
   - Weight (for pediatric patients)
2. Determine the degree of dehydration. Table P12-1 is a helpful guide to use with children.
   - Similar guidelines (excluding fontanels) can be used for adults.

TABLE P12-1 Degrees of Dehydration, Including Signs and Symptoms

Signs and symptoms	Percentage of loss of body weight		
	Mild (5%)	Moderate (10%)	Severe (15%)
Mucous membranes and lips	Dry	Very dry, cracked	Parched
Skin turgor	Normal	Slightly decreased	Tenting
Anterior fontanel	Normal	Sunken	Sunken
Eyeballs	Normal	Sunken	Sunken
Tearing	Normal	Decreased	Absent
Heart rate	Normal or slightly increased	Increased	Increased
Respirations	Normal or slightly increased	Increased	Increased
Blood pressure	Normal	Normal	Decreased
Skin perfusion	Normal, pale	Mottled, cool	Slow capillary refill time, cold, cyanotic

From: Barkin RM, Rosen P: *Emergency Pediatrics: A Guide to Ambulatory Care*, 5/e, St Louis, 1999, Mosby.

- Orthostatic vital signs in adults (these are not an accurate indicator of fluid volume status in children).
- Obtain laboratory data such as electrolytes, blood urea nitrogen, creatinine, glucose, and urinalysis.
3. Determine the cause of the diarrhea.
- It may be necessary to collect a stool sample for culture, white blood cell count, ova, and parasite testing.
- Other diagnostic procedures such as x-ray examinations, including an abdominal series, may be indicated.
- Laboratory data such as CBC with differential, blood cultures, liver function studies, amylase, and ABG levels may be useful.

ORAL REHYDRATION FOR MILD DEHYDRATION

Infants (≤1 year old)

Give clear liquids such as Pedialyte, half-strength "flattened" or "defizzed" clear soda (no caffeine), or half-strength Jell-O water offered in frequent small amounts (½ oz every 10-20 min).

Children (>1 year old)

Give clear liquids such as half-strength "flattened or de-fizzed" clear, decaffeinated soda, half-strength Jell-O water, or popsicles offered in frequent small amounts (½-1 oz every 10-20 min).

Adults

Give clear liquids such as ice chips, "flattened" or "defizzed" decaffeinated clear soda, Jell-O, or Gatorade in frequent small amounts.

IV FLUID REHYDRATION FOR MODERATE TO SEVERE DEHYDRATION

Infants and children

1. Establish a patent airway and deliver supplemental oxygen as necessary.
2. Establish two large-bore IV lines using a 22-gauge or larger IV catheter, if possible.
3. Administer a 20 ml/kg bolus of warmed normal saline or Ringer's lactate solution. Repeat crystalloid bolus as needed.
4. Initiate strict fluid intake and output monitoring.
5. Frequently monitor vital signs, pulses, skin color and tem-perature, capillary refill, and level of consciousness.

Adult

1. Establish a patent airway, and deliver supplemental oxygen as needed.
2. Establish two large-bore IV lines using 18-gauge or larger IV catheters.

IV FLUID REHYDRATION FOR MODERATE
TO SEVERE DEHYDRATION—cont'd

3. The amount of fluid replacement depends on the amount of fluid loss. For geriatric patients or patients with heart disease, rehydration should be done cautiously. In some cases it may be necessary to place a central venous line to monitor central venous pressure (Procedure 6). Normal saline or Ringer's lactate solutions are most often used for IV rehydration.
4. Initiate strict fluid intake and output monitoring.
5. Frequently monitor vital signs, pulses, skin color and temperature, and level of consciousness.

OTHER NURSING ACTIONS

1. Use antidiarrheal agents if appropriate (these are not routinely used with children because of side effects such as lethargy, nausea and vomiting, and possible respiratory depression).
2. The method of fluid replacement depends on the severity of dehydration and the patient's ability to retain fluids.

PATIENT CARE MANAGEMENT
Infants and Children

1. Instruct the parents to give clear liquids in small, frequent amounts initially and advance to normal volumes as tolerated. If the mother is breast feeding, clear liquids may be used in addition to breast milk. Examples of clear liquids include Pedialyte or Lytren (for children less than 2 years of age), decarbonated ("flattened" or "defizzed") and decaffeinated sodas, powdered drinks, gelatin, water, sports drinks, and popsicles for older children.
2. Avoid juices such as apple juice that may worsen diarrhea.
3. Instruct the parents that the child's diet may be advanced when the child can tolerate clear liquids without further diarrhea. If the infant's diet is solely formula, advance to half-strength formula and then full-strength formula as tolerated. Older children can be given bland foods such as applesauce, bananas, rice, and toast in

small quantities first and can advance to larger quantities as the child's appetite returns.

4. The child may return to a normal diet if bland foods are tolerated and the appetite returns.
5. Instruct the parents on proper dosage and administration of medications if prescribed.
6. Instruct the parents to change diapers frequently, keeping the diaper area clean and dry to prevent a skin rash and breakdown.
7. Instruct the parents on the symptoms of dehydration:
   • Decreased number of wet diapers
   • Decreased or absent tears with crying
   • Lethargy or difficult to arouse
   NOTE: Advise the parents to seek health care immediately if these symptoms occur.
8. Instruct the parents to see a physician or return to ED if the diarrhea worsens in frequency or amount or if the stool contains blood.
9. Advise follow-up with a pediatrician or pediatric nurse practitioner.

Adults

1. Instruct the patient to continue taking clear liquids for 12 to 24 hours.
2. Instruct the patient to advance to a bland diet on the second day if stool output decreases.
3. The patient should advance to a regular diet if he or she is able to tolerate bland food and stool output remains decreased.
4. Instruct the patient on proper dosage and administration of medications if prescribed.
5. Advise follow-up with private physician or clinic.

Ear Irrigation

Mark Parshall

INDICATIONS

Ear irrigation is commonly ordered for the removal of cerumen impaction or a foreign body from the external auditory canal. On occasion, both ear canals may be impacted.

CONTRAINDICATIONS

Contraindications include a ruptured tympanic membrane (TM), myringotomy tubes, and Ménière's disease. Irrigation should not be performed if the patient has vertigo. If vertigo or nystagmus develops during the procedure, the procedure should be discontinued and the physician should be notified.

EQUIPMENT

- Metal piston syringe or dental irrigation device (e.g., Water-Pik)
- 30- or 60-ml Luer-Lok syringe
- 16- or 18-gauge Teflon Angiocath sheath or a hub and clipped tubing from a butterfly (A metal needle should never be used.)
- Warm water or saline (body temperature)
- Two basins: one for irrigant and one for runoff
- Otoscope
- Ceruminolytic drops (docusate sodium,[1] Debrox, or Cerumenex)
- Towels and a gown to drape patient's clothing
- Examination gloves

INITIAL NURSING ACTIONS

1. Explain the procedure to the patient. Ask the patient to report any discomfort, vertigo, or nausea.
2. Examine both ears with an otoscope, even if only one is impacted, because this will establish a baseline for subsequent inspection.

3. If a ceruminolytic agent is being used, it should be instilled at least 10 minutes before irrigating.
4. The irrigation tip should not be advanced beyond the cartilaginous portion of the ear canal. In an adult the pinna may be pulled upward and backward (in a small child, downward and backward) to straighten the ear canal.
5. The direction of the irrigation should be toward the anterosuperior aspect of the ear canal, not at the TM (e.g., at the 1 o'clock position in the left ear and the 11 o'clock position in the right ear).[2] Irrigation can be continued until the impaction is relieved or the patient reports discomfort.
6. If a Water-Pik is used, great care must be taken to ensure that the pressure is not excessive and remains constant. For this reason a manual technique is preferred.

PATIENT CARE MANAGEMENT

1. At times a large plug will be irrigated free. If a ceruminolytic agent was used before irrigation, the impaction may tend to break up in small pieces as irrigation progresses.
2. The ear canal should be examined otoscopically at frequent intervals during the irrigation. The ear should be examined again at the conclusion of the procedure.
3. If irrigation is successful, patients generally report a marked improvement in hearing and relief from the feeling of fullness in the ear.
4. There is often some degree of redness of the ear canal after irrigation. There may even be a small amount of superficial bleeding that should stop spontaneously. At times the physician may decide to treat the inflammatory reaction as an external otitis. Frequently it resolves spontaneously within a day or two without treatment.
5. Assuming the TM is intact, some sources recommend instillation of a few drops of isopropyl alcohol or other drying agent (e.g., VoSol Otic Solution or Domeboro Otic) following irrigation.[2]
6. Recommendation of ceruminolytic agents to prevent recurrence is at the discretion of the physician. Docusate

sodium liquid, 1% solution (Colace liquid, 1%), and Debrox are available over the counter; Cerumenex is available by prescription only.

References

1. Chen DA, Caparosa RJ: A nonprescription ceruminolytic, *Am J Otol* 12:475, 1991.
2. Zivic RC, King S: Cerumen impaction management for clients of all ages, *Nurs Pract* 18(3):33, 1993.

Emergency Thoracotomy

Theresa M. Glessner

DESCRIPTION

Open thoracotomy is an emergency procedure during which the chest is opened surgically to correct exsanguinating hemorrhage or cardiac arrest from an unknown cause after blunt or penetrating trauma.

INDICATIONS

Cardiopulmonary arrest in the patient who has had signs of life (pulse, blood pressure, cardiac electrical activity, respiratory effort, or motor function of any type) just before or after arrival in the ED—the patient may have suffered blunt or penetrating trauma to the chest or abdomen.

CONTRAINDICATIONS

This procedure is *not* indicated for patients who have not had signs of life since the time of the traumatic injury or whose injury occurred >15 minutes before.

EQUIPMENT

1. Povidone-iodine solution
2. 4 × 4 sponges
3. Sterile gowns, gloves, masks, hats, and shoe covers
4. Open chest tray to include some or all of the following:
   - Finochietto-Buford rib spreader with two large blades and two small (pediatric) blades
   - Tuffier rib spreader
   - Two 9½-inch DeBakey aneurysm clamps
   - One medium Satinsky clamp
   - Six Vanderbilt clamps
   - Two 8-inch Sarot needle-holders
   - Curved Mayo scissors
   - Two Metz scissors
   - Eight large towel clamps

- One straight Liston bone cutter
- One Lebsche sternal chisel
- One mallet
- Two 9-inch DeBakey forceps
- Two 5½-inch tissue forceps
- Four sterile towel packs (six each)
- Sterile Teflon sheet (6 × 6 felt)
- Four packs of lap sponges
- Two 2-0 silk sutures
- Dacron tape
- Four 4-0 prolene sutures
- 10 2-0 Ticron suture
- No. 21 scalpel
- 3-0 prolene suture
- ¼-inch pledget
- ⅜-inch pledget
- Six 3-0 prolene sutures with strung ¼-inch pledget
- Small Satinsky clamp
- Two 9½-inch sponge forceps
- Two 8-inch Allis clamps
- Two 8-inch Gemini clamps (right angle forceps)
- Two 6-inch Gemini clamps
- Two 8-inch standard needle-holders
- Two 7-inch Sarot needle-holders
- Two Duval lung clamps
- 8-inch curved Metz scissor
- 6¾-inch straight Mayo scissors
- Six curved Kelly clamps
- Large Allison lung retractor
- Small Allison lung retractor
- Medium Richardson retractor
- Small Richardson retractor
- Two 9½-inch DeBakey forceps
- Two 7¾-inch DeBakey forceps
- Two vessel clude neuromedics
- No. 10 scalpel
- No. 11 scalpel
- Sterile Foley catheter
- Sterile internal defibrillator paddles

INITIAL NURSING ACTIONS

1. The patient must be on cardiac monitoring throughout this procedure.

2. The patient's airway must be secured by endotracheal intubation before initiation of this procedure because there is less access to the head, making bag-valve mask ventilation difficult.

3. Assist the surgeon in donning his or her sterile gown, gloves, mask, and cap. Assist in preparing the patient for the procedure; prep the patient with 4 × 4s and a povidone-iodine solution and sterilely drape the patient's thorax for the procedure.

4. Ensure that the thoracotomy tray is opened, using sterile technique, and is awaiting the surgeon when he or she is ready to perform the procedure. Using sterile technique, prepare yourself or an assistant to perform the duties of a scrub nurse—to hand the surgeon the instruments as needed. Another nurse will have to monitor the patient's vital signs and continually assess the patient during the procedure.

5. Cardiopulmonary resuscitation will have to be stopped during the time that the incision is made but will be continued internally after the chest is opened.

   Physician Actions

   • After the patient is prepped and draped, the physician makes a skin incision with the scalpel. The incision is a left thoracotomy incision made at the 4th or 5th intercostal space and can be extended to the right. Occasionally the incision is a mediastinal approach, but spreading the ribs is much easier than sawing the sternum. Next, either the sternal chisel and mallet are used to make a mediastinal opening or the fascia is cut away and the rib spreaders are used to gain access to the heart.

   • Occasionally a rib will have to be cut away, using the bone cutter, for better visualization.

   • The physician will be looking for the source of bleeding and will need lap sponges and 4 × 4s to dry the area. When the source of bleeding is found, the physician will need a variety of clamps and sutures to close the bleeder.

6. Be prepared to perform internal defibrillation; be sure that the defibrillator is in working order. Have the surgeon hand the defibrillator end of the cable to someone, so it can be properly attached to the defibrillator and be ready when the chest is open.

Physician Actions
- The internal defibrillator paddles are placed one on either ventricle, and the maximum amount of joules that can be delivered internally is 20.

7. Be ready to perform internal cardiac massage and internal defibrillation as ordered by the physician.
8. If the surgeon is successful in resuscitating the patient, be ready to proceed to the operating room for further evaluation of the patient's injuries.
9. The surgeon may place a Foley catheter in the heart for tamponade of bleeding if there is a visible hole in the heart or aorta, or it may be placed for fluid resuscitation if the heart is flat (without any circulating volume). Warm IV fluids must be given through this catheter.

Physician Actions
- If the patient is successfully resuscitated, the physician will sterilely drape the patient and proceed to the operating room; the physician will not close the chest in the emergency department.

PATIENT CARE MANAGEMENT

1. Continuously assess and monitor the trend of the patient's vital signs, noting any return of pulse, blood pressure, or cardiac electrical activity.
2. Monitor the continuing fluid resuscitation that will be ongoing during this procedure.
3. Note the amount of joules used with each internal defibrillation attempt (up to 20 joules).
4. Note any change in the patient's condition during this procedure. This may give the surgeon data to diagnose a specific problem that can be corrected.
5. The patient may need to be transported to the operating room while internal cardiac massage is ongoing. If this occurs, try to maintain sterility as much as possible. Cover the patient with a sterile sheet if possible.
6. If the patient has an indwelling Foley catheter in the heart to tamponade bleeding or for fluid resuscitation, be sure that the balloon is inflated and that it is not dislodged during the procedure or during transport.

POTENTIAL COMPLICATIONS

The most common complication of this procedure is death. Other complications include further injury to the thorax, exsanguination, and further myocardial and pleural injury.

Endotracheal Tube Insertion

George P. Glessner III

Endotracheal intubation can be accomplished orally with
the use of a laryngoscope for patients of all ages or nasally
(without the use of a laryngoscope) for adult and adolescent patients. Endotracheal intubation is used for definitive airway control in the ill and injured. The patient needing intubation may be conscious or unconscious, be
apneic, or have impaired breathing capabilities. Endotracheal intubation may require the use of induction or neuromuscular blockade (NMB) agents. Different patient situations may require modifications of the basic principles of
endotracheal intubation presented in this section.

DESCRIPTION

Endotracheal intubation requires the use of an endotracheal tube (ET).[1] The ET is a hollow, flexible, clear tube
with an opening at both ends (Figure P15-1).[2]

The distal end has an additional opening on the side, referred to as the Murphy's eye, which allows air passage if
the larger opening distal to it becomes clogged. The proximal end has a standard 15-mm adapter that connects to
ventilatory devices. ETs vary in size from 2 to 9 mm. The
size correlates to the interior diameter of the tube. All ETs
have centimeter markings on the sides at the proximal end.
These markings allow quick visual identification of the distance of the tube in the trachea.

Adult and pediatric ETs have some important differences. Adult ETs have a cuff on the outside of the distal
end that is connected by a small hollow tube to a pilot
balloon, and they have an inflation port with a one-way
valve on the proximal end. This port allows air to be injected into the low-pressure, high-volume cuff via the use
of a syringe. The pilot balloon inflates when air is in the
cuff, allowing the health care provider to determine if
the cuff is inflated. The cuff is designed to fill the void
space in the adult trachea past the vocal cords and thus
help to protect the patient from aspiration, but the cuff

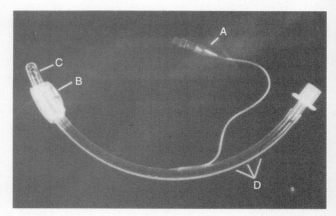

Figure P15-1   Endotracheal tube. **A,** Pilot balloon. **B,** Cuff. **C,** Murphy's eye. **D,** Centimeter markings of tube length from tip. (From Dailey R, Simon B, Young G: *The airway: emergency management,* St Louis, 1992, Mosby.)

does not prevent aspiration. The pediatric ET does not have a cuff.

The trachea of the pediatric patient is less rigid than the adult's and narrows past the vocal cords. This allows a "seal" to be created when a properly sized ET is passed through the vocal cords and into the narrow portion of the pediatric trachea. A pediatric uncuffed ET has black rings around the distal aspect of the tube where a cuff would have been. These rings are used to give visual reference for depth of insertion of the pediatric ET. Adult and pediatric endotracheal intubation is usually accomplished orally using direct visualization of the glottic opening and vocal cords with a laryngoscope.

The laryngoscope is a two-piece instrument consisting of a handle and blade. The blade is either straight or curved and varies in length, from size zero for neonates and infants to size four for large adults. Laryngoscopes are battery operated and have a source of light in the distal end of the blade that facilitates visualization of the glottic opening. A laryngoscope is not used for nasotracheal intubation.

Nasotracheal intubation is performed on spontaneously breathing adolescent or adult patients who require definitive airway control with a less invasive method or no head

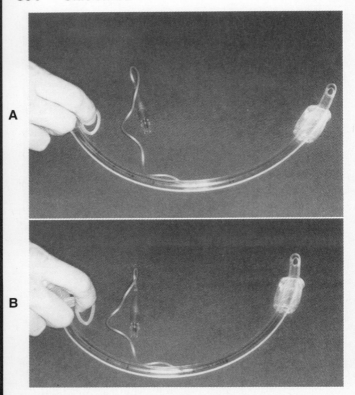

Figure P15-2 Endotrol tube. A, Relaxed position. B, Trigger pulled. Note increased angulation to direct tip of tube anteriorly. (From Dailey R, Simon B, Young G: *The airway: emergency management,* St Louis, 1992, Mosby.)

movement because of a possible spinal injury. Nasotracheal intubation is a "blind" intubation. The ET is passed through the nasal passage, past the pharynx and vocal cords, and into the trachea without direct visualization. The use of a flex-tip ET such as the Endotrol[2] (Figure P15-2) may help with the procedure. The tip of an Endotrol can be flexed with the use of a pull ring at the proximal end attached to a monofilament line that runs the length of the ET through the wall and is anchored to the end.

If a flex-tip ET is not being used to perform nasotracheal intubation, flexing the ET into a circle, inserting the distal tip into the proximal end, and placing it on ice while the patient is being prepared for intubation may help. The increased flex in the ET assists the intubator in passing the tip of the ET through the cords similar to flexing the tip of the Endotrol. The cooling of the tube helps maintain this flexed shape longer.

INDICATIONS

Orotracheal Intubation
1. Establishment, maintenance, or protection of the airway
2. Enhancement of the physiologic aspects of breathing, oxygenation, and ventilation
3. Intubation requiring a larger tube than one that can be advanced through the nasal passage

Nasotracheal Intubation
1. Dyspneic patients whose condition (e.g., chronic obstructive pulmonary disease, asthma, and pulmonary edema) could worsen or who cannot tolerate the supine position
2. Oral cavity not sufficiently accessible to permit orotracheal intubation
   - Wired jaws
   - Anatomic problems (e.g., small mouth or temporomandibular joint ankylosis)
   - Trismus (e.g., tetanus and intraoral infections)
   - Actively seizing
   - Obstructing lesions of the anterior oropharynx (e.g., tumors, Ludwig's angina, lingual swelling or hematoma, and dental abscesses)
3. Inability to attain proper sniffing position.
   - Suspected or proven unstable cervical spine injury
   - Decerebrate rigidity
   - Tetanus
   - Severe degeneration joint disease or rheumatoid arthritis of the cervical spine
4. Comatose, breathing patients (e.g., sedative overdose, cerebrovascular accidents, or head injury)
5. Situations in which NMB agents are contraindicated (e.g., hyperkalemia secondary to burns or renal failure)[2]

CONTRAINDICATIONS

Orotracheal Intubation

There are no absolute contraindications for orotracheal intubation in patients who need definitive airway control.

Nasotracheal Intubation

1. Apnea
2. Nasal or posterior pharynx obstruction
3. Children under 8 years of age (relative to size)
4. Thrombolytic therapy within 12 hours

RELATIVE CONTRAINDICATIONS

Orotracheal Intubation

There are some relative contraindications when orotracheal intubation may be difficult or could worsen or complicate an existing condition.

1. Anticipated surgical access through the mouth
2. Major maxillofacial fractures or trauma
3. Significant bleeding in the supraglottic area
4. Potential unstable cervical spine injuries
5. Epiglottitis
6. Miscellaneous (rheumatoid arthritis, ankylosing spondylitis)[3]

Nasotracheal Intubation

1. Facial fractures
2. Basilar skull fractures
3. Cribriform plate fractures
4. Clenched teeth that access to the oral cavity for suctioning
5. Anticoagulation or thrombolytic therapy
6. Neck trauma with the potential for dislodging a blood clot
7. Suspected foreign body obstruction, including epiglottitis

Battle sign, raccoon's eyes, fluid from the nose or ears, and crepitus when palpating the facial bones may be indicative of the above fractures.

EQUIPMENT

Suction equipment setup and functioning

1. Proper devices to suction the oral pharynx (e.g., a rigid tonsillar-tip suction device)

TABLE P15-1 Properly Sized Endotracheal Tubes

Age	Average weight (lb/kg)	ET size	Blade size
Premature	3/1.5	2.5, 3.0	0
Term	7.5/3.5	3.5	0
6 mo	15/7	3.5	1
1 yr	22/10	4.0	1
3 yr	33/15	4.5	1 or 2
6 yr	44/20	5.5	2
8 yr	55/30	6.0	2
11 yr	77/35	6.5	2 or 3
14 yr	99/45	7.0	3
Adult females	120 lb and up	7.0-8.0	3
Adult males	160 lb and up	8.0-9.0	3 or 4

- Suction catheters properly sized for the ET being used
2. Oxygen source
   - Bag-valve device and a properly fitting mask
   - Two properly sized ETs (Table P15-1)
   - 10-ml syringe
   - Laryngoscope handle with two differently sized blades, curved and straight
   - Properly sized stylet
   - Anesthetic, lubricating water, and soluble topical agents
3. Protective eye wear, mask, and gloves
4. Stethoscope
5. Monitors
   - Pulse oximeter (recommended but optional)
   - End-tidal CO_2 monitor or detector (recommended but optional)
   - Cardiac monitor (recommended but optional)
6. NMB agents (optional)
7. Sedation and induction agents (optional)
8. Surgical cricothyrotomy kit-may be needed if the patient cannot be successfully intubated

INITIAL NURSING ACTIONS
General Endotracheal Intubation
1. Discuss the procedure thoroughly with the conscious patient.
2. Preoxygenate the patient with 100% O_2 via bag-valve mask device for 2 to 5 minutes.

3. Start an IV access line (if not already done).

4. Assure proper noninvasive monitors are in place (e.g., electrocardiogram, blood pressure, pulse oximeter, and end-tidal CO).

5. Gather all the needed equipment and personnel.

6. Check the laryngoscope and blades to ensure that the batteries and light source are functional.

7. Prepare the ETs while keeping the distal two thirds sterile.

   A. Check the patency of the ET cuff and balloon.

   B. Insert a malleable stylet (oral intubation) into the ET, making sure that it does not extend past the distal end of the tube. Bend the ET and stylet to create a gentle curve in the tube with a sharp upward turn of the distal end at an approximate 30-degree angle (oral intubation).

   C. Lubricate the distal aspect of the ET with Xylocaine jelly or another water-soluble lubricant.

8. Ensure that universal precautions are being maintained (protective eye wear, mask, and gloves).

9. Place the patient in the proper position.

   A. Sniffing position with head resting on a folded towel (Figure P15-3).[2]

   B. If there is a possibility of a cervical spine injury, the patient is kept in neutral alignment with manual immobilization.

10. After intubation, insert a gastric tube and attach it to suction to evacuate and deflate the stomach.

11. If endotracheal intubation cannot be accomplished within 15 to 20 seconds, stop the procedure. Reoxygenate and hyperventilate the patient for 2 to 5 minutes and then reattempt intubation.

Orotracheal Intubation

1. Visualize the glottic opening and vocal cords.

   A. With the left hand, insert the blade of the laryngoscope into the right side of the mouth and sweep the tongue to the left.

   B. Lift the lower jaw and displace it up and forward at a 30- to 45-degree angle with the laryngoscope.

   • Keep the blade away from and off the teeth.

   • Do not pull back on the handle; instead, push it forward and up with a lifting motion.

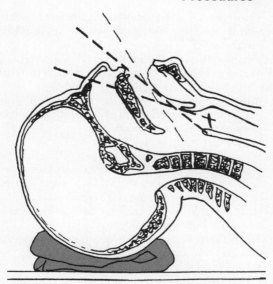

Figure P15-3 Intubating or "sniffing" position. Note approximation of three critical axes. (From Dailey R, Simon B, Young G: *The airway: emergency management,* St Louis, 1992, Mosby.)

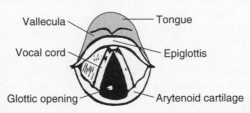

Figure P15-4 Anatomic structures seen during direct laryngoscopy.

   C. Visualize the glottic opening and the vocal cords (Figure P15-4).[3]
2. With the right hand, insert the ET into the mouth and through the glottic opening and vocal cords.
   A. Advance the ET until the cuff completely disappears through the vocal cords or one or more of the black rings on the distal end of the pediatric uncuffed ET passes through the vocal cords.

   B. Grasp the ET at the mouth with the left hand after
       setting down the laryngoscope and carefully pull
       out the stylet.
3. Inflate the cuff with a 10-ml syringe. Use only enough
   air to stop exhaled air from leaking around the cuff.
4. Check the placement of the ET.
   A. Auscultate breath sounds over the anterior and lat-
       eral aspect of the chest. Breath sounds should be
       present and equal bilaterally.
   B. Look for fogging of the ET.
   C. Watch for equal, bilateral rise and fall of the chest.
   D. Auscultate the epigastrium. Breath sounds may be
       faintly heard, but they should be less audible than
       those heard over the anterior chest. Stomach bub-
       bling should not be heard (coarse basilar rales may
       mimic air bubbling in the stomach).
   E. Assess the patient for signs of improved oxygena-
       tion and ventilation:
       • Improved skin color or capillary refill
       • Improved pulse oximetry readings (this may take
         several minutes)
       • Positive detection of end-tidal CO_2 by a colormet-
         ric CO_2 detector or a measurable reading of CO_2
         on a continuous end-tidal CO_2 monitor
   F. Note adequate compliance of the lungs while venti-
       lating the patient.
5. Note the centimeter marking at the lips or teeth and
   document.
6. Secure the ET with a commercial ET-holding device
   or adhesive tape, making sure the ET cannot be
   moved by activity such as suctioning, ventilating and
   patient movement.
   A. Secure the ET in place with adhesive tape.
       • Have someone manually secure the ET by hand.
       • Clean and dry the surface of the face.
       • Apply Mastisol or other adhesive to the skin sur-
         face of both cheeks beside the mouth.
       • With 1-inch adhesive tape, secure the ET by wrap-
         ping the middle portion of a 6-inch strip of tape
         around the ET at the level of the teeth, and se-
         cure the other portions of tape to the previously
         prepared skin surface.
   B. Follow the manufacturer's directions for commer-
       cially prepared ET holders.

Nasotracheal Intubation

1. Prepare the nare and nasal passage with 2% Xylocaine jelly or a water-soluble lubricant. A nasal pharyngeal airway may be placed and then removed to spread the topical agents evenly.
2. Gently introduce the distal end of the ET into the nare and advance it through the nasal passage into the posterior oropharynx.
   - A slight gentle twisting motion may help.
   - If passage on one side cannot be accomplished, try the opposite side.
3. Advance the ET until it reaches the glottis.
   - This usually causes the patient with an intact gag reflex to cough.
4. Advance the ET through the glottic opening. Listen with your ear at the distal end of the ET tube for breath sounds through the proximal end of the ET.
   - Gently but quickly advance the ET 5 to 6 cm through the glottic opening when the patient inhales.
5. Confirm tube placement in the same way as for oral intubation.
6. Secure the ET with a commercial holding device or adhesive tape.
   - Secure the ET in place, making sure that the tube cannot be moved by activity such as suctioning and ventilating.
   - Follow the manufacturer's directions for commercially prepared ET holders.

Rapid Sequence Induction

Rapid sequence intubation is an orotracheal intubation procedure facilitated by administration of IV induction agents and short-acting muscle relaxants. The goal is to accomplish orotracheal intubation rapidly after airway reflexes are lost.[4] The intubation procedure is the same as with orotracheal intubation

1. Administer a defasciculation dose of a nondepolarizing neuromuscular blocker to decrease intragastric pressure.
2. Administer 1 mg/kg lidocaine IV if increased intracranial pressure is suspected.
3. One person performs cricoesophageal compression throughout the remainder of the procedure until successful intubation of the trachea is confirmed.

812   Unit Three

4. If the patient is conscious, administer adequate sedation.
5. Administer a short-acting induction agent and muscle relaxant.
6. After the full effects of the agents are achieved, perform orotracheal intubation.

PATIENT CARE MANAGEMENT

1. Suction the oropharynx and ET as needed. Neither the ET cuff nor the narrowing of the pediatric trachea seals well enough to completely protect the patient from aspiration. Suctioning of the oropharynx is still required.
2. Assess and reassess the patient's ventilation, oxygenation, and perfusion status.
3. Assess for impairment of oxygenation, sometimes associated with the intubated patient.
   - Pneumothorax or tension pneumothorax
   - Dislodgment of the ET
   - Inadvertent advancement of the ET into the right mainstem bronchus
   - Clogged ET
   - Air leaks around the ET associated with a ruptured or leaking ET cuff
4. Be prepared to intervene if intubation efforts are unsuccessful.
   - Continue to assist ventilation and hyperventilate the patient with 100% oxygen.
   - Prepare and set up for surgical cricothyrotomy if intubation is unsuccessful.

References

1. Jablonski S: *Dictionary of medical acronyms and abbreviations,* Philadelphia, 1987, Hanley & Belfus.
2. Dailey R et al: *The airway: emergency management,* St Louis, 1992, Mosby.
3. American Heart Association: *Textbook of advanced cardiac life support,* Dallas, 1997, The Association.
4. Skinner M, Waldron R, Anderson M: *Normal laryngoscopy and intubation: airway management,* Philadelphia, 1996, Lippincott.

Eye Irrigation

Mark Parshall

INDICATIONS

- Decontamination of chemical injuries
- Cleansing of debris (e.g., dust) from the eyes

CONTRAINDICATIONS

- Open or impaled globe

EQUIPMENT

- Eye shower (if available)
- Ophthalmic topical anesthetic drops
- pH test strips (if acid or alkali exposure)
- 1 to 2 liters of normal saline or Ringer's lactate per eye
- Standard drip IV tubing (e.g., 10 to 15 gtt/ml)
- Hairwash tray or sink, or Chux to divert runoff
- Irrigating lens (Morgan lens) (optional)
- Lid retractors (optional)
- Towels and gloves

INITIAL NURSING ACTIONS

1. Explain the procedure to the patient.
2. Instill a topical anesthetic as prescribed by the physician.

Eye Shower

If an eye shower is available, instruct the patient to place his or her face in the middle of the two streams so that water is flushing over the eyes and lids. Instruct the patient to blink his or her eyes in the streams and look in all directions with the eyes open. Continue for at least 15 minutes.

Manual Irrigation

1. Position the patient to catch runoff and drape clothing with Chux or towels to keep from getting wet. Topically anesthetize the eyes.
2. Gently retract the lids with your nondominant hand. If the lids are swollen, an assistant may be necessary.

A Desmarres lid retractor or a retractor fashioned from a paper clip may be used if permitted by institutional policy and if the nurse is comfortable in the use of the item.[1]

3. Begin the flow of irrigant through the IV tubing, holding the distal end of the tubing in the dominant hand. The irrigant should be free flowing, not dripping. The rate can be adjusted to patient comfort.
4. Direct the flow in all directions on the anterior globe. The lower conjunctival fornix can be exposed by gentle traction on the lower lid. The palpebral conjunctiva of the upper lid can be exposed by a retractor, by gentle traction, or by eversion over an applicator swab.
5. In general, a liter of irrigant to each eye that needs irrigation is sufficient, except in the case of corrosives (strong acids or alkali), for which the amount of irrigant needed depends on the conjunctival pH (see Chapter 11).

Irrigation Via an Irrigating Contact Lens (Morgan Lens)

1. Explain the equipment to the patient and instill a topical anesthetic. Position and drape the patient.
2. Attach IV tubing to the extension on the irrigating lens.
3. Run a small amount of irrigant over the ocular surface of the lens to lubricate.
4. Ask the patient to look down. When the patient looks down, grasp the extension tubing of the lens and slip the lens under the upper lid (it should go into the upper fornix without resistance).
5. Ask the patient to look up. With your free hand, gently retract the lower lid until the lower lid is outside the margin of the lens. Release the lid so that it covers the lower part of the lens.
6. Open the flow clamp and adjust the rate to patient comfort. Irrigate at the rate of 1 to 2 liters per eye.
7. To remove the lens, ask the patient to look up. Retract the lower lid gently. The lens will pop off the ocular surface. Ask the patient to look down. When the patient looks down, slide the lens out from under the upper lid.

PATIENT CARE MANAGEMENT

1. An eye shower achieves much higher volumes at relatively lower pressure than other methods. If the ED does

not have an eye shower, often the hospital laboratory does. Use of the shower may be followed by use of an irrigating lens or by manual irrigation.

2. Apart from the eye shower, other methods of irrigation are safest if the patient is supine.

3. There are Y-connectors for the Morgan lens so that the nurse can irrigate both eyes simultaneously from one bag of irrigant and one infusion set. When the Y-connector is used, the volume of irrigant should be doubled (e.g., a minimum of 2 liters should be used if 1 liter per eye is desired). Independent setups can also be used for each eye if needed.

4. Most patients tolerate the Morgan lens well, but a few do not. The nurse should remain with the patient or close at hand in case the patient becomes restless or frightened.

5. The Morgan lens comes with clear instructions in each lens packet. It is a good idea to post the package insert wherever eye irrigation is regularly performed in the ED.

References

1. Smallwood M: Eye irrigation. In Proehl JA, editor: *Adult emergency nursing procedures,* Boston, 1993, Jones & Bartlett.

Fever Care

Mary Phillips

DESCRIPTION

Fever is one of the most common chief complaints of
patients coming to the emergency department (ED).
Fever is not a disease, but rather a nonspecific symptom
of an underlying infectious or inflammatory process.[1]
Other factors that contribute to a rise in body temperature include excessive clothing, physical exertion, and
increased environmental temperature. Fever results
when there is a rise in the core body temperature following a resetting of the body's thermostat, which is reg-
ulated by the hypothalamus. In general, for the appropriately dressed patient at rest, a rectal (core)
temperature of >100.4° F (38° C) in children and
≥99.6° F (37° C) in adults is considered a fever.
Remembering that fever is a symptom, nursing care will
focus on identification of its cause and relief of associated discomfort.

INITIAL NURSING ACTIONS

Triage Assessment and History

- General appearance and level of consciousness
- Symptoms and their duration
- Vital signs, including temperature, pulse, respirations,
  and blood pressure
- Diet and oral intake history
- Presence of rash
- Estimated urine output
- Recent exposure to illness
- Immunization status in children
- Preexisting medical conditions
- Current medications and allergies
- Time and amount of last antipyretic
- Activity level
- Weight of patient

NURSING ALERT

Fever in an immunocompromised patient, such as one receiving chemotherapy or who has acquired immunodeficiency syndrome (AIDS), should be considered an emergency and the patient should be quickly escorted to a private treatment area.

Determining the Cause of the Fever

- Anticipate a septic workup, including laboratory data such as a complete blood count with differential, electrolyte levels, glucose levels, and blood cultures. A septic workup is indicated for febrile infants <3 months old and febrile immunocompromised patients.
- Anticipate a urine culture and urinalysis.
- Anticipate a lumbar puncture to obtain cerebrospinal fluid for culture and analysis.
- Anticipate cultures from any potential focal site (e.g., wounds and central lines).
- Anticipate sputum cultures.
- Anticipate the need for chest radiography.
- Explain all diagnostic procedures to the patient.

OTHER NURSING ACTIONS

1. Administer antibiotics as ordered (dosage is based on weight in children).
2. Administer antipyretics for fever and pain reduction.

ACETAMINOPHEN AND IBUPROFEN DOSAGE

Children

Acetaminophen	15 mg/kg
Pediatric ibuprofen	10 mg/kg

Adult

Acetaminophen	650-1000 mg
Ibuprofen	400-800 mg

3. Encourage increased oral intake (clear liquids may be better tolerated).
4. Administer IV fluids if the patient's condition warrants it (e.g., severe dehydration or an inability to manage oral fluids).
5. Implement other fever reduction efforts as follows:
   • Remove excess clothing.
   • Begin sponge bathing with tepid water if the fever exceeds 104° F (40° C).
   • Prevent shivering, because shivering may increase body temperature.

PATIENT CARE MANAGEMENT

Children

1. Instruct the parent or other caregiver on the proper dosage and administration of antipyretic. A dosage chart is helpful (Table P17-1).
2. Discourage the use of aspirin because of its association with Reye's syndrome.
3. Instruct the parent or other caregiver on proper dosage and administration of antibiotics if they are prescribed. Emphasize the importance of completing antibiotic therapy.
4. Inform the parent that sponge baths with lukewarm water for 10 to 15 minutes can be used as an aid in fever reduction for fevers ≥104° F (40° C). Use a tepid-water sponge on the head, axilla, and groin.

TABLE P17-1 Proper Dosage and Administration of Acetaminophen

Age	Weight (lb)	Mg	Drops (ml)	Elixir (tsp)	Chewable tablets	Adult tablets
0-3 mo	6-11	40	0.4	¼		
4-11 mo	12-17	80	0.8	½		
12-23 mo	18-23	120	1.2	¾	1½	
2-3 yr	24-35	160	1.6	1	2	
4-5 yr	36-47	240		1½	3	
6-8 yr	48-59	320		2	4	1
9-10 yr	60-71	400		3	6	1
11 yr	72-95	480				1½

Patients 12 years and older may take two regular adult tablets (640 mg total).

5. Emphasize the prevention of shivering, since shivering increases body temperature.
6. Discourage the use of alcohol baths because of the potential for alcohol toxicity.
7. Instruct the parent or other caregiver on proper technique for taking a rectal temperature (if applicable).
8. Encourage an increased intake of oral fluids to prevent dehydration (clear liquids such as "flattened" or "defizzed" decaffeinated clear soda may be better tolerated).
9. Give follow-up instructions, including the correct procedure for obtaining culture results.
10. Give the parent or other caregiver guidelines regarding signs and symptoms that would indicate a child should be reevaluated, such as persistent fever that does not respond to antipyretics or antibiotics, a decreased level of consciousness, the development of petechiae or purpuric rash, seizure activity, and dehydration.
11. Encourage rest and the use of cool, comfortable attire.
12. Instruct the parent or other caregiver to follow up with a private physician or clinic.

Adults

1. Instruct the patient on proper dosage and administration of antipyretics and antibiotics.
2. Emphasize the need to complete antibiotic therapy.
3. Encourage increased oral intake to prevent dehydration.
4. Encourage rest and the use of cool, comfortable attire.
5. Instruct the patient to follow up with a private physician or clinic as appropriate.

References

1. Emergency Nurses' Association: *Emergency nurse pediatric course,* Park Ridge, Ill, 1998, The Association.

Fluid Administration

Donna Isfort
George P. Glessner III

DESCRIPTION

Fluid administration by IV access for volume resuscitation, maintenance fluid administration, or potential drug administration

INDICATIONS

In some cases the need for fluid administration is clear (e.g., diabetic ketoacidosis, external hemorrhage, or decreased responsiveness with dry mucous membranes or sunken fontanels). In cases where the need for fluid resuscitation is not as apparent, the combination of patient history and clinical presentation will provide adequate clues regarding the need for IV fluids. The following questions will provide additional data:

- *Vomiting and diarrhea:* If the patient has vomiting or diarrhea, how often and over what time period? With infants the number of wet diapers in a 24-hour period may be helpful information.
- *Bleeding:* Has the patient noticed any bleeding? If so, from what site and for how long? Hematuria, hematemesis, and melena may be sufficient to decrease circulating blood volume.
- *Pain:* Assess the nature of the pain using the "PQRST" method (see Chapter 4). Shoulder pain without a known shoulder injury may indicate diaphragmatic irritation from peritoneal bleeding (Kehr's sign). Abdominal pain and tenderness with anorexia may also indicate peritoneal bleeding.
- *Poor oral intake:* Patients with a history of confusion or dementia may not be able to maintain daily fluid needs. With infants, assess the amount of formula and fluids the child has taken in a 24-hour period.
- *Medical history:* Existing health problems may influence fluid and electrolytes. For example, insulin-dependent

diabetic patients are more susceptible to diabetic ketoacidosis and dehydration. Patients with congestive
heart failure may be susceptible to dehydration from
treatment of the condition, since diuretics are frequently administered.

- Does the patient have signs or symptoms of an existing
  illness that may require IV medication administration on
  an emergency basis (e.g., acute chest pain, possible dehydration in a diabetic patient, or respiratory difficulty)?
- *Environmental:* Is there a history of prolonged exposure
  to either heat or cold, or excessive sweating?
- *Diet:* Has the patient ingested fluids that may precipitate
  diuresis (e.g., alcohol or caffeine)?
- Vital Signs
  1. *Respirations:* Hyperventilation may be an early sign of
     acidosis resulting from anaerobic metabolism related
     to a decreased oxygen-carrying capacity of cells.
  2. *Heart rate:* Tachycardia may result from fever, or it may
     be a compensatory effort to maintain cardiac output
     in cases of decreased blood volume.
  3. *Blood pressure:* Hypotension is a late sign of decreased
     vascular volume. If possible, blood pressure measure-
     ment should be taken in both arms in cases of sus-
     pected hypovolemia. These measurements will not be
     equal in a patient with a leaking or dissecting aortic
     aneurysm.
- *Fever:* Fever increases metabolic needs and may induce
  dehydration.
- *Orthostatic changes:* Orthostatic vital signs may indicate hypovolemia when a change occurs in heart rate (>20
  beats/min) or systolic blood pressure (>20 mm Hg) between position changes.

NURSING ALERT

"Normal" vital signs may indicate effective but temporary
compensation to hypovolemia. Blood pressure changes occur late in hypovolemia, yet tachycardia is often an early sign
of hypovolemia in adults.

- *Injury:* Does the patient have wounds or burns that
  would allow the leakage of fluid or hematomas that
  would allow fluid accumulation?

- *Skin:* What is the color, temperature, and turgor of the patient's skin? Cool, clammy skin indicates vasoconstriction and the need to shunt blood to core organs (e.g., kidney and brain). Pale skin progressing to cyanosis indicates the decreased availability of hemoglobin. Lip margins may be faint and difficult to distinguish. Petechiae and purpura suggest thrombocytopenia and bleeding. Poor skin turgor suggests dehydration. Assess capillary refill. If refill is >2 sec (unless the patient is a geriatric individual noted to have peripheral vascular disease or hypothermia), hypovolemia may be present.

NURSING ALERT

The normal changes in skin elasticity of the geriatric population make assessment of skin turgor as a sign of hypovolemia unreliable. However, assessment of mucous membranes may be used when skin turgor is unreliable.

EQUIPMENT

- Protective gear for the caregiver
- Appropriately sized IV catheters (consider the size of the patient and the reason for fluid administration)
- IV fluids chosen according to need
- IV tubing and extension set chosen according to need
- Antiseptic solution
- Dressings for IV site
- IV additives: drugs and electrolytes
- Blood tubes if serum specimens are needed

INITIAL NURSING ACTIONS

Fluid Resuscitation

1. Initiate two large-bore IV lines (14- to 16-gauge, 1¼ inch-long catheter for adults, 22-gauge catheter or greater for pediatric patients) with Ringer's lactate or normal saline. For maximizing fluid administration, use the largest diameter tubing available. Trauma tubing is preferable. If trauma tubing is not available, use blood infusion tubing. If regular IV tubing is used, use a maxi-drip set. Obtain a specimen for a complete blood count, coagulation studies, electrolyte levels, and possible type and crossmatch simultaneously. Secure IV lines.

NURSING ALERT

Attempts to gain IV access must not interfere with efforts to correct problems with airway or breathing.

2. Consider placement of an intraosseous needle in a child if you are unable to access a vein (Procedure 22). The usual site for intraosseous infusion is the proximal tibia. The distal femur can be used in infants. Colloids, crystalloids, and medications can be administered through the intraosseous line. An intraosseous infusion site should be considered a temporary measure during emergencies and resuscitation. Once the patient is stabilized, venous access should be obtained and the intraosseous infusion line removed. This will help decrease the possibility of osteomyelitis.
3. Anticipate the need for administering blood products. Set up IV blood administration tubing and prime with normal saline (Reference Guide 3). Obtain a blood warmer or rapid infusion device. The shortest IV tubing should be used without an extension for fluid to remain warm upon entry at a slower infusion rate.
4. In conditions where cell membrane integrity is altered (e.g., sepsis or burns), massive fluid shifts occur, depleting circulating blood volume. Fluid administration is necessary, although administered fluid will also shift from the vascular space to the interstitial area to some degree. The use of natural and synthetic colloids (e.g., albumin and hetastarch, respectively) may help fluid to be mobilized from the interstitial area into the vascular space (Reference Guide 8). Pulmonary complications may occur from movement of fluid back into the vascular space if congestive heart failure is present.

Maintenance Fluid and IV Drug Administration

Insert a 20-gauge or larger IV catheter in the adult and a 24-gauge or larger IV catheter in infants and children (Table P18-1) with appropriate IV fluid as ordered. See Reference Guide 9 for fluid administration formulas.

TABLE P18-1 Maintenance IV Fluids

Solution type	Examples	Uses
Isotonic	0.9% NS	Expands intravascular volume
		Used for dehydration (e.g., diabetic ketoacidosis, hyperosmolar nonketotic coma) and for packed red blood cell administration
	Ringer's lactate	Expands intravascular solution (Ringer's lactate) volume
		Used for maintenance when patient is at risk for free water loss
Hypotonic	NS 0.45% NS 0.2%	Shifts water into intracellular spaces
	Dextrose 5% and water (D_5W)	Useful in preventing dehydration and assessing renal status
		D_5W may be used for adult patients for mixing IV medications
		Used for maintenance fluid when patient is at risk for free water loss
Hypertonic	Dextrose 5% in NS	Shifts fluid from intracellular to extracellular space
	Dextrose 10% in NS	Use in water intoxication states created by too much hypotonic fluid administration
	Dextrose 10% in water	Used for maintenance fluid to promote diuresis
	Dextrose 5% in 0.45 NS	
	Dextrose 20% in water	

NS, Normal Saline.

PATIENT CARE MANAGEMENT

Goals in patient care management are as follows:
1. IV lines remain patent for fluid administration.
2. The level of consciousness improves or remains at a Glasgow Coma Scale score of 15 or at baseline.
3. Urine output is adequate for weight.

4. Hemorrhage decreases or the patient is transported quickly to the operating suite.

5. Acidosis improves, as demonstrated by arterial blood gas levels.

Reassessment must occur frequently because of subtle and rapid changes that may occur.

1. *Respiratory:* Rapid, deep breathing may indicate oxygen deprivation from inadequate hemoglobin. This same pattern may be associated with acidosis in diabetic patients, suggesting dehydration (see Chapter 8).

2. *Breath sounds:* It is crucial that available hemoglobin receives oxygen for transport to tissues. Unilateral, diminished, or absent breath sounds indicate an underlying pulmonary problem that may need immediate treatment to enhance perfusion (e.g., placement of a chest tube or readjustment of an endotracheal tube). Basilar crackles may indicate underlying pulmonary or heart disease, predisposing the patient to fluid overload with minimal volume replacement. Crackles may be present if the patient received too much volume replacement in the prehospital setting or at a transferring facility.

3. *Oxygen saturation:* Decreased oxygen saturation may indicate a decrease in circulating hemoglobin and not primary respiratory decompensation.

4. *Neck veins:* Flat neck veins are associated with hypovolemia. Distended neck veins indicate hyperperfusion, increased pulmonary hypertension, or decreased cardiac contractility.

5. *Peripheral pulses:* Peripheral pulses may be difficult to palpate in hypovolemia or existing arterial insufficiency.

6. *Heart tones:* In cases of hypovolemia, the apical pulse may be rapid and distant. A bounding, shifted apical pulse suggests heart failure and a decreased ability to circulate blood volume effectively. The presence of a murmur suggests hyperperfusion whether because of a metabolic state (e.g., pregnancy or adolescence) or because of fluid administration.

7. *Abdomen:* Although the abdomen is not traditionally viewed as an organ assessed for perfusion data, in cases of suspected hypovolemia the abdomen should be examined as a potential bleeding source. A rigid abdomen that is tender to palpation, with absent bowel sounds and with or without ecchymotic areas, suggests peritoneal bleeding.

8. *Level of consciousness:* Restlessness and irritability are the first indications of decreasing blood volume. Lethargy and decreased responsiveness occur later. Central nervous system changes are related to decreased cerebral oxygenation. A Glasgow Coma Scale score (see Reference Guide 10 for Adult and Reference Guide 18 for Child and Infant) should be documented and monitored throughout the emergency department (ED) stay.

9. *Urine output:* Expected urine output in a normovolemic state for patients up to 30 kg is 40 ml/kg/24 hr (2 ml/kg/hr) and for patients over 30 kg it is 1200 ml/kg/24 hr (17 to 18 ml/kg/hr). Specific gravity should be checked to assess the concentration of urine to preserve circulating fluid volume. A specific gravity >1.015 may be indicative of decreased fluid volume or an increase in solutes causing osmotic diuresis. Decreased urine output indicates either compensation induced by antidiuretic hormone in cases of hypovolemia or acute or chronic renal failure. Acute renal failure can be induced by hypovolemia. Acute renal failure may also occur in cases of transfusion reaction. Hematuria may occur in transfusion reactions. It may also indicate the need for colloid replacement.

10. *Stools:* Monitor the number, amount, consistency, and color of stools. Constipation may suggest dehydration. Diarrhea may indicate the need for fluid administration. Melena (tarry stools) may indicate the need for colloid administration.

11. Monitor for signs of fluid overload.

SIGNS OF FLUID OVERLOAD

- Dyspnea, crackles on auscultation
- Tachycardia, distended neck veins
- Diaphoresis, edema
- Increased central venous pressure and pulmonary wedge pressure, if measurement is available

12. Monitor hemodynamic readings, if they are available.
13. Monitor for signs and symptoms of a blood transfusion reaction (Reference Guide 4).

DISCHARGE IMPLICATIONS

Most patients requiring fluid resuscitation will not be discharged from the ED. In cases where patients have received IV fluids for minor hypovolemia and have responded favorably to treatment, the following areas should be addressed:

1. Patients may have a delayed (7 to 10 days) reaction to blood transfusion. Delayed reactions are mild and do not require treatment. In delayed reactions, bilirubin levels rise, producing jaundice and possible frothy, dark urine.
2. Symptoms of fluid overload may not appear immediately after IV fluid administration. The development of edema, dyspnea, and tachycardia may indicate the decreased ability of the heart to manage the circulating blood volume. Patients should be instructed to see their primary care provider or return to the ED if symptoms develop.
3. If vomiting, fever, or diarrhea returns, patients should increase their fluid intake, take prescribed antidiarrheal, antiemetic drugs, and return to the ED or their primary care provider if no improvement occurs.
4. Adult respiratory distress syndrome, disseminated intravascular coagulation, or multiple organ dysfunction may develop on a delayed basis after fluid administration, particularly in high-risk populations (e.g., geriatric patients with heart disease). Patients should be instructed to return to the ED if the following symptoms develop: respiratory distress, dyspnea, cough, decreased urination, hematuria, bleeding from mucous membranes, or fever.

Gastric Tube Insertion and Lavage

Kim Sparks

DESCRIPTION

Gastric intubation is a procedure performed commonly in the emergency department. Gastric intubation involves the insertion of a tube, through either the nose or the mouth, into the stomach for gastric evacuation or lavage.

INDICATIONS

1. Empty gastric contents and suppress vomiting caused by an ileus or mechanical obstruction.
2. Remove toxic substances.
3. Prevent gastric dilation and aspiration in patients with major trauma.
4. Instill radiopaque contrast media.
5. Perform therapeutic or diagnostic gastric lavage. Lavage facilitates removal of blood and clots with patients who have upper gastrointestinal bleeding.

CONTRAINDICATIONS

1. Insertion of a gastric tube in patients who have ingested a caustic substance (e.g., acid or lye) may cause further esophageal damage.
2. A gastric tube should not be inserted nasally in patients who have massive facial trauma or a basilar skull fracture. In such cases the tube should be inserted orally.

EQUIPMENT

- *Gastric tube:* Gastric tubes are also known as Levin, Salem-sump, Ewald, and Levacuator tubes. The Salem-sump tube has a vent lumen that allows for controlled suction force at the drainage openings. The sump tube is also less likely to be lodged against the stomach wall.

NURSING ALERT

The size and type of tube used depends on the reason for placement. For adult patients who have active upper gastrointestinal bleeding, a large-bore tube (32 to 36 Fr) should be inserted through the mouth.

- Water-soluble lubricant
- 60-ml piston or catheter-tip syringe
- Emesis basin
- Tape
- Stethoscope
- Suction equipment
- Gloves
- Normal saline

INITIAL NURSING ACTIONS

1. Explain the procedure to the patient.
2. If the patient is alert, place the patient in a higher Fowler's position.

NURSING ALERT

Maintain spinal immobilization in trauma patients. Have suction readily available. Be prepared to logroll the patient if vomiting occurs.

Nasogastric Placement

- Measure the distance of insertion by placing the tip of the tube at the patient's nose and following the length of the tubing to the ear and then from the ear to the xiphoid process. Mark the tubing at this point.
- Examine the nose and select the larger nare.
- Lubricate the end of the tube with a water-soluble lubricant. Occasionally, lidocaine jelly is used to lubricate the tube and anesthetize the nasal tract.
- Insert the tube into the nostril at a 60- to 90-degree angle to the plane of the face.
- Once the tube is in the oropharynx, have the patient flex the head forward slightly and swallow several times. If possible, have the patient swallow a few sips of water through a straw. Advance the tube (while the patient swallows) to the previously marked point.

NURSING ALERT

If the tube slips into the trachea, violent coughing will ensue. Withdraw the tube into the oropharynx and try again to advance the tube into the esophagus and stomach.

Orogastric Placement

- If the patient is alert, place the patient in a high Fowler's position. If a lavage is to be performed, place the patient on the left side in a slight Trendelenburg position to promote the return of lavage fluid and to prevent aspiration.
- Measure the distance of insertion by placing the tip of the tube at the lips. Follow the length of the tubing to the angle of the jaw and then from the jaw to the xiphoid process. Mark the tubing at that point.
- If the patient is uncooperative, place a bite block in the mouth to prevent the patient from biting the tube.
- Lubricate the tip of the tube, and pass it gently over the tongue, aiming down and back toward the pharynx.
- Flex the patient's head forward, and advance the tube when the patient swallows.

NURSING ALERT

Do not flex the head if there is the possibility of a cervical spine injury.

3. Verify proper placement by aspirating gastric contents and by injecting 20 to 30 cc of air (with piston or catheter-tip syringe) into the tube while listening over the stomach with a stethoscope.
4. Secure the tube with tape or a gastric tube holder. Do not tape the tube to the forehead because this places pressure on the nares.

PATIENT CARE MANAGEMENT

1. Connect the tube to suction as prescribed by the physician.
2. Lavage may be needed for patients who have upper gastrointestinal bleeding or ingestion of toxic substance.
   - Pour normal saline solution into a container. For patients who have GI bleeding, the use of iced saline is controversial. Some clinicians prefer using room-

temperature tap water on the grounds that it breaks up clots better and it does not lower core body temperature as much.
- Instill 150 to 200 ml (the actual volume is controversial) of fluid in an adult patient by a piston or catheter-tip syringe. Gently withdraw the fluid with the syringe and discard the fluid into a measured basin. For pediatric patients 10 ml/kg of lavage solution is used.
- Continue the lavage until the fluid returns clear or an endoscopy is performed. Prepackaged gastric lavage kits that can be connected to suction are commercially available.
3. Consider providing the patient with anesthetic throat lozenges or spray to relieve throat discomfort from the tube.

Head Injury

Lisa Creech

DESCRIPTION

Patients sustaining mild head injuries will often be discharged from the emergency department (ED). Discharge teaching is imperative, and the nurse must ensure that the patient and family understand signs and symptoms that warrant immediate return to the ED. Proper education may help patients and family members assess the need for return to the hospital.

INDICATIONS

Generally, patients who have no loss of consciousness or a loss of consciousness lasting <5 minutes will be discharged from the hospital. Discharge instructions should include both monitoring for symptoms of a worsening head injury and symptoms associated with postconcussion syndrome.

INITIAL NURSING ACTIONS

The patient and family should be alerted to signs and symptoms that warrant return to the hospital. Instruct the patient and family that it will be necessary for a responsible person to remain with the patient for the first 24 hours following the injury to observe and monitor for the following:
- Obvious pupillary changes (e.g., one large, one small)
- Blurred vision
- Vomiting more than three times or forceful vomiting
- Severe headache
- Slurred speech
- Gait or balance disturbance
- Noticeable new weakness of either arm or leg
- Unusual behavior
- Confusion
- Severe lethargy or unusual drowsiness[1]

The patient should be awakened every 2 hours, or as determined by the physician, to ensure that he or she is arousable to a normal state of alertness.[2]

NURSING ALERT

Patients and families should be instructed to call or return to the ED immediately if any of the above are noted. In addition, alcohol and other sedative medication should be avoided for 24 hours. Activity levels should be kept to a minimum for 48 hours. Acetaminophen and ibuprofen are acceptable measures for pain control unless contraindicated.

PATIENT CARE MANAGEMENT

Postconcussion syndrome is a generalized term used to describe a specific group of symptoms following a head injury. These symptoms may persist for weeks to months. It has been estimated that nearly 50% of all patients sustaining mild head injuries will develop some degree of postconcussion syndrome.[3] Complaints vary among individuals, but those most commonly noted include headache, mood changes, forgetfulness, and visual changes. Because treatment is palliative, families must understand the need for follow-up care after discharge from the ED.

References

1. Oman S, Drury T: Head trauma. In Ritt S et al, editors: *Emergency nursing,* ed 2, Philadelphia, 1995, WB Saunders.
2. Bartkowski H: Head trauma. In Saunders C, Ho M, editors: *Current emergency diagnosis and treatment,* Norwalk, Conn, 1992, Appleton & Lange.
3. Evans RW: The post concussion syndrome and the sequelae of mild head injury. In *The neurology of trauma,* vol 10, Philadelphia, 1992, WB Saunders.

Intracranial Pressure Monitoring

Patty Sturt

Intracranial pressure (ICP) monitoring provides continuous data regarding the pressure exerted within the cranial vault. Direct measurement of ICP is best achieved by use of an intraventricular catheter placed into the lateral ventricle. The intraventricular catheter also allows withdrawal of cerebrospinal fluid (CSF) to control ICP. The normal ICP is 0 to 15 mm Hg. In addition, it is possible to calculate the cerebral perfusion pressure (CPP) if the ICP is known. The CPP is an indirect measurement of cerebral blood flow and is calculated by subtracting the ICP from the mean arterial pressure. Normal CPP is considered 60 to 100 mm Hg. Monitoring the ICP may provide evidence of intracranial hypertension before serious signs and symptoms appear, thus permitting earlier intervention. ICP monitoring is based on the concept of converting CSF pressure into electrical current and displaying it on a monitor.

INDICATIONS

The decision of which patients should be monitored for ICP varies among physicians.[1] Patients with certain pathophysiologic conditions may be considered candidates for ICP monitoring. These pathophysiologic conditions include the following:
1. Head injury
2. Intracerebral hematoma
3. Subarachnoid hemorrhage
4. Space-occupying lesions
5. Central nervous system infections
6. Toxic or metabolic encephalopathies
7. Cerebral edema
8. Hydrocephalus
9. Ischemic and hypoxic insults

A depressed level of consciousness with a Glasgow Coma Scale (GCS) score ≤8 in any of the above conditions is a commonly used indicator for ICP monitoring. ICP monitoring may also be indicated for patients who are clinically difficult to assess because of paralytic agents.

CONTRAINDICATIONS

1. Coagulation abnormalities
2. Generalized cerebral edema resulting in small, compressed ventricles

INTRAVENTRICULAR CATHETER SETUP, INSERTION, AND MONITORING

Description

The intraventricular catheter is most commonly placed into the anterior horn of the lateral ventricle of the nondominant hemisphere. The right hemisphere is considered the nondominant hemisphere in most humans. The catheter is inserted through a burr hole for the purposes of the following:

1. Monitoring intracranial pressure
2. Removal of CSF for culture and laboratory specimens
3. Removal of CSF to control and reduce ICP

The catheter is inserted by a neurosurgeon.

Equipment

- Razor
- Betadine scrub brush or container of sponges with povidone-iodine solution
- Lidocaine with or without epinephrine for injection
- 5- to 10-ml syringe and different sizes of needles for injection
- IV pole attached to the bed
- Pressure module and monitor
- Stopcock
- Transducer
- 12-inch pressure tubing
- One bottle of nonbacteriostatic normal saline (NS)
- 10-ml syringe with 18-gauge needle for drawing up NS
- Luer-Lok
- Betadine ointment, sterile eye patch, and 3-inch tape for dressing over insertion site
- Intraventricular catheter and external drainage collection system

The ICP insertion tray includes the following:

- Iodine cup

- Twist drill
- Needle-holder
- Sharp, blunt scissors
- Knife handle and scalpel
- 4 × 4 sponges
- 16- and 18-gauge ventricular needles
- 10-ml syringe

Initial Nursing Actions

1. Fill a 10-ml syringe with sterile nonbacteriostatic NS for injection.
2. Attach the open end of the transducer to the side port of the stopcock.
3. Attach 12-inch pressure tubing to the other side port of the stopcock.
4. Attach a 10-ml syringe of NS to the vertical port of the stopcock.
5. Turn the stopcock off to the transducer and flush the pressure tubing.
6. Turn stopcock off to the pressure tubing and flush the transducer. Turn the stopcock on to the transducer and tubing.
7. Remove the syringe and place the Luer-Lok on the open end of the stopcock. Aseptic technique should be used when assembling and flushing the system. **Never use a transducer with a flush system.**
8. Attach the transducer to the pressure cable. The pressure cable should be connected to a pressure module on the monitor.
9. Tape the transducer to a towel roll to maintain the position of the transducer at the correct level.
10. Elevate the head of the bed. The neck should be kept in a neutral position. Place a protective barrier under the head.
11. The physician will shave the hair around the insertion site and prep the area with a Betadine brush or sponges soaked with povidone-iodine solution. The physician should wear a mask and sterile gloves. Depending on the patient's condition and the urgency of the situation, lidocaine may be injected to anesthetize the insertion site. Using a twist drill, a burr hole is made anterior to the coronal suture. A catheter over

a guidewire is inserted, aimed at the inner canthus of the eye. The guidewire is withdrawn. Using aseptic technique, the end of the external drainage collection system is connected to the catheter via a port or valve. Attach the pressure tubing from the transducer to the other end of the port. The distal end of the catheter is sutured to the scalp.

12. Record the opening pressure.
13. Maintain the transducer at the level of the foramen of Monro (Figure P21-1).
14. Place Betadine ointment (as directed by the physician) over the insertion site. Cover the site with a sterile eye patch or gauze and tape the patch or gauze in place.
15. Using the cord provided, suspend the external drainage collection system from the IV pole attached to the bed. The drip chamber is usually placed 10 to 20 cm above the level of the foramen of Monro.
16. CSF should be drained intermittently or continuously, as prescribed. With intermittent drainage, the system is turned on to drainage when the ICP reaches a certain level. The physician usually orders drainage of CSF when the ICP is 20 mm Hg or greater.

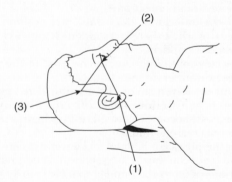

Figure P21-1   Location of foramen of Monro for transducer placement. Map an imaginary equilateral triangle from (1) the external auditory meatus, to (2) the outer canthus of the eye, to (3) behind the hairline. Point 3 is the location of the foramen of Monro. (From Stillwell S: *Mosby's critical care nursing reference,* St Louis, 1996, Mosby.)

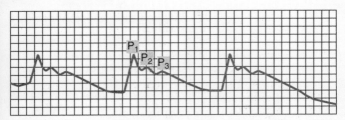

Figure P21-2   ICP waveform. (From Stillwell S: *Mosby's critical care nursing reference,* St Louis, 1996, Mosby.)

17. The system should be turned off to drainage when an ICP reading is obtained for documentation.[2] Pressure vented toward the collection system and away from the transducer may cause an artificially low ICP.

Patient Care Management

1. Avoid kinks in the drainage system.
2. Evaluate and document the clarity, color, and amount of CSF drainage.
3. Notify the physician if there is no CSF drainage in the presence of intracranial hypertension.
4. Ensure the integrity of the system to prevent the entrance of air and infection.
5. "Zero" the transducer every shift, after position changes, or when there is a sudden change in the ICP reading or waveform.
6. Prophylactic antibiotics may be ordered by the physician to prevent brain infection.
7. Monitor the waveform on the monitor. The waveform consists of at least three peaks (Figure P21-2). As ICP increases, P_2 becomes elevated. If P_2 is higher than P_1, suspect decreased compliance.
8. Notify the physician if abnormal waveforms are noted. A-waves (plateau waves) are seen with sudden transient elevations of 50 to 100 mm Hg that last 5 to 20 minutes. B-waves (sawtooth waves) are seen with increases in ICP of up to 50 mm Hg and occur every 30 seconds to 2 minutes. B-waves indicate an unstable ICP.[3]
9. See Table P21-1 for possible problems that can occur with ICP monitoring and for the appropriate nursing actions.

TABLE P21-1 Checklist for ICP Monitoring

Problem	Action
No waveform	Check power to monitor and to trace
	Check gain setting
	Check all connections
	Check for air bubbles in system
High pressure reading	Check transducer level placement
	Check calibration and rezero
	Evaluate patient:
	Check airway
	Check ventilator settings
	Check arterial blood gases for hypoxemia, hypercarbia
	Check head of bed (15-30 degrees)
	Check position of head (do not rotate head)
	Check extremities (limit flexion in lower extremities and hips)
	Check excessive muscle activity (administer muscle relaxants, paralyzing agents as ordered)
	Check abdominal distention
	Check noxious stimuli and remove
	Check temperature
	Check PAP, CO, SvO_2, and BP
	Check electrolytes
Low pressure reading	Check transducer level placement (Figure P20-1)
	Check for otorrhea and rhinorrhea
	Check for dislodged catheter and notify physician if cathether is dislodged
	Check if 15-20 mm Hg positive pressure exists (with use of external ventriculostomy)

BP, Blood pressure; *CO*, cardiac output; *PAP*, pulmonary artery pressure; *SvO_2*, pulmonary artery oximetry.

CAMINO ICP SYSTEM SETUP, INSERTION, AND MONITORING

Description

The Camino catheter contains a miniature transducer located at the distal end of a fiberoptic catheter to sense ICP. A fluid-filled external transducer system is not used, since the transducer is placed directly into the brain parenchyma.

Equipment

- Sterile gloves
- Camino OLM intracranial kit, which contains the following items: a sterile transducer-tipped pressure monitoring catheter, Camino bolt, compression cap, drill bit, stylet, Allen wrench, zero adjustment tool, and strain relief sheath (Figure P21-3)
- Camino disposable twist drill procedure kit, which contains the following items: the hand drill, scalp retractor, needle-holder, Metzenbaum scissors, 18-gauge spinal needle, forceps, scalpel with handle, normal saline ampules, 1% lidocaine, sponges, medicine cups, Betadine swabs, syringes, and needles of various sizes
- Camino V420 direct pressure monitor with power cord and pole mount[4]
- Pole stand

Initial Nursing Actions

1. After the physician chooses the insertion site, the area is shaved and prepped in a sterile fashion with Betadine solution. The area is then draped with sterile towels. The physician injects the area with lidocaine and makes an incision to the bone with the scalpel. The drill bit is secured to the hand drill, and a twist drill hole is made through the skull. The hole is irrigated with normal saline, and an 18-gauge spinal needle is used to open the dura. The Camino bolt is screwed into the skull. The stylet is inserted through the dura to clear the passage for the Camino catheter. The Camino bolt is then irrigated with nonbacteriostatic sterile saline.

2. The catheter is removed from the sterile package. Firmly attach the transducer connector to the preamp connector (Figure P21-4).

3. If the Camino 420 display does not read "zero" after a short system self-check, use the tool from the catheter kit to turn the zero adjustment on the bottom side of the transducer connector until the Camino 420 display reads "zero." Once this is accomplished, it is not necessary to zero the system again (Figure P21-5).

4. The physician inserts the Camino catheter into the bolt. A waveform should appear if the V420 is connected to a bedside monitor. The compression cap on the bolt is turned to lock the catheter in place. The physician then

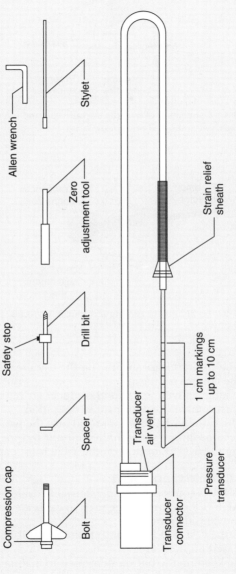

Compression cap

Bolt

Spacer

Safety stop

Drill bit

Zero
adjustment tool

Allen wrench

Stylet

Transducer
air vent

Transducer
connector

Pressure
transducer

1 cm markings
up to 10 cm

Strain relief
sheath

Figure P21-3 Camino OLM intracranial kit. (Courtesy Camino Laboratories.)

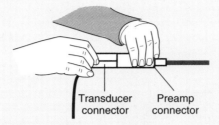

Figure P21-4   Connection of transducer connector and preamp connector. (Courtesy Camino Laboratories.)

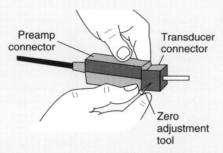

Figure P21-5   Technique for zeroing transducer. (Courtesy Camino Laboratories.)

slides the strain release sheath (on the catheter) down onto the compression cap.
5. Do not attach anything to the transducer air vent. The vent must remain open for proper operation.
6. After the catheter has been inserted into the patient, select the appropriate scale on the monitor by repeatedly pressing the SCALE button on the V420 front panel.[4]

Patient Care Management
1. If the V420 is connected to an external bedside monitor, the CAL STEP button may be used to calibrate or balance the bedside monitor.
   - Press the CAL STEP button repeatedly until "zero" is displayed on the V420.
   - While keeping the button depressed to maintain "zero," simultaneously zero the bedside monitor.

- Release the CAL STEP button. The CAL STEP does not affect the transducer calibration.
2. The V420 can be connected to a 427 recorder as follows:
   - Connect the V420 interface cable to the V420 monitor accessory receptacle.
   - Insert the V420 power cable into the V420 power cord receptacle.
   - Insert the power cord into its receptacle on the back of the 427 recorder. Then insert the plug into a grounded outlet.
   - Turn on the power by moving the circuit breaker switch to its "up" position.
   - To record waveforms, press the 25 mm/sec button. The recording will continue until the STOP button is pressed.[4]
3. Monitor the waveforms as described under Patient Care Management with intraventricular catheters.

References

1. Richmond TS: Intracranial pressure monitoring, *AACN Clin Iss* 4(1):148-160, 1993.
2. McQuillan KA: Intracranial pressure monitoring technical imperatives, *AACN Clin Iss* 2(4):624-636, 1991.
3. Barker E: Avoiding increased intracranial pressure, *Nursing* 20(5):64Q-64RR, 1990.
4. Camino Laboratories: *Camino user information guide,* San Diego, Calif.

Intraosseous Infusion

George P. Glessner III

DESCRIPTION

Intraosseous infusion is used for fluid and medication administration in infants and children 8 years of age or less when attempts at venous access have been unsuccessful. There is minimal risk of complications if the procedure is performed properly and appropriately. Colloids, crystalloids, and medications that can be administered intravenously can be administered intraosseously. The proximal tibia is the usual site for intraosseous cannulation. The distal femur of an infant can also be used. Intraosseous access is a temporary measure and should be replaced with venous access as soon as possible.[1]

INDICATIONS

- The indications for intraosseous cannulation and infusion are the same as for venous cannulation (Procedure 18).
- Intraosseous cannulation is indicated in an emergency after unsuccessful attempts have been made to establish venous access.

CONTRAINDICATIONS

- When the intraosseous site is in an extremity with a recent or possible acute fracture
- Bone disorders
- Marrow-toxic drugs

EQUIPMENT

- Appropriate IV administration set and IV fluid
- Spinal needles with stylets, bone marrow needles, or standard 16- or 18-gauge hypodermic needles (hypodermic needles sometimes bend or break)

INITIAL NURSING ACTIONS

1. Assemble the necessary equipment.
2. Prepare the site with a povidone-iodine solution. The

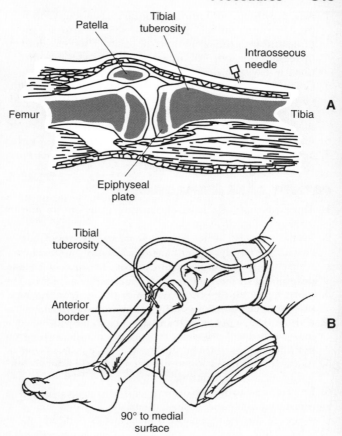

Figure P22-1   A, Insertion. B, Intraosseous infusion technique. (A from Barkin RM, Rosen P: *Emergency pediatrics: a guide to ambulatory care,* ed 5, St Louis, 1999, Mosby; B Reproduced with permission © *Pediatric Advanced Life Support,* 1997 (70-1091). Copyright American Heart Association.

   usual site is 1 to 3 cm or approximately two finger-breadths below and medial to the tibial tuberosity.
3. Stabilize the leg and insert the syringe needle into the anterior-medial aspect of the leg perpendicularly or pointed slightly inferiorly to avoid the epiphyseal plate (Figure P22-1, *A*).

4. Advance the needle until the bone is reached. With firm pressure and control, advance the needle through the bone and into the bone marrow cavity. This is evidenced by feeling the "pop" of the needle entering the bone marrow cavity.
5. Correct placement of the intraosseous cannula can be confirmed by aspirating bone marrow into the attached syringe. Follow the aspiration with irrigation of the needle to prevent an occlusion by the bone marrow.
6. Attach the appropriate IV administration set and fluid.
7. Secure both the leg and the intraosseous cannula to prevent dislodgment (Figure P22-1, *B*).

PATIENT CARE MANAGEMENT

1. To ensure patency, assess the intraosseous site frequently for signs of infiltration.
2. Prepare for and anticipate the need to gain venous access as soon as the patient's condition has stabilized or resuscitation is complete. This minimizes the chance of developing osteomyelitis.
3. Assist with gaining venous access by means of a saphenous vein cutdown or central venous cannulation.
4. If the intraosseous needle becomes clogged with bone marrow and will not clear, replace the needle with a similar needle passed through the same hole in the bone.
5. Assess for the development of infection and administer antibiotics when ordered.
6. Be prepared to secure the leg to prevent excessive movement that may cause dislodgment.
   • Secure the leg to a padded IV board or padded full leg splint.

References

1. Chameides L, Hazinski MF, editors: *Pediatric advanced life support*, Dallas, 1997, American Heart Association.

Lumbar Puncture

Barbara Blake

DESCRIPTION

A lumbar puncture (LP) involves insertion of a hollow needle with a stylet into the subarachnoid space between the L3 and L4 or L4 and L5 vertebrae to obtain cerebrospinal fluid (CSF) for diagnostic purposes.

INDICATIONS

In the ED setting, an LP may be performed to do the following:

- Obtain CSF for microscopic examination or culture and sensitivity (This may be necessary in cases where meningitis or encephalitis is suspected [Chapter 14].)
- Determine the presence of blood in the CSF (Blood in the CSF is suggestive of subarachnoid hemorrhage.)
- Measure CSF pressure.
- Instill blood, medications (such as antibiotics), or radiopaque contrast material into the subarachnoid space.

CONTRAINDICATIONS

- The patient has a local infection of the lumbar area.
- A spinal cord mass lesion is suspected.
- The patient is receiving anticoagulant therapy.
- There are signs of increased intracranial pressure from a suspected intracranial mass (e.g., brain abscess, lesion, tumor, or posterior fossa lesion). In these cases a CT scan should be performed before the LP, since fluid drainage may cause herniation (Chapter 14).

EQUIPMENT

Prepackaged sterile, disposable LP trays are commercially available. If the tray is not available, gather the following items:

- Sterile gloves
- 1% lidocaine (some physicians prefer 1% lidocaine with epinephrine)

- Antiseptic solution such as povidone-iodine solution
- Sterile towels or drapes
- Sterile gauze sponges
- Four sterile collection tubes
- 3- to 5-ml syringe
- 22- or 25-gauge needle, 1½ inches in length for lidocaine infiltration
- Pressure manometer with a three-way stopcock
- Spinal needles with stylet
  - Adults: 20- to 22-gauge, 3 to 3½ inches
  - <1 year: 22-gauge, 1½ inches
  - >1 year: 22-gauge, 2½ inches
- Small adhesive dressing for puncture site
- Stool or chair for physician to sit on during procedure

INITIAL NURSING ACTIONS

1. Explain the procedure to the patient.
2. Obtain informed consent. Written consent can be obtained in accordance with the hospital policies.
3. Position the patient. Proper positioning is necessary to perform an LP.
   - *Lying position:* Assist the patient to the lateral decubitus position with the shoulders and pelvis perpendicular to the stretcher. Instruct the patient to curl his or her back by drawing the knees up to the abdomen and flexing the neck forward. Place a small pillow under the head to keep the spine in the horizontal position. Assist the patient in maintaining this position during the procedure by placing your hands or arms behind the neck and knees (Figure P23-1).
   - *Sitting or upright position:* Assist patients to a sitting position on the side of the examination table. Have the patient curl his or her back by placing the head and arms over a padded bedside table. If the patient is an infant, place the infant in an upright position with the thighs flexing up to the abdomen and the neck flexed forward. Stabilize the infant against your upper torso and immobilize the extremities with your hands (Figure P23-2).

NURSING ALERT

Avoid hyperflexion of the neck in infants because this may lead to airway obstruction. Observe for signs of respiratory distress.

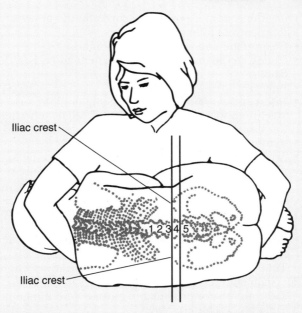

Figure P23-1   Position for lumbar puncture. The desired sites are the interspaces between L3 and L4, or L4 and L5. (From Kelley SJ: *Pediatric Emergency Nursing*, 2/e, 1994, Appleton & Lange.)

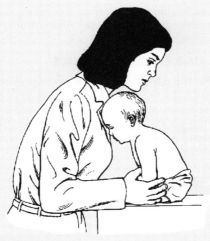

Figure P23-2   Position for lumbar puncture of an infant.

4. Once the patient is positioned correctly, the physician will proceed as follows:
   - Cleanse the skin with antiseptic solution.
   - Place a sterile drape under the patient and across the back.
   - Inject the area with 1% lidocaine.
   - Insert and slowly advance the needle until the subarachnoid space is entered (a "pop" will be felt when the space is entered).
   - Remove the stylet to observe for flow of CSF.
   - Attach a stopcock and manometer to the needle to measure opening CSF pressure. Normal pressure is between 70 and 180 mm H_2O. Have the patient slowly relax the legs and neck to prevent falsely elevated readings (the nurse may need to assist the patient to a relaxed position).
   - Remove the manometer and collect CSF in the four collection tubes.
     Tube no. 1 is usually for culture and sensitivity, Gram stain, and red blood cell count.
     Tube no. 2 is for protein and glucose determinations.
     Tube no. 3 is for cytology.
     Tube no. 4 is for cell count.
   - Reinsert the stylet and remove the needle.
5. The nurse or physician will place a small adhesive dressing over the puncture site.
6. Cleanse antiseptic solution from the back.
7. Send specimens to the laboratory for studies ordered by the physician.

PATIENT CARE MANAGEMENT

1. Document the patient's reaction to the procedure, the specimen disposition, and the appearance of the CSF. For example, was the CSF clear, cloudy, or blood tinged?
2. Instruct the patient to lie prone for at least 2 hours or per physician's instructions to decrease the chance of a spinal headache.
3. A lumbar puncture or spinal headache may occur afterward from CSF leakage. A blood patch (injection of autologous blood into the epidural space) may be required.

Medicolegal Evidence

Patty Sturt

DESCRIPTION

Forensic laboratories have been established to serve a vital need in the criminal justice system. Their purpose is to scientifically analyze physical evidence that may be used in a court case. However, analysis of the evidence is only possible when the evidence has been collected and preserved in the correct manner. Emergency department nurses play a vital role in the collection and preservation of evidence from patients.

"Physical evidence" denotes material objects and can include hair, fibers, blood, body secretions, glass, bullets, or almost anything that can be collected or deposited. Physical evidence is helpful in proving that a crime has been committed.

INDICATIONS

Indications for the collection and preservation of medicolegal evidence may include cases involving suspected suicide, homicide, physical assault, sexual assault (Procedure 27), and driving under the influence of alcohol or illegal drugs.

INITIAL NURSING ACTIONS

1. Medicolegal evidence should be collected and preserved, keeping in mind specific state laws and following the hospital's policies and guidelines.
2. ALWAYS maintain the chain of evidence. The chain of evidence is simply documentation of who has possession of the evidence at all times. Transfer of evidence from one health care professional to another should be documented. This documentation should include the person that received the evidence and the time. In most cases the evidence is handed over to a police or law enforcement officer. The law enforcement officer should sign a document that indicates that he or she received the evi-

dence and the time the evidence was received. This chain of evidence can be kept on the patient's medical record (chart) or a chain of evidence form. Evidence may be rendered invalid in court if the chain of evidence is not maintained and recorded.

3. If the evidence is placed in a lock box or refrigerator, document the name of the individual who placed the evidence in the lock box and the time the evidence was placed there.

4. The following principles should be followed with the collection and preservation of clothing:

   • Articles of clothing may provide useful information about the weapon and help distinguish entrance from exit wounds. Clothing fibers will deform in the direction of the passing projectile. Gunpowder residues and soot will deposit on clothing as they do on skin. Residue that is invisible to the naked eye may be seen with forensic laboratory staining techniques. Some bullets may leave a lead or lubricant residue that is termed "bullet wipe." Do not cut or rip through bullet holes when cutting clothing for removal. Allow the garment to air dry (if wet) before packaging. Place paper or cardboard over and under the bullet hole and fold the garment over twice. Place the garment in a paper bag. Do not use plastic bags.

   • Stains on clothing (such as semen, blood, grass, or soil) may provide crucial evidence. Blood stains may help to identify the suspected assailant. Make sure that all stains are dry. If the stain is wet, it must be air dried. Package each item of clothing separately to avoid contamination. Do not use plastic bags, since plastic retains moisture and thus permits bacterial and fungal growth. Avoid unnecessary handling of any garment with stains.

   • A law enforcement officer may request clothing for analysis of fibers. Fibers on clothing may be microscopically examined for the type, dye content, or weave content. This may be useful evidence if the fibers found match the fibers of the suspected assailant's clothing or fibers at the scene of the crime from carpet or other objects.

NURSING ALERT

Each bag of clothing collected for evidence should be labeled with the patient's name, hospital identification number, date, time, and the name of the person collecting the clothing for evidence.

5. A bullet can be examined in a forensic laboratory to determine whether it was fired from a specific firearm by comparing striated marks or microscopic marks with the aid of a microscope. Bullets should be handled with gloves and surgical instruments covered with gauze to ensure the preservation of these microscopic markings. For the collection and preservation of bullets, wrap each one in clean soft tissue paper and place it in a rigid container such as a sterile specimen cup. Place a label on the container to include the patient's name and hospital identification number, the date and time of collection, and the name of the person collecting the bullet.

6. Many guns have gaps around the firing chamber through which residue can escape and coat the hand that fired it. The first priority of the nurse is always resuscitation of the patient. When possible, paper bags may be placed over the hands to prevent the removal of gunshot residue. Many state forensic laboratories provide law enforcement officers with gunshot residue kits to use for obtaining the residue for analysis. This information may be useful for determining if the patient fired a weapon.

7. Occasionally, syringes and other drug paraphernalia may be found on a patient. Generally, if you cannot see residue in the syringe or paraphernalia, there is not enough to identify the substance. The needle should be capped or taped and placed in a rigid container. Always mark the container with "Contains Syringes" in bold lettering.

8. The following principles should be followed when collecting of blood for alcohol or drug identification and levels for medicolegal purposes:
   • Follow the hospital policy regarding the collection of blood for medicolegal purposes. Many state forensic laboratories have specific kits for the collection of blood.

- Use nonalcoholic swabs when prepping the skin for obtaining blood.
- Label each blood tube with the patient's name and hospital identification number, the date and time of collection, and the name of the person collecting the specimen.

PATIENT CARE MANAGEMENT

Never leave evidence in an area of the emergency department where it can be tampered with by patients or visitors.

Pericardiocentesis

Janet Coyle

DESCRIPTION

A pericardiocentesis is performed by placing a needle or catheter into the pericardial space and aspirating fluid and blood from the pericardial sac. Decreasing the amount of fluid that has accumulated within the pericardial sac may allow for improved filling of the heart and increased contractility.

INDICATIONS

1. Cardiac tamponade
2. Aspiration of fluid for cytology and microbiology evaluation
3. Increasing pericardial effusion

EQUIPMENT

- Cardiac monitor
- Resuscitation medications and equipment
- Povidone-iodine solution
- Local anesthetic (lidocaine 1% without epinephrine)
- Needles of various sizes
- 10-ml syringe
- Sterile 4 × 4 gauze pads
- Razors
- Sterile gowns, gloves, and drape
- Masks and hair covers
- Sterile specimen containers
- Three-way stopcock
- 60-ml syringe
- Suture material
- Hemostat
- Sterile IV tubing
- Sterile drainage collector
- Catheter adapter
- 1-inch tape
- Occlusive dressing

- Sterile alligator clamps
- ECG machine
- Pericardiocentesis needle 16- to 18-gauge, 9 to 15 cm in length (may be a spinal needle or a through-the-needle or an over-the-needle type catheter per physician's preference)

INITIAL NURSING ACTIONS

1. Position the patient with the head of the bed elevated approximately 30 degrees. The reverse Trendelenburg position may be used.
2. Explain the procedure to the patient.
3. Initiate cardiac monitoring.
4. Establish a large-bore peripheral IV for fluid, blood, or medication administration as ordered.
5. Monitor the patient throughout the procedure. Observe the patient closely for changes in cardiac rhythm, dys-rhythmias, and elevation of the PR and ST segment from baseline. These changes indicate that the catheter or needle is in contact with the epicardium. Conduction of electrical activity from the epicardium through the pericardiocentesis needle is most accurately assessed by attaching a sterile alligator clamp to the pericardiocen-tesis needle and connecting it to the V lead on an ECG. If time allows, this is recommended.
6. If a catheter is left in place for potential reaspiration when the procedure has been completed, attach the catheter to the collection device using the sterile IV tub-ing and a catheter adapter. Secure all connections with tape. Place a Luer-Lok cap over the stopcock opening. Occasionally in critical situations, the physician may use a hemostat to clamp the catheter to the chest wall.
7. Cover the insertion site with an occlusive dressing after the catheter has been secured or after it has been removed.
8. Coil extra tubing from the collection system and place it on the bed.

NURSING ALERT

If CPR is in progress, continue chest compressions until nee-dle insertion is initiated.

NURSING ALERT

Isolated pericardial effusion fluid will not clot rapidly, whereas blood inadvertently aspirated from within the cardiac chambers will clot rapidly. Remember that clotting times may vary greatly, depending on the presence of preexisting diseases that alter clotting factors, medical and surgical interventions that reduce clotting factors, hemorrhage, and the use of anticoagulants.

Traumatic cardiac tamponade may result from rapid hemorrhage into the pericardial space. The blood may clot within the pericardial sac, making aspiration impossible, or may clot rapidly after aspiration.

PATIENT CARE MANAGEMENT

1. Assess vital signs, peripheral perfusion, heart sounds, and cardiac rhythm every 15 minutes for 1 hour, then advance according to the patient's condition. If invasive monitoring has been initiated, such as a pulmonary artery catheter or central venous catheter, these pressures should also be assessed. Notify the physician if symptoms of pericardial tamponade reoccur (e.g., jugular vein distention, respiratory distress, and hypotension).
2. Monitor and record blood and fluid drainage within the collection system every 15 minutes for 1 hour, then continue to monitor and record drainage hourly.
3. If clots develop within the collection tubing, gently squeeze the tubing between your fingers and advance the clot into the collection chamber.

Pulmonary Arterial Catheter

Theresa M. Glessner

DESCRIPTION

Pulmonary artery (PA) catheters are IV catheters inserted through a large central vein (femoral, internal jugular, or subclavian) into the right side of the heart with the tip of the catheter extending into the PA. The purpose of this catheter is to directly measure pressures in the right side of the heart, indirectly measure pressures in the left side of the heart, and measure cardiac output.

INDICATIONS

1. Monitoring of fluid status
2. Right or left heart failure
3. Shock states
4. Titration of vasoactive drugs

CONTRAINDICATIONS

Any bleeding disorder or coagulation disorder is a reason to consider the risk versus the benefit of using a pulmonary arterial catheter. There are no absolute contraindications to this procedure.

EQUIPMENT

- PA catheter (Figure P26-1)
- Introducer kit
- Local anesthetic
- Gloves
- Povidone-iodine solution
- Transducer setup with pressure bag—need two transducers or a cardiac bridge to monitor CVP readings
- Monitor with pressure capability and appropriate cables
- Cardiac output monitor with appropriate cable and cardiac output setup—includes IV solution, tubing, and 10-ml syringe (if using thermodilution technique)
- 4 × 4 gauze

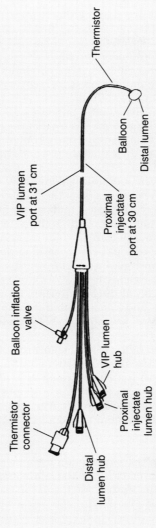

Figure P26-1 Swan-Ganz venous infusion port (VIP) thermodilution catheter. (Courtesy Baxter Health Care Corporation, Edwards Critical-Care Division, Irvine, Calif)

- Sterile normal saline for flushing ports and 10-ml syringes and needles for each port

INITIAL NURSING ACTIONS

1. Ensure that this procedure is thoroughly explained to the patient and his or her family before initiation and that informed consent has been obtained.
2. Assemble the transducer and flush system. Completely flush through the system, eliminating all air bubbles. Ensure that the pressure bag is inflated to 300 mm Hg.
3. Assemble the cardiac output measurement system and flush through this system. Ensure that the computation constant for the cardiac output computer is appropriate for the size of the catheter used and the temperature of the diluent.
4. Ensure that all the monitoring equipment is functional and "zero" the transducer(s) at the phlebostatic axis (4th or 5th intercostal space, midaxillary line), remembering to turn the stopcock off to the patient side and open to air (atmosphere).
5. Ensure that the patient's electrocardiogram (ECG) is being continuously monitored for ventricular arrhythmias (ventricular tachycardia, PVCs, and ventricular fibrillation can occur during insertion through the right ventricle), and remain with the patient throughout the procedure, providing verbal support and comfort measures.
6. Before insertion of the catheter, ensure that the catheter is flushed. Use the flush system for the PA port and the CVP port (either separately or bridged) to flush these ports respectively. Use a 10-ml syringe of saline to flush the infusion port. Also, ensure patency of the balloon by inflating it and allowing it to deflate passively.

Physician Actions

- Initially, the physician palpates the area where the catheter is placed to locate the landmarks for insertion such as the sternal notch and the clavicle.
- After donning a mask, sterile gloves, a sterile gown, and a cap, the physician preps and sterilely drapes the area where the catheter will be placed.
- The area is anesthetized with a local anesthetic such as 1% lidocaine.

- The physician next locates the blood vessel with a large needle and syringe. Once there is blood return, the syringe is removed and a wire is threaded through the needle. The needle is then removed and a large catheter called an introducer is threaded over the wire. The physician may need to make a skin incision in order to pass the introducer through the skin and into the vessel.
- The physician is now ready to float the PA catheter through the introducer (which was just inserted). The PA catheter must have the sterile sleeve placed over it before being placed into the patient.
- When the physician has the catheter advanced approximately 10 to 15 cm, the balloon should be inflated by the nurse (or whoever is helping).
- Once the catheter is floated to a wedge position, the physician will ask for the balloon to be deflated.

7. During insertion of the catheter, monitor the ECG for dysrhythmias, especially while passing the catheter through the right ventricle, because irritation of the ventricle can cause ventricular arrhythmias—ventricular tachycardia, PVCs, and ventricular fibrillation.

8. Immediately after insertion of the catheter, perform a portable chest x-ray examination to verify line placement and to rule out a pneumothorax caused by insertion of the introducer.
    - When the physician is satisfied with the catheter placement, it is sutured in place and dressed sterilely.

9. Continuously monitor the PA pressure (and the central venous pressure if the ports are monitored with separate transducers).

10. Record all hemodynamic parameters—CVP, PAP, PCWP, CO/CI, SVR, and other parameters—according to department protocol.

11. After the catheter is sutured in place, apply a sterile, deep-line dressing using strict aseptic technique. Secure the catheter to the patient with tape to prevent catheter dislodgment from the weight of the catheter or accidental pulling on the catheter.

PATIENT CARE MANAGEMENT

1. Assess and monitor the trend of the patient's vital signs and hemodynamic parameters and note improvement or deterioration.

2. Record all hemodynamic parameters every hour or per department protocol and notify the physician of any significant changes in the patient's condition.

3. Ensure that transducer(s) are zeroed to atmosphere at least every shift or per department protocol.

4. Monitor the insertion site for infection and change the dressing every 72 hours or per unit protocol.

5. Monitor PA waveform for signs of catheter migration. If the catheter floats in (distally), the waveform changes to a permanent wedge waveform. If the catheter floats out (proximally), the waveform shows a right ventricular tracing (Figure P26-2). Notify the physician if either occurs. Both are dangerous conditions.

6. Continuously monitor the patient's ECG. Ventricular arrhythmias may indicate catheter migration into the right ventricle. The physician floating the catheter back into the pulmonary artery can correct this.

7. Change pressure tubing, including bridge systems and Luer-Loks, every 72 hours or per department protocol. Use strict aseptic technique for this, including gloves and a mask. Ensure that all stopcocks have sterile Luer-Loks on each unused port.

8. If blood specimens are being withdrawn through the PA catheter system, ensure that the system is thoroughly flushed after each blood draw to prevent clot formation in the catheter.

9. Ensure that the system pressure bag is always inflated to 300 mm Hg to prevent clot formation and to ensure a crisp waveform at all times.

10. Ensure that the balloon passively deflates after each wedge reading. If it does not, attempt to manually deflate the balloon with the syringe. If the normal resistance is not felt when inflating the balloon, and the balloon does not passively deflate, the balloon is probably ruptured and should not be reinflated at any time until the catheter is replaced.

11. If using an SvO_2 or Oximetrix PA catheter (Figure P26-3), ensure the following:
    - The SvO_2 monitor and cables are available and functional.
    - The optical connector is attached to the cable and monitor and is calibrated before removing the catheter from the package.
    - The SvO_2 system is calibrated using the in vivo method every 24 hours or per department protocol.

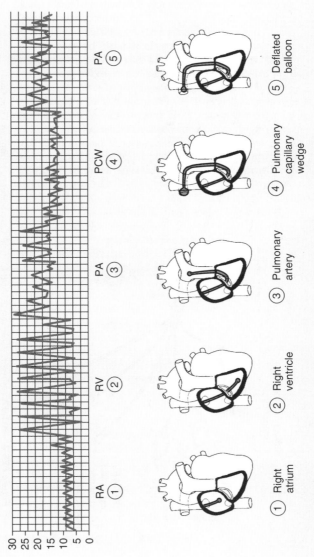

Figure P26-2 PA waveforms: RA, RV, PA, wedge. (Courtesy Abbott Critical Care Systems, Mountain View, Calif)

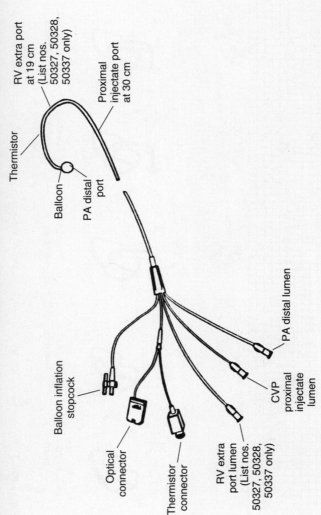

Figure P26-3 SvO$_2$ PA catheter. (Courtesy Abbott Critical Care Systems, Mountain View, Calif)

TABLE P26-1 Troubleshooting

Problem	Cause	Solution
Bleed back	Loose connections	Check connections
	Open stopcock	Check system
	Crack in transducer or connection	
Dampened waveform	Air bubbles	Check connections
	Clot	Flush system
	Loose connections	Check system
No waveform	Transducer not properly connected to monitor	Check system
False readings	Transducer not properly zeroed or not at the phlebostatic axis	Zero transducer always zero at the phlebostatic axis

POTENTIAL COMPLICATIONS

1. Pneumothorax from deep-line insertion
2. Bleeding at the site
3. A life-threatening arrhythmia
4. Puncture of a great vessel or the heart with the catheter
5. Poor catheter placement
6. Balloon breakage during insertion

For troubleshooting of problems, see Table P26-1.

Sexual Assault Evidence Collection

Patty Sturt

DESCRIPTION

Rape and sexual assault are crimes that remain prevalent in our society. Emergency department (ED) nurses need to be aware of their role in the care of these patients. The primary role of the nurse includes (1) minimizing further physical and psychologic trauma of the victim and (2) collecting and preserving medicolegal evidence for potential use in the legal system.

Sexual assault nurse examiner programs are available in many states. These programs train nurses in the forensic aspects of the care of the sexual assault patient. Obtaining a history, assessing the patient, collecting and preserving medicolegal evidence, and testifying as an expert witness are some of the responsibilities of the sexual assault nurse examiner.

INDICATIONS

Patients who come to the ED reporting they have been raped or sexually assaulted

CONTRAINDICATIONS

The chances of finding physical evidence decrease in direct proportion to the time that has elapsed between the assault and examination. Generally, if the assault took place more than 48 hours before the examination, it is unlikely that trace evidence will still be present on the patient. However, evidence may still be gathered by documenting any findings obtained during the examination such as lacerations, bruises, bite marks, and statements about the assault. In addition, counseling on prophylaxis for sexually transmitted diseases (STDs) and community support services should be provided.

EQUIPMENT

- Speculum (Have different sizes available. If vaginal trauma is present, a small speculum may be needed to prevent additional discomfort.)

- Sexual assault evidence collection kit-if this is not available, obtain the following:
  - Paper bags (for clothing)
  - Comb
  - 8 to 12 packaged cotton-tipped applicators
  - Microscopic slide with slide cover and container
  - Two blood tubes with an anticoagulant
  - Several envelopes and zip-locking bags
  - Labels with the patient's name and hospital identification number and the date, time of evidence collection, and specimen (evidence collected)
- *Chlamydia* and gonorrhea cultures
- Personal care items such as toothbrush, toothpaste, and soap for the patient's use after the sexual assault examination

INITIAL NURSING ACTIONS

1. Some sexual assault victims suffer life-threatening injuries. Always assess and treat life-threatening injuries first.
2. Place the patient in a private area away from other patients and visitors. Never allow a sexual assault victim to wait in the lobby.
3. Approach the patient in a nonjudgmental manner, conveying empathy and concern. Sexual assault victims experience psychologic trauma, although the effects of this trauma may be more difficult to recognize than the physical trauma. Each person has his or her own way of coping with sudden stress. Victims can appear calm, indifferent, submissive, jocular, angry, withdrawn, or even uncooperative and hostile toward those who are trying to help. All of these responses are within the range of anticipated reactions. These patients should be treated with special consideration to help alleviate the psychologic trauma associated with sexual assault.
4. Explain the plan of care, which includes identifying injuries, collecting medicolegal evidence, STD and pregnancy prophylaxis, and support service referrals.
5. If the patient does not have a friend or family member present, ask if there is someone he or she would like to call. Offer to call the rape crisis center that serves the area. Many rape crisis centers will send a counselor to the ED.

NURSING ALERT

Every effort should be made to have one primary nurse assigned to the patient. Sexual assault victims often experience shame, guilt, and fear. The patient is more likely to express his or her concerns and cooperate with the examination if a rapport is established with one nurse.

6. Obtain consent for treatment in the ED and for the collection of medicolegal evidence. If adult victims are reluctant to sign a consent form for the collection of evidence, they should be assured that evidence will NOT obligate them to pursue prosecution of their case.

7. Notify police per hospital policy and state laws. Sexual assault victims should be gently encouraged to report the assault and cooperate in the police investigation. However, they may refuse to do so out of fear or embarrassment or for other reasons.

8. Follow the hospital policy regarding the collection of sexual assault medicolegal evidence. In some institutions the nurse can collect the appropriate clothing, saliva swabs, and hair and blood specimens.

9. Have the patient undress and put on a hospital gown while standing on a sheet or pad. Hair, grass, fibers, or other evidence may fall from the clothing while the patient undresses. Carefully fold the pad (or sheet) and place it in a paper bag with a label or in the sexual assault evidence collection kit. Collect the panties and place them in a small paper bag. Seal the bag with tape. Attach a patient label to the outside of the bag. *Rationale:* The panties can be analyzed for seminal fluid, spermatozoa, or foreign debris.

10. Other pieces of clothing should be collected if they are damaged or torn or if there are stains such as blood or semen. Each piece of clothing collected should be air dried (if wet) and placed in a separate paper bag. Attach a patient label to each bag.

NURSING ALERT

Plastic bags should not be used, since they retain moisture that can deteriorate evidence.

11. Obtain four saliva swabs. Place all four in the patient's mouth and instruct the patient to saturate them with saliva. The patient should not have anything to eat, drink, or smoke for a minimum of 15 minutes before obtaining the saliva swabs. Allow the swabs to air dry. Place the swabs in an envelope. Tape the envelope and label. *Rationale:* The saliva swabs are used to determine if the patient secretes properties of his or her blood group (secretor status).

12. Have the patient pull at least 15 head hairs from different locations on the scalp. Place the hairs in a zip-locking bag and label the bag accordingly. *Rationale:* Hair may have been transferred from the suspect to the victim. Hair can be analyzed using a comparison microscope. It is best to use pulled hair because the roots can also be analyzed for comparison purposes.

13. Place either the pad provided in the evidence kit or a paper towel under the patient's perineal area. Thoroughly comb the pubic hair with downward strokes. Place the comb on the paper and gently fold the paper to retain the comb and any evidence. Place this in an envelope, tape the envelope, and label the envelope accordingly.

14. Pull (or have the victim pull) at least 15 pubic hairs from different locations. Place the hairs in a zip-locking bag. Seal the bag and label. *Rationale:* The pulled pubic hairs are used for comparison with hairs found at the crime scene or on the assailant's body.

15. Obtain one to two tubes of blood for medicolegal purposes. Many crime laboratories prefer blood tubes with an anticoagulant. Place a patient label on each tube. *Rationale:* The purpose of this is to determine the victim's blood groups. Blood groups include ABO type and properties or groupings of certain proteins. This may be useful in identifying the victim's blood if it is found on the suspect or at the crime scene. Determining the victim's blood group makes it possible to determine if the victim secretes properties of his or her blood groups in body secretions such as saliva. Other blood should be obtained at this time if ordered by the physician. Blood and urine screens for toxicology should be performed if the victim states that he or she was drugged by the assailant or if the victim's med-

ical condition appears to warrant toxicology screening for optimal patient care. For patients at risk for pregnancy, a urine or blood test should be performed to rule out preexisting pregnancy.

16. Many sexual assault kits contain special blood cards or blotters that are used to determine DNA status.

17. Assist the physician with the collection of evidence during the pelvic examination. Four vaginal swabs should be collected. Use one of these swabs to prepare a smear on the slide. Allow the vaginal swabs to air dry. Place them in an envelope. Tape the envelope and label it accordingly. Place the vaginal smear in a slide holder, tape it closed, and label it. These should be collected if a vaginal assault occurred. The slide should not be fixed or stained. Write "vaginal" on the frosted end of the slide. *Rationale:* The vaginal swabs and smear are analyzed for spermatozoa and blood groups. If the assailant is a secretor, properties of his blood may be found in the vaginal swabs. The alleged assailant (if known) will have blood drawn to test for his blood groups. If there is a match between the swabs and his blood groups, it can serve as medicolegal evidence in court.

18. Four anal swabs should be collected if anal assault occurred.

19. Four buccal swabs should be collected if an oral-genital assault occurred. Swab along the buccal area and gum line.

PATIENT CARE MANAGEMENT

1. The physician or nurse should document the patient's description of the assault. This should include any oral, vaginal, or rectal penetration.

2. Document and describe any bruises, lacerations, bite marks, or other signs of trauma. Body diagrams are useful in describing the location and type of injury.

3. The date of the patient's last menstrual period and the patient's contraceptive history should be recorded.

4. Administer antibiotics for STD prophylaxis as ordered by the physician.

5. Treatment for the prevention of pregnancy should be discussed with the patient. Overall, two tablets orally and repeated in 12 hours may be prescribed. This

should be given only if a urine or blood pregnancy test is negative. Inform the patient that nausea and vomiting may occur. Small, frequent meals may decrease the nausea.

6. Refer the patient to a rape crisis center or sexual assault counselor for counseling.

7. Refer the patient to a gynecology clinic for follow-up STD and pregnancy testing and possible HIV testing. HIV testing of sexual assault victims in the ED is controversial. Emergency departments do not routinely provide confidential individual HIV counseling. For this reason the patient can be referred to a clinic or office that performs the test and provides counseling.

8. Provide clean clothing for the patient. Assist the patient in finding transportation home.

9. Maintain the chain of evidence at all times. If at all possible, one nurse should assist with the evidence collection and maintain possession of the evidence until it is signed over to a law enforcement officer.

Splint Application

Betty Gaudet Nolan
Carlos B. Coyle

DESCRIPTION

Splinting is a technique used to immobilize or stabilize an injured extremity. Immobilization decreases pain, swelling, muscle spasm, bleeding into the tissue, and the risk of fat emboli. Immobilization can also prevent a closed fracture from converting to an open fracture.

INDICATIONS

Splinting is indicated anytime there is trauma to an extremity with evidence of deformity, angulation, crepitus, edema, ecchymosis, significant pain, an open soft-tissue injury, an impaled object, or neurovascular compromise.[1]

EQUIPMENT

• Splinting material that is appropriate for the injury
The following are four general categories of splints:
1. *Soft nonrigid splints:* Pillows, blankets, cravats, sling and swathe (Figure P28-1)
2. *Hard rigid and semirigid splints:* Aluminum, wooden boards, molded plastic, plaster, fiberglass, and vacuum splints
3. *Pneumatic-inflatable splints:* Air splints and pneumatic antishock garments (PASG)
4. *Traction splints:* Hare, Sager, and Thomas splints
Other equipment may include tape, padding material, and elastic bandages (Ace wraps).

INITIAL NURSING ACTIONS

1. Explain the procedure to the patient.
2. Prepare the patient for splinting by removing clothing over the injury site, dressing any open wounds, removing jewelry, and completing a baseline neurovascular assessment (distal and proximal pulses, color, temperature, movement, sensation, and capillary refill of the digits).

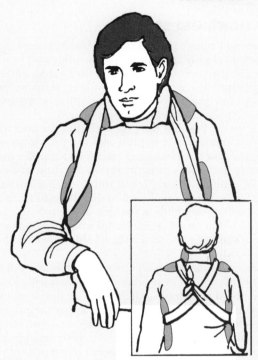

Figure P28-1   Posterior and anterior views of clavicle strap with a cravat.

3. Use padding over bony prominences.
4. For nonjoints, immobilize the injured area along with the joint above and below the site.
5. Splint the joint in the position found unless the distal pulse is diminished or absent. When no pulse is palpable, apply sustained and gentle traction along the long axis of the extremity, distal to the injury, until the pulse can be palpated.[1] If any resistance is encountered, discontinue the process and splint in the position found.
6. Splints should not be tight enough to be constrictive.
7. Check the neurovascular status before and after splinting. Recheck the neurovascular examination if the splint is removed or reapplied or if the extremity is repositioned.

SOFT NONRIGID SPLINTS

Soft nonrigid splints such as pillows, blankets, and cravats are often used to splint injuries of the ankle and foot. Pillows are also used in conjunction with a sling and swathe to help immobilize a dislocated shoulder. Blankets, pillows, and straps in conjunction with a long spine board are often used to help stabilize pelvic fractures.

- *Pillow splints:* Position the pillow around the area to be splinted and secure the splint with several cravats or tape.
- *Sling and swathe for stabilizing clavicle and scapular fractures:* Place the patient's extremity across the chest in a position of comfort. Place a cravat under the patient's extremity. Tie the pointed ends at the elbow to form a cradle. Tie the other ends at the side of the patient's neck. Tie two wide cravats together and wrap them around the patient's upper torso and affected side to secure the sling to the body.
- *Blanket and pillow pelvis splinting:* A combination of blankets or pillows can be used in conjunction with a long spine board and straps to help stabilize pelvic fractures. Blankets and pillows can be placed as padding around the patient's pelvic area and then secured with straps to a long spine board. The combination of the padding and securing straps should help prevent movement of the fractured pelvis.

HARD RIGID AND SEMIRIGID SPLINTS

Hard rigid and semirigid splints are used to splint a variety of long bone fractures.

- Aluminum, wooden, plastic, and fiberglass splints: Aluminum, wooden, plastic, and fiberglass splints are applied generally in the same manner. Pad the splint, and ensure that it is long enough to extend above and below the joints of the suspected fracture site. Apply gentle traction above and below the fracture site. Place the splint under the extremity. Secure the splint to the extremity using an elastic bandage. Fingers and toes should be left out of the bandage so that circulation can be checked.
- Vacuum splints: Vacuum splints are used to splint a variety of fractures. Vacuum splints are available for full body immobilization, dislocated shoulders, joints, arms, and legs.

They conform to the affected extremity or full body and essentially are a moldable rigid splint. They are applied in a manner similar to the other rigid splints and are often secured with straps that are connected to the splint. The splints become rigid when the air is removed by attaching a pump to the valve. Some splints require the valve to be closed to prevent loss of vacuum. To remove the splint, open the valve and allow it to refill with air.

PNEUMATIC-INFLATABLE SPLINTS

Air splints are used to splint fractures of the forearm and lower leg. PASGs are often used to help stabilize pelvic and femur fractures.

- Air splints: Air splints are administered by applying gentle traction above and below the suspected fracture site and sliding the splint under the extremity. Secure and inflate the splint until finger pressure can dent it only slightly. Release the gentle traction only after the splint has been inflated. Observe the splint for loss of pressure. Remember that temperature and altitude changes can affect pressure inside an air splint. Observe the extremity for signs of compartment syndrome.
- Pneumatic antishock garments: PASGs can be used to help stabilize pelvic and femur fractures. When using the PASG for splinting the pelvis, apply the garment in the usual manner and inflate all three compartments to approximately 20 mm Hg. The effectiveness of the PASG for splinting pelvic fractures is controversial. For femur fractures only the affected leg sections need to be inflated.

PREASSEMBLED PLASTER SPLINTS

Certain splinting can be done with preassembled plaster splints with incorporated padding, such as those made by Orthopedic Casting Laboratory (OCL). They come in 2-, 3-, 4-, and 6-inch widths.

General Preparation Steps for OCL Splinting Material

1. Prepare the OCL splint with a template (a cutting guide for different splints). Wear goggles to prevent plaster from getting into your eyes.
2. Immerse the splint in cool water.
3. Squeeze and remove excess water.

4. Stretch and smooth out on a towel.
5. Apply the foam side to skin and wrap the splint.

Application of Common Splints
Posterior short leg splint (ankle)

1. Measure (from the toes to below the knee) and cut a 4- or 6-inch wide roll (Figure P28-2, *A*). (Figure P28-2, *A* to *D*, shows application of a posterior short leg splint.)
2. Place the foot at a 90-degree angle to the leg.
3. Apply the roll posteriorly, folding back the plaster at the toes (Figure P28-2, *B*).
4. Tuck in the fold at the heel area. Secure the fold with an elastic bandage (Figure P28-2, *C*).
5. Flare back the plaster below knee, secure the plaster with an elastic bandage, and position and hold the foot at a 90-degree angle to the leg until the plaster is set (Figure P28-2, *D*).[2]

Volar cock-up splint

1. Measure from the base of the fingers to below the elbow and cut a 3- or 4-inch-wide roll.
2. Apply and secure the roll to the volar side (inner aspect) of the arm and palm, positioning the wrist in a 15- to 30-degree dorsiflexion (Figure P28-3).

Ulnar gutter (boxer) splint

1. Use a template to cut a 3- or 4-inch roll measuring from the fingertips to just below the elbow.
2. Fold the roll to form the desired gutter, and place the flap in the palm of the hand (Figure P28-4).
3. Pad between buddied fingers. Position the hand with the fingers in "position of function" at a 50-degree flexion at the metacarpophalangeal joint, a 15- to 20-degree flexion at the interphalangeal joint, and the wrist in a neutral position.[3]

Sugar tong splint

- *Forearm:* Measure from the knuckles over the flexed elbow and around the back to the hand at the midpalmar crease.
- *Humerus:* Measure from the acromion process down the humerus, around the elbow, and up to the axilla.
- Using a 3- or 4-inch wide roll, apply the splint with the elbow at 90-degree flexion and secure the splint with an elastic bandage (Figure P28-5).[2]

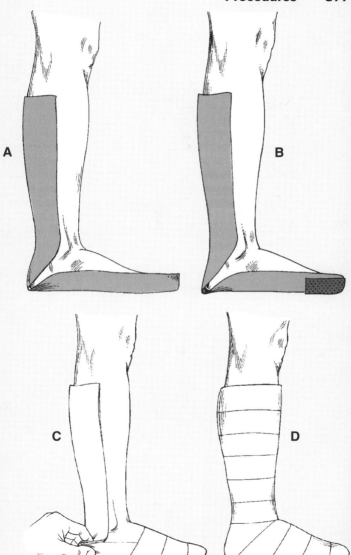

Figure P28-2 Application of posterior short leg splint.

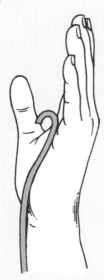

Figure P28-3   Application of volar cock-up splint.

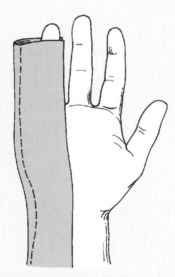

Figure P28-4   Placement of ulnar gutter splint to form desired gutter.

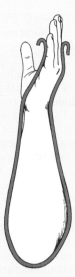

Figure P28-5 Application of sugar tong splint.

PATIENT CARE MANAGEMENT

1. Instruct the patient to keep the splint clean and dry.
2. Plaster requires 12 to 24 hours to dry. Prevent impression of the plaster during this time, or it may become misaligned, causing pressure sores to develop.
3. If plaster becomes wet, it will crumble and not harden again.
4. Look for changes in fingers or toes—coolness, dusky color, swelling, or a decrease in sensation.
5. Report pain that increases and does not respond to pain medication.
6. Elevate the limb to decrease swelling and pain, and apply cold packs as directed.
7. Do not put sharp objects inside the splint for scratching.
8. Instruct the patient on crutch walking as needed (Procedure 9).

TRACTION SPLINTS

Description

Traction splints are designed to reduce muscle spasms of the injured leg.

Indications

Traction splints are used to align and stabilize a midshaft femur or proximal tibial fracture.

Contraindications

Traction splints should not be used for fractures of the distal fibula, distal tibia, ankle, foot, or upper extremity.

Equipment

Various types of traction splints are available, including the Thomas half ring, Hare traction, and Sager traction splint.

Initial Nursing Actions

1. Remove any constrictive clothing or jewelry.
2. Assess pedal pulses, skin color and temperature, capillary refill, sensation, and movement in the foot of the injured leg.
3. Generally, two clinicians (and optimally three) are needed to apply a traction splint. The first clinician applies manual traction by holding the lower leg and pulling with both hands. Manual traction must be maintained until the splint is in place.

Hare traction splint or Thomas splint application

1. Assemble the equipment (Figure P28-6).
2. Adjust the length of the splint using the patient's uninjured leg as a guide. Place the padded ischial bar (Hare) or padded ring (Thomas) next to the patient's iliac crest, and extend the distal end of the splint by loosening the sleeve-locking device. The end of the splint should be approximately 10 inches past the heel of the foot (Figures P28-7 and P28-8).
3. Tighten the sleeve-locking device.
4. Open all support straps (those that support the thigh and lower leg) or tie four cravats with overhand knots spaced evenly throughout the splint.
5. With manual traction still being applied, slide the splint under the affected extremity until the padded ischial strap or ring is against the ischial tuberosity.
6. Pad the groin area with gauze or other suitable material. Secure the ischial strap.
7. Place the ankle hitch under the heel of the foot and cross the side straps over the top of the foot.

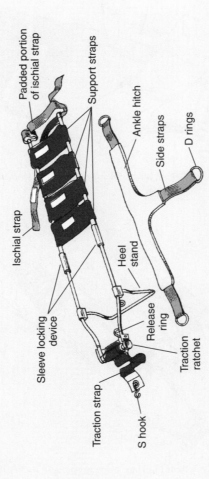

Figure P28-6 Hare traction equipment.

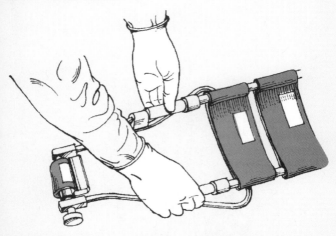

Figure P28-7   Adjusting length of splint with sleeve-locking device.

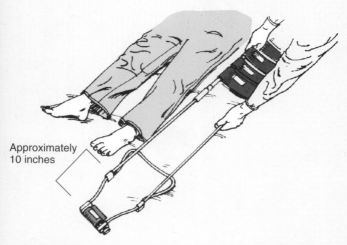

Approximately
10 inches

Figure P28-8   Extending Hare traction splint 10 inches past foot.

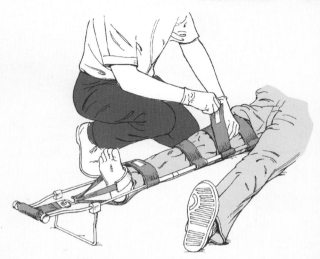

Figure P28-9   Application of strap.

8. Pull the release ring on the traction ratchet and release the traction strap. Connect the D rings of the ankle hitch to the S hook of the traction strap.

9. Apply mechanical traction by turning the ratchet knob until the splint equals manual traction.[4] The clinician holding traction should feel the gentle release of pressure as the splint assumes the traction.

10. Extend the heel stand into place to elevate the leg.

11. Secure the Velcro straps or cravats, two above and two below the knee. Do not place straps over the suspected fracture site (Figure P28-9).

12. Assess the pedal pulses, skin color and temperature, capillary refill, sensation, and movement in the foot of the splinted extremity.

Sager traction splint application

1. Assemble equipment.

2. Place the splint medial to the injured extremity with the padded bar resting against the inner aspect of the thigh (Figure P28-10).

3. Adjust the length until the wheel of the pulley is level with the heel of the patient.

4. Secure the thigh strap.

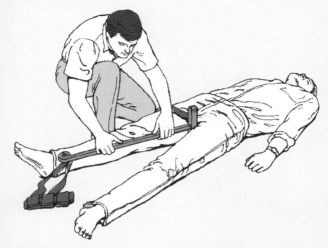

Figure P28-10 Application of Sager traction splint to medial aspect of injured leg.

5. Wrap the ankle harness snugly above the ankle, and secure the strap under the heel.
6. Shorten the loop of the ankle harness by threading the strap through the D buckle.
7. Release the lock on the splint, and pull the shaft out until the desired amount of traction tension is noted on the marking of the pulley wheel. The amount of traction should equal approximately 10% of the patient's body weight.
8. Secure straps at the thigh, knee, and lower leg.
9. Strap ankle and foot together to prevent rotation of the injured extremity (Figure P28-11).
10. Reassess pedal pulses, skin color, temperature, capillary refill, sensation, and movement in the foot of the injured extremity.

Patient Care Management
1. Continue to monitor the neurovascular status of the injured extremity at frequent intervals.
2. Maintain traction until definite stabilization, such as the insertion of a Steinmann pin, is initiated.

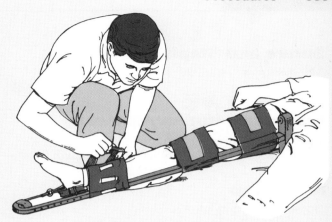

Figure P28-11 Application of straps.

3. If pedal pulses are absent or there are other significant changes in the neurovascular status, inform the physician. The amount of traction may need to be slightly decreased or increased.

References

1. Emergency Nurses Association, *Trauma nurse core course,* ed 4, Chicago, 1995, The Association.
2. *OCL splinting manual,* Eudora, Kan, 1992, M-PACT Management.
3. Proehl JA: *Adult emergency nursing procedures,* Boston, 1993, Jones & Bartlett.
4. Grant HD, Murray RH, Bergeron JD: *Emergency care,* Englewood Cliffs, NJ, 1990, Prentice-Hall.

Suture and Staple Removal

Betty Gaudet Nolan

DESCRIPTION (SUTURE REMOVAL)

Removal of nonabsorbable sutures is performed on a wound that shows signs of healing with no gaps in the skin integrity.

INDICATIONS

The amount of time stitches stay in place depends on several factors such as the laceration, type of wound closure, age and health of the patient, and presence of infection (see the "Timing of Suture Removal" box).

EQUIPMENT

- Suture removal kit (forceps, scissors, 4 × 4 gauze)
- Normal saline or an antiseptic solution
- Dressings as needed

TIMING OF SUTURE REMOVAL	
Location	**Time (days)**
Eyelid	3
Cheek	3-5
Nose, forehead, neck	5
Ear, scalp	5-7
Trunk	7-10
Arms and legs	7-10
Hands and feet	7-14
Joints	10-14

The above timeframes are general guidelines. Modifications of these recommendations should be tailored to individual needs. Older patients or patients with a chronic illness may have delayed healing times. Leaving sutures in too long increases the risk of abscess and scar formation. Premature removal of sutures may result in wound disruption and delayed healing.

INITIAL NURSING ACTIONS

1. Explain the procedure to the patient.
2. Gently clean the suture line with normal saline; use hydrogen peroxide if there is dried blood.
3. With forceps, grasp the suture knot and gently pull upwards.
4. Cut the stitch as close to the skin as possible, and pull the stitch out. Avoid pulling the outside suture through the skin to decrease contamination of the underlying tissue.
5. Document the number of stitches removed.
6. When removing continuous sutures, cut the stitches on one side of the suture line and remove them through the opposite side.
7. Clean the site as before. Apply a small dressing if there is any bleeding or per physician order.

PATIENT CARE MANAGEMENT

1. Instruct the patient to watch for signs and symptoms of infection such as redness, swelling, pus, red streaks, increased pain or tenderness, or unexplained fever.
2. Remind the patient to keep the wound clean until it is completely healed and not to pick at crusts or scabs; they will fall off naturally.

DESCRIPTION (STAPLE REMOVAL)

Staple removal is performed on a wound that shows signs of healing with no gaps in the skin integrity.

INDICATIONS

The amount of time staples stay in place depends on the part of the body affected (e.g., head and neck, 3 to 5 days; chest and abdomen, 5 to 7 days; lower extremities, 7 to 10 days).

EQUIPMENT

- Staple removal kit (staple extractor and gauze)
- Normal saline or an antiseptic solution
- Dressings as needed

INITIAL NURSING ACTIONS

1. Gently clean the staple line with normal saline; use hydrogen peroxide if dried blood is present.

2. Place the nose of the extractor device beneath the center of the staple.
3. Squeeze down with the thumbs to lift the edges of the staple up until it is reformed.
4. When the extractor is fully closed and the staple reformed, lift the extractor from the skin.

PATIENT CARE MANAGEMENT

1. Instruct the patient to watch for signs and symptoms of infection such as redness, swelling, pus, red streaks, increased pain or tenderness, or unexplained fever.
2. Remind the patient to keep the wound clean until it is completely healed and not to pick at crusts or scabs; they will fall off naturally.

Thoracentesis and Paracentesis

Mary Rose Bauer

THORACENTESIS

Thoracentesis is a procedure used to evacuate air or fluid and to obtain sterile fluid specimens from the pleural space. This procedure can be performed at the bedside using sterile technique.

INDICATIONS

1. Accumulation of fluid (pleural effusion) because of an inflammatory or infectious process
   - Removal of fluid from the pleural cavity may be done for therapeutic or diagnostic purposes.
2. Accumulation of air (pneumothorax) because of chest trauma or trauma of the visceral pleura
   - Removal of air will facilitate lung expansion. However, tube thoracostomy is the treatment of choice.

CONTRAINDICATIONS

1. The patient's respiratory status is compromised because of certain conditions such as ruptured diaphragm or emphysema. (These patients have a higher incidence of a pneumothorax secondary to lung perforation.[1])
2. Coagulopathy[1] should be corrected before this procedure, unless there is severe respiratory failure.[2]
3. Pleural adhesions increase the risk of perforation of the lung.[1]

EQUIPMENT

- Sterile drapes
- Antiseptic solution (povidone-iodine solution commonly used)
- Several sizes of needles for aspiration (may use 18- or 20-gauge spinal needles, or 16-gauge, 3-inch needle) or through-the-needle catheters (Through-the-needle

catheters are preferable in patients who must remain in the supine position.)

- 60-ml and 10-ml syringes
- 25-gauge, ⅝-inch and 22-gauge, 1½-inch needles
- Local anesthetic (1% lidocaine usually used)
- Mask
- Sterile gloves
- Three-way stopcock
- 4 × 4 gauze sponges
- Three sterile specimen tubes
- Drainage tube and 500-ml vacuum bottle or collection bag (If this is unavailable, you may substitute IV tubing and a 500-ml bag of normal saline. Spike and drain the bag of fluid. Then invert the bag, maintaining sterility, and connect the sterile tubing to the three-way stopcock for drainage collection.)
- Puncture site bandage

NOTE: Preassembled kits containing much of this equipment are available in many settings.

INITIAL NURSING ACTION

1. Diagnostic x-ray examination is generally performed before the procedure to determine the highest level of the effusion.
2. Explain the procedure to the patient.
3. Ideally, the patient should be placed in a seated position, leaning slightly forward, with his or her back to the person performing the procedure. This can be accomplished by having the patient lean forward over a padded bedside table or the back of a chair. If the patient must be supine, the lateral approach may be used. For this approach the affected side should face the person performing the procedure with the arm extended above the head for accessibility of site.
4. Prepare the site using antiseptic solution. For the removal of pleural fluid, the insertion site is the midscapular or posterior axillary line at a level below the top of the fluid.[1] Use the 2nd intercostal space, midclavicular line, for a pneumothorax.
5. Instruct the patient to refrain from coughing throughout the procedure.

NOTE: At this point the physician drapes the patient with sterile towels, exposing the site of the insertion. When the physician inserts the needle and there is a return of fluid, the nurse connects the tubing (maintaining sterility) to the stopcock and fastens the tubing securely.

6. Provide verbal support and comfort measures during the procedure.

7. Sterility should be maintained throughout the procedure, and the sterile connection should not be broken to ensure the specimen is not contaminated. Record the amount, appearance, and consistency of all fluid obtained during the procedure.

8. Following the procedure, apply pressure to the site to prevent bleeding. Apply a small dressing to the puncture site. Obtain a chest x-ray examination.

9. All specimens should be appropriately labeled and sent to the laboratory for analysis as ordered by the physician. Among the commonly ordered tests are a Gram stain, culture and sensitivity, cell count, cytology, pH, specific gravity, acid-fast staining, lactic dehydrogenase, and total protein tests.

PATIENT CARE MANAGEMENT

1. Monitor vital signs every 15 minutes for 1 hour, every 30 minutes for 2 hours, and then every hour until the patient is stable.

2. Monitor the patient for signs and symptoms of complications such as pneumothorax, hemothorax, pulmonary edema, hypoxia, respiratory distress, and, later, infection. Symptoms may include dizziness, increased respirations, uncontrollable cough, tightness in the chest, frothy blood-tinged sputum, tachycardia, and shortness of breath.

3. Continue to assess for pain, tenderness, redness, or drainage from the site.

PARACENTESIS

Paracentesis is a procedure for removing fluid from the peritoneal space using a large-bore needle and closed drainage system. It may be performed to obtain specimens used in the diagnosis of certain conditions or as a preparation for other procedures.

INDICATIONS

1. Accumulation of fluid or pressure in the abdominal cavity because of trauma or a disease process
   - Aspiration of fluid in the peritoneal space for analysis and culture
   - Drainage of fluid to relieve intraabdominal pressure
2. Preparation for other procedures such as peritoneal dialysis or surgery

CONTRAINDICATIONS

1. Coagulopathy or thrombocytopenia should be corrected before this procedure to prevent bleeding.
2. The patient has severe bowel distention.
   - Placement of a nasogastric tube or rectal tube may be required for decompression before the procedure.
3. The patient has had previous abdominal surgery.

EQUIPMENT

The equipment for paracentesis is the same as the equipment for thoracentesis listed earlier in this chapter.

INITIAL NURSING ACTIONS

1. Explain the procedure to the patient.
2. The bladder must be emptied before the procedure, either by voiding or by placement of a catheter.
3. Raise the head of the bed to a 45-degree angle (if tolerated). Allow at least 10 minutes for fluid to pool in the abdominal cavity.
4. Prepare the insertion site by cleansing the abdomen between the umbilicus and the symphysis pubis, including both lower quadrants, with antiseptic solution.

NOTE: At this point the physician drapes the patient with sterile drapes, exposing the site of the insertion. Attach a collection device to the tubing and three-way stopcock. After insertion of the catheter and aspiration with syringe, connect the stopcock and tubing to the catheter.

5. Be sure to record the amount, color, and consistency of all drainage.
6. Continue to assess vital signs during the procedure.
7. Apply pressure to the site for approximately 5 minutes, and place a small sterile dressing on the puncture site following the procedure.

8. Label all specimens appropriately, and send them to the laboratory for testing per physician request.

PATIENT CARE MANAGEMENT

1. Monitor the patient for pain or discomfort. Provide comfort measures.
2. Monitor vital signs every 30 minutes for 2 hours, then every hour until vital signs are stable.
3. Check the dressing for signs of leakage, bleeding, tenderness, swelling, or redness.

References

1. Gray MJ, Littleton AD: Thoracentesis. In Proehl JA, editor: *Adult emergency nursing procedures*, Boston, 1993, Jones & Bartlett.
2. Knighton D, Locksley RM, Mills J: Emergency procedures. In Saunder CE, Ho MT, editors: *Current emergency diagnosis and treatment*, Norwalk, Conn, 1992, Appleton & Lange.

Vascular Access Devices

Patty Sturt

In recent years major advances have been made in vascular access devices (VADs). These devices are placed in patients who require frequent, prolonged, or repeated fluid or drug administration such as chemotherapy, antibiotics, or hyperalimentation. Emergency nurses may encounter patients with various VADs, including peripherally inserted central catheters (PICCs), central venous tunneled catheters, and implanted ports. Blood products can be administered through these devices.

PERIPHERALLY INSERTED CENTRAL CATHETERS

PICCs are available in sizes ranging from 23- to 16-gauge. The catheter length varies from 3 to 24 inches. The catheters are inserted into the antecubital region with the tip resting at the superior vena cava or another major vessel. Correct tip location is confirmed by a chest x-ray examination after placement of the catheter. These catheters can remain in place for several weeks to several months.

INITIAL NURSING ACTIONS

1. *Obtaining blood:* It may be difficult to obtain blood from a PICC with a very small lumen because the catheter tends to collapse on aspiration. Flushing the catheter with 5 to 10 ml of normal saline before aspirating makes it easier to obtain blood from PICCs with larger lumens. When obtaining blood, discard the first 3 ml. Use another syringe to obtain blood specimens. Pull back on the syringe plunger gently and slowly for best results.
2. *Flushing:* Flush the line after infusing any agent or obtaining blood. The flush should consist of 5 to 10 ml of normal saline followed by 1 ml of heparin solution (100 U/ml). Use a 10-ml syringe for flushing. Smaller syringes generate higher pressures that can cause a

catheter rupture. PICC lines not being used for fluid administration are usually flushed every 12 hours with 3 ml of normal saline followed by 1 ml of heparin solution. Follow the manufacturer's recommendations for flushing.

3. *Infusing fluid and medications:* Avoid excessive pressure when infusing fluids or IV push medications. Excessive pressure may tear the catheter. Fluids and medications should not be forcefully injected through a PICC. To start an infusion, connect a 1-inch or shorter needle (or needleless adapter) to the IV tubing and insert the needle into the PICC latex port.

4. *Dressing:* Keep a transparent occlusive dressing over the entrance site. Many PICC lines are not sutured in place. They are secured with strip tape and an occlusive dressing. Take care not to dislodge the catheter when changing the dressing.

CENTRAL VENOUS TUNNELLED CATHETERS

Central venous tunneled catheters are also referred to as long-term indwelling catheters or right atrial catheters. Two examples of such catheters are the Hickman catheter (Figure P31-1) and the Groshong catheter (Figure P31-2). The catheter tip is placed in the superior vena cava proximal to the right atrium. The catheter is tunneled under the skin and exits at the 4th to 5th intercostal space onto the chest.

INITIAL NURSING ACTIONS

Hickman Catheter

1. *Obtaining blood:* Stop infusions for 1 minute before obtaining blood. Prep the injection cap with an antiseptic swab. Insert a 20-gauge, 1-inch needle or a needleless syringe device into the injection cap. Open the clamp, slowly withdraw 5 ml of blood, and discard the blood. Use another syringe and needle to obtain the needed blood. NOTE: A vacuum blood collection system may be used to withdraw the waste (discard) sample and lab samples. Use at least a 5-ml tube to obtain the waste sample.

2. *Flushing:* Clean the injection cap with an antiseptic swab. Irrigate the catheter with 10 ml of normal saline between drug infusions and after drawing blood. Flush

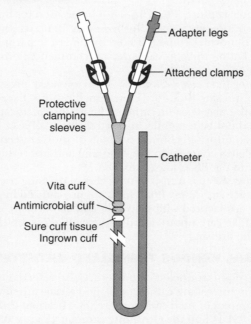

Figure P31-1 Hickman dual-lumen catheter.

with 2.5 to 3 ml of heparin solution in a 10-ml syringe after using the catheter and once a day to keep the
catheter patent. A concentration of 100 U/ml of heparin solution is commonly used for adults. Other heparin concentrations (10 to 1000 U/ml, amount of solution adjusted as appropriate for dosage) may be used
depending on the patient's medical condition and laboratory values. If more than one lumen is present, flush
each lumen. Inject the heparin slowly. Withdraw the
needle from the injection cap as the last 0.5 cc of solution is infused. Close each clamp.
3. *Infusing fluids:* For continuous IV fluid administration,
remove the male adapter (injection cap) from the hub
of the catheter and connect the IV tubing. Unclamp the
catheter and start IV infusion.
4. *Dressing:* Use a transparent occlusive dressing.

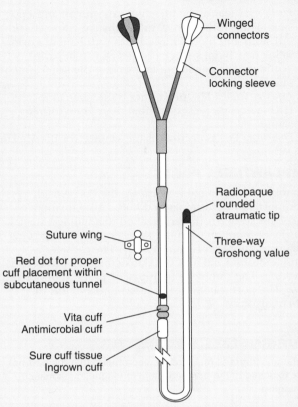

Figure P31-2 Groshong dual-lumen catheter.

Groshong Catheter

1. *Obtaining blood:* The procedure is the same as for the Hickman catheter except that the Groshong catheter does not have a clamp because of the closed distal tip. A small slit near the tip stays closed under normal conditions, which prevents the backflow of blood. It is often helpful to pull back the plunger 1 to 2 ml, to pause for a 2-second count, then slowly to withdraw blood. A vacuum blood collection system may be used as described with the Hickman catheter.

2. *Flushing:* Cleanse the injection cap with an antiseptic swab. Flush with 10 to 20 ml of normal saline after drug infusions and blood draws. Flush with 5 ml of normal saline in a 10-ml syringe each week (no heparin). Withdraw the needle while injecting the last 0.5 ml of saline.

3. *Infusing fluids:* The procedure is the same as for the Hickman catheter, except that there is no catheter clamp.

4. *Dressings:* The procedure is the same as for the Hickman catheter.

IMPLANTABLE PORTS

Examples of implantable ports are the Port-A-Cath Mediport and Bard Implanted Ports. An implantable port consists of a catheter attached to a stainless steel, plastic, or titanium chamber that contains a self-sealing silicone diaphragm (Figure P31-3). The catheter is completely internal with the skin acting as a protective covering. The catheter's tip is placed in the superior vena cava. The port usually lies near the 2nd and 4th rib subcutaneously.

NURSING ALERT

Manufacturers of metal ports recommend that the port not be exposed to the magnetic field in magnetic resonance imaging.

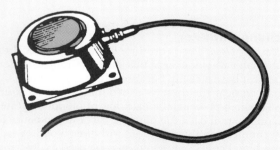

Figure P31-3   Implantable port.

INITIAL NURSING ACTIONS (ACCESSING THE PORT)

1. Open sterile gloves, and use the glove package as a sterile field. Place the following on the sterile field:
   * Alcohol and povidone-iodine swabs
   * 90-degree noncoring VAD needle (Huber, Lifeport)
   * Clear occlusive dressing
   * 20-gauge, 1-inch needle or needleless syringe device
   * Eye patches
   * Male Luer-Lok with injectable diaphragm
   * 10-ml syringe
   * Extension tubing

NURSING ALERT

The VAD needles vary in size from 22- to 19-gauge and in length from ⅝ to 1½ inch. Use the larger gauge if the patient requires blood products.

2. Put on sterile gloves.
3. Cleanse the skin over the injection port with one to three alcohol swabs, using circular motions with each swab. Allow the alcohol to dry.
4. Cleanse the same area with povidone-iodine swabs. Let the area dry for 1 to 2 minutes. Omit the povidone-iodine swab if the patient has a known allergy or skin sensitivity to the agent.
5. Connect a male Luer-Lok to extension tubing.
6. Connect extension tubing to the 90-degree VAD needle (some needles come with attached extension sets).
7. Draw 10 ml of normal saline. Remove air bubbles.
8. Insert the needle of the syringe into the Luer-Lok, and flush the extension tubing and VAD needle.
9. Feel the injection site (port) with one hand.
10. Place a thumb on one side of the port and an index finger on the other to stabilize the port.
11. With the other hand, hold the needle perpendicular to the skin. Firmly insert the needle through the skin into the port until it touches the bottom of the chamber. Do not rock or move the needle from side to side during insertion (Figure P31-4).

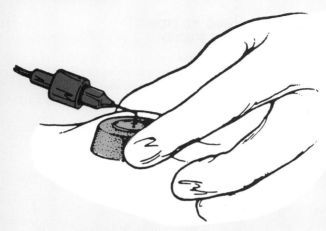

Figure P31-4 Accessing the port.

12. Unclamp extension tubing.
13. Gently pull back on the plunger of the syringe until you see blood. If there is no blood return with aspiration, have the patient raise his or her arms, cough, or turn sideways. If there is still no blood return, remove the needle and try again with a new needle.
14. Flush the port with normal saline.
15. Clamp the extension set. Place one sterile eye patch under and one above the 90-degree VAD needle. Cover with an occlusive dressing such as Tegaderm. The dressing and infusion components should be changed every 24 to 48 hours during infusion therapy.

NURSING ALERT

If the patient is to receive long-term IV fluids or blood products, connect the IV tubing directly to the extension tubing. If the patient is to receive IV fluids and be discharged from the ED, the IV tubing can be connected to the Luer-Lok by a needle. Contact the patient's physician, hospice, or home health nurse (if appropriate) to determine if the VAD needle and extension tubing should stay in place for IV fluids or medication while the patient is home.

16. *Starting an infusion:* Connect primed IV tubing into the extension tubing. Unclamp the extension tubing. Start infusion.

17. *Disconnecting an infusion:* Draw up 10 ml of normal saline in a syringe and 3 to 5 ml of heparinized solution (100 U/ml for adults and 10 U/ml for children) in a separate syringe. Use at least a 10-ml syringe. Clamp the extension tubing. Remove IV tubing. Inject normal saline and then heparinized solution into a male Luer-Lok. Clamp the extension set while flushing the last 0.5 ml of solution.

18. *Obtaining blood:* Unclamp the extension set. Withdraw 3 to 5 ml of blood from a Luer-Lok, and discard the blood. Obtain the needed blood with another syringe and needle. Flush with 10 to 20 ml of normal saline and continue IV infusion. If not infusing, additional flushing is necessary. Inject 10 to 20 ml of normal saline. Administer heparinized solution in the same manner as when discontinuing infusion.

19. *Removing a VAD needle:* Remove the dressing. Cleanse the end of the Luer-Lok with an antiseptic swab. Insert a needle containing a 10-ml syringe with heparinized solution into the Luer-Lok. Stabilize the port with a thumb and index finger. Push in the solution. Begin pulling the needle out while pushing in the last 0.5 ml.

20. *Flushing requirements:* When not accessed, the port should be flushed every 4 weeks with 5 ml of heparinized (100 U/ml for adults, 10 U/ml for children) solution.

Wound Care

Julia Fultz

DESCRIPTION

Wound care begins once life- and limb-threatening conditions have been treated. The goals of wound care are to minimize the risk of infection; prevent scarring; ensure adequate pain control while the wound is being evaluated, cleaned, repaired, and dressed; and ensure that the patient or the patient's caregiver understand the discharge instructions for wound care.

INDICATIONS

Wound care is provided to any area of the skin where its integrity has been damaged.

EQUIPMENT

- Protective gear—gloves, gown, goggles, and mask
- Sterile gloves
- Analgesics (e.g., lidocaine, bupivacaine, tetracaine, epinephrine, and cocaine as single or mixed solutions)
- Needles (25- and 27-gauge) to inject anesthetic
- 20- to 35-ml syringe
- 18-gauge intravenous catheter
- Normal saline
- Skin disinfectant
- Razor with recessed blade or clean scissors
- Instruments for debridement
- Triple antibiotic ointment
- Suture material
- Wound tape
- Sterile gauze
- Mesh gauze rolls for securing dressings
- Microporous tape

INITIAL NURSING ACTIONS

1. Bleeding may need to be controlled by direct pressure or a pressure bandage and elevation.

2. Review the patient's medical history for diseases that may affect healing (e.g., diabetes, peripheral vascular disease, and immunosuppression), allergies, and tetanus status (Reference Guide 24). Although a true allergy to local anesthetics is uncommon, obtaining a good history will help prevent an allergic reaction. There are two families of "caine" anesthetics, the ester and the amide families. Esters include procaine, tetracaine, and benzocaine. The amide family includes lidocaine and bupivacaine. There is no cross-reactivity between the two families.[1]

3. Radiographs may be ordered if the presence of a foreign body is suspected. However, if the suspected foreign body is organic (e.g., wood), xerograms, computed tomography scans, or ultrasonograms may be ordered because organic substances will not be seen on standard radiographs unless they displace tissues enough to produce a radiolucent shadow.[1]

4. Inform the patient of the procedure, and ensure patient comfort.

5. Ensure adequate pain control. Anesthesia must be adequate for exploration of the wound to determine wound depth, presence of foreign matter, and damage to underlying tissue and structures, for preparation of the wound (debridement and cleansing), and for wound closure if needed. If IV conscious sedation is used, monitor the patient according to the procedure for IV conscious sedation (see Procedure 8). A topical anesthetic may be chosen for the repair of small lacerations (<5 cm), especially for children. A solution of tetracaine, epinephrine (adrenaline), and cocaine (TAC) is placed directly in the wound, or a cotton ball or cotton-tipped applicator is soaked in the TAC solution and placed into the wound. TAC is never applied to mucous membranes (because of the rapid absorption from the membranes) or to wounds of the nose, ears, penis, digits, or eyelids (because of the vasoconstrictive properties of the epinephrine and cocaine). EMLA (lidocaine 2.5%, prilocaine 2.5%) cream may be applied to the affected area but must be left in place for 1 hour to achieve anesthesia.

6. Clip hair in proximity to the wound. Using a razor damages the hair follicle, providing an area for bacterial entrance and growth. If a razor must be used for hair re-

moval, use one with a recessed blade. Areas that provide an anatomic landmark useful in alignment of the wound edges, such as the eyebrows, should not be removed.

7. Disinfect the skin surrounding the wound with either povidone-iodine (Betadine) or chlorhexidine (Hibiclens). Both of these agents are fast acting with a broad spectrum of antimicrobial activity.[1] Great care must be taken to prevent either of these substances from entering the wound because they impair the wound's defenses against infection.[1]

8. The physician caring for the patient debrides the wound, removing foreign matter and tissue that is non-viable. Revision of the round edges may be needed to allow better closure of the wound and to minimize the potential for scarring. With puncture wounds a regional block may be needed to anesthetize the area well enough to allow an excision of the wound for proper exploration and cleaning.[2] Wound care may differ according to the severity of the wound.

9. After the wound has been debrided, it must be irrigated with copious amounts (at least 200 ml)[2] of normal saline under pressure. Cleansing the wound before closure is one of the most important steps in minimizing wound infection (Table P32-1). Normal saline (NS) is the wound irrigant of choice because it is inexpensive, easy to prepare, and nontoxic to the wound's defense mechanisms.[1] Irrigating the wound with NS under high pressure (18-gauge IV catheter, with the needle removed, connected to a 20- to 35-ml syringe) within 1 in of the wound is the most effective method of removing bacteria. Irrigation with bulb syringes, scrubbing the wound, or soaking the wound in an antiseptic solution will not clean the wound effectively.[1] Abrasions may have dirt and gravel embedded in the dermis. Once anesthetized, the area requires meticulous cleaning to prevent an unsightly scar. Scrubbing in a circular pattern with a soft-bristled brush moistened with saline may be necessary to remove the debris.[2]

10. Primary closure of wounds may be accomplished with wound tape, sutures, or staples (Table 19-1). Certain types of wounds, such as some puncture wounds, some animal and human bites, and some avulsions, may be left to close by themselves.

Procedures **905**

TABLE P32-1 Wound Cleansing Agents

Agents	Antimicrobial activity	Mechanics of actions	Tissue toxicity	Indications and contraindications
Povidone-iodine solution (iodine complexes) (Betadine)	Available as a 10% solution with polyvinyl-pyrrolidine (povi-done) containing 1% free iodine; has broad rapid-onset antimicrobial activity	Potent germicide in low concentrations	Will decrease polymorphonuclear cell migration and life span at concentration >1% May cause systemic toxicity at higher concentrations; questionable toxicity at 1% concentration Toxic to open wounds	Probably a safe and effective wound cleanser at a 1% concentration 10% solution is effective to prepare the skin about the wound
Povidone-iodine surgical scrub	Same as the solution	Same	Toxic to open wounds	Best as a hand cleanser; never use in open wounds
Nonionic detergents (Pluronic F-68, Shur-Clens)	Ethylene oxide is 80% of its molecular weight It has no antimicrobial activity	Wound cleanser	No toxicity to open wounds, eyes, or IV solutions	Appears to be an effective, safe wound cleanser

Continued

TABLE P32-1   Wound Cleansing Agents—cont'd

Agents	Antimicrobial activity	Mechanics of actions	Tissue toxicity	Indications and contraindications
Hydrogen peroxide	3% solution in water has brief germicidal activity	Oxidizing agent that denatures protein	Toxic to open wounds	Should not be used on wounds after the initial cleansing; may be used to clean intact skin
Hexachlorophene (pHisoHex) (polychlorinated bisphenol)	Bacteriostatic (2% to 5%) Greater activity against gram-positive organisms	Interruption of bacterial electron transport and disruption of membrane-bound enzymes	Little skin toxicity; scrub form is damaging to open wound	Never use scrub solution in open wounds. Very good preoperative hand preparation
Alcohols	Low-potency antimicrobial most effective as a 70% ethyl and 70% isopropyl alcohol solution	Denatures protein	Will kill irreversibly and function as a fixative	No role in routine care
Phenols	Bacteriostatic >0.2% Bactericidal >1% Fungicidal 1.3%	Denatures protein	Extensive tissue necrosis and systemic toxicity	Never use >2% aqueous phenol or >4% phenol plus glycerol

11. Apply a sterile dressing when indicated. Dressings should be impermeable to bacteria and prevent evaporation of water (drying of the wound causes a scab that delays healing). They can also provide pressure to the wound site, minimizing edema and bleeding. Dressings may include petroleum-covered gauze placed over the wound and covered with a coarse mesh gauze, an occlusive transparent film dressing such as Tegaderm or Op-site, or a semiocclusive, semipermeable dressing such as Epi-lock or Biobrane. Dressings can be secured in place with mesh gauze rolls or microporous tape. Do not secure dressings with tape circumferentially because of the constrictive result if the extremity swells.

12. Wounds in proximity to joints must be immobilized to prevent excessive stress on the wound.

PATIENT CARE MANAGEMENT

1. Administer antibiotics if ordered. Antibiotic treatment is usually reserved for exceptional circumstances, including cat bites, some hand wounds, intraoral lacerations, and some punctures to the foot, and for cases in which early signs of infection are already present with human bites to the hand.[1]

2. Immunize the patient against tetanus if needed (Reference Guide 24).

3. Elevate the extremity for the first 24 hours and apply ice packs to decrease edema. Use a barrier between the ice pack and the skin.

4. Immobilize the extremity, especially if the wound is near or over a joint, until the sutures are removed.

5. Injuries that are high risk for infection must be evaluated in 48 hours.

6. Give the patient discharge instructions that include daily wound care, signs and symptoms of infection, suture removal dates (Procedure 29), and telephone numbers (e.g., private physician, clinics, emergency department) for follow-up appointments.

References

1. Simon B: Principles of wound management. In Rosen P et al, editors: *Emergency medicine concepts and clinical practice*, ed 4, St Louis, 1998, Mosby.
2. Larson JL, Wischman J: Tissue integrity: surface trauma. In Neff JA, Kidd PS, editors: *Trauma nursing: the art and science*, St Louis, 1993, Mosby.